Lecture Notes in Networks and Systems

Volume 376

The series "Lecture Notes in Networks and Systems" publishes the latest developments in Networks and Systems—quickly, informally and with high quality. Original research reported in proceedings and post-proceedings represents the core of LNNS.

Volumes published in LNNS embrace all aspects and subfields of, as well as new challenges in, Networks and Systems.

The series contains proceedings and edited volumes in systems and networks, spanning the areas of Cyber-Physical Systems, Autonomous Systems, Sensor Networks, Control Systems, Energy Systems, Automotive Systems, Biological Systems, Vehicular Networking and Connected Vehicles, Aerospace Systems, Automation, Manufacturing, Smart Grids, Nonlinear Systems, Power Systems, Robotics, Social Systems, Economic Systems and other. Of particular value to both the contributors and the readership are the short publication timeframe and the world-wide distribution and exposure which enable both a wide and rapid dissemination of research output.

The series covers the theory, applications, and perspectives on the state of the art and future developments relevant to systems and networks, decision making, control, complex processes and related areas, as embedded in the fields of interdisciplinary and applied sciences, engineering, computer science, physics, economics, social, and life sciences, as well as the paradigms and methodologies behind them.

Indexed by SCOPUS, INSPEC, WTI Frankfurt eG, zbMATH, SCImago.

All books published in the series are submitted for consideration in Web of Science.

For proposals from Asia please contact Aninda Bose (aninda.bose@springer.com).

More information about this series at https://link.springer.com/bookseries/15179

M. Shamim Kaiser · Anirban Bandyopadhyay ·
Kanad Ray · Raghvendra Singh · Vishal Nagar
Editors

Proceedings of Trends in Electronics and Health Informatics

TEHI 2021

Springer

Editors
M. Shamim Kaiser
Jahangirnagar University
Dhaka, Bangladesh

Anirban Bandyopadhyay
National Institute for Materials Science
Tsukuba, Japan

Kanad Ray
Amity University
Jaipur, India

Raghvendra Singh
Pranveer Singh Institute of Technology
Kanpur, India

Vishal Nagar
Pranveer Singh Institute of Technology
Kanpur, India

ISSN 2367-3370 ISSN 2367-3389 (electronic)
Lecture Notes in Networks and Systems
ISBN 978-981-16-8825-6 ISBN 978-981-16-8826-3 (eBook)
https://doi.org/10.1007/978-981-16-8826-3

This Springer imprint is published by the registered company Springer Nature Singapore Pte Ltd.
The registered company address is: 152 Beach Road, #21-01/04 Gateway East, Singapore 189721, Singapore

Organization

Chief Patron

Vinay Kumar Pathak	Vice Chancellor, APJAKTU, Lucknow
Pranveer Singh	Chairman, PSIT, Kanpur

Patron

Sanjeev Kumar Bhalla	Director, PSIT, Kanpur

Conference Chairs

Dr. Chi-Sang Poon	Massachusetts Institute of Technology, USA
Dr. Anirban Bandyopadhyay	National Institute for Materials Science, Japan
Dr. Kanad Ray	Amity University, Rajasthan, India

Steering Committee

Anirban Bandyopadhyay	National Institute for Materials Science, Japan
Anirban Dutta	The State University of New York at Buffalo, USA
Chi-Sang Poon	Massachusetts Institute of Technology, USA
J. E. Lugo	University of Montreal, Canada
Jocelyn Faubert	University of Montreal, Canada
Kanad Ray	Amity University Rajasthan, India
Luigi M. Caligiuri	The University of Calabria, Italy

Mufti Mahmud	Nottingham Trent University, UK
M. Shamim Kaiser	Jahangirnagar University, Bangladesh
Subrata Ghosh	Northeast Institute of Science and Technology, India
Shamim Al Mamun	Jahangirnagar University, Bangladesh

Advisory Committee

Boaz Tsaban	Bar-Ilan University, Israel
Sreeram Dhurjaty	AD2BW, Rochester, NY
Alex Khang	Data Scientist, Portfolio Manager GRITEx, Vietnam
Mikael Syvajarvi	Manager at JMS center of Research Utilization, Sweden
Balwinder Raj	NIT Jalandhar, India
Shyam Lal	NIT Karnataka
Bharat Gupta	NIT Patna
D. S. Yadav	IETE Lucknow
Pramod Singhal	MITS Gwalior
Manoj Kumar Shukla	REC Kannauj
Mrutyunjay Rout	NIT Jamshedpur
Vinay Kumar	MNNIT Allahabad, Prayagraj
R. K. Chauhan	MMMUT, Gorakhpur, India
Anand Sharma	MNNIT Allahabad, Prayagraj, India
D. K. Tripathi	REC Sonbhadra, India
Dharmendra Kumar	MMMUT, Gorakhpur, India
Satish Kumar Singh	IIIT Allahabad, Prayagraj
B. D. K. Patro	REC Kannauj
Arun Kumar Singh	REC Kannauj
Shamim Akhter	JIIT, Noida
Vishal Mehta	PSIT, Kanpur
Manmohan Shukla	PSIT, Kanpur
Yogesh Chandra	PSIT, Kanpur
Ashish Chakraborty	PSIT, Kanpur
Atul Kumar Srivastava	PSIT, Kanpur
Nitin Srivastava	PSIT, Kanpur
Anshuman Tyagi	PSIT, Kanpur
Piyush Bhushan	PSIT, Kanpur
Sumit Chandra	PSIT, Kanpur

Organizing Chairs

Raghvendra Singh	Head, ECE, PSIT, Kanpur
Vishal Nagar	Head, CSE, PSIT, Kanpur, cs@psit.ac.in

Organizing Co-chairs

M. Shamim Kaiser	IIT, JU
Satyasundara Mahapatra	PSIT
Vivek Kumar	PSIT
Manish Kumar	PSIT
Raghuraj Singh Suryavanshi	PSIT

Organizing Committee

Abhishek Singh Rathor	ECE, PSIT
Gaurav Sahu	ECE, PSIT
Akash Porwal	ECE, PSIT
Rohit Tripathi	ECE, PSIT
Ajay Garg	ECE, PSIT
Sandeep Kumar	ECE, PSIT
Sudhir Kumar Singh	ECE, PSIT
Ravi Kumar	ECE, PSIT
Megha Dixit	ECE, PSIT
Sangama Singh Bhadauria	ECE, PSIT
Anjali Gupta	ECE, PSIT
Sandeep Sharma	CSE, PSIT
Gaurav Bajpai	CSE, PSIT
Kumar Saurabh	CSE, PSIT
Rajeev Kumar Singh	CSE, PSIT
Sunil Kumar	CSE, PSIT
Amit Tiwari	CSE, PSIT
Deepak Gupta	CSE, PSIT
Dhaneshwar Kumar	CSE, PSIT
Praveen Kumar Rai	CSE, PSIT
Rajat Verma	CSE, PSIT
Ankit Jain	ECE, PSIT

Registration Chairs

Shivani Dixit	PSIT, Kanpur
Pratibha Singh	PSIT, Kanpur
Charu Awasthi	PSIT, Kanpur

Finance Chairs

Harsh Dev	PSIT, Kanpur
Raghuraj Singh Suryavanshi	PSIT, Kanpur
Tanmai Kulshrestha	PSIT, Kanpur

Finance and Audit Chairs

Raghvendra Singh	PSIT, Kanpur
Vishal Nagar	CSE, PSIT, Kanpur
Utkarsh Pandey	ECE, PSIT
Ashutosh Pandey	CSE, PSIT

Website and Social Media Chairs

Rohit Saxena	CSE, PSIT
Gyanendra Tiwari	CSE, PSIT
Nishant Tripathi	ECE, PSIT
Utkarsh Pandey	ECE, PSIT

Transportation and Hospitality Chairs

Pradeep Gupta	ECE, PSIT
Chandrahas Mishra	CSE, PSIT

Technical Program Committee Chairs

Anirban Bandyopadhyay	National Institute for Materials Science, Japan

Technical Program Committee Co-chairs

Manish Kumar	PSIT
Varun Shukla	PSIT
Prashant Kumar Mishra	PSIT

Atul Srivastava	PSIT

Technical Program Committee Members

Aparna Dixit	PSIT, Kanpur
M. A. Jalil	KUET, Bangladesh
Mukesh Arora	SKIT, Jaipur
Sarfaraz Nawaz	SKIT, Jaipur
Tanmai Kulshrestha	PSIT, Kanpur
Ashish Shukla	GLAU, Mathura
Chandra Shankar Porwal	JSSA, Noida
Prashant Kumar Mishra	PSIT, Kanpur
Atul Srivastava	PSIT, Kanpur
D. S. Kushwaha	PSIT, Kanpur
Shailendra Kumar Sinha	PSIT, Kanpur
Abhishek Singh	PSIT, Kanpur
Nidhi Shukla	PSIT, Kanpur
Ruchi Chaurasia	PSIT, Kanpur

Publication Chair

Dr. Kanad Ray	Amity University Rajasthan, India

Publicity Chair

Shamim Al Mamun	IIT, JU, BD

Technical Review Committee

Kavi Kumar	UTM, Malaysia
Nabihah Ahmad	UTM, Malaysia
S. P. Tiwari	IIT Dhanbad, India
Su Rong	NTU, Singapore
Said Broumi	University of New Mexico, USA
Pal Madhumangal	Vidyasagar University, India
F. Suresh Singh	University of Kerala, India
Sabariah Saharan	UTHM, Malaysia

Arif Jalil	UTM, Malaysia
Muhammad Arifur Rahman	Jahangirngar University, Bangladesh
Sajjad Waheed	MBSTU, Bangladesh
Md. Zahidur Rahman	GUB, Bangladesh
Muhammad Golam Kibria	ULAB, Bangladesh
Md. Majharul Haque	Deputy Director, Bangladesh Bank
Samsul Arefin	CUET, Bangladesh
Md. Obaidur Rahman	DUET, Bangladesh
Mustafa Habib Chowdhury	IUB, Bangladesh
Marzia Hoque-Tania	Oxford University, UK
Antesar Shabut	CSE, Leeds Trinity University, UK
Md. Khalilur Rhaman	BRAC University, Bangladesh
Md. Hanif Seddiqui	University of Chittagong, Bangladesh
M. M. A. Hashem	KUET, Bangladesh
Tomonori Hashiyama	The University of Electro-Communications, Japan
Wladyslaw Homenda	Warsaw University of Technology, Poland
M. Moshiul Hoque	CUET, Bangladesh
A. B. M. Aowlad Hossain	KUET, Bangladesh
Sheikh Md. Rabiul Islam	KUET, Bangladesh
Manohar Das	Oakland University, USA
Kaushik Deb	CUET, Bangladesh
Carl James Debono	University of Malta, Malta
M. Ali Akber Dewan	Athabasca University, Canada
Belayat Hossain	Loughborough University, UK
Khoo Bee Ee	Universiti Sains Malaysia, Malaysia
Ashik Eftakhar	Nikon Corporation, Japan
Md. Tajuddin Sikder	Jahangirnagar University, Bangladesh
Mrs. Shayla Islam	UCSI, Malaysia
Antony Lam	Mercari Inc. Japan
Ryote Suzuki	Saitama University, Japan
Hishato Fukuda	Saitama University, Japan
Md. Golam Rashed	Rajshahi University, Bangladesh
Md Sheikh Sadi	KUET, Bangladesh
Tushar kanti Shaha	JKKNIU, Bangladesh
M. Shazzad Hosain	NSU, Bangladesh
M. Mostafizur Rahman	AIUB, Bangladesh
Tabin Hassan	AIUB, Bangladesh
Aye Su Phyo	Computer University Kalay, Myanmar
Md. Shahedur Rahman	Jahangirnagar University
Lu Cao	Saitama University, Japan
Nihad Adnan	Jahangirnagar University
Mohammad Firoz Ahmed	Jahangirnagar University
A. S. M. Sanwar Hosen	JNU, South Korea
Mahabub Hossain	ECE, HSTU, Bangladesh
Md. Sarwar Ali	Rajshahi University, Bangladesh

Risala T. Khan	Jahangirnagar University, Bangladesh
Mohammad Shahidul Islam	Jahangirnagar University, Bangladesh
Manan Binte Taj Noor	Jahangirnagar University, Bangladesh
Md Abu Yousuf	Jahangirnagar University, Bangladesh
Md Sazzadur Rahman	Jahangirnagar University, Bangladesh
Rashed Mazumder	Jahangirnagar University, Bangladesh
Md. Abu Layek	Jagannath University, Bangladesh
Saiful Azad	Universiti Malaysia Pahang, Malaysia
Mostofa Kamal Nasir	MBSTU, Bangladesh
Mufti Mahmud	NTU, UK
A. K. M. Mahbubur Rahman	IUB, Bangladesh
Al Mamun	Jahangirnagar University, Bangladesh
Al-Zadid Sultan Bin Habib	KUET, Bangladesh
Anup Majumder	Jahangirnagar University, Bangladesh
Atik Mahabub	Concordia University, Canada
Bikash Kumar Paul	MBSTU, Bangladesh
Md. Obaidur Rahman	DUET, Bangladesh
Nazrul Islam	MIST, Bangladesh
Ezharul Islam	Jahangirnagar University, Bangladesh
Farah Deeba	DUET, Bangladesh
Md. Manowarul Islam	Jagannath University, Bangladesh
Md. Waliur Rahman Miah	DUET, Bangladesh
Rubaiyat Yasmin	Rajshahi University, Bangladesh
Sarwar Ali	Rajshahi University, Bangladesh
Rabiul Islam	Kulliyyah of ICT, Malaysia
Dejan C. Gope	Jahangirnagar University, Bangladesh
Sk. Md. Masudul Ahsan	KUET, Bangladesh
Mohammad Shahriar Rahman	ULAB, Bangladesh
Golam Dastoger Bashar	Boise State University, USA
Md. Hossam-E-Haider	MIST, Bangladesh
H. Liu	Wayne State University, USA
Imtiaz Mahmud	Kyungpook National University, Korea
Kawsar Ahmed	MBSTU, Bangladesh
Kazi Abu Taher	BUP, Bangladesh
Linta Islam	Jagannath University, Bangladesh
Md. Musfique Anwar	Jahangirnagar University, Bangladesh
Md. Sanaul Haque	University of Oulu, Finland
Md. Ahsan Habib	MBSTU, Bangladesh
Md. Habibur Rahman	MBSTU, Bangladesh
M. A. F. M. Rashidul Hasan	Rajshahi University, Bangladesh
Md. Badrul Alam Miah	UPM, Malaysia
Mohammad Ashraful Islam	MBSTU, Bangladesh
Mokammel Haque	CUET, Bangladesh
Muhammad Ahmed	ANU, Australia
Nazia Hameed	University of Nottingham, UK

Publication Committee

Preface

The 1st International Conference on Trends in Electronics and Health Informatics, TEHI 2021, was held from December 16 to 17, 2021. The conference was hosted by Pranveer Singh Institute of Technology, Kanpur, Uttar Pradesh, India. The TEHI conference series has established itself as the world's premier research forum on electronics and health informatics, which is an emerging interdisciplinary and multidisciplinary research field with joint efforts from artificial intelligence and soft computing, healthcare informatics, IoT and data analytics, electronics and communication technologies. The conference's objective is to bring together researchers, educators, and business professionals involved in related fields of research and development. This volume compiles the peer-reviewed papers presented at the meeting.

The conference on TEHI 2021 attracted 133 full papers from 10 countries in five tracks. These tracks include—artificial intelligence and soft computing, healthcare informatics, IoT and data analytics, electronics and communication. The submitted papers underwent a single-blind review process, soliciting expert opinion from at least two experts: at least two independent reviewers, the track co-chair, and the respective track chair. Following rigorous review reports from the reviewers and the track chairs, the technical program committee has selected 63 high-quality full papers from 09 countries that were accepted for presentation at the conference. Due to the COVID-19 pandemic, the organizing committee decided to host the event in hybrid mode. The research community reacted amazingly in this challenging time.

The volume is insightful and fascinating for those interested in learning about electronics and health informatics that explores the dynamics of exponentially increasing knowledge in core and related fields. We are thankful to the authors who have made a significant contribution to the conference and have developed relevant research and literature in artificial intelligence and soft computing, healthcare informatics, IoT and data analytics, electronics and communication.

We would like to express our gratitude to the organizing committee and the technical committee members for their unconditional support, particularly the chair, the co-chair, and the reviewers. Special thanks to the Prof. Vinay Kumar Pathak, Hon'ble Vice Chancellor, Dr. A. P. J. Abdul Kalam Technical University, Lucknow; Pranveer Singh, Hon'ble Chairman, PSIT, Kanpur; and Dr. Sanjeev Kumar Bhalla, Director,

PSIT, Kanpur, for their thorough support. TCCE 2021 could not have taken place without the tremendous work of the team and the gracious assistance. We would like to thank IEEE UTHM Student Branch. We are grateful to Aninda Bose, Ms. Sharmila Mary Panner Selvam, and other team members of Springer Nature for their continuous support in coordinating this volume publication. We would also like to thank Mr. Md. Mahfuzur Rahman of DIU and Milon Biswas of BUBT for continuous support. Last but not least, we thank all of our contributors and volunteers for their support during this challenging time to make TEHI 2021 a success.

Dhaka, Bangladesh
Jaipur, India
Tsukuba, Japan
Kanpur, India
Kanpur, India
October 2021

M. Shamim Kaiser
Kanad Ray
Anirban Bandyopadhyay
Raghvendra Singh
Vishal Nagar

Contents

Editors and Contributors

About the Editors

Dr. M. Shamim Kaiser is currently working as Professor at the Institute of Information Technology of Jahangirnagar University, Savar, Dhaka-1342, Bangladesh. He received his Bachelor's and Master's degrees in Applied Physics Electronics and Communication Engineering from the University of Dhaka, Bangladesh, in 2002 and 2004, respectively, and the Ph.D. degree in Telecommunication Engineering from the Asian Institute of Technology, Thailand, in 2010. His current research interests include data analytics, machine learning, wireless network and signal processing, cognitive radio network, big data and cyber-security, renewable energy. He has authored more than 100 papers in different peer-reviewed journals and conferences. He is Associate Editor of the *IEEE Access Journal*, Guest Editor of *Brain Informatics Journal* and *Cognitive Computation Journal*. Dr. Kaiser is Life Member of Bangladesh Electronic Society; Bangladesh Physical Society. He is also Senior Member of IEEE, USA, and IEICE, Japan, and Active Volunteer of the IEEE Bangladesh Section. He is Founding Chapter Chair of the IEEE Bangladesh Section Computer Society Chapter. Dr. Kaiser organized various international conferences such as ICEEICT 2015–2018, IEEE HTC 2017, IEEE ICREST 2018 and BI2020.

Anirban Bandyopadhyay is Senior Scientist in the National Institute for Materials Science (NIMS), Tsukuba, Japan. He completed Ph.D. from Indian Association for the Cultivation of Science (IACS), Kolkata 2005, December, on supramolecular electronics; 2005–2007: ICYS Research Fellow NIMS, Japan; 2007–now, permanent Scientist in NIMS, Japan; 10 patents on building artificial organic brain, big data, molecular bot, cancer and Alzheimer drug, fourth circuit element, etc.; 2013–2014 Visiting Scientist in MIT, USA, on biorhythms; World Technology Network, WTN Fellow, (2009–continued); Hitachi Science and Technology Award 2010, Inamori Foundation Award 2011–2012, Kurata Foundation Award, Inamori Foundation Fellow (2011), Sewa Society International SSS Fellow (2012), Japan; SSI Gold medal (2017).

Kanad Ray (Senior Member, IEEE) received the M.Sc. degree in physics from Calcutta University and the Ph.D. degree in physics from Jadavpur University, West Bengal, India. He has been Professor of Physics and Electronics and Communication and is presently working as Head of the Department of Physics, Amity School of Applied Sciences, Amity University Rajasthan (AUR), Jaipur, India. His current research areas of interest include cognition, communication, electromagnetic field theory, antenna and wave propagation, microwave, computational biology and applied physics. He has been serving as Editor for various Springer book series. He was Associate Editor of the *Journal of Integrative Neuroscience* (The Netherlands: IOS Press). He has been Visiting Professor to UTM and UTeM, Malyasia and Visiting Scientist to NIMS, Japan. He has established MOU with UTeM Malaysia, NIMS Japan and University of Montreal, Canada. He has visited several countries such as Netherlands, Turkey, China, Czechoslovakia, Russia, Portugal, Finland, Belgium, South Africa, Japan, Singapore, Thailand, Malaysia, etc., for various academic missions. He has organized various conferences such as SoCPROS, SoCTA, ICOEVCI, TCCE as General Chair and Steering Committee Member.

Dr. Raghvendra Singh is currently working as Associate Professor at Pranveer Singh Institute of Technology, Kanpur Uttar Pradesh India. He received Bachelor's and Master's degrees in Electronics and Communication Engineering from UPTU University, Lucknow, National Institute of Technology, Jaipur, in 2004 and 2011, respectively, and Ph.D. degree in Wireless communication using Implantable and Wearable Antennas from JKLU, Jaipur, in 2019. His research includes wireless body area network for health care, microwave communication and antennas for WBAN. He has authored more than 21 papers in different peer-reviewed journals and conferences and 6 book chapters in reputed publishing houses. He is guiding many research scholars in the capacity of Guide. Dr. Raghvendra Singh is Life Member of ISTE and Member of IEEE.

Dr. Vishal Nagar is currently working as Professor at Pranveer Singh Institute of Technology, Kanpur Uttar Pradesh India. He received Bachelor's and Master's degrees and Ph.D. degree in Computer Science and Engineering in 2004, 2008 and 2012, respectively. His interest in research includes multicast routing in the field of computer network, machine learning and blockchain. He has authored more than 35 papers in different peer-reviewed journals and conferences and 5 book chapters in repudiated publishing houses like Springer and Wiley publications. He is guiding many research scholars in the capacity of Guide and Co-guide from various universities. He has experience of organizing National and International Conferences. Dr. Nagar is Life Member of the Computer Society of India and IEEE.

Contributors

Abdullah-Al-Mahmod Department of ICE, Bangladesh University of Professionals, Dhaka, Bangladesh

Zeeshan Adeen Department of Computer Engineering, Jamia Millia Islamia, New Delhi, India

Bharat Bhushan Agarwal Department of Computer Science and Engineering, IFTM University, Moradabad, India

Priyanka Agarwal Department of Electronics Engineering, Harcourt Butler Technical University, Kanpur, Uttar Pradesh, India

Rashi Agarwal Department of Information Technology, University Institute of Engineering and Technology, Chhatrapati Shahu Ji Maharaj University, Kanpur, India

Musheer Ahmad Department of Computer Engineering, Jamia Millia Islamia, New Delhi, India

Mosabber Uddin Ahmed University of Dhaka, Dhaka, Bangladesh

Sabbir Ahmed Institute of Information Technology, Jahangirnagar University, Savar, Dhaka, Bangladesh

Shamim Ahmed Bangladesh University of Business and Technology, Dhaka, Bangladesh

Nahid Ibne Akhter Bangladesh University of Professionals, Dhaka, Bangladesh

Ahmed Alkhayyat Department of Computer Technical Engineering, College of Technical Engineering, Islamic University, Najaf, Iraq

Karl Andersson Pervasive and Mobile Computing Laboratory, Luleå University of Technology, Skellefteå, Sweden

Mohammad Amir Ansari Integral University, Lucknow, India

Amit Arora DAV Institute of Engineering and Technology, Jalandhar, Punjab, India

Deepak Arora Amity University Uttar Pradesh, Lucknow Campus, Lucknow, India;
Pranveer Singh Institute of Technology, Kanpur, Uttar Pradesh, India

Vaibhav J. Babrekar Professor Ram Meghe Institute of Technology and Research, Badnera, Amravati, India

Deepak Balodi BBD Engineering College, Lucknow, India

Anirban Bandyopadhyay International Center for Materials and Nanoarchitectronics (WPI-MANA) and Research Center for Advanced Measurement and Characterization (RCAMC), National Institute for Materials Science (NIMS), Tsukuba, Japan

Mimun Barid University of South Asia, Dhaka, Bangladesh

Norazlina Bateni Faculty of Engineering, Universiti Malaysia Sarawak, Kota Samarahan, Malaysia

Isha Batra Computer Science and Engineering, Lovely Professional University, Phagwara, Punjab, India

Saima Beg Department of Electronics and Communication Engineering, Integral University, Lucknow, India

S. K. Bhalla Department of Electrical Engineering, PSIT, Kanpur, U.P., India

Sanjeev Kumar Bhalla Department of Electronics and Communication Engineering, PSIT-Pranveer Singh Institute of Technology, Kanpur, India

Milon Biswas Bangladesh University of Business and Technology, Dhaka, Bangladesh

Sudipto Chaki Bangladesh University of Business and Technology, Dhaka, Bangladesh

Satarupa Chakrabarti School of Computer Engineering, KIIT University, Bhubaneswar, India

Pritam Chakraborty St. Mary Technical Campus Kolkata, Kolkata, West Bengal, India

Ashish Kumar Chakraverti Department of Information Technology, Pranveer Singh Institute of Technology, Kanpur, UP, India;
Department of Computer Science and Engineering, Pranveer Singh Institute of Technology, Kanpur, India

Akansha Chandravanshi Department of ECE, School of Studies of Engineering & Technology, Guru Ghasidas Vishwavidyalaya Bilaspur (C.G.), Bilaspur, India

Ruchi Chaurasia Pranveer Singh Institute of Technology, Kanpur, India;
Integral University, Lucknow, India

Ravindra Raman Cholla Department of Computer Science and Engineering, Bapatla Engineering College, Guntur, India

Kuldeep Chouhan Department of Computer Science and Engineering, I.T.S Engineering College, Greater Noida, India

Achintya Das Kalyani Government Engineering College, Kalyani, West Bengal, India

Manish Deshmukh Department of ECE, School of Studies of Engineering & Technology, Guru Ghasidas Vishwavidyalaya Bilaspur (C.G.), Bilaspur, India

Shirish M. Deshmukh Professor Ram Meghe Institute of Technology and Research, Badnera, Amravati, India

Namrata Dhanda Department of Computer Science & Engineering, Amity University Uttar Pradesh, Lucknow Campus, Lucknow, India

Shivani Dixit Department of Electronics and Communication Engineering, Pranveer Singh Institute of Technology, Kanpur, Uttar Pradesh, India

Akhilesh Kumar Dubey Koneru Lakshmaiah Education Foundation (Deemed to be University), Guntur, Andhra Pradesh, India

Tanusree Dutta Organizational Behavior and Human Resource Management, Indian Institute of Management, Ranchi, India

Jocelyn Faubert Faubert Lab, School of Optometry, University of Montreal, Montreal, QC, Canada

Md. Foyjul Haque Somrat Department of ICE, Bangladesh University of Professionals, Dhaka, Bangladesh

Daisuke Fujita International Center for Materials and Nanoarchitectronics (MANA), Research Center for Advanced Measurement and Characterization (RCAMC), NIMS, Tsukuba, Ibaraki, Japan

Subrata Ghosh Chemical Science & Technology Division, CSIR North East Institute of Science andTechnology, Jorhat, Assam, India;
Academy of Scientific and Innovative Research (AcSIR), Ghaziabad, Uttar Pradesh, India

Pradeep K. Gupta Pranveer Singh Institute of Technology Kanpur, Kanpur, U.P., India

Rupali Gupta Department of Electronics and Communication Engineering, Integral University, Lucknow, India

Sumit Kumar Gupta Department of ECE, School of Studies of Engineering & Technology, Guru Ghasidas Vishwavidyalaya Bilaspur (C.G.), Bilaspur, India

Md. Manzurul Hasan American International University-Bangladesh (AIUB), Dhaka, Bangladesh

Md. Farhad Hossain Institute of Information Technology, Jahangirnagar University, Savar, Dhaka, Bangladesh

Mohammad Shahadat Hossain Department of Computer Science and Engineering, University of Chittagong, Chittagong, Bangladesh

Shahadat Hossain City University, Dhaka, Bangladesh

Lee Yee Hui Department of Electrical and Electronics, Faculty of Engineering, Universiti Malaysia Sarawak, Kota Samarahan, Malaysia

Farooq Husain SSITM Aligarh, Aligarh, U.P., India

Roshan Jahan Integral University Lucknow, Lucknow, India

Ankit Jain Department of Electronics and Communication Engineering, PSIT, Kanpur, U.P., India

Sandeep Kumar Jain ECE, I.K. Gujral PTU, Jalandhar, Punjab, India

M. A. Jalil Department of Physics, Faculty of Science, Universiti Teknologi Malaysia, Skudai, Johor, Malaysia

M. Josephine Mary Juliana Puducherry Technological University, Puducherry, India

Md. Alomgir Kabir Department of Electrical, Electronic and Communication Engineering, Military Institute of Science and Technology, Dhaka, Bangladesh

Ruchi Kadwane Department of Electronics and Communication Engineering, LNCTU, Bhopal, Madhya Pradesh, India

M. Shamim Kaiser Institute of Information Technology, Jahangirnagar University, Savar, Dhaka, Bangladesh;
Applied Intelligence and Informatics (AII), Wazed Miah Science Research Centre (WMSRC), Jahangirnagar University, Savar, Dhaka, Bangladesh

Sushil Kakkar ECE Department, Bhai Gurdas Institute of Engineering and Technology, Sangrur, Punjab, India

Baljeet Kaur ECE, GNDEC, Ludhiana, Punjab, India

Imran Ullah Khan Department of Electronics & Communication Engineering, Integral University, Lucknow, India

Zohaib Hasan Khan Integral University, Lucknow, India

Naimur Rahman Kidwai Integral University, Lucknow, India

Kuryati Kipli Department of Electrical and Electronics, Faculty of Engineering, Universiti Malaysia Sarawak, Kota Samarahan, Malaysia

Rani Kiran Department of Electronics & Communication Engineering, Integral University, Lucknow, India

Daya Krishnanda Microwave Physics Laboratory, Department of Physics and Computer Science, Dayalbagh Educational Institute, Agra, Uttar Pradesh, India

Tanmai Kulshreshtha Pranveer Singh Institute of Technology, Kanpur, India

Anil Kumar Department of ECE, ASET, Amity University, Uttar Pradesh, Noida, UP, India

Ashish Kumar Department of Computer Science and Engineering, I.T.S Engineering College, Greater Noida, India

Avishisht Kumar Integral University, Lucknow, India

Manish Kumar Pranveer Singh Institute of Technology, Kanpur, India

Shailendra Kumar Integral University, Lucknow, India

Tapesh Kumar Swami Keshvanand Institute of Technology, Management & Gramothan, Jaipur, Rajasthan, India

Vivek Kumar Department of Electronics and Communication Engineering, Pranveer Singh Institute of Technology, Kanpur, India

Aisya Amelia Abdul Latip Faculty of Engineering, Universiti Malaysia Sarawak, Kota Samarahan, Malaysia

Kasumawati Lias Faculty of Engineering, Universiti Malaysia Sarawak, Kota Samarahan, Malaysia

J. Eduardo Lugo Faubert Lab, School of Optometry, University of Montreal, Montreal, QC, Canada;
Facultad de Ciencias Fisico-Matematicas, Benem´Erita Universidad Aut´Onoma de Puebla, Col. San Manuel Ciudad Universitaria, Puebla, Mexico

Mufti Mahmud Department of Computer Science, Nottingham Trent University, Nottingham, UK

Mehul Mahrishi Swami Keshvanand Institute of Technology, Management & Gramothan, Jaipur, Rajasthan, India

Arun Malik Computer Science and Engineering, Lovely Professional University, Phagwara, Punjab, India

Shweta Mallick Department of Computer Science and Information Technology, WCTM, Gurgaon, Haryana, India

Dayang Azra Awang Mat Department of Electrical and Electronics, Faculty of Engineering, Universiti Malaysia Sarawak, Kota Samarahan, Malaysia

Khashayar Misaghian Faubert Lab, School of Optometry, University of Montreal, Montreal, QC, Canada

Sarojananda Mishra Department of Computer Science Engineering and Applications, Indira Gandhi Institute of Technology, Sarang, India

Surya Prakash Mishra Department of Computer Science and Information Technology, SHIATS, Allahabad, India

Md. Shahadat Hossain Moon Bangladesh University of Professionals, Dhaka, Bangladesh

Nasirul Mumenin Bangladesh University of Professionals, Dhaka, Bangladesh

Vishal Nagar Department of Computer Science & Engineering, Pranveer Singh Institute of Technology, Uttar Pradesh, Kanpur, India

R. Nakkeeran Pondicherry University, Puducherry, India

Sarfaraz Nawaz Swami Keshvanand Institute of Technology, Management & Gramothan, Jaipur, Rajasthan, India

Nabil Neggaz Université Des Sciences et de la Technologie d'Oran Mohamed Boudiaf, USTO-MB, Oran, Algeria;
Faculté Des Mathématiques et Informatique, Département d'Informatique Laboratoire Signal IMage PArole (SIMPA), Oran, Algeria

Biswarup Neogi JIS College of Engineering, Kalyani, West Bengal, India

Silvia Binte Nur Institute of Information Technology, Jahangirnagar University, Savar, Dhaka, Bangladesh

M. A. Palomino-Ovando Facultad de Ciencias Físico-Matemáticas, Benemérita Universidad Autónoma de Puebla, Puebla Pue., Mexico

Utkarsh Pandey Department of Electronics and Communication Engineering, Pranveer Singh Institute of Technology, Kanpur, India

Chandrahash Patel Research Scholar, Centre for Studies in Science Technology and Innovation Policy (CSSTIP), School of Social Sciences (SSS), Central University of Gujarat, Gandhinagar, India

Binaya Kumar Patra Department of Computer Science Engineering and Applications, Indira Gandhi Institute of Technology, Sarang, India

Sanjay Kumar Patra Department of Computer Science Engineering and Applications, Indira Gandhi Institute of Technology, Sarang, India

Anindya Pattanayak Organizational Behavior and Human Resource Management, Indian Institute of Management, Ranchi, India

Prasant Kumar Pattnaik School of Computer Engineering, KIIT University, Bhubaneswar, India

Shiva Prakash Department of Information Technology and Computer Application, Madan Mohan Malaviya University of Technology, Gorakhpur, India

Piyush Pranjal Management Department, O.P. Jindal Global University, Sonipat, India

Shweta Rani ECE Department, GZSCCET, Maharaja Ranjit Singh Punjab Technical University, Bathinda, Punjab, India

Kumud Ranjan Pal Seharabazar C. K. Institution, Seharabazar, Bardhaman, West Bengal, India

Abhishek Singh Rathour Department of Electronics and Communication Engineering, Pranveer Singh Institute of Technology, Kanpur, India

CH. Ravikumar Computer Science and Engineering, Lovely Professional University, Phagwara, Punjab, India

Kanad Ray Amity School of Applied Sciences, Amity University Rajasthan, Kant KalwarJaipur, Rajasthan, India

Navleen S. Rekhi IKG Punjab Technical University, Kapurthala, Punjab, India; DAV Institute of Engineering and Technology, Jalandhar, Punjab, India

Syed Hasan Saeed Integral University, Lucknow, India

Siti Kudnie Sahari Department of Electrical and Electronics, Faculty of Engineering, Universiti Malaysia Sarawak, Kota Samarahan, Malaysia

Pathik Sahoo International Center for Materials and Nanoarchitectronics (WPI-MANA) and Research Center for Advanced Measurement and Characterization (RCAMC), National Institute for Materials Science (NIMS), Tsukuba, Japan

Gaurav Sahu Department of Electronics and Communication Engineering, Pranveer Singh Institute of Technology, Kanpur, India

Mohammad Abdus Salam Department of ICE, Bangladesh University of Professionals, Dhaka, Bangladesh;
Institute of Information Technology, Jahangirnagar University, Savar, Dhaka, Bangladesh

Rohana Sapawi Department of Electrical and Electronics, Faculty of Engineering, Universiti Malaysia Sarawak, Kota Samarahan, Malaysia

Soumya Sarkar Marketing Management, Indian Institute of Management, Ranchi, India

Komal Saxena Microwave Physics Laboratory, Department of Physics and Computer Science, Dayalbagh Educational Institute, Agra, Uttar Pradesh, India;
International Center for Materials and Nanoarchitectronics (MANA), Research Center for Advanced Measurement and Characterization (RCAMC), NIMS, Tsukuba, Ibaraki, Japan

Rohit Saxena Amity University Uttar Pradesh, Lucknow Campus, Lucknow, India; Pranveer Singh Institute of Technology, Kanpur, Uttar Pradesh, India

Shampa Sengupta Department of Information Technology, MCKV Institute of Engineering, Liluah, Howrah, West Bengal, India

Aditya Pratap Shahi Department of Mechanical Engineering, B. N. College of Engineering and Technology, Lucknow, India

Preeta Sharan Department of ECE, The Oxford College of Engineering, Bengaluru, India

Kamal Kumar Sharma Pranveer Singh Institute of Technology, Kanpur, India

M. Shukla Department of Electronics Engineering, Harcourt Butler Technical University, Kanpur, Uttar Pradesh, India

Varun Shukla Department of Electronics and Communication Engineering, Pranveer Singh Institute of Technology, Kanpur, Uttar Pradesh, India

Yusra Siddiqui Department of Electronics & Communication Engineering, Integral University, Lucknow, India

Jagroop S. Sidhu DAV Institute of Engineering and Technology, Jalandhar, Punjab, India

Deepak Kumar Singh VSB Purvanchal University, Jaunpur, Uttar Pradesh, India

Jaikaran Singh Department of Electronics and Communication Engineering, LNCTU, Bhopal, Madhya Pradesh, India

Jasjit Singh IKG Punjab Technical University, Kapurthala, Punjab, India

Parulpreet Singh Lovely Professional University Jalandhar, Jalandhar, India

Pawan Singh Amity School of Engineering and Technology, Amity University Uttar Pradesh, Lucknow Campus, Lucknow, India

Pushpendra Singh Amity School of Applied Science, Amity University Rajasthan, Kant KalwarJaipur, Rajasthan, India;
International Center for Materials and Nanoarchitectronics (WPI-MANA) and Research Center for Advanced Measurement and Characterization (RCAMC), National Institute for Materials Science (NIMS), Tsukuba, Japan

Raghvendra Singh Department of Electronics and Communication Engineering, PSIT-Pranveer Singh Institute of Technology, Kanpur, U.P., India;
A.P.J Abdul Kalam Technical University, Lucknow, India;
Department of Computer Science and Engineering, IFTM University, Moradabad, India

Ravendra Singh Department of Computer Science and Engineering, IFTM University, Moradabad, India

Shailendra Singh Department of Electronics and Communication Engineering, PSIT-Pranveer Singh Institute of Technology, Kanpur, India

Sudhir Kumar Singh Pranveer Singh Institute of Technology, Kanpur, India;
Integral University, Lucknow, India

Amit Singha Jahangirnagar University, Dhaka, Bangladesh

Kunal Sinha Assistant Professor, Centre for Studies in Science Technology and Innovation Policy (CSSTIP), School of Social Sciences (SSS), Central University of Gujarat, Gandhinagar, India

Shailendra Kumar Sinha Pranveer Singh Institute of Technology, Kanpur, India

Nidhi Srivastava Amity Institute of Information Technology, Amity University Uttar Pradesh, Lucknow Campus, Lucknow, India

Prateek Srivastava Amity Institute of Information Technology, Amity University Uttar Pradesh, Lucknow Campus, Lucknow, India

Vikas Srivastava Lovely Professional University Jalandhar, Jalandhar, India; Pranveer Singh Institute of Technology, Kanpur, India

Gnanou Florence Sudha Puducherry Technological University, Puducherry, India

Tahmina Akter Sumi Department of Computer Science and Engineering, University of Chittagong, Chittagong, Bangladesh

Aleena Swetapadma School of Computer Engineering, KIIT University, Bhubaneswar, India

E. Sánchez-Mora Instituto de Física "Luis Rivera Terrazas", Benemérita Universidad Autónoma de Puebla, Puebla, Mexico

Nurul Mirza Afiqah Tajudin Department of Electrical and Electronics, Faculty of Engineering, Universiti Malaysia Sarawak, Kota Samarahan, Malaysia

Iffat Tamanna Bangladesh University of Business and Technology, Dhaka, Bangladesh

B. B. Tiwari VBS Purvanchal University, Jaunpur, Uttar Pradesh, India

M. Toledo-Solano CONACYT-Facultad de Ciencias Físico-Matemáticas, Benemérita Universidad Autónoma de Puebla, Puebla Pue., Mexico

Manish Madhav Tripathi Integral University Lucknow, Lucknow, India

Nishant Tripathi School of Electronics and Electrical Engineering, Lovely Professional University, Phagwara, India;
Department of Electronics and Communication Engineering, Pranveer Singh Institute of Technology, Kanpur, India

Rajesh Kumar Tyagi Department of CSE, Amity School of Engineering and Technology, Amity University Haryana, Manesar, Gurgaon, India

Sabbir Ahmed Usmani Department of ICE, Bangladesh University of Professionals, Dhaka, Bangladesh

Deepak Kumar Verma Department of CSE, Greater Noida Institute of Technology, Greater Noida, Uttar Pradesh, India

Garima Verma Department of Computer Science, Pranveer Singh Institute of Technology, Kanpur, India

Rajat Verma Department of Computer Science & Engineering, Amity University Uttar Pradesh, Lucknow Campus, Lucknow, India

Archana Yadav Department of ECE, ASET, Amity University, Uttar Pradesh, Noida, UP, India

Salmah Mohamad Yusoff Faculty of Cognitive Sciences and Human Development, Universiti Malaysia Sarawak, Kota Samarahan, Malaysia

Artificial Intelligence and Soft Computing

A Heuristic Approach for Analyzing Some Reading Behaviors of Online News Viewers Using RF and KNN

Shahadat Hossain, Md. Manzurul Hasan, and Mimun Barid

Abstract This paper focuses on the factors that motivate readers to get their news online by analyzing readers' reading behaviors. It sheds light on the variety of electronic press media, especially on various online news hubs. We have gathered several opinions regarding reading news online. We use the K-nearest neighbor (KNN) algorithm and the random forest (RF) algorithm for the analysis [1, 13]. In addition, a heuristic approach is hereby unveiled to analyze the activities of online news viewers. As a result, we find some factors that influenced the readers most to read news online, which assist the news agencies in understanding how newsreaders are behaving on online news platforms. Furthermore, we have results on the relative contributions, which show that these models are more accurate in predicting the factors inspiring the readers to surf news online than that of no existing one to the best of our knowledge. Additionally, as far as observed in previous literature, our paper have directed a new path on the subject matter besides some mentionable results.

Keywords Electronic media · Random forest (RF) · Newspaper · K-nearest neighbor (KNN)

The original version of this chapter was revised: Figures 5c and 5d has been included. A correction to this chapter is available at https://doi.org/10.1007/978-981-16-8826-3_57

S. Hossain (✉)
City University, Dhaka, Bangladesh

Md. M. Hasan
American International University-Bangladesh (AIUB), Dhaka, Bangladesh
e-mail: manzurul@aiub.edu

M. Barid
University of South Asia, Dhaka, Bangladesh

M. S. Kaiser et al. (eds.), *Proceedings of Trends in Electronics and Health Informatics*, Lecture Notes in Networks and Systems 376,
https://doi.org/10.1007/978-981-16-8826-3_1

1 Introduction

The dramatic advancement of technology in the last few decades has changed the world significantly. The digital world is now the primary source of knowledge of all kinds, whether personal, national, or international. In contrast, some days back, physical newspapers were thought to be storehouses of knowledge. Electronic media are gradually replacing the traditional ways of getting news from all regions. As a result, the degree of reliance issue on online news agencies is increasing day by day. We live in a society where all things are interconnected using the Internet. Most of the whats we read is now available online, which was not true at actual a few decades ago. The newspaper serves as a global knowledge center. So, newspaper publishers are acutely conscious of the importance of serving their readers. They can conduct daily reviews of the viewers' perceptions on reading online news. According to Zickuhr et al. [21], 43% of news audiences in America read news online.

Along with the printed newspapers, online news portals are being launched. For daily news viewers, this is the most followed source of information. An online news source must have certain features and attributes to attract viewers. Some news organizations have methods for transmitting or publishing online versions [18]. There is dissatisfaction with these news portals among readers and viewers, impacting news viewers' reading habits. This study focuses on the factors that influence newsreaders' behavior. Pertaining to social media, a significant number of people follow these online news portals. These people have some prior experience in reading online content. They make decisions to follow the news portals based on that. In this analysis, the perceptions of 264 people are analyzed and observed using machine learning approaches. We are using a relevant machine learning approach on a small dataset, which results in better outcomes. This paper's relative contribution is to explore a field of data analysis concerning online news reading habits. The objectives of this study are the following.

- To evaluate the impacts of supervised learnings on online news reading habits.
- To observe the performances of the RF models and KNN classifiers.
- To explain how the online news media have effects over readers' news reading habits.

The remaining paper is accordingly arranged. Section 2 includes related papers on reading habits for news. Next, the methodologies are presented in Sect. 3. In Sect. 4, the experiments, along with our models, are finally demonstrated. Finally, Sect. 5 shows the results and observations, while Sect. 6 shows the future directions and conclusion.

2 Related Work

Richard et al. [7] illustrated the impacts of individual trust on news media and how various levels of trust influence news viewers' participatory activities. They also looked at how different levels of trust could impact the mainstream or unconventional news media. Jonathan et al. [9] studied the possibility of topic-based innovator detection in social media and tested their built model on large-scale Twitter data. Their model outperformed other models that had previously been used. Finally, a broad-based analysis has been completed by Qihao et al. [12] to find the contents of inspiring online news. They found that some forms of expression can predict inspiring news. Furthermore, they showed how long you could see an article on the most-shared list.

Min-lind et al. [20] developed the first multi-label lazy learning algorithm, ML-KNN, which is based on the well-known K-nearest neighbor algorithm. They improved their approach by evaluating it on three different multi-label learning problems. Next, Isabelle et al. [14] conducted a survey and discovered that although reading comments do not impact the news brands, negative comments can be disruptive. Finally, Annika et al. [4] surveyed data from a common type of news media in Sweden, and the findings indicate that socioeconomic statuses have significant impacts on news readings.

Lee et al. [5] conducted an article review and discovered that user inputs have huge influences on news outputs as well as on changing users' sensitivities and responses against the news. Furthermore, the effects of accidental exposures have significant impacts on users so that they can recall the news contents [16]. Sanne et al. [15] carried out an experimental study in which they used an eye-tracking experiment to determine the impacts of readers' visual attention to the news (printed or online). The results revealed that printed news contributes to diverse learnings, while Web sites only contribute to introductory learning. Anja et al. [19] performed a study on European readers and discovered that automated and combined journalism are trustworthy and dependable alternatives to human-created materials. Finally, Manuel et al. [8] demonstrated the influences of authorships by experimenting on Spanish adults and found differences among authorships and exclusive media-depending news. For various dimensions of contemporary research on big data, machine learning, etc., some papers may be recommended like [11, 17].

3 Methodology

This section depicts the essential aspect of the analysis. The description of the dataset and its preprocessing have been completed and recorded. In this analysis, machine learning models and algorithms are being used.

3.1 Sample Collection and Data Preprocessing

We survey 264 people from different backgrounds using the online platform Google form. The question set has been chosen based on the author-reader impact model

Table 1 Participants' profile sample ($N = 264$)

Question	Count	Percentage
Age		
≤30	254	96.22
>30	10	3.78
Gender		
Male	222	84.10
Female	42	15.90
Regularity of reading news		
Regular reader	201	76.14
Irregular reader	63	23.86

[9] and on research regarding consumers' behaviors analysis in F-commerce [11]. Table 1 shows a key description of the participants. After collecting the raw data from the survey, we use data preprocessing techniques such as converting nominal data to numerical data, shortening attribute names, and removing missing data. The evaluation of machine learning algorithms has a lot to do with why a specific machine learning algorithm does not perform unbalanced data. When using machine learning, dataset imbalance may cause unbalanced learning. Therefore, we use the synthetic minoring oversampling approach (*SMOTE*) from the Python *imbalanced learning* package to balance the dataset.

3.2 Random Forest Algorithm

Random forest algorithm is used for supervised learning since it reduces dataset from over-fitting, developed by Ho [10]. It is used for classification as well as for regression. This algorithm selects the features and row samples from the dataset. Presume we have a dataset D, and RF chooses $d(d_1, d_2, d_3, ..., d_n)$ training data samples from D where $d < D$. Individual decision tree model exists for each sample set d which is $M(M_1, M_2, M_3, ...M_n)$. From these M, the average model is created for predictions for the testing dataset.

3.3 K-nearest Neighbor

Fix [6] developed the *KNN* algorithm in 1952, and Altman [3] improved it later on. It is a method of nonparametric classification. The training samples are the input to *KNN*, and the output depends on the method (classification or regression) that we use. These types are specified when we use *KNN*. The new member is classified in the

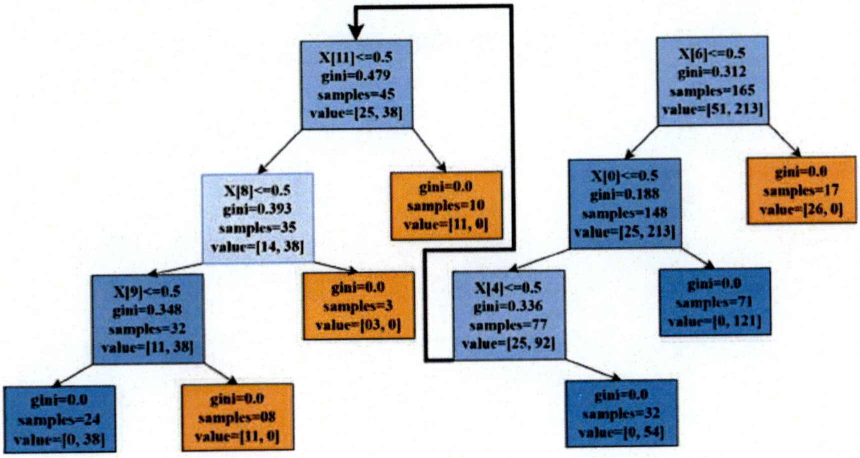

Fig. 1 Proposed random forest decision tree model.

KNN classifier by maximization vote of neighbor, where $k(k = 1, 2, 3, 4, 5, ...)$ is a positive integer. This k represents the nearest neighbor's number. *KNN* regression returns the average value of k nearest neighbors for each new member. The Euclidean distance of the current class value of samples is used to fit the training samples into the model. It uses the nearest distance from the training sample points to predict the class of the testing dataset.

4 Experiment with Models

On our dataset, we use a data cleaning process. The nominal data is converted into numerical data and shuffled the dataset 150 times in data preprocessing before implementing the random forest algorithm. We have scaled our data for KNN using the *StandardScaler* method from *Scikit-learn* library.

We have then split the shuffled dataset into two sub-datasets using the *train_test_split* method from the *sklearn* library. They are training (63%) and testing (37%) datasets. We fit the training dataset into the RF model after splitting. The result metrices are developed and observed using the *sklearn* library. The RF algorithm has created a total number of 20 identical decision trees. We represent one of those trees in Fig. 1. A node in our RF model tree contains some details. In the node, *gini* displays the likelihood of a random sample which is gradually reducing up to the leaf node [2]. The number of observations in a node is measured by the *sample*.

The *class* specifies the highest classification for nodes which is simplified to leaf nodes for the final prediction. We have applied the KNN to the scaled dataset for classification and observed its results. Similarly to RF, we have divided the dataset into testing (63%) and training (37%) datasets. The training data is being fitted in

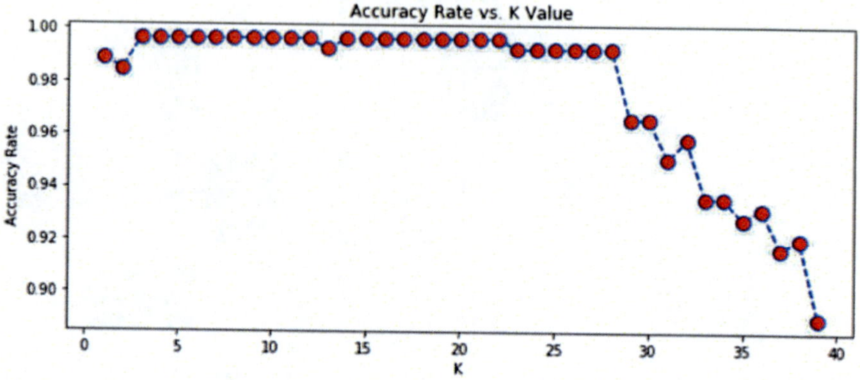

Fig. 2 Accuracy rate versus K-values

the classifier with $k = 1$. Then, using testing data, we make predictions based on our class attribute.

To generate the KNN classifier's performance metrices, we use the *Scikit-learn* library. The classifier is trained by varying the value of $k(1–40)$, and the error rate is calculated. The error rates are then plotted into a graph for comparison concerning the various values of k. Though the analyses are not for a massive dataset, we have empirical assumptions on what the news audiences perceive. According to Fig. 2, our KNN model performed robustly (99%) when the value of k is between 4 and 20. After that range, the accuracy decreases and then increases when $k = 30$. In $k = 40$, the accuracy of this classifier decreased by up to 84%.

5 Results and Observations

We identify some relevant results based on our model's performance and data analysis. This section records all of the model's performance parameters. For example, we utilize several figures and tables. For the measurements in both models, we utilize the *Scikit-learn* package. Values from the data are presented in Fig. 3. True positive (TP) is shown by 00 and for false positive (FP) is 01, false negative (FN) indicates 00, and true negative (TN) is indicated by 10 in Fig. 3.

Both models have shown outstanding results. In terms of accuracy, random forest and KNN achieved 93% and 99%, respectively. However, RF has outperformed KNN in terms of sensitivity. The sensitivity for RF is 99% and for KNN is 96% (Table 2).

We also find out the features' importance that may influence our model for predictions, and some features impact our RF model. For example, from Fig. 4, a feature named fake news in an online news portal has the highest importance in the RF model. This information indicates that the RF model is using this feature as an important

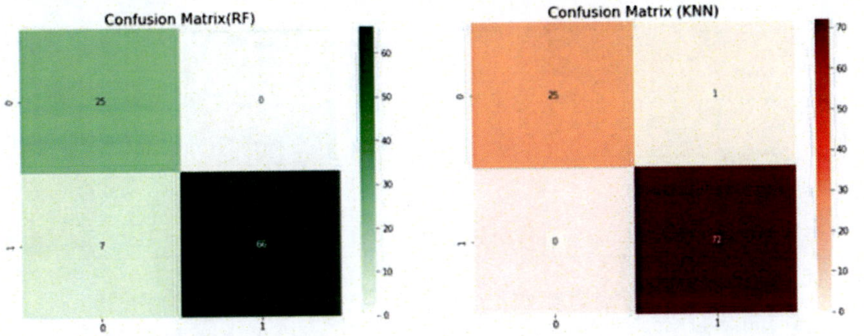

(a) Confusion Matrix of Random Forest Model

(b) Confusion Matrix of K-Nearest Neighbour

Fig. 3 Confusion matrix of random forest and KNN

Table 2 Result table

	Random forest decision tree (%)	K-nearest neighbor (%)
Accuracy	93	99
Precision	89	99
Sensitivity	99	96
Specificity	90	99

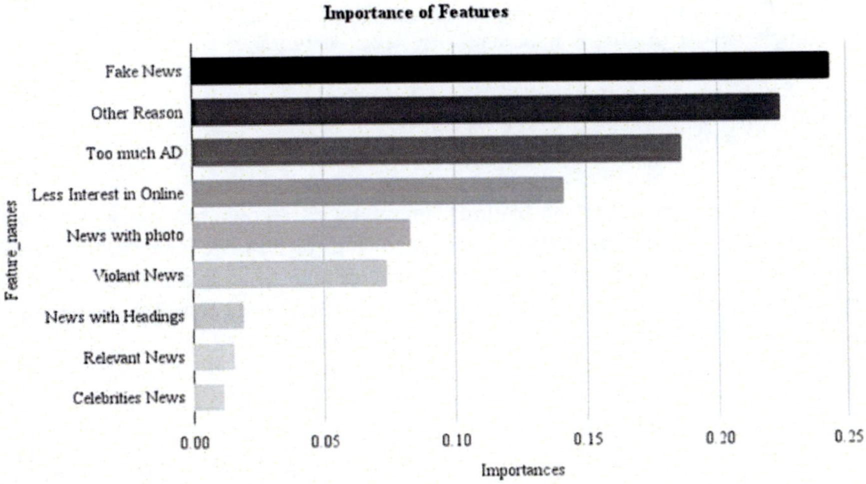

Fig. 4 Importance of features

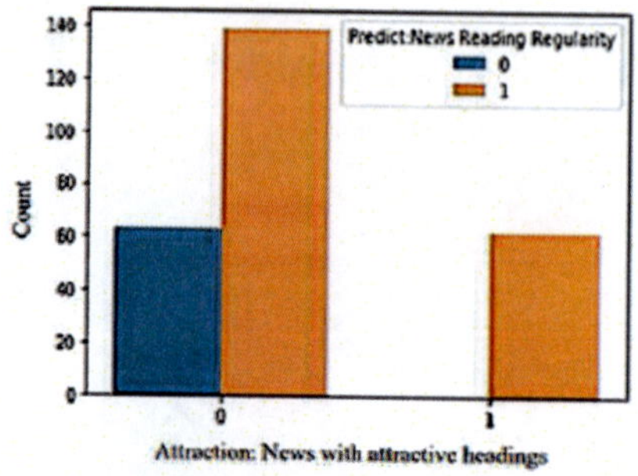

(a) Bar chart for news reading regularity under news with attractive headings: real vs. prediction

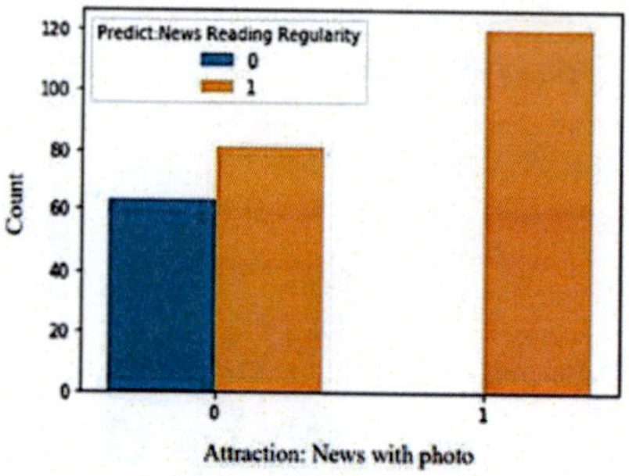

(b) Bar chart for news reading regularity under news with photo: real vs. prediction

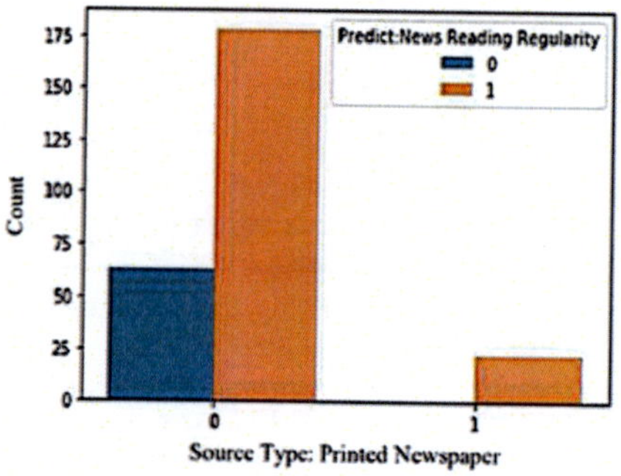

(c) Bar chart for news reading regularity under printed newspaper: real vs. prediction

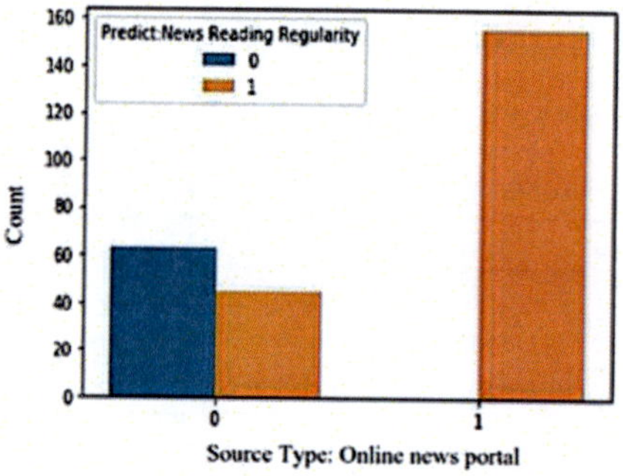

(d) Bar chart for news reading regularity under online news source: real vs. prediction

Fig. 5 Different bar chart analyses of predicted data

for predictions. The rest of the features' importance is shown gradually in the bar chart (Fig. 4). Although our dataset contains various factors, we have demonstrated the effects of few critical factors on the frequencies with which respondents read the news. In Fig. 5, we show the outcomes of the class that have been chosen and compared to the other variables using *matplotlib*, a Python plotting library. In this case, the X-axis represents the factor, while the Y-axis represents the total count based on our class attribute. Figure 5a represents the participants who read the news daily without concern for the news heading. On the other hand, a small group of respondents considers attractive news headlines while reading the news. The participants are being driven to the news by the pictures, whereas others are not (Fig. 5b).

Figure 5c indicates that traditional printed newspapers have no impact on regularity behind the reading habits of our participants. Figure 5d reveals that almost all daily news viewers read news from online news portals. We can illustrate any of the similar figures shown in Fig. 5. In all figures, orange bars indicate regular readings, whereas blue bars indicate the counts of inconsistent readings. Irregular news viewers are unconcerned regardless of the sources and attractions toward components. That is why there is no response against this issue. Hence, the blue color bar is 0 beside the orange color bar for 1 in X-axis, which can easily be observed in all the figures of Fig. 5.

6 Future Research Directions and Conclusion

We have introduced a novel concept along with a new dimension to research. This research reveals the wide-ranging environments in which researchers can explore different machine learning methods on larger datasets. The study's potential direction is to forecast news coverage features that might influence the readers most.

The reading patterns of newsreaders should be studied so that news publishers would recognize the readers' behaviors and publish their news contents accordingly. We have studied various machine learning models on the dataset of online news viewers and have found it to be robust. This study may encourage fellow researchers to walk along with the new era. Lastly, in our electronic age, we would like to emphasize that further more research works on online news reading habits must be attentioned by the researchers in the same community with a view to keen decision-making.

References

1. Afsana F, Asif-Ur-Rahman M, Ahmed MR, Mahmud M, Kaiser MS (2018) An energy conserving routing scheme for wireless body sensor nanonetwork communication. IEEE Access 6:9186–9200
2. Ali J, Khan R, Ahmad N, Maqsood I (2012) Random forests and decision trees. Int J Comput Sci Issues (IJCSI) 9(5):272
3. Altman NS (1992) An introduction to kernel and nearest-neighbor nonparametric regression. J Am Stat 46(3):175–185
4. Bergström A, Strömbäck J, Arkhede S (2019) Towards rising inequalities in newspaper and television news consumption? A longitudinal analysis. J Eur J Commun 34(2):175–189
5. Eun-Ju L, Tandoc EC Jr (2017) When news meets the audience: how audience feedback online affects news production and consumption. J Hum Commun Res 43(4):436–449
6. Fix E, Hodges JL Jr (1952) Discriminatory analysis-nonparametric discrimination: small sample performance. California Univ Berkeley, Tech. rep
7. Fletcher R, Park S (2017) The impact of trust in the news media on online news consumption and participation. Digit J 5(10):1281–1299
8. Goyanes M, Artero JP, Zapata L, The effects of news authorship, exclusiveness and media type in readers' paying intent for online news: an experimental study. Journalism 0(0):1464884918820741 (0). 10.1177/1464884918820741
9. Herzig J, Mass Y, Roitman H (2014) An author-reader influence model for detecting topic-based influencers in social media. In: Proceedings of 25th ACM conference on hypertext and social media, HT '14, Santiago, Chile. ACM, pp 46–55. 10.1145/2631775.2631804

10. Ho TK (2002) A data complexity analysis of comparative advantages of decision forest constructors. Pattern Anal Appl 5(2):102–112. https://doi.org/10.1007/s100440200009
11. Hossain S, Hasan MM, Hossain T (2020) An analytical study of influencing factors on consumers' behaviors in facebook using ANN and RF. In: Proceedings of international conference on intelligent computing & optimization (ICO). AISC, vol 1324. Springer, Cham, pp 744–753
12. Ji Q, Raney AA, Raney SH, Dale KR, Oliver MB, Reed A, Seibert J, Raney AA (2019) Spreading the good news: analyzing socially shared inspirational news content. J Journalism Mass Commun Q 96(3):872–893
13. Kaiser MS et al (2018) Advances in crowd analysis for urban applications through urban event detection. IEEE Trans Intell Transp Syst 19(10):3092–3112
14. Krebs I, Lischka JA (2019) Is audience engagement worth the buzz? the value of audience engagement, comment reading, and content for online news brands. J Journalism 20(6):714–732
15. Kruikemeier S, Lecheler S, Boyer MM (2018) Learning from news on different media platforms: an eye-tracking experiment. J Polit Commun 35(1):75–96
16. Lee JK, Kim E (2017) Incidental exposure to news: predictors in the social media setting and effects on information gain online. Comput Hum Behav 75:1008–1015. https://doi.org/10.1016/j.chb.2017.02.018
17. Mahmud M, Kaiser MS, McGinnity TM, Hussain A (2021) Deep learning in mining biological data. Cognit Comput 13(1):1–33
18. Mahmud M, Kaiser MS, Hussain A, Vassanelli S (2018) Applications of deep learning and reinforcement learning to biological data. IEEE Trans Neural Netw Learn Syst 29(6):2063–2079
19. Wölker A, Powell TE (2018) Algorithms in the newsroom? News readers' perceived credibility and selection of automated journalism. J Journalism, pp 86–103. 10.1177/1464884918757072
20. Zhang M, Zhou Z (2007) ML-KNN: A lazy learning approach to multi-label learning. Pattern Recognit 40(7):2038–2048. https://doi.org/10.1016/j.patcog.2006.12.019
21. Zickuhr K, Rainie L, Purcell K, Madden M, Brenner J (2012) Younger Americans' reading and library habits. J Pew Internet Am Life Project

Automatic Image Classification and Abnormality Identification Using Machine Learning

Ravendra Singh and Bharat Bhushan Agarwal

Abstract Magnetic resonance imaging (MRI) is a non-invasive technology for examining, diagnosing, and treating tumor regions in the medical field. An early detection of a brain tumor can save a patient's life if appropriate therapy is given. The correct detection of tumors in MRI slices is a difficult problem, and this suggested approach can effectively classify and segment the tumor region. In the field of computer vision, machine learning has played a critical role. It has numerous uses in the realm of illness detection, particularly in the diagnosis of brain tumors. Relevant features are extracted from each segmented tissue to improve the accuracy and quality rate of the support vector machine (SVM)-based classifier in brain tumor identification. The experimental results of the recommended technique on magnetic resonance brain imaging have been examined and validated for performance and quality analysis. An SVM classifier was used to identify brain tumors.

Keywords Support vector machine (SVM) · Radial basis function (RBF) · Magnetic resonance imaging

1 Introduction

In recent years, the medical industry has benefited from the development of information technology and e-health care systems, which allows clinical experts to give better health care to patients. The challenge of segmenting sick brain tissues and normal brain tissues such as gray matter (GM), white matter (WM), and cerebrospinal fluid (CSF) from magnetic resonance (MR) images is solved in this study using a feature extraction technique and a support vector machine (SVM) classifier. Tumors are divided into two categories: benign and malignant. The benign tumor, which begins in the membranes surrounding the brain and spinal cord, is the most common form. Benign tumors do not spread throughout the brain and are simple to cure. Tumors that are malignant are cancerous and can spread to other parts of the body. The patient has

R. Singh (✉) · B. B. Agarwal
Department of Computer Science and Engineering, IFTM University, Moradabad, India

M. S. Kaiser et al. (eds.), *Proceedings of Trends in Electronics and Health Informatics*, Lecture Notes in Networks and Systems 376,
https://doi.org/10.1007/978-981-16-8826-3_2

a better chance of survival if the tumor is detected early. The most common imaging procedure for diagnosing brain cancers is magnetic resonance imaging (MRI). The magnetic field principle underpins MRI. The input data in an MRI system is multidimensional. In the diagnosis of brain cancers, segmentation is crucial. It distinguishes the suspicious (tumor) region from the MR image background. Tumors are described as the uncontrolled proliferation of cancerous cells in any part of the body, but a brain tumor is defined as cancerous cells growing uncontrollably in the brain. There are two types of brain tumors: benign and malignant. The structure of a benign brain tumor is uniform, and it does not contain active (cancer) cells, whereas the structure of a malignant brain tumor is non-uniform (heterogeneous), and it contains active (cancer) cells. Cells that are active low-grade tumors, such as gliomas and meningiomas, are classed as a benign tumor, but high-grade tumors, such as glioblastomas and astrocytoma's, are classified as malignant tumors. Different magnetic resonance imaging (MRI) sequence pictures, such as T1-weighted MRI, T2-weighted MRI, fluid-attenuated inversion recovery (FLAIR) weighted MRI, and proton density-weighted MRI, are used in this study for diagnosis. A benign brain tumor has a uniform structure and does not contain active (cancer) cells, whereas a malignant brain tumor has a non-uniform (heterogeneous) structure and does contain active (cancer) cells. These are active cells. Low-grade tumors like gliomas and meningiomas are benign, whereas high-grade tumors like glioblastomas and astrocytoma's are malignant. This study uses a variety of magnetic resonance imaging (MRI) sequence photographs for diagnosis, including T1-weighted MRI, T2-weighted MRI, fluid-attenuated inversion recovery (FLAIR) weighted MRI, and proton density-weighted MRI ability to diagnose a brain tumor at an early stage is critical for better therapy. Once a brain tumor is detected clinically, a radiological examination is required to determine its location, size, and influence on the surrounding areas. The optimal treatment, whether surgery, radiation, or chemotherapy, is chosen based on this information.

2 Background Study

Medical image segmentation for brain tumor detection using magnetic resonance (MR) images or other medical imaging modalities is a critical step in determining the best treatment option at the correct time. Many techniques have been proposed for classifying a brain tumor in MR images, including fuzzy clustering means (FCM), support vector machine (SVM), artificial neural network (ANN), knowledge-based techniques, and the expectation–maximization (EM) algorithm technique, which are some of the most popular techniques used for region-based segmentation and thus to extract the important information from medical imaging modalities. In our suggested method, we use two pixel-based segmentation methods. Histogram statistics and k-means clustering are two examples. The histogram approach uses single or many thresholds to pixel-by-pixel classify an image. Analyzing the histogram for peak values and identifying the lowest point, which is often located between two successive peak values of the histogram, is a simple way to establish the gray value threshold t.

The histogram statistics method can produce good results if a histogram is bi-modal. The k-means clustering algorithm divides data into k groupings and is commonly utilized. Clustering is the process of putting data points with comparable feature vectors in one cluster and data points with dissimilar feature vectors in another. Fusion-based: Detecting the tumor by superimposing the victim's train image over a test image of the same age group. (1) Due to the varying proportions of both photographs, the overlapping produces complication. (2) The procedure is time-consuming. Canny-based edge detection: A better technique to tackle the challenge of detecting edges is to employ Canny-based edge detection. (1) Color photographs are not supported. (2) As a result, the time it takes to find the best answer increases.

3 Methodology

The proposed method has used an image processing technique to detect and classify brain tumors. The proposed method consists of various steps to get the final results. MRI image has been acquired in the first step and preprocessing the image for the next step. In the second step, segmentation of the image is done by k-mean clustering. In a final step, for the prediction of accuracy, support vector machine is applied. All these steps are discussed in the next sections.

3.1 Phase 1: Preprocessing

In initial consideration, an MRI image is taken for making it ready to act as an input for the algorithm. After completing this step, the resizing [1] of the two-dimensional image is done. The purpose of the reshaping of an image is to make it uniform by converting it into a dimension of the same size. The next process which is involved here is a conversion of a two-dimensional image into a grayscale format [2]. The purpose of this conversion is to lessen the complexity of a typical RGB image. The flowchart of brain tumor detection (proposed) is illustrated in Fig. 1.

3.2 Phase 2: Feature Extraction

The extraction of the brain tumor requires the separation of the brain MR images into two regions [3]. One region contains the tumor cells of the brain, and the second contains the normal brain cells [4]. The MR image contains a large amount of information that is required, so the feature extraction has been applied to the MR image and relevant features have been retrieved from an image that described an image completely. The proposed method uses discrete wavelet transform (DWT) procedure for retrieving the features from an image. DWT reveals both time and frequency

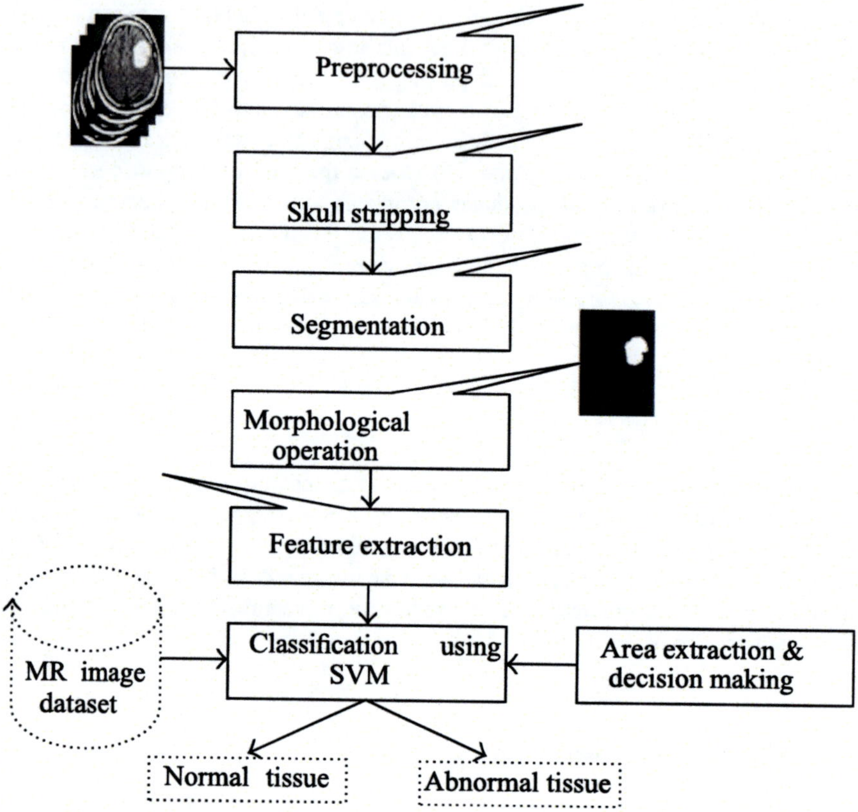

Fig. 1 Proposed methodology for detection and classification

information. For MR images, 2D-DWT [5, 6] is used as MR images which are of two dimensions. The DWT works on the filters of high and low passes. In the first step, both the filters have been used along with the columns of the MR image after downsampling. Once downsampling has been done, the bandwidth of the MR image is half and the redundant features are left. MR image characteristics have not been lost as Nyquist criteria reproduces the full signal from the half information. After downsampling, the low and high pass filters are implemented along with rows of the MRI. In the DWT [7], high pass filters provide an edge of MR image and low pass filters provide an approximation of MR image. The first obtained band is the LL sub-band that provides the approximation of MR images. The horizontal features of the MR image are retrieved from the LH sub-band, and the vertical features of an image are extracted from the HL sub-band. The diagonal features of the MR image are extracted from HH.

3.3 Phase 3: Classification

After evaluating its classification accuracy with KNN, the classification phase divides the input test image into normal and abnormal classes. Kernel support vector machines (KSVMs) are used for classification. The resultant normal and abnormal images of the categorized image are displayed.

The support vector machine (SVM) is a recently introduced powerful supervised classifier and accurate learning tool. Over neural networks and RBF classifiers, SVM has proven to be more efficient. To separate two sets of data in feature space, SVM employs an optimal linear separating hyperplane. The lowest margin between the two sets is maximized to get this ideal hyperplane. As a result, the hyperplane that emerges will rely solely on boundary training patterns known as support vectors. SVM works by performing a nonlinear mapping of an input vector into a high-dimensional feature space that is hidden from both the input and output. Figure 2 depicts the construction of an ideal hyperplane for separating the features [8]. An SVM's output is a linear combination of training samples projected onto a high-dimensional feature space using the kernel function [5].

SVM is based on the statistical learning theory's structured risk minimization principle. Its core goal is to reduce the margins between classes and the true cost by controlling empirical risk and classification capacity [9] (Fig. 3).

SVM with linear kernel function and radial basis function (RBF) is used in this study to classify images into two categories: "normal" and "abnormal." The labels for these classes are "1" and "2," respectively, meaning "normal" and "abnormal." Decisions about pattern recognition or classification made in the context of medical diagnosis have consequences that go beyond statistical metrics of accuracy and validity. We need to provide a clinical or diagnostic interpretation of pattern vector-based statistical or rule-based decisions [10–17]. The alternatives are as follows: When a test results in a true positive (TP) or a "hit," it means the patient has the condition. When a test is negative for a subject who does not have the condition, it is referred to as a true negative (TN). When a test is negative for a patient who has the disease of

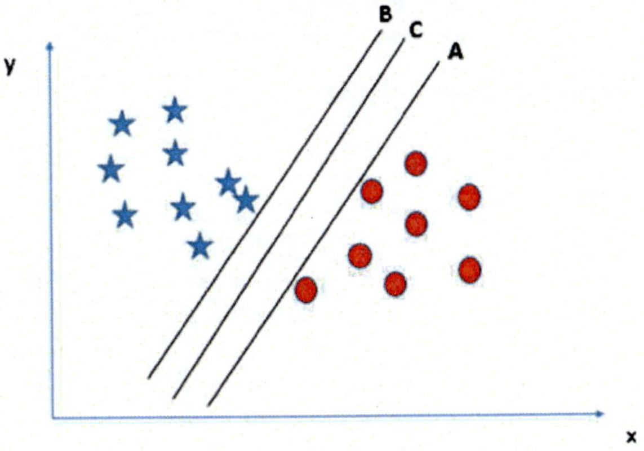

Fig. 2 Hyperplanes (A, B, and C)

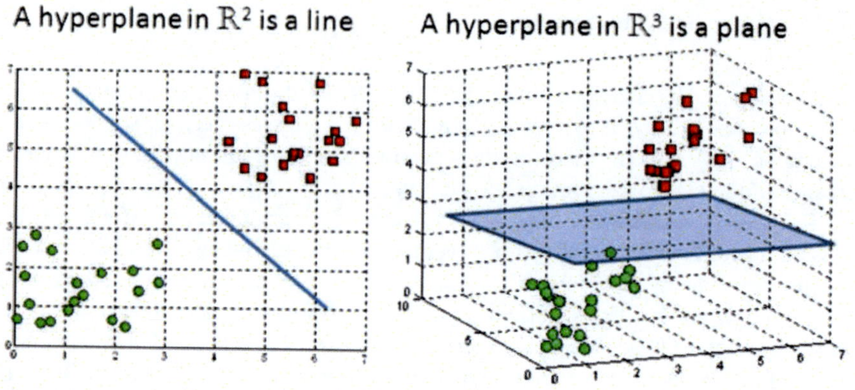

Fig. 3 Hyperplanes in 2D and 3D feature space

concern, it is considered to be a false negative (FN) or a "miss," implying that the test has missed the case. A false positive (FP) or false alarm occurs when a test results in a positive result even when the person being tested does not have the disease [18–22].

4 Result Discussion

The KSM classifier is used to classify the test input image. The ROI detection in an anomalous class image is shown in Fig. 4. A confusion matrix was used to calculate the classification accuracy. The confusion matrix for SVM (Linear) and SVM (RBF) is given in Tables 1 and 2.

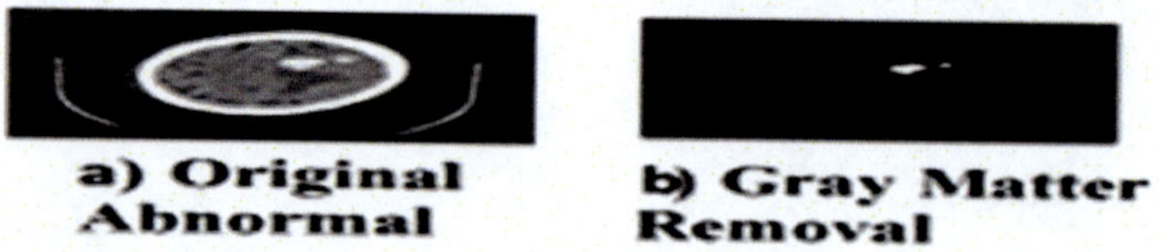

Fig. 4 Abnormality detection

Table 1 Confusion matrix of SVM classifier with linear kernel

	Normal	Abnormal	Total
Normal	21	7	28
Abnormal	12	15	27

Table 2 Confusion matrix of SVM classifier with RBF kernel

	Normal	Abnormal	Total
Normal	22	4	26
Abnormal	4	21	25

5 Conclusion

This work provides an object identification prototype based on SVMs that can achieve real-time performance while maintaining excellent detection accuracy. The research proposed an accurate method for automatically classifying and detecting abnormalities in MRI images. The KSVM classifier with a 90% classification rate is used to classify the input MRI picture as normal or abnormal. This system will be improved by extending it to detect abnormalities in multimodal brain pictures and increasing the classification rate. Furthermore, regardless of the window size, amount of support vectors, or image size, the same prototype can be utilized for multiple applications.

References

1. Mohsin S (2011) Concentration of the specific absorption rate around deep brain stimulation electrodes during MRI. Prog Electromagn Res 121:469–484
2. Najadat H, Jaffal Y, Darwish O, Yasser N (2011) A classifier to detect abnormality in CT brain images. In: Proceedings of the International multiconference of engineers and computer scientists, pp 16–18
3. Kharrat A, Gasmi K, Ben Messaoud M, Benamrane N, Abid M (2010) A hybrid approach for automatic classification of brain MRI using genetic algorithm and support vector machine. Leonardo J Sci 17(1):71–82
4. Tagluk ME, Akin M, Sezgin N (2010) Classıfication of sleep apnea by using wavelet transform and artificial neural networks. Expert Syst Appl 37(2):1600–1607
5. Zhang Y-D, Lenan Wu (2008) Weights optimization of neural network via improved BCO approach. Prog Electromagn Res 83:185–198
6. Xu Y, Guo Y, Xia L, Wu Y (2008) An support vector regression based nonlinear modeling method for SiC MESFET. Prog Electromagn Res 2:103–114
7. Yeh JY, Fu JC (2008) A hierarchical genetic algorithm for segmentation of multi-spectral human-brain MRI. Expert Syst Appl 34(2):1285–1295
8. Kumar S, Dabas C, Godara S (2017) Classification of brain MRI tumor images: a hybrid approach. Procedia Comput Sci 122:510–517
9. Rejani Y, Thamarai Selvi S (2009) Early detection of breast cancer using SVM classifier technique. arXiv preprint arXiv:0912-2314
10. Mohrekesh M, Akbari M, Soroushmehr SR, Nasr-Esfahani E, Karimi N, Samavi S, Najarian K (2018) Left ventricle segmentation in cardiac MR images using fully convolutional network. In: 2018 40th Annual international conference of the IEEE engineering in medicine and biology society (EMBC), pp 1275–1278
11. Godara S, Singh R, Kumar S (2016) A novel weighted class based clustering for medical diagnostic interface. Indian J Sci Technol 9(44)
12. Iqbal A, Jeoti V (2012) A novel wavelet-Galerkin method for modeling radio wave propagation in tropospheric ducts. Prog Electromagn Res B 36:35–52

13. Singh K, Verma S (2012) Detecting brain MRI anomalies by using SVM classification. Int J Eng Res Appl (IJERA) 2:724–726
14. Ulagamuthalvi V, Sridharan D (2012) Automatic identification of ultrasound liver cancer tumor using support vector machine. In: International conference on emerging trends in computer and electronics engineering, pp 41–43
15. Mathew JA, Khan AM, Niranjan UC (2011) Algorithms to find the thresholds for the abnormality extraction of the MRI slice images of a GUI based intelligent diagnostic imaging system. In: International conference on VLSI, communication & instrumentation (ICVCI), Proceedings published by International Journal of Computer Applications (IJCA), pp 18–23
16. Hiremath PS, Bannigidad P, Hiremath M (2011) Digital microscopic image analysis of virus particles. Int J Mach Intell 4: 180–184
17. Qurat-Ul-Ain, Latif G, Kazmi SB, Jaffar MA, Mirza AM (2010) Classification and segmentation of brain tumor using texture analysis. In: Recent advances in artificial intelligence, knowledge engineering and databases, pp 147–155
18. Zhang YD, Wu L (2008) Weights optimization of neural network via improved BCO approach. Prog Electromagn Res 83:185–198
19. Hiremath PS, Humnabad Iranna Y, Pujari JD (2007) Classification of squamous cell carcinoma based on color and textural features in microscopic images of esophagus tissues. J Comput Sci 3(7):566–573
20. Gao Z, Po L, Jiang W, Zhao X, Dong H (2007) A novel computerized method based on support vector machine for tongue diagnosis. In: 2007 Third international IEEE conference on signal-image technologies and internet-based system. IEEE, pp 849–854
21. Selvaraj H, Thamarai Selvi S, Selvathi D, Gewali L (2007) Brain MRI slices classification using least squares support vector machine. IC-MED 1(1):21–33
22. Mancas M, Gosselin B, Macq B (2005) Tumor detection using Airways asymmetry. In: IEEE-EMBS 2005, 27th annual international conference. Engineering in Medicine and Biology Society

A Review of Speech Sentiment Analysis Using Machine Learning

Tapesh Kumar, Mehul Mahrishi, and Sarfaraz Nawaz

Abstract Over recent decades, sentiment analysis has been progressive. A lot of effort focused on text analysis using techniques of text mining. However, audio sentiment analysis is still in the developing phase in the academic community. In this recommended study, we examine different transcripts of speech sentiment also with speaker recognition to assess speakers' emotions. The study of the sentiment of speech in many businesses, such as customer service, health care, and education, represents a major issue.

Keywords Emotion detection · Machine learning · Sentiment analysis · Speech recognition · Text analysis

1 Introduction

Sentiment analysis is an analysis of the individual's mood or attitude to an event, a debate on issues, or in general. In various applications, sentiment analysis is used, in which human thoughts based on their conversation are understood. A computer has to know who interacts and what is being said to understand the mind/mood of individuals in the discussion so that we develop a system for voice and speech recognition first and conduct a sentimental analysis of data acquired from previous procedures. Audio content like songs, discussions, political disputes was transformed into text by the research community. And, the community has also been researching audio analysis [15–17], which included more than one speaker, to investigate customer service calls. Since the conversation involves more than one speaker, analyzing the audio recordings becomes tedious (Fig. 1).

Speech sentiment analysis generally has four main phases:

1. **Speech recognition**: Speech recognition is a computer or program's capacity to detect words and phrases in people's language and convert them to a machine-readable format, which may be used to further process them. Tools like Sphinx-4 [9, 10, 20], Bing Speech, Google Speech Recognition can also be used.

T. Kumar (✉) · M. Mahrishi · S. Nawaz
Swami Keshvanand Institute of Technology, Management & Gramothan, Jaipur, Rajasthan, India

M. S. Kaiser et al. (eds.), *Proceedings of Trends in Electronics and Health Informatics*, Lecture Notes in Networks and Systems 376,
https://doi.org/10.1007/978-981-16-8826-3_3

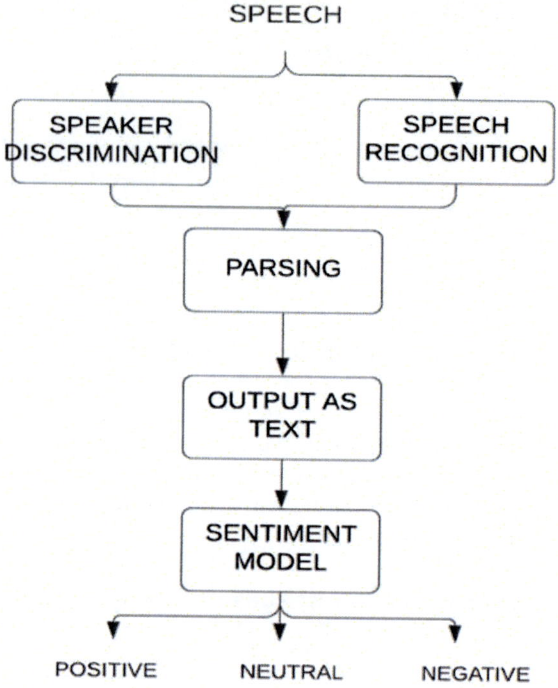

Fig. 1 Speech sentiment analysis

2. **Speaker recognition**: Speaker recognition is the identification of a person based on the variations and uniqueness of the voice. For nearly eight decades, it has received considerable attention from the scholarly community [18]. The signal speech comprises many aspects that can provide linguistic, emotional, speaking data [3]. The recognition of the speaker uses the voice signal's special properties.
3. **Feature extraction**: To obtain greater accuracy, the extraction of the unique discriminating feature of the speaker is crucial. In the following step, the correctness of this phase is crucial since it provides the input for the next phase. Some feature extraction approaches are the MFCC, LPC, LSF, PLP, and DWT, which have been utilized to extract relevant voice-recognizing information from signals [11, 12].
4. **Feature matching**: Speech recognition engines match the word identified by one of the following methods to any known word. Hidden Markov model (HMM), dynamic time warping (DTW), deep belief network are some feature matching methods.

2 Recent Works on Speech Sentiment Analysis

In the last several years, many academics have created speech sentiment analysis frameworks and tools. Some recent novel techniques and advancements in these techniques are presented in this section. Lu Zhiyun et al. proposed in a study [6] that pre-trained ASR model characteristics be used to solve the downstream analysis of the sentiments of speech. The end-to-end ASR features were shown to include acoustic and textual speech information and to provide improved results. They utilized RNN as a sentiment classifier with self-attention that also facilitates straightforward display using weights to understand model predictions. They utilized an IEMOCAP dataset and a new, large-scale SWBD-sentiment dataset to analyze. This technique increases the state-of-the-art accuracy of IEMOCAP from 66.6 to 71.7% and achieves an accuracy of 70.10% on SWBD-sentiment.

In research [7], J. Luo et al. suggested enhancing the accurate analysis of sentiment when a dataset already has a specific quantity of data and long sentences, a novel data augmentation method based on sequence generative adversarial networks (SeqGAN) may be used. SeqGAN is a penalty-based tool for high-quality and versatile text data generation. For the conduct of sentencing compression in the SeqGAN training data, long short-term memory (LSTM) networks with attention mechanisms are utilized. The words of feeling for compressed data are kept in a sentiment dictionary. In addition, they suggested a technique of data screening to provide precise information from the data collected. Usability is increased by 24.6% after applying the recommended sentence reduction, and originality on average is improved by 4.8%. In comparison with the standard EDA process, the diversity of data generated by the framework is improved by an average of 58.4%. In some of the benchmark sentiment analysis data, the data provided by the suggested system enhance the classification precision of 1%.

Al-Azani et al. [1] analyze the possible contribution to video analysis in the morphologically rich Arabic language by the various modes and how they are linked to video analysis. In addition, video analytics have an improved technique to anticipate the speaker's feelings in multi-dialect Arabic by combining textual, auditive, and visual modalities. Various characteristics are retrieved to represent each modality, including prosodic and spectral acoustic features that describe audio, neural word insertion for transcript audio, and the rich visual flow descriptors. Two machine learning classifiers are being trained with the retrieved features to provide a baseline. Then, multi-level fusion checks the efficacy of different combinations of modalities (feature, score, and decision). The testing findings show that the suggested combination technique can lead to a precise prediction of speech with a precise feeling of more than 94%.

In a study, Seo et al. [19] proposed heterogeneous modality transfer learning (HMTL) for the use of the knowledge of aligned text data to transfer learning to improve the performance of the audio-visual sentimental analysis. To decrease the gap between the target modalities and the source in the embedded area for multi-modal representation, the strategy utilizes decoder and opposite methods. This approach experimentally outperforms recent audio-visual analysis of unimodal and bimodal performance.

The tree-structured regional model of CNN-LSTM consisting of two sections: regional CNN and LSTM to foresee valence-arousal (VA) text ratings for dimensional sentiment analysis is proposed in this work by Wang et al. [21]. In contrast to traditional CNN, the regional CNN suggested employs a section of the text as a region, splitting the input text into multiple areas to extract, weigh, and evaluate valuable information in each region according to its contribution to VA. Such regional information is incorporated progressively across LSTM regions for VA prediction. By bringing together regional CNN and LSTM, the prediction method may incorporate both local (regional) information inside sentences and long-range sentence reliance. A technique for a regional division to find task-related words and sentences to include structured information into VA prediction is presented to further enhance performance [4]. Experimental findings on different firms demonstrate that the suggested technique exceeds the methods presented in the earlier studies of lexicon, regression, conventional NN, and other structured NN.

Zhang et al. [23] presented a WIS (KGCapsAN) network, knowledge-guided capsule attention network, which is developed for aspect-based sentiment analysis. This is a two-part approach: a Bi-LSTM network and a capsule payload system. By attention mechanism, the capsule care network implements the routing technique. In addition, the capsule was guided by two previous information: syntactic structures and n-gram structures. Extensive trials on six datasets are done, and the findings demonstrate that this technique produces the latest.

T. Manshu et al., in a paper [13], suggest a prior-knowledge information hierarchical attention network (HANP) for the CDSC project. Unlike other current techniques, by incorporating prior information, HANP may simultaneously get both domain-independent and domain-specific properties. Further, the HANP also has a hierarchical layer of representation with a care mechanism to allow the HANP to record keywords and phrases in connection to feeling. In addition, a direct view of previous sentimental knowledge may be provided in the suggested paradigm. Experiments of the datasets of the Amazon review show that the suggested HANP can exceed state-of-the-art techniques substantially.

In a study by Kaushik et al. [5], they indicate that the baseline approach is ineffective to extract audio feelings. Alternatively, a novel architecture is suggested for sentiment detection utilizing keyword spotting (KWS). A text-based sentiment classifier will automatically be employed in the new architecture to identify the most helpful and discriminatory keyword words that carry feelings and then serve as a KWS term list. In addition, iterative feature optimization is presented to minimize the model complexity while retaining an effective classification accuracy to get a compact yet discriminative sentiment term [14]. In a unique integrated wording, a novel hybrid ME-KWS joint measuring process is designed to model text and audio-based characteristics. Two new datasets for audio-based sentiment identification are being built for assessment, notably a database for YouTube sentiment, and an updated corpus dubbed the UT Opinion audio archive. These datasets feature audio that is captured in real-world circumstances with real opinions. Audio taken from videos on youtube.com and UT Opinion corpus are analyzed for the suggested approach. Experimental findings demonstrate that the proposed system based on KWS exceeds the standard architecture of ASR substantially to detect sentiments for difficult jobs.

The work by Maghilnan et al. [8] provides a generalized approach, which uses an audio conveying two persons as input and examines the content and identity of the speaker by translating the audios automatically into text and recognizing the speaker. In this study, they suggested an easy approach for carrying out the activity specified. The system works well with the artificially produced dataset, collects a bigger dataset, and increases the system's scalability.

Due to the restricted textual properties of short messages, short text characteristics that should be extracted from several viewpoints and many combinations of sentiments are needed to gain information about hidden feelings. A new sentiment analysis model based on a multi-channel convolutionary neural network (MCNN-MA) is proposed by Feng et al. [2]. This model combines word characteristics with part of the speech, location characteristics, and syntactic dependence characteristics into three new combined properties independently, instilling them in the convolutionary multi-channel neural network. Finally, two Chinese short text datasets have been experimented with. The findings from the experiments indicate that the MCNN-MA model has a greater classification precision and comparatively cheap time-to-train costs compared to others.

The sentiment lexicon that gives word feeling information plays a vital part in the process of sentiment analysis. Most lexicons of emotion now only contain one feeling of polarity per word and neglect the ambiguity of sentiments. In paper, Yin et al. [22] have suggested the construction of a vocabulary of feelings based on POS chunks, specifically CP-chunks, which would solve the ambiguity of lexical feelings. Their objective is to develop the lexicon of feeling. Because the context POS affects the word polarity and intensity, CP-chunks is used as a device for the computation of sentiments. The classification job of text sentiment evaluates this approach. The results of the experiments show that the applicability for both the positive and negative polarity corpora is more steady and balancing, and the precision for the sentiment classification of a field-specific corpus approaches 82% in comparison with the previous methods.

3 Results

Many innovative models are available. Here are the results of several reasonable models. Lu Zhiyun et al. suggested the use of pre-trained features from end-to-end ASR models in the solution of SWBD-sentiment, improved state-of-the-art IEMOCAP accuracy from 66.6 to 71.7%, and achieved an accuracy of 70.10% with over 49,500 statements. J Luo et al. developed a new data augmentation framework based on sequential generative adversarial networks (SeqGAN), which increased usability by 24.6% and improved the novelty by 4.8% on average following the use of the suggested sentence compression. S. Al-Azani et al. proposed an enhanced video analysis approach to predict the multi-dialect of speaker sentiment in Arabic language in three dimensions, i.e., text, speech and video, and findings show that the approach proposed to combine different ways of prediction of the speaker's feelings may lead to more accurate prediction with over 94% accuracy. J. Yu et al. proposed the ESAFN, and the findings demonstrate that ESAFN can outperform various unimodal and multi-modal highly competitive techniques.

4 Research Gap

The thorough literature survey states that a lot of research is already in progress in the categorization of speech into various classes. Furthermore, numerous tools and techniques are proposed by researchers for sentiment analysis of the speech in the English language, whereas the case is very restrictive in regional and local languages like Hindi. This research intends to work on speech sentiment and emotion analysis, particularly for the Hindi language. The analysis will be done on all three dimensions of media, i.e., text, speech, and video. The study will be very useful for analyzing sentiments in podcasts, speeches, and videos that are available in the Hindi language.

5 Conclusion and Future Scope

The sentiments analysis is based on text or audio sensations. The key focus of this work is a review of the sentimental analysis paradigm comprising. Analytics of the sentiment is an emerging subject of textual, audio, and computer language studies and has attracted significant interest in recent years. Future work should explore improved opinion approaches and product attributes extraction and new classification models capable of handling the property of the ordered labels in the grading of inferences. In the future, applications should also be created utilizing the sentiment analysis findings.

References

1. Al-Azani S, El-Alfy ESM (2020) Enhanced video analytics for sentiment analysis based on fusing textual, auditory and visual information. IEEE Access 8:136843–136857. https://doi.org/10.1109/ACCESS.2020.3011977
2. Feng Y, Cheng Y (2021) Short text sentiment analysis based on multi-channel CNN with multi-head attention mechanism. IEEE Access 9:19854–19863. https://doi.org/10.1109/ACCESS.2021.3054521

3. Herbig T, Gerl F, Minker W (2010) Fast adaptation of speech and speaker characteristics for enhanced speech recognition in adverse intelligent environments. In: 2010 sixth international conference on intelligent environments, pp 100–105. https://doi.org/10.1109/IE.2010.26
4. Horovitz S, Ohayon Y (2020) Boocture: automatic educational videos hierarchical indexing with ebooks. In: 2020 IEEE international conference on teaching, assessment, and learning for engineering (TALE), pp 482–489 (2020). https://doi.org/10.1109/TALE48869.2020.9368461
5. Kaushik L, Sangwan A, Hansen JHL (2017) Automatic sentiment detection in naturalistic audio. IEEE/ACM Trans Audio Speech Lang Process 25(8):1668–1679. https://doi.org/10.1109/TASLP.2017.2678164
6. Lu Z, Cao L, Zhang Y, Chiu CC, Fan J (2020) Speech sentiment analysis via pre-trained features from end-to-end ASR models. In: ICASSP 2020—2020 IEEE international conference on acoustics, speech and signal processing (ICASSP). pp. 7149–7153. https://doi.org/10.1109/ICASSP40776.2020.9052937
7. Luo J, Bouazizi M, Ohtsuki T (2021) Data augmentation for sentiment analysis using sentence compression-based Seqgan with data screening. IEEE Access 9:99922–99931. https://doi.org/10.1109/ACCESS.2021.3094023
8. Maghilnan S, RajeshKumar M (2017) Sentiment analysis on speaker specific speech data. In: 2017 international conference on intelligent computing and control (I2C2), pp 1–5
9. Mahmud M, Kaiser MS, Hussain A (2020) Deep learning in mining biological data. arXiv preprint arXiv:2003.00108
10. Mahmud M, Kaiser MS, Hussain A, Vassanelli S (2018) Applications of deep learning and reinforcement learning to biological data. IEEE Trans Neural Netw Learn Syst 29(6):2063–2079
11. Mahmud M et al (2018) A brain-inspired trust management model to assure security in a cloud based Iot framework for neuroscience applications. Cogn Comput 10(5):864–873
12. Mahrishi M, Morwal S (2020) Index point detection and semantic indexing of videos a comparative review. Advances in intelligent systems and computing AISC Springer
13. Manshu T, Bing W (2019) Adding prior knowledge in hierarchical attention neural network for cross domain sentiment classification. IEEE Access 7:32578–32588. https://doi.org/10.1109/ACCESS.2019.2901929
14. Mehul M, Sudha M, Nidhi D, Hanisha N (2021) A framework for index point detection using effective title extraction from video thumbnails. Int J Syst Assur Eng Manag. https://doi.org/10.1007/s13198-021-01166-z
15. Pang B, Lee L (2004) A sentimental education: sentiment analysis using subjectivity summarization based on minimum cuts. In: Proceedings of the 42nd annual meeting of the association for computational linguistics (ACL-04). Barcelona, Spain, pp 271–278. https://doi.org/10.3115/1218955.1218990, https://aclanthology.org/P04-1035
16. Pang B, Lee L (2005) Seeing stars: exploiting class relationships for sentiment categorization with respect to rating scales. In: Proceedings of the 43rd annual meeting of the association for computational linguistics (ACL'05). Association for computational linguistics, Ann Arbor, Michigan, pp 115–124. https://doi.org/10.3115/1219840.1219855, https://aclanthology.org/P05-1015
17. Pang B, Lee L, Vaithyanathan S (2002) Thumbs up? Sentiment classification using machine learning techniques. In: Proceedings of the 2002 conference on empirical methods in natural language processing (EMNLP 2002). Association for computational linguistics, pp 79–86. https://doi.org/10.3115/1118693.1118704, https://aclanthology.org/W02-1011
18. Salvador S, Chan P (2004) Fastdtw: toward accurate dynamic time warping in linear time and space
19. Seo S, Na S, Kim J (2020) Hmtl: heterogeneous modality transfer learning for audio-visual sentiment analysis. IEEE Access 8:140426–140437. https://doi.org/10.1109/ACCESS.2020.3006563
20. Walker W, Lamere P, Kwok P, Raj B, Singh R, Gouvea E, Wolf P, Wölfel J (2004) Sphinx-4: a flexible open source framework for speech recognition. Sun microsystems

21. Wang J, Yu LC, Lai KR, Zhang X (2020) Tree-structured regional CNN-LSTM model for dimensional sentiment analysis. IEEE/ACM Trans Audio Speech Lang Process 28:581–591. https://doi.org/10.1109/TASLP.2019.2959251
22. Yin F, Wang Y, Liu J, Lin L (2020) The construction of sentiment lexicon based on context-dependent part-of-speech chunks for semantic disambiguation. IEEE Access 8:63359–63367. https://doi.org/10.1109/ACCESS.2020.2984284
23. Zhang B, Li X, Xu X, Leung KC, Chen Z, Ye Y (2020) Knowledge guided capsule attention network for aspect-based sentiment analysis. IEEE/ACM Trans Audio Speech Lang Process 28:2538–2551. https://doi.org/10.1109/TASLP.2020.3017093

Performance Evaluation of Enhancement Algorithm for Contrast Distorted Images

Navleen S. Rekhi, Jasjit Singh, Jagroop S. Sidhu, and Amit Arora

Abstract The digital cameras have played the crucial role for the revolutionary growth of digital platform. The digital cameras capture the high-resolution images. But still, it is prone to the noise that might be due to improper acquisition settings, light conditions or any other noise artifacts. In this paper, our work was focused to improve the contrast and preserving the brightness in digital images. Firstly, the illumination was estimation through 2D-discrete wavelet transform. From the obtained value, logarithmic scale was calculated. The logarithmic scale is used to expand the dark scales in the image. With the obtained scale parameter, adaptive gamma correction was implemented. The nature of gamma was automated through logarithmic scale for each input image. The experiments were conducted on the TID2008 database. In comparison to the published algorithms, our proposed method had proved to be effective. The performance of the proposed method was measured from peak SNR, absolute mean brightness error, image quality index and entropy.

Keywords Contrast enhancement · Gamma correction · Discrete wavelet transform

1 Introduction

With great demand of mobile phones and social media platforms, the digital images have been extensively used both at personal and professional applications, for example, the usage of images in medical field to monitor health, in forensics and many other allied platform. Due to imperfection in acquisition settings of digital cameras, the quality of image deteriorated. Also, the limited exposure to light conditions decreases the dynamic range of intensity scale. Hence, it is necessary to enhance the contrast for better visual quality of the image. By enhancement, it is the process of

N. S. Rekhi (✉) · J. Singh
IKG Punjab Technical University, Kapurthala, Punjab, India

N. S. Rekhi · J. S. Sidhu · A. Arora
DAV Institute of Engineering and Technology, Jalandhar, Punjab, India

M. S. Kaiser et al. (eds.), *Proceedings of Trends in Electronics and Health Informatics*, Lecture Notes in Networks and Systems 376,
https://doi.org/10.1007/978-981-16-8826-3_4

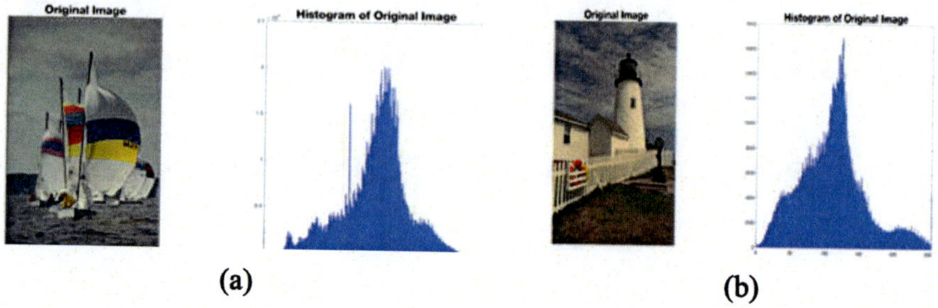

Fig. 1 Image with varying dynamic range, **a** boat, **b** tower

stretching the contrast to improve dynamic range. The two types of the enhancement, viz., visual and the machine interpretation are used for processing [1]. Mostly, the various techniques on visual properties had been developed for image enhancement. It could be clearly observed from Fig. 1 that dynamic range of tower is better as compared to boat. Because the pixel distribution of boat is narrow and lies at the middle range of intensity scale. Mostly, if the dynamic range is inclined to right, left or in middle like in boat is said to have low contrast. Similarly, tower has the better dynamic range than the boat. Due to this variability in the dynamic range, the contrast enhancement become the challenging task in image processing. Such variation produces nonlinearity in the pixel distribution. It is required to maintain the equilibrium between contrast and brightness in the image.

2 Related Work

The most of the digital images are low in dynamic range. Such conditions may be the result of low light conditions or incorrect aperture settings of digital camera. This rises the nonlinearity and causes the loss of relevant information content in the images. To address the challenge of nonlinearity, researchers had proposed different techniques to improve the quality of image. Traditionally, histogram equalization (HE) is popular technique due to its ease of use. But the limitation of HE is either it transforms the image to over or under enhancement. To overcome, many researchers proposed the modified HE [2–5] by preserving its brightness and thus improving the contrast of the image. The purpose of modification was to widen the dynamic range of the images. However, the HE does not provide sufficient information on the composition of fine details and edges.

The illustration of Figs. 2 and 3 showed the results obtained from conventional histogram equalization and the median–mean-based HE proposed by Singh and Kapoor [6]. The author proposed a median–mean-based clipped histogram for automatically improvement in the contrast. As seen from Figs. 2 and 3, the approach of HE had widened the dynamic range of intensity scale. But, the insignificant

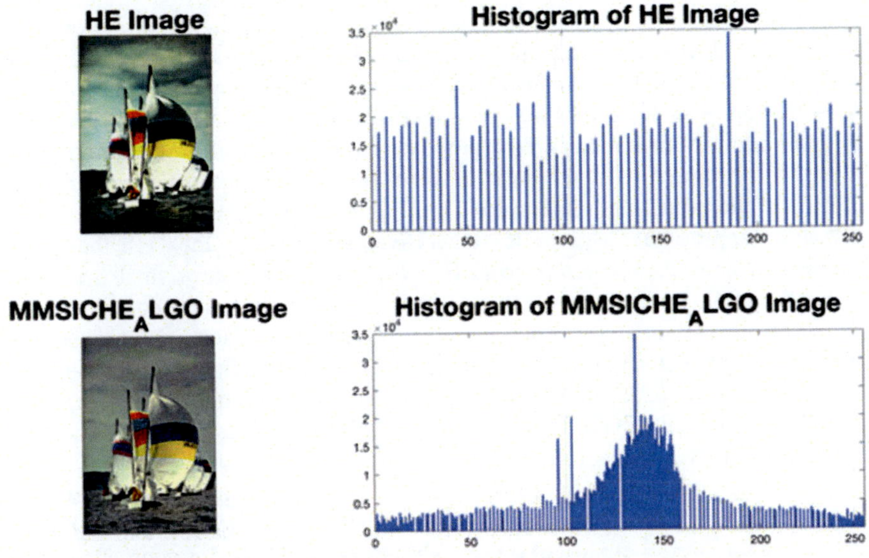

Fig. 2 Result of boat: Conventional HE (top) and mean–median-based HE (bottom)

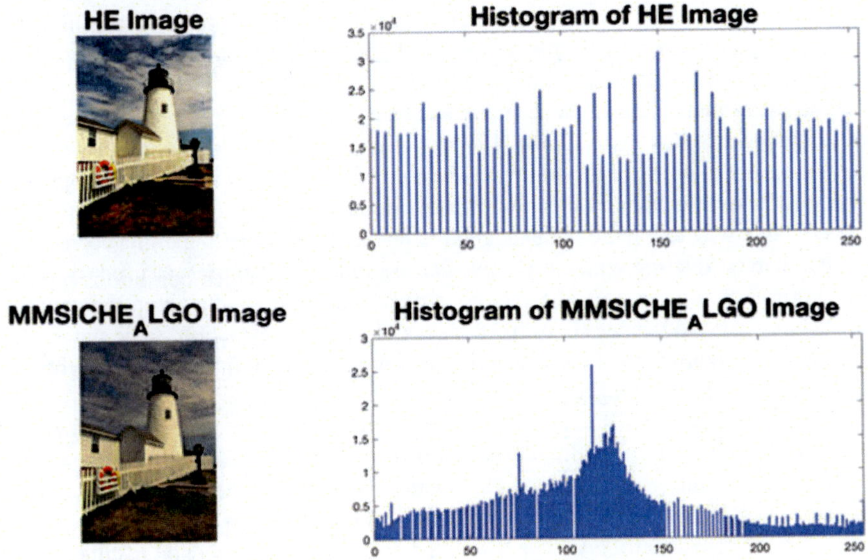

Fig. 3 Result of house: conventional HE (top) and mean–median-based HE (bottom)

contrast enhancement degraded the visual quality of picture. The effect of color saturation is clearly observed from Figs.2 and 3. Similarly, with the approach of MMSICHE, the significant improvement was observed in contrast. But uneven illumination resulted in the loss of information content in the image. Similarly, Naushad Ali and Abdullah-Al-Wadud [7] have proposed the boosting algorithm for correction in over-enhancement. With the boost of minor regions obtained after applying HE, clipping of the values was implemented to suppress the quantum jumps.

Another approach is the global and local HE methods. In the global HE, the overall picture is enhanced, whereas in local HE, with the utilization of small windows, the quality of picture is improved. Tian and Cohen [8] proposed the combination of global and local HE to preserve the naturalness in the image. Saruchi [9] proposed an overall enhancement using a sigmoid mapping function. The sigmoid is an S-shaped non-linear transformation function for compressing the dynamic range. Therefore, it is effective for contrast enhancement. Additionally, fast quadratic HE [10] was the extension suggested by Saurabh Patel.

The author claimed that the method was computationally faster as compared to global HE and local HE. Other than HE, discrete wavelet transform is also useful tool to improve the overall quality of image. Muslim et al. [11] had proposed the noise reduction using discrete wavelet transform (DWT) and Gaussian low-pass filter. The DWT was used to filter the high frequency content and for the other part, Gaussian low-pass filter was implemented. The algorithm was designed for medical images.

In the recent times, the implementation of gamma has been extensively used for contrast improvement. It is a nonlinear approach to enhance the quality of image. Due to over-enhancement, the increase in noise level becomes the major drawback of this approach. However, Huang [12] proposed a weighted distribution mapping of the histogram to improve the contrast. The algorithm designed is limited in approach and mostly over-enhanced the low contrast images. Cao et al. [13] had proposed the effective way to handle the exaggerated enhancement due to gamma correction. Rather than correlating with cumulative density function, gamma was used for negative portion of the images. The modulated value of gamma alleviated the contrast for better quality of image. For effectiveness of gamma correction, scale parameter is required to computed such that along with the contrast improvement, brightness is to preserved in the image.

The motivation for this paper is to design an adaptive scale parameter for gamma that could effectively manipulate the contrast in the image. Moreover, the robust algorithm is required to preserve the mean brightness in the image. The consequent sections of the paper are organized to deal the problems mentioned above. In Sect. 3, a proposed method will be discussed. In Sect. 4, experimental results will be demonstrated. Lastly, conclusion of the proposed algorithm will be interpreted.

3 Proposed Method

The proposed algorithm, performance evaluation of enhancement algorithm for contrast distorted images (PEAC), is categorized into three steps: preprocessing, discrete wavelet transform and estimation of scale parameter. The flow diagram of the proposed method is shown in Fig. 4. Firstly, the linear contrast stretching of available raw (RGB) image was obtained. Then, the image was transformed to hue, saturation and value (HSV) scale. Secondly, the multiscale partition was implemented using discrete wavelet transform. From this, the estimation of illumination was computed using logarithmic scale. Lastly, the gamma correction was implemented for contrast improvement in the images.

3.1 *Channel Stretching*

Let us assume, F(u,v) = [R(u,v),G(u,v),B(u,v)] where R is the red, G is the green and B is the blue component of the original color image. For individual channel, the minimum and maximum values of pixel are computed. Such values defined the limits of contrast stretch in preprocessing stage.

Hence, the contrast was stretched to provide uniform distribution in color space. The magnitude of scaling function was obtained as follows:

$$R_{(u,v)} = \frac{R_{(u,v)} - \min\left[R_{(u,v)}\right]}{\max\left[R_{(u,v)}\right] - \min\left[R_{(u,v)}\right]} \quad (1)$$

With individual channel stretching, our approach of contrast stretched images (Fig. 5) showed better results. Since, it was difficult to process the information for individual colors. Hence, we converted the RGB space to HSV channel (H—hue, S—saturation and V—value). The value 'V' has the brightness content in the image.

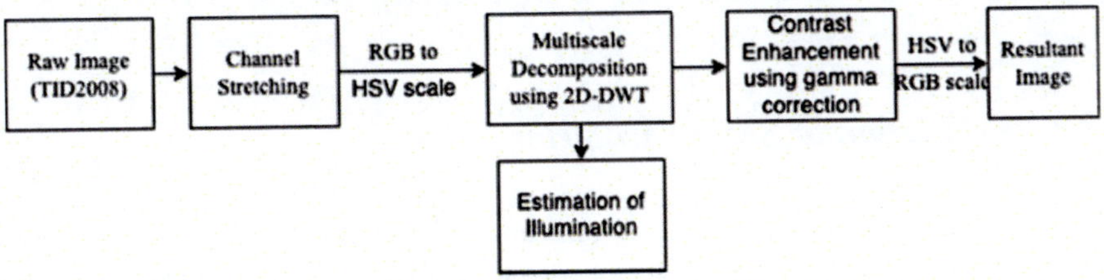

Fig. 4 Flow diagram of the proposed method

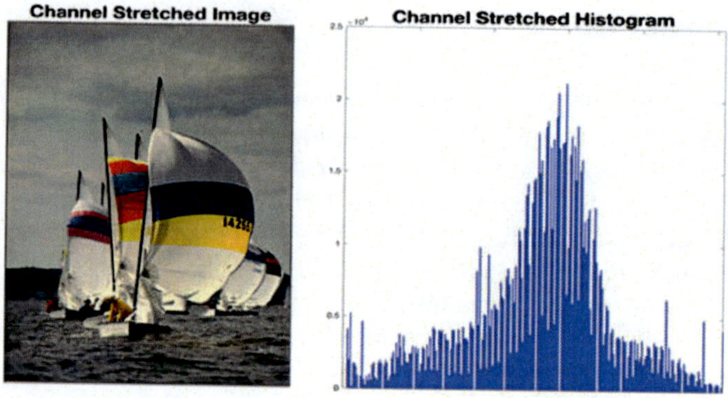

Fig. 5 Resultant images from contrast stretch boat

3.2 Multiscale Decomposition

The main motivation of the PEAC was to obtain the scale parameter for gamma correction. At the beginning stage, we focused on estimating the illumination content by downscaling the information content in the image. The reason was to estimate the brightness content in the image. Many researchers proposed the techniques like histogram splitting, based on mean intensity [14] or through the median intensity [15] or the combination of both like proposed by Singh and Kapoor [6].

With the profound studies [16, 17], our work was implemented on multiscale discrete wavelet transform (2D-DWT). The 2D-discrete wavelet transform was implemented at a scale level of 2 with mother wavelet as 'symlet.' The choice of decomposition and mother wavelet was based on intensive hit and trial method on various images.

Figure 6 illustrated the decomposition of original image into low-pass and high-pass filter coefficients. At a scale level of '2,' the low-pass coefficients is further decomposed into low-pass–low-pass (LL), low-pass–high-pass (LH), high-pass–low-pass (HL) and high-pass–high-pass (HH) coefficients.

3.3 Estimation of Scale Parameter

The maximum likelihood estimation of illumination was calculated from low-pass coefficients obtained from 2D-discrete wavelet transform. Since, for the scale value of gamma less than '0.5,' yield the non-uniform brightness and greater than '1' will decrease the contrast. The estimation of gamma scale is calculated. Hence, to automate using the relation as mentioned below:

$$\xi = \frac{J - \mu}{\log_{10}(1 + \mu)} \tag{2}$$

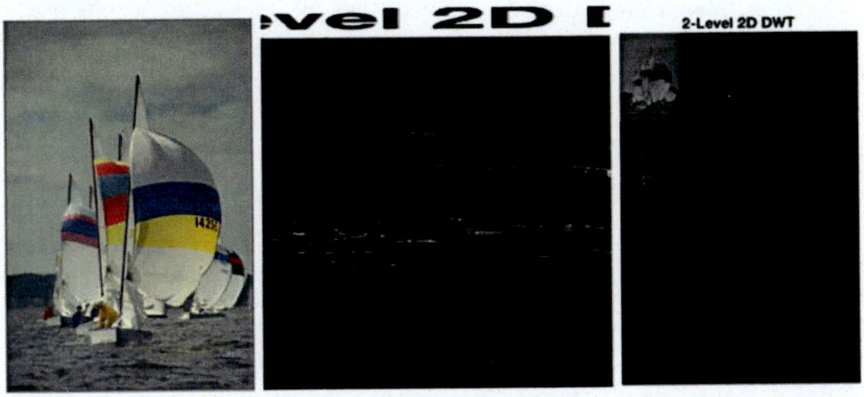

Fig. 6 Two-level decomposition of original image using 2D-DWT

Table 1 Step-by-step procedure of proposed technique

Stepwise Procedure of implementation of PEAC algorithm
(i) *Preprocessing the original image using contrast stretch as mentioned in* Eq. (1)
(ii) *Conversion of original RGB into HSV transformation*
(iii) *Keeping the hue and saturation constant, decompose the 'V' component using 2D-DWT at a scale level of '2'*
(iv) *Compute the scale parameter from the LL coefficients obtained at a scale level of '2' using* Eq. (2)
(v) *Further, obtain the final gamma scale value using* $\xi^{(0.005)}$
(vi) *At final stage, obtain the enhanced image while converting back to RGB image*

where 'ξ' denotes the scale parameter, and 'J' is the maximum intensity scale.

However, the value 'ξ' was not sufficient enough to scale the contrast in the image. Hence, a constant value of steepness was chosen as 0.005. Any value less than or greater the steepness bounced the output to a contrast distorted image. Lastly, the image was converted back to its original channel space, viz., RGB scale (Table 1).

4 Performance Evaluation

The quantitative performance was evaluated through peak SNR [18], absolute mean brightness error [19], entropy and perceptual-based quality index [20]. The database used for evaluation is TID 2008 [21]. Figure 7a illustrated the preservation of information through entropy. If the resultant entropy is closer to original entropy, more will be the preservation of information. The proposed method entropy is obtained as 7.36, which is more close to the original (7.29), as compared to other methods (CHE is 5.86, and for MMBSIC, 7.17).

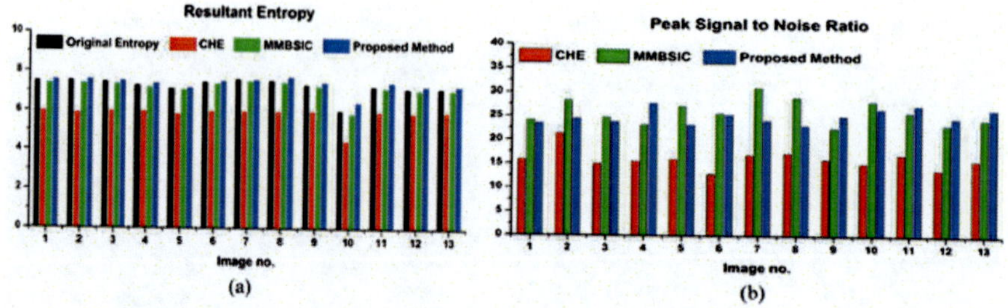

Fig. 7 Comparison of proposed method with CHE, MMBSIC, **a** resultant entropy, and **b** PSNR

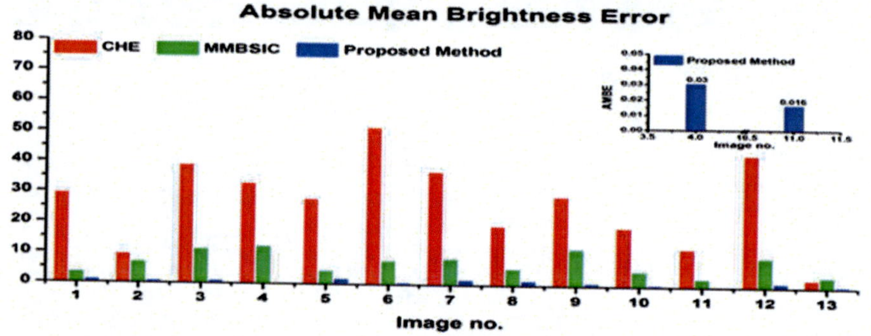

Fig. 8 Comparison of AMBE with conventional HE, median–mean-based HE and proposed method

The another metric, AMBE, is evaluated to estimate the preservation of mean brightness. Lower the value of AMBE, better will be the brightness preservation. As shown in Fig. 8, the proposed method calculated the average AMBE of 0.827. In case of MMBSIC, it was 7.07 and that of conventional HE 16.09. The AMBE calculated is irrespective of noise content in the image. Hence, the peak SNR is used to estimate the suppression of noise in the image. More is the value of PSNR, lesser will be the noise content in the enhanced image. The PSNR is computed from original and enhanced image. From Fig. 7b, compared to MMBSIC of 26 db, the proposed method had 25.1 db. In our case, with improvement of contrast, brightness was to be well preserved. Hence, it could be observed that for the rare lesser value of PSNR, the brightness (AMBE) preserved in the enhanced image is far better in comparison to the HE-based methods.

Additionally, the visual comparison of the enhanced image is Fig. 9 for better insight of the PEAC. The proposed method is further compared with state-of-the-art techniques developed by Arriaga-Garcia et al. [22] and Veluchamy and Subramani [23]. Arriaga-Garcia et al. [22] developed the contrast stretching algorithm using a sigmoid function, whereas Veluchamy and Subramani [23] implemented the improved HE computed from other nonlinear transformation as gamma correction.

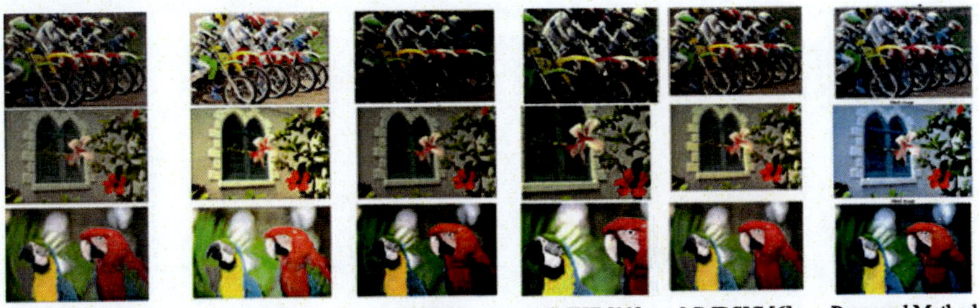

Fig. 9 Comparison of enhanced images obtained from recent and proposed method

Table 2 Comparison of methods for different metrics

Method\Metrics	Entropy	PSNR	AMBE	Image Quality
CS	5.83	16.09	24.1	0.43
MMBSIC [6]	7.16	**26.11**	7.02	0.93
ACS [22]	6.28	19.37	113.67	0.78
Proposed method	**7.37**	25.11	**0.82**	**0.97**

With over-enhancement in CHE, poor contrast in ACS, AGCHE (adaptive gamma-based CHE), and MMBSIC, the PEAC had shown the optimal balance in contrast and mean brightness in the enhanced images.

Moreover, quality of image is also measured to quantify the degradation. Higher the value of perception-based quality index, more consistent would be the quality of image. In our method, the average quality index of 0.978 was observed. Table 2 showed the comparison of different methods with proposed technique. Except PSNR, measure of information, AMBE and perception-based quality index is better in the PEAC.

5 Conclusion and Future Scope

The enhancement method (PEAC) proposed is a combination of discrete wavelet transform and nonlinear transformation (gamma) function to effectively improve the contrast and preserved the mean brightness in the image. The uniformity in distribution of pixel across intensity scale measures the better contrast in the images. The uniformity of pixel distribution (Fig. 2), obtained from CHE and MMBSIC, had degraded the quality of the image. But from Fig. 10, with high contrast, PEAC had shown the improvement in detail and better visual quality in the image. Most of the work is focused on modification of conventional HE. In our work, while preserving the simplicity, the approach of implementing gamma had shown better results in both qualitative and quantitative measures.

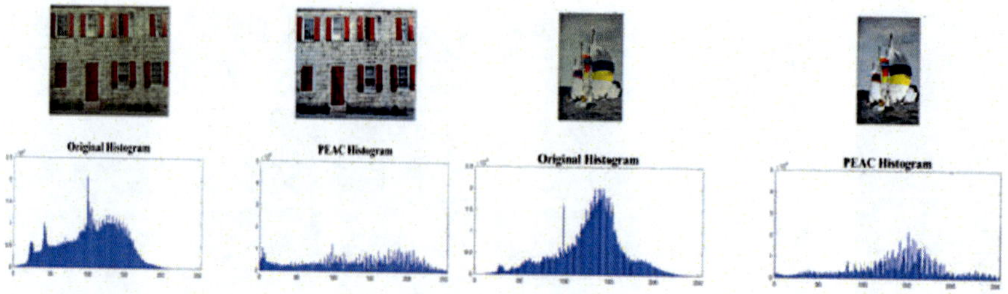

Fig. 10 Resultant images obtained from proposed method

Due to its minimum AMBE and better PSNR, the proposed method can found its suitability in restoration of contrast and brightness distorted images. In future studies, the method will be implemented to dark images. Moreover, the approach will be modified to automatically select the gamma scale for individual images.

References

1. Gonzalez RC, Woods RE, Eddins SL (2000) 1 Image g
2. Ibrahim H, Pik Kong N (2007) Brightness preserving dynamic histogram equalization for image contrast enhancement. IEEE Trans Consum Electron 53:1752–1758. https://doi.org/10.1109/TCE.2007.4429280
3. Lal S, Chandra M (2014) Efficient algorithm for contrast enhancement of natural images. Int Arab J Inf Technol 11:95–102
4. SinghBagri N, Sharma S, Sahu S (2012) Images enhancement with brightness preserving using MRHRBFN. Int J Comput Appl 40:22–26. https://doi.org/10.5120/4976-7231
5. Santhi K, Wahida Banu RSD (2015) Adaptive contrast enhancement using modified histogram equalization. Optik 126:1809–1814. https://doi.org/10.1016/j.ijleo.2015.05.023
6. Singh K, Kapoor R (2014) Image enhancement via median-mean based sub-image-clipped histogram equalization. Optik 125:4646–4651. https://doi.org/10.1016/j.ijleo.2014.04.093
7. Naushad Ali MM, Abdullah-Al-Wadud M (2012) Image enhancement using a modified histogram equalization. Presented at the computer applications for web, human computer interaction, signal and image processing and pattern recognition. https://doi.org/10.1007/978-3-642-35270-6_3
8. Tian QC, Cohen LD (2018) A variational-based fusion model for non-uniform illumination image enhancement via contrast optimization and color correction. Signal Process 153:210–220. https://doi.org/10.1016/j.sigpro.2018.07.022
9. Saruchi S (2012) Adaptive Sigmoid function to enhance low contrast images. Int J Comput Appl 55:45–49. https://doi.org/10.5120/8747-2634
10. Patel S, Goswami M (2014) Comparative analysis of histogram equalization techniques. Proceedings of 2014 International conference on contemporary computing and informatics, IC3I 2014, vol 1, pp 167–168. https://doi.org/10.1109/IC3I.2014.7019808
11. Muslim HSM, Khan SA, Hussain S, Jamal A, Qasim HSA (2019) A knowledge-based image enhancement and denoising approach. Comput Math Organ Theory 25:108–121. https://doi.org/10.1007/s10588-018-9274-8
12. Huang SC, Cheng FC, Chiu YS (2013) Efficient contrast enhancement using adaptive gamma correction with weighting distribution. IEEE Trans Image Process 22:1032–1041. https://doi.org/10.1109/TIP.2012.2226047

13. Cao G, Huang L, Tian H, Huang X, Wang Y, Zhi R (2018) Contrast enhancement of brightness-distorted images by improved adaptive gamma correction. Comput Electr Eng 66:569–582. https://doi.org/10.1016/j.compeleceng.2017.09.012
14. Kim YT (1997) Contrast enhancement using brightness preserving bi-histogram equalization. IEEE Trans Consum Electron 43:1–8. https://doi.org/10.1109/30.580378
15. Zuo C, Chen Q, Sui X (2013) Range limited Bi-histogram equalization for image contrast enhancement. Optik 124:425–431. https://doi.org/10.1016/j.ijleo.2011.12.057
16. Bhandari AK, Soni V, Kumar A, Singh GK (2014) Cuckoo search algorithm based satellite image contrast and brightness enhancement using DWT-SVD. ISA Trans 53:1286–1296. https://doi.org/10.1016/j.isatra.2014.04.007
17. Boraste PD, NPKP (2015) Image enhancement using DWT. Int J Eng Comput Sci 4:10509–10515. ISSN: 2319-7242
18. Horé A, Ziou D (2010) Image quality metrics: PSNR vs. SSIM. In: Proceedings of International conference on pattern recognition, pp 2366–2369. https://doi.org/10.1109/ICPR.2010.579
19. Chen SD, Ramli AR (2003) Minimum mean brightness error bi-histogram equalization in contrast enhancement. https://doi.org/10.1109/TCE.2003.1261234
20. Shokrollahi A, Mahmoudi-Aznaveh A, Mazloom-Nezhad Maybodi B (2017) Image quality assessment for contrast enhancement evaluation. AEU-Int J Electron C 77:61–66. https://doi.org/10.1016/j.aeue.2017.04.026
21. Ponomarenko N, Lukin V, Zelensky A, Egiazarian K, Astola J, Carli M, Battisti F (2009) TID2008-A database for evaluation of full-reference visual quality assessment metrics. Adv Mod Radioelectronics 10:30–45
22. Arriaga-Garcia EF, Sanchez-Yanez RE, Ruiz-Pinales J, Garcia-Hernandez Ma de G (2015) Adaptive sigmoid function bihistogram equalization for image contrast enhancement. https://doi.org/10.1117/1.jei.24.5.053009
23. Veluchamy M, Subramani B (2019) Image contrast and color enhancement using adaptive gamma correction and histogram equalization. Optik 183:329–337. https://doi.org/10.1016/j.ijleo.2019.02.054

MHGSO: A Modified Hunger Game Search Optimizer Using Opposition-Based Learning for Feature Selection

Zeeshan Adeen, Musheer Ahmad, Nabil Neggaz, and Ahmed Alkhayyat

Abstract Feature selection (FS) is one of the crucial pre-processing tasks in many data mining, machine learning, and pattern recognition applications. It facilitates limiting the feature count, dimensionality of datasets, and overfitting. Feature selection methods are developed to explore the benefits with good accuracy outcomes. This paper proposes a novel modification to the conventional Hunger Games Search optimization using the concept of opposition-based learning (OBL) to solve the FS problem. Here, the opposition-based learning enables the searching ability of HGSO to determine the optimal solution by looking in random directions and in the opposite directions as well, simultaneously. Moreover, three binarization approaches, namely transfer function (TF), great value priority (GVP), and angle modulation (AM), have been incorporated with modified HGSO and investigated to study the effective feature selection ability of the modified optimizer. The simulation results have been obtained using standard datasets for accuracy, fitness value, and a number of features, along with a convergence curve for each dataset. The obtained results demonstrate better performance compared to the Support Vector Machine (SVM) approach over most of the datasets for effective feature selection.

Keywords Feature selection · Modified hunger games search · Opposition-based learning · Optimization techniques

---

Z. Adeen · M. Ahmad (✉)
Department of Computer Engineering, Jamia Millia Islamia, New Delhi 110025, India

N. Neggaz
Université Des Sciences et de la Technologie d'Oran Mohamed Boudiaf, USTO-MB, BP1505, El M'naouer, 31000 Oran, Algeria

Faculté Des Mathématiques et Informatique, Département d'Informatique Laboratoire Signal IMage PArole (SIMPA), Oran, Algeria

A. Alkhayyat
Department of Computer Technical Engineering, College of Technical Engineering, Islamic University, Najaf 54001, Iraq

M. S. Kaiser et al. (eds.), *Proceedings of Trends in Electronics and Health Informatics*, Lecture Notes in Networks and Systems 376,
https://doi.org/10.1007/978-981-16-8826-3_5

1 Introduction

Due to the advancement of data on the internet, the dimension of the datasets has grown tremendously, thus increasing the complexity of machine learning models and making data analysis difficult. Feature selection (FS) is one way of reducing the dimensions of the datasets. FS is a process of selecting a subset of features without compromising the original sense of data. There are two main categories into which feature selection algorithms can be divided, namely filter-based and wrapper-based approaches. The filter-based approach to feature selection is independent of the learning algorithm, while the wrapper-based approach to feature selection is tied to the learning algorithm [1]. An optimization algorithm or a learning algorithm is used to decide whether a feature subset is suitable or not in the wrapper-based approach for feature selection. A problem having N features has a complexity of O (2^N), making feature selection a non-polynomial hard problem [2]. Traditional optimization algorithms are incapable of solving complex optimization problems. To tackle these complex optimization problems, many meta-heuristic algorithms have been developed. In Ref. [3], the authors try to solve binary problems using particle swarm optimization (PSO) based on angle modulation. A binary coded ant colony optimization (ACO) has been used in Ref. [2] for feature selection. The authors suggested a grey wolf optimization algorithm (GWO) based feature selection approach to classifying coronary artery disease in Ref. [4]. The authors of Ref. [5] proposed a correlation-based feature selection technique using the PSO algorithm. In Ref. [6], the authors suggested feature selection using PSO in intrusion detection. The feature selection model based on the PSO algorithm and SVM classification to diagnose erythemato-squamous disease has been suggested in Ref. [7].

In Ref. [8], the use of deep learning for mining biological data has attracted several researchers due to their efficiency in terms of classification and significant extracted features. Whereas Ref. [9] investigates a feature selection model based on the artificial bee colony (ABC) algorithm and SVM classification for disease identification. In Ref. [10], the authors proposed a minimum redundancy, maximum relevance feature selection approach based on the PSO algorithm and SVM classification. Hunger Games Search Optimization has recently been proposed as a means of solving a global optimization problem. So, the majority of swarm algorithms suffer from failing to converge to local optima. With the theory of "No free lunch", we attempt to solve the problem of feature selection using a modified Hunger Games Search optimization (MHGSO) algorithm. This algorithm is proposed to solve the feature selection problem. The major contributions of this paper are focused on the following:

- The proposed MHGSO is a novel variant of the binary wrapper feature selection algorithm.
- Several binarization techniques are applied to obtain the optimal solution more rapidly and with better accuracy.

- A novel operator is integrated into basic HGSO based on opposition-based learning (OBL).
- Testing high dimensional datasets using MHGSO and realizing a comparative study with the state for FS problem.

The structure of our paper is organized as follows: Sect. 2 explains basic HGSO, the Opposition-based learning operator, some techniques of binarization, and the modified version of HGSO. Section 3 depicts the obtained results in terms of fitness, accuracy, and the selected number of features.

2 Proposed Modified Hunger Games Search Using OBL

Hunger Games Search is an optimization algorithm recently developed by Yang et al. in 2021 [11]. It is inspired by the social behavior of animals, and hunger is the strong motivating force behind their behavior and decisions. The following section demonstrates the mathematical model of the HGSO algorithm. The way an animal approaches food is mathematically modeled by the given equation. The equation is divided into two categories. The first part stimulates the movement of animals that are self-dependent and do not cooperate with other animals. The second part stimulates those animals which move in cooperation with other animals and follows Eq. (1) (Fig. 1):

$$\overrightarrow{X(t+1)} = \begin{cases} \overrightarrow{X(t)} \cdot (1 + \text{randn}(1)) & r_1 < l \\ \overrightarrow{W_1} \cdot \overrightarrow{X_b} + \vec{R} \cdot \overrightarrow{W_2} \cdot \left| \overrightarrow{X_b} - \overrightarrow{X(t)} \right| & r_1 > l, r_2 > E \\ \overrightarrow{W_1} \cdot \overrightarrow{X_b} - \vec{R} \cdot \overrightarrow{W_2} \cdot \left| \overrightarrow{X_b} - \overrightarrow{X(t)} \right| & r_1 > l, r_2 < E \end{cases} \tag{1}$$

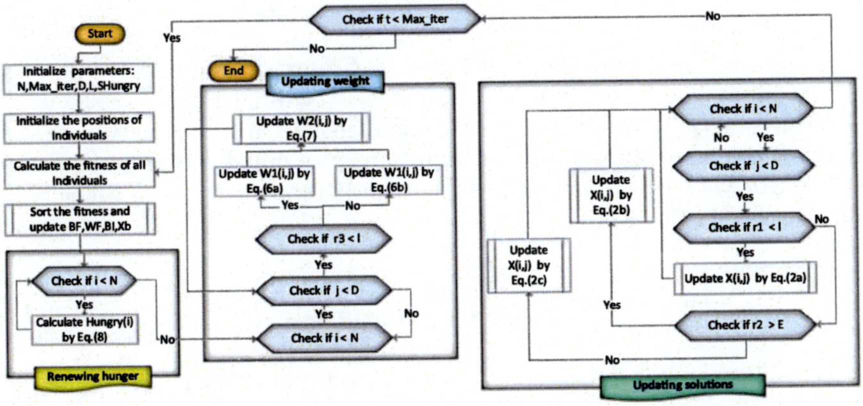

Fig. 1 Conventional hunger games search optimization

where, $\overrightarrow{X(t)}$ is the individual's location, $\overrightarrow{X_b}$ is the position of the best individual, and $\overrightarrow{W_2}$ are weights of hunger, r_1 and r_2 are random numbers ranging between 0 and 1, t is the current iteration, randn(1) generates normally distributed random number. l is a parameter of the HGSO algorithm designed to improve the algorithm. E is a variation control parameter, which is defined as Eq. (2):

$$E = \mathrm{Sech}(|F(i) - BF|) \tag{2}$$

where $F(i)$ denotes the fitness value (cost function value) of each individual, $i \in 1, 2, 3 \ldots n$ is the best fitness value of the current iteration. Sech is a hyperbolic function defined in Eq. (3).

$$\mathrm{Sech}(x) = \frac{2}{e^x + e^{-x}} \tag{3}$$

$\vec{R}$ is a random vector between $[-a, a]$ and is applied to restrict the activity range as given in Eqs. (4, 5).

$$\vec{R} = 2 \times a \times \mathrm{rand} - a \tag{4}$$

$$a = 2 \times \left(1 - \frac{t}{\max_{\mathrm{iter}}}\right) \tag{5}$$

where $\max_{\mathrm{iter}}$ is the total number of iterations and rand is a random number between [0,1]. The starvation characteristics of each individual are simulated by the given equations. The formulas for $\overrightarrow{W_1}$ and $\overrightarrow{W_2}$ are expressed in Eqs. (6) and (7), respectively.

$$\overrightarrow{W_1(i)} = \begin{cases} \mathrm{hungry}(i) \cdot \frac{N}{\mathrm{SHungry}} \times r_4 & r_3 < l \\ 1 & r_3 > l \end{cases} \tag{6}$$

$$\overrightarrow{W_2(i)} = (1 - \exp(-|\mathrm{hungry}(i) - \mathrm{SHungry}|)) \times r_5 \times 2 \tag{7}$$

where hungry(i) denotes the hunger value for each population, SHungry is the sum of the hunger of all individuals, N is the total number of individuals, r_3, r_4, and r_5 are independent random numbers between 0 and 1. The hunger of each individual is simulated by the Eq. (8)

$$\mathrm{hungry}(i) = \begin{cases} 0 & \mathrm{AllFitness}(i) == \mathrm{BF} \\ \mathrm{hungry}(i) + H & \mathrm{AllFitness}(i)! = \mathrm{BF} \end{cases} \tag{8}$$

where AllFitness(i) is the fitness value of each individual. The hunger of the best individual is set to 0 in every iteration, while a new hunger factor H is added to other individuals' hunger. The formula for H is given below in Eqs. (9), (10).

$$\text{TH} = \frac{F(i) - \text{BF}}{\text{WF} - \text{BF}} \times r_6 \times 2 \times (\text{UB} - \text{LB}) \tag{9}$$

$$H = \begin{cases} \text{LH} \times (1 + r) & \text{TH} < \text{LH} \\ \text{TH} & \text{TH} \geq \text{LH} \end{cases} \tag{10}$$

where $F(i)$ denotes the fitness value, BF and WF and denotes the best and worst fitness values in the current iteration, respectively, UB and LB represents the upper and lower bound of the feature space respectively, r_6 is a random number between [0, 1]. LH is the lower limit of H.

2.1 *Proposed MHGSO*

In this paper, an opposition-based learning (OBL) modification is added to the HGSO algorithm. As for any population-based optimization algorithm, the first step is to randomly initialize the population. This random population can be far or close to the optimal solution, which can therefore increase or decrease the optimization time. The idea of opposition-based learning is to calculate the position opposite to the initial random position and pick the one closer to the optimal solution [12]. The opposite positions are calculated using the mathematical model of the OBL operator in Eq. (11).

$$\overline{X}(t) = UB + LB - X(t) \tag{11}$$

After getting the initial population, we move toward the feature selection part. For feature selection, a wrapper-based method has been applied in which a classification algorithm is used for training and validating at each iteration, and then the MHGSO algorithm is applied to select the best set of features. The MHGSO algorithm is used to pick the best set of features and, in turn, increase the classification accuracy. The feature selection problem is a binary problem. Either a feature is selected or ignored. A selected feature is represented by 1 and the feature that is not selected is represented by 0. As the MHGSO algorithm works in continuous search space, three different binarization techniques have been applied to the MHGSO algorithm to map continuous values into corresponding binary values.

2.1.1 Transfer Function (MGHSO-TF)

This technique was introduced by Kennedy [13] for the binary version of the PSO algorithm. A transfer function (TF) is used to map the continuous values to the probabilities of changing a bit into a binary number. The most common transfer functions are S-shaped and V-shaped functions. The sigmoidal function is used in our study. These probabilities are then converted to binary vectors using the formula in Eq. (12).

$$x_{\text{new}} = \begin{cases} 1 \text{ if rand} \leq T(x) \\ 0 \quad \text{otherwise} \end{cases} \tag{12}$$

2.1.2 Great Value Priority (MGHSO-GVP)

The technique of great value priority (GVP) was introduced in Ref. [14], where a particle swarm optimization algorithm is used to solve a quadratic assignment problem. In this technique, a permutation vector is calculated using an initial solution. The first element of this permutation vector will store the position of the heaviest element. The second element will store the position of the second heaviest element and so on. Then the permutation vector is mapped to a binary vector using the formula in Eq. (13) (Fig. 2).

Proposed MHGSO using OBL

Initialize the parameters N, Max_iter, l, Dand SHungry.
Initialize the positions of individuals X_i(i=1,2,...,N)
While ($t \leq Max\_iter$)
    for i=1 to N
Apply OBL operator on the population X using Eq. (11)
Calculate the fitness of all indivisuals $t \leq Max\_iter$
Determine the best N solutions
    Endfor
Update BF, WF, X_b, B
Calculate the Hungry by Eq. (8)
Calculate the W_1 by Eq. (6)
Calculate the W_2 by Eq. (7)
for each individual
Calculate E by Eq. (2)
Update R by Eq. (4)
Update position by Eq. (1)
End for
$t = t + 1$
End while
Return BF& X_b

Fig. 2 Proposed modified HGSO algorithm using opposition-based learning

$$x_{\text{new}} = \begin{cases} 1 & p_j > p_{j+1} \\ 0 & \text{otherwise} \end{cases} \tag{13}$$

2.1.3 Angle Modulation (MHGSO-AM)

This method was first introduced by Franken [15]. This technique uses a trigonometric function having four parameters (*a*, *b*, *c*, *d*) used in the telecommunication industry [16] and governed as Eq. (14).

$$g(x) = \sin(2\pi(x - a) \times b \times \cos(2\pi \times c \times (x - a))) + d \tag{14}$$

In this approach, the four-dimensional vector (*a*, *b*, *c*, *d*) is optimized using the optimization algorithm. The parameters are substituted back after each iteration and then the function is sampled at equal intervals using the value x to generate a corresponding binary vector.

3 Results and Discussions

Five datasets from the UCI data source and three datasets from the Scikit-learn (SKT) package listed in Table 1 have been selected for experimentation. 80% of the dataset is used for training the classification algorithm, and 20% of the dataset is used for validation. As a classification algorithm, a Support Vector Machine is used.

Table 1 Datasets selected for study

Name	Sample size	Number of features	Number of classes	Source
Wine	178	13	3	SKT-L
Handwritten	1797	64	10	SKT-L
Spambase	4601	57	2	UCI
Image	2100	19	7	UCI
Cardiotocography	2126	24	2	UCI
Biodegradation	1055	41	2	UCI
Steel	1941	33	2	UCI
Breast Cancer	569	30	2	SKT-L

3.1 Evaluation Criterions

We have selected some parameters for MHGSO as the number of iterations (Max_iter = 100), the size of the population ($N = 10, L = 0.08$, LH = 10,000). The classification accuracy is calculated using the given formula in Eq. (15).

$$\text{Accuracy} = \frac{T_p + T_n}{T_p + T_n + F_p + F_n} \tag{15}$$

where, T_p (True Positive) denotes test sample which belongs to positive class and is correctly identified as positive by the classification model; T_n (True Negative) denotes test sample which belongs to negative class and is correctly identified as negative; F_p (False Positive) denotes test sample which belongs to negative class and is incorrectly identified as positive by the classification model; and F_n (False Negative) denotes test sample which belongs to positive class and is incorrectly identified as negative. The main aim of the feature selection problem is to use a smaller number of features and attain higher accuracy. Therefore, the objective function used for optimization is given as Eq. (16).

$$F(i) = (0.99 \times (1 - \text{accuracy}(i))) + \left(0.01 \times \left(\frac{\text{number of feature selected}}{\text{total number of features}}\right)\right) \tag{16}$$

3.2 Simulation Results

The proposed algorithm is implemented in Python on a personal computer that runs on an Intel (R) Core (TM) i5-8250U CPU @ 1.60 GHz with 8 GB RAM under the Windows 10 operating system. Tables 2, 3 and 4 presents the results from our MHGSO for classification, fitness value, and the selected number of features of different algorithms. It is evident from the data in Table 2, that the proposed algorithms show better accuracy than simple SVM for most of the dataset. MHGSO-TF shows the highest accuracy for seven out of eight datasets. MHGSO-AM shows the highest accuracy for a breast cancer dataset. MHGSO-GVP shows less accuracy as compared to the other two algorithms for most of the datasets. For the handwritten dataset, MHGSO-TF shows 99.17% accuracy as compared to 97.5% accuracy by SVM. For the breast cancer dataset, the classification accuracy exceeded 99% using MHGSO-AM. Table 3 shows satisfactory fitness values for all datasets by the different algorithms of our MHGSO.

It is also clear from Table 4 that MGHSO-GVP selects the least number of features as compared to the other two algorithms for most of the datasets. But, it shows less classification accuracy as compared to the other two and thus has a higher fitness

Table 2 Classification accuracy of different algorithms

Dataset	SVM	MHGSO-TF	MHGSO-GVP	MHGSO-AM
Wine	**1.00000**	**1.00000**	**1.00000**	**1.00000**
Handwritten	0.97500	**0.99167**	0.98333	0.98889
Spambase	0.93160	**0.94137**	0.92834	0.93594
Image	0.93095	**0.95238**	0.95000	0.93809
Cardiotocography	0.95070	**0.96244**	0.94836	0.96244
Biodegradation	0.88625	**0.90521**	0.89099	0.90047
Steel	**1.00000**	**1.00000**	0.96658	**1.00000**
Breast Cancer	0.98245	0.98245	0.98245	**0.99123**
Average	0.95712	**0.96694**	0.95626	0.96463

Bold values showing higher and better accuracies

Table 3 Fitness value of different algorithms

Dataset	SVM	MHGSO-TF	MHGSO-GVP	MHGSO-AM
Wine	0.0100	**0.00308**	**0.00308**	0.00385
Handwritten	0.07398	**0.01559**	0.02072	0.01850
Spambase	0.07772	**0.06576**	0.07568	0.07149
Image	0.07836	**0.05293**	0.05371	0.06655
Cardiotocography	0.05880	**0.04426**	0.05571	0.04551
Biodegradation	0.12261	**0.09945**	0.11182	0.10438
Steel	0.01000	0.00454	0.03763	**0.00182**
Breast Cancer	0.02737	0.02070	0.02104	**0.01202**
Average	0.05735	**0.03828**	0.04742	0.04052

Bold values showing higher and better accuracies

Table 4 Selected feature number of different algorithms

Dataset	SVM	MHGSO-TF	MHGSO-GVP	MHGSO-AM
Wine	13	**4**	**4**	5
Handwritten	64	47	**27**	48
Spambase	57	44	**27**	46
Image	19	11	**8**	10
Cardiotocography	24	17	**11**	20
Biodegradation	41	23	**16**	24
Steel	33	15	15	**6**
Breast Cancer	30	**10**	11	**10**
Average	35.13	21.38	**14.87**	21.12

Bold values showing higher and better accuracies

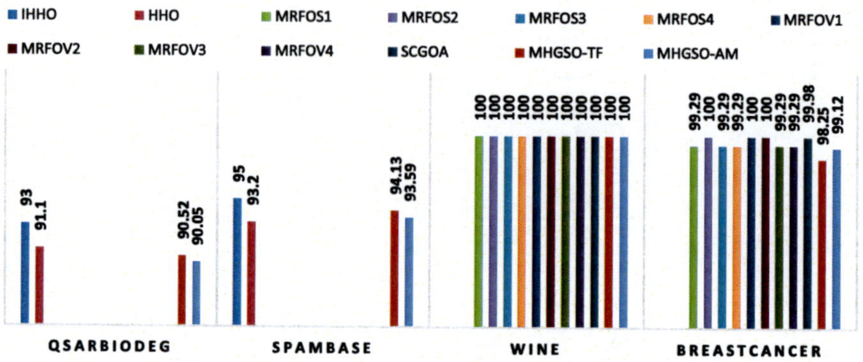

Fig. 3 Comparative study with some algorithms of state-of-the-art

value. For the wine and breast cancer datasets, the number of features selected by all three algorithms is less than one-third of the original number of features. For the breast cancer and steel datasets, the MGHSO-AM algorithm selected the least number of features along with the highest classification accuracy, resulting in the least fitness value. MGHSO-TF shows the least fitness value as compared to the other two because of higher classification accuracy and a smaller number of selected features.

4 Comparative Study with Some Techniques from Literature

In order to access the performance of the different variants of MHGSO, we compare the performance in terms of accuracy with some works from literature including improved HHO (IHHO) [17], basic HHO [17], S and V MRFO [18], and SCGOA. Figure 3 illustrates the comparative results. It is clear that MHGSO provides a competitive result, especially for Wine dataset, Spambase, and Breast Cancer.

5 Conclusion

This paper presented a modification of the recent Hunger Games Search optimization algorithm using the concept of opposition-based learning. The opposition-based learning technique allows you to search for a solution near to optimal by using random solutions as well as opposite-direction solutions simultaneously. The OBL technique helps HGSO to search for the optimal solution in less time. The modified HGSO using OBL is also incorporated with various binarization techniques to solve the feature selection problem. The simulations have been done using the eight standard datasets to evaluate the performance of the modified HGSO algorithm for solving the FS problem. It has been found that the performance outcomes of the modified algorithm are pretty good and better than the SVM technique in terms of classification accuracy, fitness values, and a number of features. Hence, the modified algorithm can be applied to several problems, like task scheduling, knapsack problems, traveling salesman problems, etc.

References

1. Too J et al (2018) A new competitive binary grey wolf optimizer to solve the feature selection problem in EMG signals classification. Computers 7(4):58
2. Wan Y et al (2016) A feature selection method based on modified binary coded ant colony optimization algorithm. Appl Soft Comput 49: 248–258
3. Pampara G, Franken N, Engelbrecht AP (2005) Combining particle swarm optimisation with angle modulation to solve binary problems. In: 2005 IEEE congress on evolutionary computation, vol 1. IEEE
4. Al-Tashi Q, Rais H, Jadid S (2018) Feature selection method based on grey wolf optimization for coronary artery disease classification. In: International conference of reliable information and communication technology. Springer, Cham
5. Singh S, Singh AK (2018) Web-spam features selection using CFS-PSO. Procedia Comput Sci 125:568–575
6. Ahmad I (2015) Feature selection using particle swarm optimization in intrusion detection. Int J Distrib Sensor Netw 11(10):806954
7. Abdi MJ, Giveki D (2013) Automatic detection of erythemato-squamous diseases using PSO–SVM based on association rules. Eng Appl Artif Intell 26(1):603–608
8. Mahmud M, Shamim Kaiser M, Martin McGinnity T, Hussain A (2021) Deep learning in mining biological data. Cogn Comput 13(1):1–33
9. Subanya B, Rajalaxmi RR (2014) Feature selection using artificial bee colony for cardiovascular disease classification. In: 2014 International conference on electronics and communication systems (ICECS). IEEE
10. Unler A, Murat A, Chinnam RB (2011) mr2PSO: a maximum relevance minimum redundancy feature selection method based on swarm intelligence for support vector machine classification. Inf Sci 181(20):4625–4641
11. Yang Y, Chen H, Heidari AA, Gandomi AH (2021) Hunger games search: visions, conception, implementation, deep analysis, perspectives, and towards performance shifts. Expert Syst Appl 177:114864
12. Tizhoosh HR (2005) Opposition-based learning: a new scheme for machine intelligence. In: International conference on computational intelligence for modelling, control and automation and international conference on intelligent agents, web technologies and internet commerce (CIMCA-IAWTIC'06), vol 1. IEEE
13. Kennedy J, Eberhart RC (1997) A discrete binary version of the particle swarm algorithm. In: 1997 IEEE International conference on systems, man, and cybernetics. Computational cybernetics and simulation, vol 5. IEEE
14. Lv C, Zhao H, Yang X (2011) Particle swarm optimization algorithm for quadratic assignment problem. In: Proceedings of the International conference on computer science and network technology (ICCSNT '11), pp 1728–1731
15. Franken N (2004) PSO-based coevolutionary game learning. Master's thesis, Department of Computer Science, University of Pretoria, South Africa
16. Proakis JG et al (1994) Communication systems engineering, vol. 2. Prentice Hall, New Jersey

17. Sihwail R, Omar K, Ariffin KAZ, Tubishat M (2020) Improved Harris Hawks optimization using elite opposition-based learning and novel search mechanism for feature selection. IEEE Access 8:121127–121145
18. Ghosh KK, Guha R, Bera SK, Kumar N, Sarkar R (2021) S-shaped versus V-shaped transfer functions for binary Manta ray foraging optimization in feature selection problem. Neural Comput Appl 1–15

Analysis of Hyperspectral Image Denoising Using Deep Neural Network (DNN) Models

Vaibhav J. Babrekar and Shirish M. Deshmukh

Abstract Image denoising is considered a common preprocessing step in the analysis and interpretation of hyperspectral images. Nevertheless, most of the methods developed and used previously was adopted for HSI denoising exploit architectures originally developed for grayscale and RGB images which limit the processing of high-dimensional HSI data cubes. As rich spectral information is present in HSI which is to be fully exploited considering the high degree of spectral correlation between adjacent bands in HSIs which gives in resulting poor image denoising, HSI denoising is the most important preprocessing step before the image is being classified. End to end mapping is needed between the clean and noisy images for the dataset by the deep learning method. Conventional low-rank methods lack flexibility for considering the correlation between different HSI which results to loss of information. This paper gives a brief review and analysis of the state-of-the-art available methods for hyperspectral image de-noising with the major advancements, benefits and obstacles in denoising an HSI. Due to limited availability of real time dataset of HSI and equipment expenses, researchers rely on the freely available hyperspectral datasets. This research proposes Hyperspectral image denoising for efficient classification of objects on the earth surface.

Keywords Hyperspectral image denoising · Remote sensing · Deep neural networks · HSI classification · Feature extraction

1 Introduction

HSI is extensively used in numerous applications such as agriculture planning, urban locality planning, monitoring the changes occurring in environment, anomaly detection. Because of some factors, these images are usually tarnished with noise which are type casted in regions of salt and pepper, stripes, Gaussian or dead-line noise, which is primary cause of the degradation of HSIs [1, 2]. Hyperspectral imaging

V. J. Babrekar (✉) · S. M. Deshmukh
Professor Ram Meghe Institute of Technology and Research, Badnera, Amravati 444607, India

M. S. Kaiser et al. (eds.), *Proceedings of Trends in Electronics and Health Informatics*, Lecture Notes in Networks and Systems 376,
https://doi.org/10.1007/978-981-16-8826-3_6

spectrometers are specially used for collecting the information among the electromagnetic spectrum in many of the contiguous and narrow bands which produces high-dimensional images with more than hundreds of spectral bands. Spectral variations in an HSI are to be focused more compared to spatial variations. By enlarging spectral dimension of a pixel, objects on the earth surface can be underlined because it contains a unique and characteristic spectral signature. In the process of image acquisition, a substantial amount of noise gets usually introduced in the data which gives resulting interclass variability and interclass similarity. This noise degradation is primarily due to instrumental acquisition limitations and atmospheric distortions [3]. To overcome these issues, denoising of images must be used as a preprocessing step for the removal of noise before the analysis of HSI. Many techniques adopted for HSI denoising were originally developed for the gray scale and RGB images which do not guarantee accurate results which can lead to the loss of rich spectral information contained in HSI.

1.1 Convolutional Neural Network for HSI Denoising

The growth in publishing the research articles over the years shows how much attention grabbing this subject is. HSI-SDeCNN is a method that was advantageous in some ways like providing the fast solution to the HSI denoising problem which exploits a down sampling kernel that allows the network to perform faster without losing performance. This method is also beneficial allowing to control the back-and-forth between denoising performance and details preservation. This makes the network more flexible and more adaptive to multilevel noise in which avoiding the need to train a different model for different noise levels [3]. Making denoising of the image at only one band can be said as disadvantageous because noise generally differs from band to band. Hyperspectral images belong to the remote sensing domain in which these images are used in applications such as classification, detection of target and spectral unmixing [4]. Due to instrumental malfunctioning and atmospheric effects, HSIs often get corrupted by various noises such as random noise, strip noise and dead pixels. For improving the degraded quality of HSI, it is critical to reducing the noise. Hence, there is a need of taking the spectral and spatial constraints for image denoising. A deep residual network which is a combined spatial-spectral features and multiscale features is used to recover the HSI from noise or called noise-free HSI approach. This approach uses nonlinear end-to-end mapping between the corrupted noisy image and the clean reference image with two-dimensional spatial and three-dimensional spatial-spectral combination training network [4].

1.2 Total Variation and Block Matching

For improving the peak signal to noise ratio (PSNR), BM3D is combined with CNN which also improves the denoising performance and has the feature learning ability. When this hyperspectral data is transmitted in the medium, due to the factors involved in acquisition, this data is contaminated by various noises, i.e., impulse noise, stripes and deadlines which is unavoidable and degrades the image quality. Because of the complexity, the analysis of HSI such as target detection, image classification and compressive sensing got effected and disturbed. Therefore, hyperspectral image restoration is a challenging but necessary preprocessing step in remote sensing [5]. The image denoising method based on two-dimensional band by band denoising is the most fundamental among the various methods of denoising [4].

1.3 Deep Learning Methods

Hyperspectral images (HSIs) are ordinarily corrupted by various sorts of noises and their mixture leading to the degradation in acquired image standard which further restricts the applications deployment. The generation of noise is consequential from many aspects, including sensor noise and the atmospheric effect [6]. The HSIs also are termed hyperspectral data cubes as given in Fig. 1; plots on the highest right-hand side show the fields of pixels containing parameters of soil, vegetation, and water. A schematic overview of the spectral characteristics of hyperspectral data is given in Fig. 2 [7]. Large data sets are appropriate for signifying the performance of learning systems. Nevertheless, for hyperspectral images, it is often tough to obtain

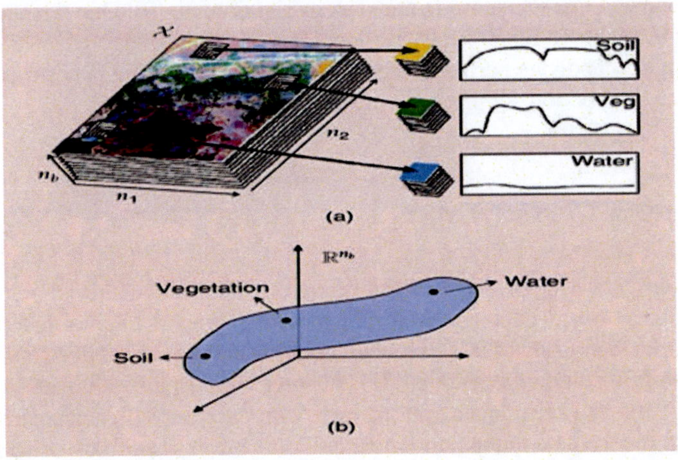

Fig. 1 **a** Hyperspectral imaging concept, **b** hyperspectral vectors represented in a low-dimensional manifold [2]

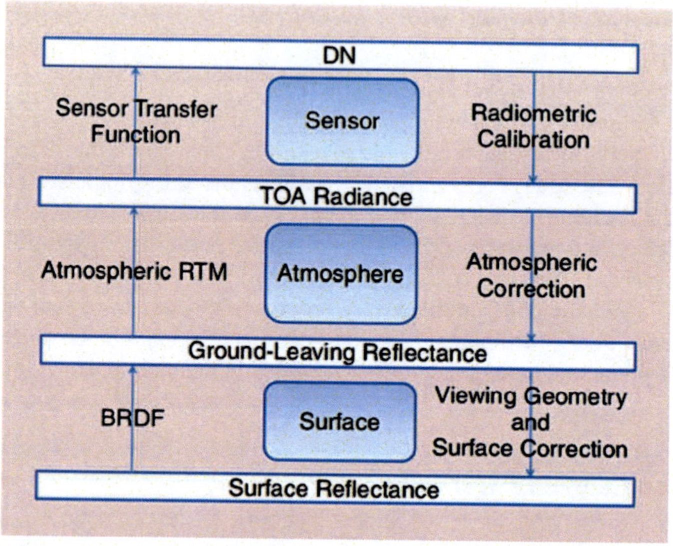

Fig. 2 Spectral characterization of hyperspectral data [2]

such a large data set [8]. Deep learning not only provides great potential in regards to removal of complex spectral cum spatial noise but also thrives for greater contribution toward HSI. From the requirements of HSI, the context information needs to be extracted in regards to provide for pixel information surrounding the pixel under test in HSI and this is denoted a crucial step. Hence, when there is a challenge of image denoising, effective receptive field is of great importance. When HSI denoising model preserves the correlation of adjacent spectral bands, it is proven to be achieving better performance and extracts more features in spatial domain [9]. One method for HSI denoising available in literature is non-local low-rank tensor approximation. While considering its denoising performance in terms of more spectral bands then benefits less and the time period significantly increases [10].

1.4 Spectral Characteristics

The need for recovering denoising techniques has brought about the natural introduction of different image denoising algorithms, with having its unique characteristics. Total variation denoising (TVD) is a beginning for noise removal developed to hold sharp edges in the underlying signal. It is characterized as an optimization problem [3]. One of the key techniques that has provided success in hyperspectral dimensionality to reduce data embed nonlinear and nonconvex manifolds noise is that of local manifold. This technique is composite of matrix construction based on affinity rules. Affinity knowledge is based on two backbones which are selection of neighbor as well its weight composite. Each step comes with a challenge, where in the first step of neighbor selection is restricted to spectral variability in terms of uneven data distribution in regards to original image followed by illumination noise that is again uneven in regards to sensor placement inducing angular noise. The second step of weight definition not only is limited by singular spectral correlation prejudice with the first step definition [4]. It is difficult to preserve both spectral and spatial structures as well as there is a requirement of removing mixed type of noises in HSI denoising which is a challenging task [11]. One of the methods for HSI denoising which is recently attracting the considerable attention because of its performance is discriminative model learning [5].

HSI denoising is important and fundamental task for improving the performance of classification, spectral unmixing, and hence, it is a preprocessing step before subsequent application. In hyperspectral image data, there is local and global redundancy in spatial domain which generally preserves the details and texture of image. Another valuable property is correlation of spectral domain which can be utilized for obtaining good results [6]. Image can be recovered from noisy image with dictionary and sparse codes corresponding to it. The process of HSI denoising is shown in Fig. 3 [10]. In this study article, our contribution is mentioned as:

1. Collection of different HSI datasets and analysis of image denoising models.
2. The commonly used HSI denoising methods are evaluated on objectives.
3. The main challenges and flow of HSI denoising.

In Sect. 2, the literature survey of available denoising methods. In Sect. 3, comparative analysis of over the decade available denoising methods and research gap identified. In Sect. 4, the performance parameters included. In last section, we concluded the paper.

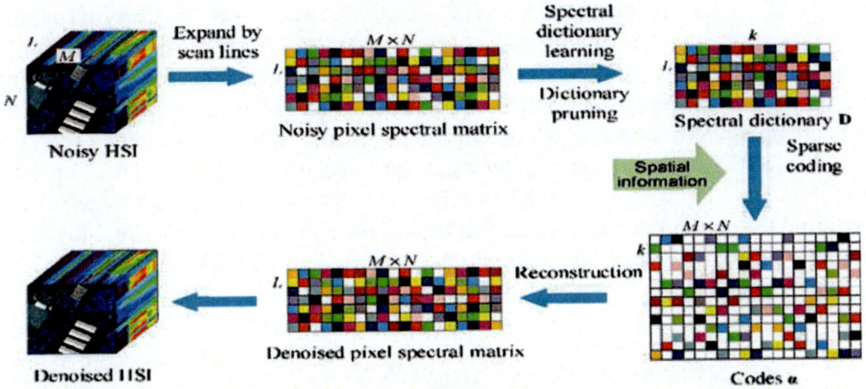

Fig. 3 HSI denoising based on spectral dictionary learning and sparse coding [10]

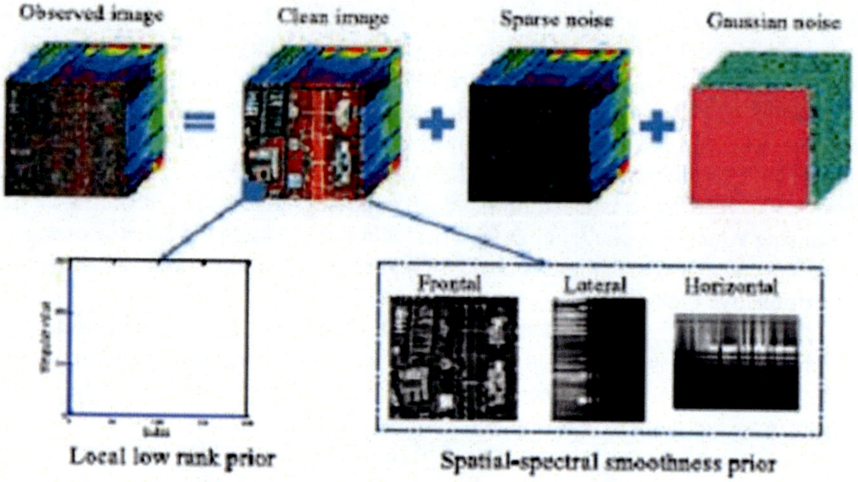

Fig. 4 Degradation of HSI and prior steps for obtaining clean HIS [12]

2 Literature Review

2.1 *Total Variation and Deep Learning-Based Approaches*

Many researchers have worked for the development of algorithms or techniques for HSI denoising to get the precise noise-free images for classification. The detail literature review of the existing systems is discussed below. Figure 4 shows how observed HSI get degrades and what prior steps are involved for clean HSI.

An HSI single denoising CNN (HSI-SDeCNN) model resourcefully takes into consideration both the spatial and spectral information which is primary source contained in HSIs [13]. An innovative deep learning-based method for HSI denoising is anticipated by Qiangqiang Yuan et al. which includes learning a nonlinear end-to-end mapping between the noisy image and the clean one with a combined spectral-spatial DCNN. The proposed network is assigned with both spatial and spectral information simultaneously. Additionally, for capturing both multiscale spatial and spectral feature and to fuse diverse feature representations for recovering the image, multiscale feature extraction and multilevel feature representation are used [14].

2.2 *Denoising Algorithms Using CNN*

In regards to novel methodology, learning algorithm needs to utilize linear and robust data representation which primarily needs to provide hierarchical selection. This method makes sure that variation in complex spectral data representation can be eliminated which provides normalization in regards to weights reconstructing neighbor selection [4]. The aim of non-LRMA method is to decompose the HSI which is degraded by not only noise but also the representation of ranked-based matrix weights. This method takes support of Lagrangian multipliers which provides improvements in terms of nonconvex surrogate function [11]. The feed-forward denoising convolutional neural network (DnCNN) can hold the improvement in very deep manner, learning set of rules and regularization method resulting into image denoising. For boosting-up, the process and performance of image denoising residual learning and batch normalization are used. Gaussian noise can be dealt by CNN models without knowing the noise level. By using residual learning strategy, DnCNN is able to remove latent clean image in hidden layers [5]. Among the HSI denoising algorithms presented in past decades, one can have classification in terms of natural images having either band or pixel characterization yet it remains restricted for spectral correlation. Overcoming this restriction is desired for having good quality of denoised image. Some methods also destroy the spectral correlation which produces extra distortion. Hence, there is a need to consider spectral and spatial dimensions simultaneously [6].

3 Research Analysis and Researchgap Identification

Table 1 shows the state-of-the-art HIS denoising methods over the decade with technology used, their applications and required improvement according to us.

4 HSI Denoising Performance Parameters

Performance of HSI denoising methods is most important indices in denoising. Researchers focused in evaluation of different objectives over the years. For HIS denoising few prominent methods that are adopted are.

4.1 The Mean Square Error

The difference in regards to original and captured image in context of average is defined as the mean square error (MSE). Lower the value of MSE, better the quality of image.

$$\text{MSE} = \frac{1}{N}||1 - L||$$

Table 1 Research analysis and research gap identification

Author	Reference	Year	Method used	Technology used	Application	Research gap identified
Yang et al	[15]	2021	SSLR-SSTV	Spatial-spectral TV	HSI noise removal	Cost of computation and time is little bit more
Wang et al	[16]	2021	Low-rank denoising model based on Tensor-based non-local,	Low-rank tensor decomposition, sparse prior information	Denoising of HSI	Less prior information included and running speed to be improved
Wang et al	[17]	2021	MLR-SSTV	Regularization weighted nuclear norm to estimate the more accurate low-rank tensor	HSI dead line noise removal	To remove dead line noise completely, modified LR tensor and l1 norm of SSTV is needed
Wei et al	[12]	2020	3DQRNN	3D convolution and quasi-recurrent pooling function for local and global correlation along spectrum	HIS restoration accuracy and computation time	Focused on few image sequences only, can be made generalized for any dataset
Leng et al	[14]	2019	HSID-CNN	Nonlinear end-to-end mapping based on deep learning between the noisy and clean HSIs	Image restoration with multiscale feature extraction and multilevel feature representation	Less efficient in terms of mixed noise removal and spectral distortion
Shan et al	[18]	2019	DD-CNN	Structural similar-ity index metric (SSIM)	Correlation between the target specific noisy images and the input clean reference images	This method shows significant advantages when larger the noise in the image
Dev et al	[3]	2017	Least square approach	Different wavelet filters	Image denoising and retaining the features	Gives better results but doesn't smoothen the image at par

(continued)

Table 1 (continued)

Author	Reference	Year	Method used	Technology used	Application	Research gap identified
Leng et al	[19]	2020	Adaptive multiscale segmentations	Intra–inter-scale discrimination index	Image segmentation and classification	It is hard to choose effective and complementary scales
Zhang et al	[20]	2020	TV-NLRTD	Alternating direction method of multipliers (ADMM) algorithm	HSI restoration by combining non-local LR tensor decomposition and total variation regularization	Doesn't provide better results with varying band intensities assigning the weights
Liu et al	[21]	2019	3DADCNN	Spatial-spectral feature extraction and enlarging receptive field	To denoise the corrupted image by mixed type of photon and thermal noise	Only limited to photon and thermal noise but not mixed noise
He et al	[22]	2019	Unified spatial-spectral paradigm for HSI denoising	Non-local low-rank denoising and iterative regularization	HSI denoising based on non-local low-rank tensor approximation	Cannot find non-local similarity between hyperparameters
Fernandez-Beltran et al	[23]	2018	DEpLSA	Dual-depth architecture	Estimating both the endmember and abundances from remotely sensed hyperspectral imagery	Limitations in terms of computational time, estimation of ideal sparsity factor for the input image, finding the number of endmembers
Hong et al	[4]	2017	Manifold learning methodology based on locally linear embedding	Localmanifold learning	Hyperspectral dimensionality reduction	Manifold learning is applied only to small scale data

(continued)

Table 1 (continued)

Author	Reference	Year	Method used	Technology used	Application	Research gap identified
Chen et al	[11]	2017	Non-LRMA	Reformulating the approximation problem using non-convex regularizer	LRMA-basedHSI denoising	Time consuming and less accurate method of denoising
Gao et al	[24]	2017	HyDRoS	RPCA and BM3D	Mineral Mapping	Proposed denoiser is slower owing to the process of outlier removal by RPCA
Wu et al	[25]	2016	TWNNM	Total variation regularization (TV)	Hyperspectral image mixed denoising	The noise levels are different over bands hence a noise-adjusted parameter setting is needed, also this is effective for only edge preserving
Hong et al	[26]	2018	LeMA	Semi supervised cross-modality learning Framework and ADMM	Land cover and land use classification	Limited ability while facing highly nonlinear heterogenous data for Morphological profiles
Yang et al	[27]	2018	BM3D-Net	Clock matching 3D filtering technique	Gray-scale and color image denoising also with depth map denoising	Limited applications in color image deblurring, super resolution and video denoising but not applicable in general
Zhang	[11]	2017	Residual learning of deep CNN	Residual learning and batch normalization are utilized	Denoising of Gaussian noise, super-resolution of single image and JPEG image deblocking	Not applicable on denoising of images with real complex noise and other general image restoration tasks

(continued)

Table 1 (continued)

Author	Reference	Year	Method used	Technology used	Application	Research gap identified
Gong et al	[28]	2019	NLRATV	Non-local patch-based rank constraint	HSI denoising with 3D anisotropic total variation	Can be extended to the tensor form to explore the 3D rank-constrain methods for HSIs noise reduction

4.2 Peak Signal to Noise Ratio (PSNR)

It is determined through MSE keeping in mind that a ratio between maximum original signal and MSE is to be maintained in terms of engineering aspiration. Higher the value of PSNR, better is the quality of image.

$$\text{PSNR} = 10 * \log_{10}\left(\frac{(\max(I))^2}{\text{MSE}}\right)$$

4.3 Structural Similarity Index Matrix (SSIM)

This quantity measures the perceptual difference of two similar images. This perceptual difference depends upon parameters such as contrast and luminance. Higher the value of SSIM, better the quality of image.

$$\text{SSIM}_{(u,v)} = \frac{(2_{\mu I \mu L} + Q_1)(2_{\sigma IL} + Q_2)}{(\mu_I^2 + \mu_L^2 + Q_1)(\sigma_I^2 + \sigma_L^2 + Q_2)}$$

where average gray values and variance patches are represented by I and L. Covariance is provided by IL, and finally, positive constant representation is provided by Q1 and Q2 typically around 0.01.

4.4 Root Mean Square Error (RMSE)

The change between predictions expected and observed is defined by RMSE which is of square scale of MSE. In terms of equation, it is realized in regards of two of the prominent image metrics (P, Q) is:

$$\text{RMSE} = \sqrt{\text{MSE}(P, Q)} = \sqrt{\sum_{p=1}^{m}\sum_{q=1}^{n}(P_{pq} - Q_{pq})^2}$$

4.5 *Feature Similarity (FSIM and FSIMc)*

The evaluation that covers gray scaling in images along with color luminance in images is covered by FSIM. As the first step, it calculates the local similarity and categories them in based on similarity scores.

$$\mathrm{FSIM} = \frac{\sum_{x\in\Omega} \mathrm{SL}(x) \cdot \mathrm{PCm}(x)}{\sum_{x\in\Omega} \mathrm{PCm}(x)}$$

$$\mathrm{FSIMc} = \frac{\sum_{x\in\Omega} \mathrm{SL}(x) \cdot [\mathrm{Sc}(x)]^{\lambda} \cdot \mathrm{PCm}(x)}{\sum_{x\in\Omega} \mathrm{PCm}(x)}$$

4.6 *The Signal to Noise Ratio (SNR)*

Relation of noise in ratio and proportion to original image is defined as SNR which is formulated as:

$$SNR = 10 \log_{10} \frac{\|L\|}{\|I - L\|}$$

A paper that provides a spectral angle mapper (SAM) along with Erreur Relative Globale Adimensionnelle de Synthèse (ERGAS) [26] for the provisions that PSNR and SSIM calculations is achieved easily. As utilization of SSIm and PSNR is prima facial for CNN-based image denoising, these two methods make them popular because of their ease, and these are considered to be tested and valid [29].

5 Discussion

A total of 45 reference papers included in this review article, out of that 30 research papers belong to the HSI denoising. In this review article, sensible efforts were made including all research articles which belong to HSI denoising but it is obvious that some papers might have been skipped. Some sample pictures and methods of remote sensing and HSI are shown in Fig. 5. A graph shown in figure indicates the number of papers and publication year for the articles belong to HSI denoising available in Fig. 6. It can be perceived from figure that researchers have recently adopted neural networks and machine learning for research in HSI denoising. This article covers generalized research that needs to adopt a practical experimentation to enhance exploration of HSI by denoising. This research can be better understood by graph indicating the types of images that have well-known dataset adopted by the HSI denoising systems which is available in Fig. 7.

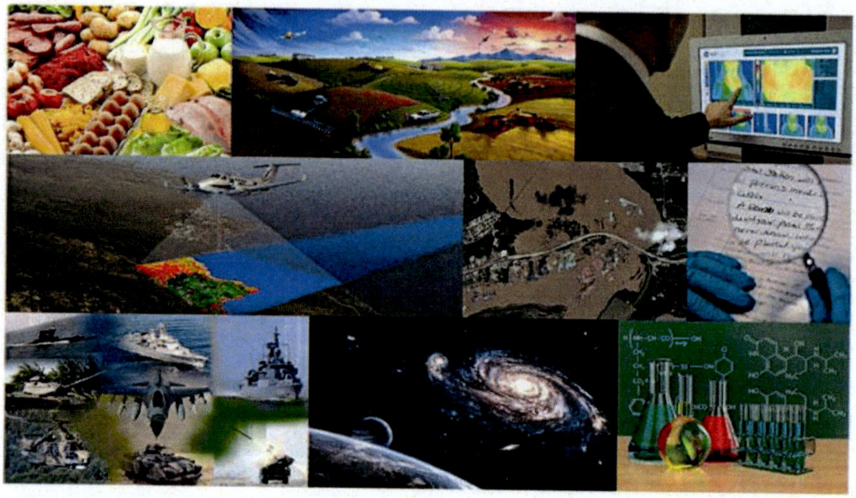

Fig. 5 Few of sample images in famous datasets used by the researchers

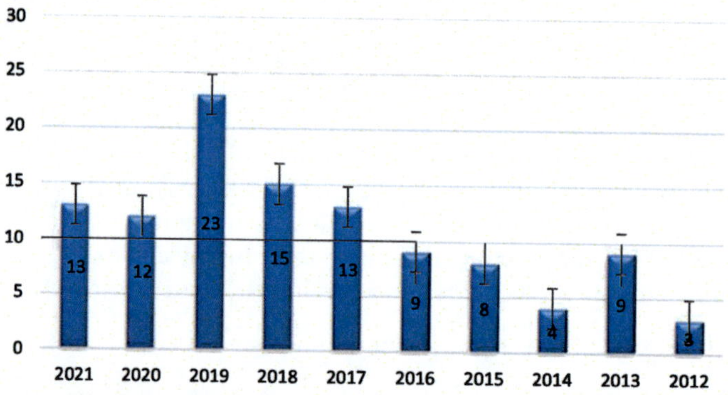

Fig. 6 Number of papers published yearly on HSI denoising (Papers from Google)

6 Conclusion

Recently, the CNN, DNN and ANN are becoming very useful in HSI denoising. The survey of different neural network-based hyperspectral image denoising methods is proposed in this study. Few of these methods made use of the originator and discriminator for mining and clean image creation. The inventive step implemented by the researchers was to try diverse noise which contains impulse Gaussian noise. This noise can be made to reduce by using several careful deep convolutional networks which are commonly used in most of the HSI denoising performing articles. The reason behind the worldwide acceptance of these methods is because of their popularity and effective denoising results. The concluding remarks for this review can be

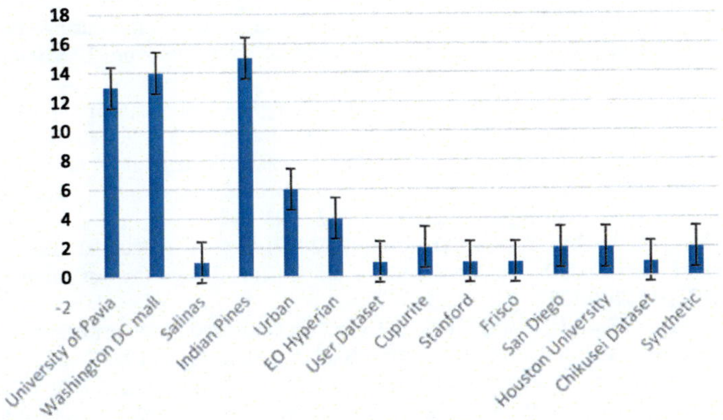

Fig. 7 Dataset used by the researchers over the years (According to references)

concise as below: From the reported literature, till then it can be said that the neural networks can remove most types of noise from HSI and advance the capability in image denoising. Some of the reported literature showed higher performance of neural networks architecture for HSI denoising. The architecture of neural networks is customizable for removal of noise creating patterns which can remove the blockage of vanishing gradients. Most of the studies used the pretraining of neural networks; however, properties of noise are continuous in nature and require a denoising model which is built from graze. For this, task of building model from beginning requires high computation cost in terms of space and time.

References

1. Rasti B, Scheunders P, Ghamisi P, Licciardi G, Chanussot J (2018) Noise reduction in hyperspectral imagery: overview and application. Remote Sens. https://doi.org/10.3390/rs10030482
2. Bioucasdias JM, Plaza A, Camps-valls G, Scheunders P, Nasrabadi NM, Chanussot J (2013) Bioucasdias2013, no. June, 2013
3. Dev VS, Rajan S, Sowmya V, Soman KP (2017) Hyperspectral image denoising: a least square approach using wavelet filters. https://doi.org/10.1109/ICACCI.2017.8125941
4. Chen Y, Guo Y, Wang Y, Wang D, Peng C, He G (2017) Denoising of hyperspectral images using nonconvex low rank matrix approximation. IEEE Trans Geosci Remote Sens 55(9):5366–5380. https://doi.org/10.1109/TGRS.2017.2706326
5. Sun L, Jeon B, Zheng Y, Wu Z (2017) A novel weighted cross total variation method for hyperspectral image mixed denoising. IEEE Access 5:27172–27188. https://doi.org/10.1109/ACCESS.2017.2768580
6. Lu T, Li S (2015) Gradient-guided sparse representation for hyperspectral image denoising. Int Geosci Remote Sens Symp 2015:1128–1131. https://doi.org/10.1109/IGARSS.2015.7325969
7. Zhang M, Li W, Du Q (2018) Diverse region-based CNN for hyperspectral image classification. IEEE Trans Image Process 27(6):2623–2634. https://doi.org/10.1109/TIP.2018.2809606

8. Li W, Wu G, Zhang F, Du Q (2017) Hyperspectral image classification using deep pixel-pair features. IEEE Trans Geosci Remote Sens 55(2):844–853. https://doi.org/10.1109/TGRS.2016.2616355
9. Song X, Wu L, Hao H, Xu W (2019) Hyperspectral image denoising based on spectral dictionary learning and sparse coding. Electronics 8(1). https://doi.org/10.3390/electronics8010086
10. Wang M, Wang Q, Chanussot J, Li D (2021) Hyperspectral image mixed noise removal based on multidirectional low-rank modeling and spatial-spectral total variation. IEEE Trans Geosci Remote Sens. https://doi.org/10.1109/TGRS.2020.2993631
11. Zhang K, Zuo W, Chen Y, Meng D, Zhang L (2017) Beyond a Gaussian denoiser: residual learning of deep CNN for image denoising. IEEE Trans Image Process. https://doi.org/10.1109/TIP.2017.2662206
12. He W, Zhang H, Shen H, Zhang L (2018) Hyperspectral image denoising using local low-rank matrix recovery and global spatial-spectral total variation. IEEE J Sel Top Appl Earth Obs Remote Sens 11(3):713–729. https://doi.org/10.1109/JSTARS.2018.2800701
13. Maffei A, Haut JM, Paoletti ME, Plaza J, Bruzzone L, Plaza A (2020) A single model CNN for hyperspectral image denoising. IEEE Trans Geosci Remote Sens. https://doi.org/10.1109/TGRS.2019.2952062
14. Yuan Q, Zhang Q, Li J, Shen H, Zhang L (2019) Hyperspectral image denoising employing a spatial-spectral deep residual convolutional neural network. IEEE Trans Geosci Remote Sens 57(2):1205–1218. https://doi.org/10.1109/TGRS.2018.2865197
15. Yang F, Chen X, Chai L (2021) Hyperspectral image destriping and denoising using stripe and spectral low-rank matrix recovery and global spatial-spectral total variation. Remote Sens 13(4):1–19. https://doi.org/10.3390/rs13040827
16. Wang G, Han H, Carranza EJM, Guo S, Guo K, Xiao K (2020) Tensor-based low-rank and sparse prior information constraints for hyperspectral image denoising. IEEE Access 8:102935–102946. https://doi.org/10.1109/ACCESS.2020.2996303
17. Wei K, Fu Y, Huang H (2021) 3-D Quasi-recurrent neural network for hyperspectral image denoising. IEEE Trans Neural Netw Learn Syst. https://doi.org/10.1109/TNNLS.2020.2978756
18. Shan W, Liu P, Mu L, Cao C, He G (2019) Hyperspectral image denoising with dual deep CNN. IEEE Access. https://doi.org/10.1109/ACCESS.2019.2955810
19. Leng Q, Yang H, Jiang J, Tian Q (2020) Adaptive multiscale segmentations for hyperspectral image classification. IEEE Trans Geosci Remote Sens. https://doi.org/10.1109/TGRS.2020.2971716
20. Zhang H, Liu L, He W, Zhang L (2020) Hyperspectral image denoising with total variation regularization and nonlocal low-rank tensor decomposition. IEEE Trans Geosci Remote Sens 58(5):3071–3084. https://doi.org/10.1109/TGRS.2019.2947333
21. Liu W, Lee J (2019) A 3-D atrous convolution neural network for hyperspectral image denoising. IEEE Trans Geosci Remote Sens 57(8). https://doi.org/10.1109/TGRS.2019.2901737
22. He W, Yao Q, Li C, Yokoya N, Zhao Q (2019) Non-local meets global: an integrated paradigm for hyperspectral denoising. Proc IEEE Comput Soc Conf Comput Vis Pattern Recognit 2019:6861–6870. https://doi.org/10.1109/CVPR.2019.00703
23. Hong D, Yokoya N, Zhu XX (2017) Learning a robust local manifold representation for hyperspectral dimensionality reduction. IEEE J Sel Top Appl Earth Obs Remote Sens 10(6):2960–2975. https://doi.org/10.1109/JSTARS.2017.2682189
24. Gao L, Yao D, Li Q, Zhuang L, Zhang B, Bioucas-Dias JM (2017) A new low-rank representation based hyperspectral image denoising method for mineral mapping. Remote Sens 9(11):1–20. https://doi.org/10.3390/rs9111145
25. Wu Z, Wang Q, Wu Z, Shen Y (2016) Total variation-regularized weighted nuclear norm minimization for hyperspectral image mixed denoising. J Electron Imaging 25(1):013037. https://doi.org/10.1117/1.jei.25.1.013037

26. Hong D, Yokoya N, Ge N, Chanussot J, Zhu XX (2019) Learnable manifold alignment (LeMA): a semi-supervised cross-modality learning framework for land cover and land use classification. ISPRS J Photogramm Remote Sens 147:193–205. https://doi.org/10.1016/j.isprsjprs.2018.10.006
27. Yang D, Sun J (2018) BM3D-Net: a convolutional neural network for transform-domain collaborative filtering. IEEE Signal Process Lett 25(1):55–59. https://doi.org/10.1109/LSP.2017.2768660
28. Gong T, Wen D, He T (2020) A non-local rank-constraint hyperspectral images denoising method with 3-D anisotropic total variation. J Phys Conf Ser 1438(1). https://doi.org/10.1088/1742-6596/1438/1/012024
29. Setiadi DRIM (2021) PSNR vs SSIM: imperceptibility quality assessment for image steganography. Multimed Tools Appl 80(6):8423–8444. https://doi.org/10.1007/s11042-020-10035-z

Significance of Source Information in Hypernasality Detection

Akhilesh Kumar Dubey, Deepak Kumar Singh, and B. B. Tiwari

Abstract This work analyzes the peak to side-lobe ratio (PSR) around each glottal closure instant (GCI) in the Hilbert envelope (HE) of linear prediction (LP) residual as an excitation source-based cue for the hypernasality detection. PSR is defined as the ratio of peak value around GCI to the mean of sample values around GCI in the 3 ms range of HE of LP residual. The coupling between nasal and oral tract occurs during the production of voiced sound in hypernasal speech. The air leakage from nasal tract affects the abruptness of glottal closure, which in turn affects the peak strength around the GCIs. The nasal tract adds zeros in the spectrum of voiced sound. Since the LP model is poor in modeling the zeros in the spectrum, the zeros get filtered in the LP residual signal. This increases the side-lobe strength around the peak in the HE of LP residual. Hence, the PSR gets affected in hypernasal speech. Classification between pre-known normal and hypernasal sound based on a threshold value of PSR gives the accuracy of 70.49, 78.19, 63.15, 60.67, and 67.27% for high vowel, low vowel, glides, liquids, and voicebar sounds, respectively.

Keywords Hypernasality · Peak to side-lobe ratio · Glottal closure instants (GCIs) · Hilbert envelope (HE) of LP residual

1 Introduction

The cleft lip and palate (CLP) is a facial and oral birth defect in children. The velopharyngeal insufficiency causes the coupling of the nasal tract with the oral tract, which nasalizes the CLP speech. The excesses nasality heard during the production of voice sounds is called hypernasality [8]. Hypernasality reduces the intelligibility

---

A. K. Dubey (✉)
Koneru Lakshmaiah Education Foundation (Deemed to be University), Vaddeswaram, Guntur, Andhra Pradesh 522502, India
e-mail: dubey18oct@kluniversity.in

D. K. Singh · B. B. Tiwari
VSB Purvanchal University, Jaunpur, Uttar Pradesh 222002, India

M. S. Kaiser et al. (eds.), *Proceedings of Trends in Electronics and Health Informatics*, Lecture Notes in Networks and Systems 376,
https://doi.org/10.1007/978-981-16-8826-3_7

of the CLP speech [7]. The detection and severity rating of hypernasal speech helps the plastic surgeons and speech pathologists in the diagnosis of individuals with CLP. Mostly, the subjective evaluation of hypernasality is done by experience speech pathologists. The objective evaluation is done by the device called nasometer, which determines the percentage of nasalance in speech. The subjective judgment may be biased, and the nasometer device may be inconvenience for children and does not work for stored speech data [1]. Hence, the acoustic analysis cues based on the speech processing have been proposed for the objective evaluation of hypernasal speech.

In the literature, hypernasality is detected by the acoustic analysis of nasalized vowels present in hypernasal speech. The most important cues for the nasalized vowels are: the presence of extra pole-zero in the first formant region and broadening of first formant [19]. Based on these cues, many researchers attempted for the hypernasality detection in CLP speech. In [2], the difference between the low-pass and band-pass profiles of the Teager energy operator is used for hypernasality detection. The distance between the low- and high-order linear prediction cepstral coefficients is used as a parameter to estimate hypernasality in [15]. The voice low tone to high tone ratio in [9] and the detection of extra nasal formant with the help of high spectra resolution group delay method are used in [19] for the hypernasality detection. In [10], the combination of frame-based feature MFCC plus Teager energy operator profile is used for detection. In [13, 17], two set of features, one based on acoustic, noise, and cepstral analysis and other based on nonlinear dynamic features, is used for the hypernasality detection in CLP. The combination of nonlinear dynamic features plus entropy measurements is used as a feature in [14]. The energy distribution ratio and GMM-based classification of hypernasality severity are proposed in [6]. In [5], the raising and falling slope amplitude reductions are proposed as a cue for hypernasal speech. In [3], a high-resolution spectro-temporal method called zero time windowing is used to detect the extra nasal peak and for the severity analysis of hypernasal speech in [4].

All the above attempts for hypernasality detection are based on the analysis of vowel spectrum, to capture the changes in vocal tract response in CLP speech compared to normal speech. Some attempts have been done to capture the change in excitation source response in CLP speech. In hypernasal speech, the loudness of sound reduces. This happens due to acoustic damping in the nasal tract. Analog model studies in [5] have demonstrated that the overall sound energy of the vowels is reduced as a consequence of nasal coupling. An effective representation of the excitation source response can be derived from the linear prediction (LP) residual signal. The peak around the glottal closure instant (GCI) in Hilbert envelope (HE) of LP residual may, hence, get affected in the hypernasal speech. As the coupling of nasal cavity introduces the extra zeros in the spectrum and the LP model is poor in modeling the zeros in the spectrum, the extra zeros get filtered in the residual signal of hypernasal speech. The extra zeros in residual will enhance the side-lobes around the peak, making it more noisy. Figures 1a, b show the normal vowel speech waveform and its HE of LP residual signal, respectively, and (c), (d) show the hypernasal vowel speech waveform and its HE of LP residual signal, respectively. The peak strength in case of normal vowel is more compared to the hypernasal vowel,

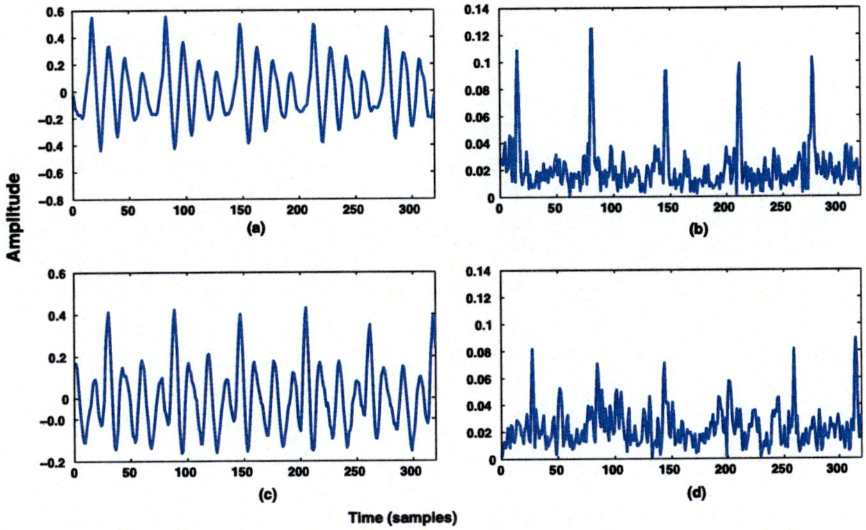

Fig. 1 Illustration of peak and side-lobe in HE of LP residual signal of normal and hypernasal vowel. **a, b** Normal vowel speech waveform and its HE of LP residual signal, respectively and **c, d** Hypernasal vowel speech waveform and its HE of LP residual signal, respectively

whereas the side-lobe strength is more in case of hypernasal vowel. This observation motivates us to analyze the PSR around each GCI in the HE of LP residual signal as an excitation source-based acoustic cue for the hypernasality detection. The analysis is done not only for the vowels, but also for the semivowels (glides and liquids) and voicebar. It is expected that the glottal closure will be more abrupt in normal vowels compared to hypernasal vowels which has nasal leakage. Hence, the peak strength will decrease in hypernasal vowels. Since the side-lobe strength will increase in hypernasal vowels due to extra zeros, the PSR should decrease in hypernasal speech. In the case of semivowels and voicebar, the decrease in pressure inside the mouth due to nasal leakage may increase the trans-glottal pressure; hence, the more abrupt glottal closure may happen. This will increase in peak strength in hypernasal speech. Here also, the side-lobe strength will increase due to extra zeros. Since the both the quantity in PSR is increasing, the net effect will depend on which quantity increases more. Since the PSR gives the distinctive characteristics for the normal and hypernasal speech, it can be proposed as a excitation source-based cue for the hypernasality detection.

The rest of the paper is organized as follows. In Sect. 2, excitation source analysis in hypernasal speech is done. Section 3 gives the excitation source-based cue for hypernasality. Section 4 gives the experimental result, and finally, Sect. 5 contains the summary and conclusion of the work.

2 Excitation Source Analysis in Hypernasal Speech

The excitation source information can be derived from a given speech segment of a particular sound unit (vowels, semivowels, or voicebar) using the inverse LP filtering. The inverse filtering using the LP coefficients suppresses the vocal tract information and mostly contains information about the excitation source in the form of residual signal. The large amplitude fluctuations, either in positive or negative polarity, in the LP residual are the location of GCIs. The difficulty due to polarity change can be overcome by using the HE of LP residual. The HE $h_e(n)$ of LP residual signal $e(n)$ is defined as $h_e(n) = \sqrt{e^2(n) + e_h^2(n)}$ where $e_h(n)$ is the Hilbert transform of the $e(n)$ and computed as $e_h(n) = IDFT\{E_h(k)\}$ where

$$E_h(k) = \begin{cases} -jE(k), & k = 0, 1, ...(\frac{N}{2}) - 1 \\ jE(k), & k = (\frac{N}{2}), (\frac{N}{2}) + 1, ..., (N-1) \end{cases} \tag{1}$$

$E(k)$ is the DFT of the residual signal $e(n)$, and N is the number of points for computing DFT.

Normal speech segments of 20 ms and its HE of LP residual for vowel, semivowel, and voicebar are shown in Figs. 2a–c and d–f, respectively. Similarly, hypernasal speech segments of 20 ms and its HE of LP residual for vowel, semivowel, and

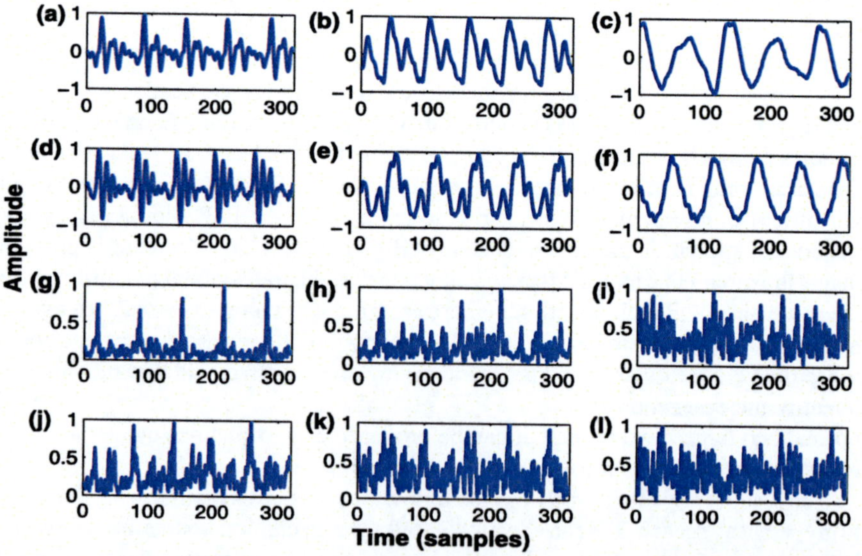

Fig. 2 Illustration of difference in nature of excitation source in vowels, semivowels, and voicebar for the normal and hypernasal speech. **a–c** show 20 ms normal vowel, semivowel, and voicebar signal and **g–i** show its HE of LP residual, respectively. Similarly, **d–f** show 20 ms hypernasal vowel, semivowel, and voicebar signal, and **j–l** show its HE of LP residual, respectively

voicebar are shown in (g–i) and (j–k), respectively. Here, the LP residual is derived by performing LP analysis on speech signal of frame size 20 ms with the frame shift of 10 ms. The sampling frequency of 16 kHz and LP order of 18 is used in this analysis. It can be observed that the peak strength is low in the HE of the residual signal for hypernasal vowel compared to normal vowel. This is due to sharp glottal closure in normal vowel compared to hypernasal vowel. In case of semivowels and voicebar, the glottal closure is more sharp in hypernasal speech, so the peak strength is more in the corresponding HE of residual signal. We can also observe that the hypernasal speech sounds are more noisy in nature due to the addition of extra zeros; hence, the side-lobes in corresponding HE of the residual signal have the more strength compared to normal speech. Hence, the PSR may give the cue for hypernasality detection.

3 Excitation Source-based Cue for Hypernasality

For the excitation source-based cue for hypernasality, we analyzed the PSR around each GCI location of normal as well as the hypernasal speech. The HE of LP residual signal for high vowel, low vowel, glides, liquids, and voicebar is obtained. The peak locations in HE of LP residual signal are detected by searching the maximum peak around the GCIs, obtained from ZFF signal [12]. A frame of size 3 ms is then selected from HE of LP residual centered around each peak. Each frame is normalized by dividing the each sample value by the maximum value in that frame. The equal number of such frames of all type of the sounds of normal and hypernasal speech is superimposed and plotted in Fig. 3. Figs. 3a–e show the 3 ms frame of superimposed HE of LP residual signal of different sounds of normal speech and (f–j) for the hypernasal speech. We can observe that the central window height in the hypernasal speech is small compared to the normal speech for the case of high vowel and low vowel and large for the glides, liquids, and voicebar. The central window height represents the peak strength in the HE of LP residual. We can also observe the increase in the side-lobe strength in all types of hypernasal sounds compared to normal sound. Since the peak strength and the side-lobes, both get modified in case of hypernasal speech, their ratio, peak to side-lobe ratio (PSR), which is used for the different task in the speech analysis [16, 18], can be used as the cue for the hypernasality detection.

3.1 Peak to Side-lobe Ratio

The coupling of the nasal cavity with the oral cavity during the production of hypernasal speech may change the peak strength as well as the side-lobe strength in the HE of LP residual of the signal. The peak strength gets modified due to the change in intra-oral pressure inside the mouth and the side-lobe strength, due to the addition

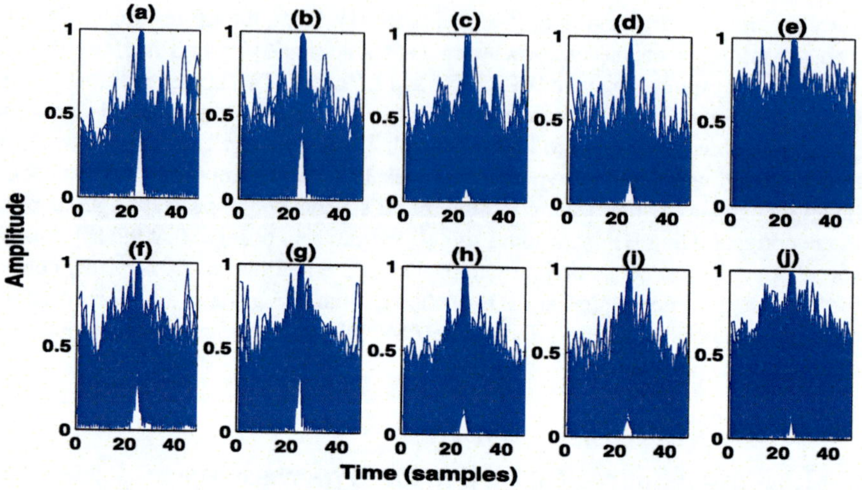

Fig. 3 3 ms duration of superimposed segments of HE of LP residual in the vicinity of impulse-like excitations for **a** High vowels, **b** Low vowels, **c** Glides, **d** Liquids, **e** Voicebar in normal speech. **f** High vowels, **g** Low vowels, **h** Glides, **i** Liquids, **j** Voicebar in hypernasal speech

of nasal zeros in the spectrum which gets filtered in HE of LP residual signal. Hence, we can analyze the peak to side-lobe ratio around the epoch location as an excitation source-based cue for the hypernasality detection. The peak strength is the maximum value in the HE of LP residual around each GCIs, whereas the side-lobe strength is taken as the mean of the all the values from 2 to 3 ms in the 3 ms frame centered around the peak of the HE. The ratio of these two quantities is defined as the peak to side-lobe ratio (PSR) at particular GCI. The PSR for the whole voiced sound is the mean of all PSR at all GCI locations.

4 Experiments

4.1 Database

The database used in this analysis consists of 10 normal and 10 CLP recorded children speech. All the children belong to the 7–13 years of the age. Both boys and girls children participated in the recording. The severity rating of hypernasality in CLP children is moderate to severe. Table 1 shows the voiced sound type and corresponding words used for the recording. The utterances are repeated three times in three different sessions by each children. The recording is done in sound-treated room. The sampling frequency was 44.1 kHz, 16 bits in WAV format. The manual annotation of vowels, glides, liquids, and voicebar from the words is done using the Wavesurfer tool [11]. The speech is down-sampled at 16 kHz for the further analysis.

Table 1 Voiced sound and corresponding words used for recording

Voiced sound	Word
High vowel /i/	/kiki/
Low vowel /a/	/kaka/
Glides /w/, /y/	/wawa/, /yaya/
Liquids /l/, /r/	/lala/, /rara/
Voicebar /b/, /d/, /g/	/baba/, /dada/, /gaga/

4.2 *Peak to Side-lobe Ratio Analysis in Hypernasal Speech*

To analyze the nature of peak to side-lobe ratio in hypernasal speech compared to the normal speech, we first analyzed the individual nature of both peak strength and side-lobe separately. The analysis is done for high vowel, low vowel, glides, liquids, and voicebar sounds. This analysis is done to find the dominant nature of the individual quantities. Figures 4a–e show the box plot comparing the peak strength at each GCI in all high vowel, low vowel, glides, liquids, and voicebar sounds, respectively, in normal and hypernasal speech present in the database. From Figs. 4a, b, we can observe that the peak strength decreases in both the vowels of the hypernasal speech compared to normal speech, as we have hypothesized. The reason for the decrement may be the abrupt glottal closure in normal vowels and smooth closure in hypernasal speech due to the nasal tract leakage path. We can also observe from Figs. 4c–e, the increase in the peak strength in the hypernasal speech compared to the normal speech in the case of glides, liquids, and voicebar sounds. The vocal fold vibration in the semivowels, (glides and liquids), and voicebar sounds is not that much strong as in the case of vowel sounds. This is due to more intra-oral pressure inside the mouth and, hence, less trans-glottal pressure. In case of hypernasal semivowels and voicebars, the intra-oral pressure reduces and, hence, the trans-glottal pressure increases, which increases the vocal folds vibration. Now, the glottal closure in hypernasal semivowels and voicebars is more abrupt comparable to the normal semivowels and voicebars. This may be the reason for the increase in the peak strength in hypernasal semivowels and voicebars. Figures 4f–j show the box plot comparing the side-lobe strength around each GCI in high vowel, low vowel, glides, liquids, and voicebar, respectively, in normal and hypernasal speech present in the database. The side-lobe strength increases in all cases for the hypernasal speech. The reason for the increment is the filtering of extra zeros in the residual signal, due to poor modeling of the LP model for the zeros in the spectrum. The nature of PSR will depend on the nature of the both the peak strength as well as the side-lobe strength.

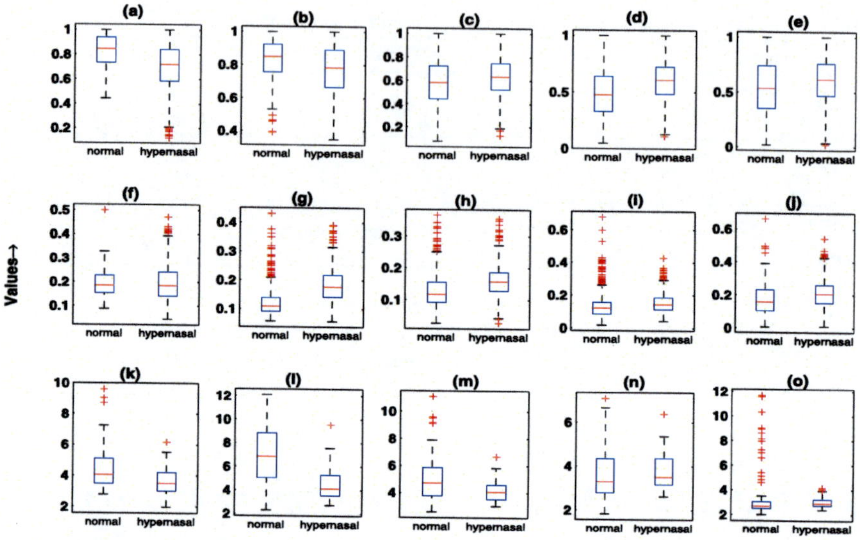

Fig. 4 Comparison of peak strength and mean of side-lobe in normal and hypernasal speech. **a–e** show the comparison of peak strength, **f–j** show the comparison of side-lobe strength, and **k–o** show the comparison of PSR value in normal and hypernasal high vowel, low vowel, glides, liquids, and voicebar respectively

Figures 4k–o show the box plot comparing the PSR in high vowel, low vowel, glides, liquids, and voicebar, respectively, in normal and hypernasal speech present in the database. Since the peak strength decreases and the side-lobe strength increases in case of hypernasal high and low vowel, so their PSR value also decreases as shown in Figs. 4k–l, respectively. In the case of glides, both the peak strength and the side-lobe strength increase, but the side-lobe strength increases more compared to the peak strength. Hence, the PSR value decreases in hypernasal glides case also, as shown in Fig. 4m. Similarly, for the case of liquids and voicebar also, both the peak strength and the side-lobe strength increase, but the peak strength increases more compared to side-lobe strength. Hence, the peak to side-lobe ratio increases in hypernasal liquids and voicebar as shown in Figs. 4n–o, respectively. Since PSR value is showing a distinct nature for normal and hypernasal speech, this excitation-based source cue can be used further for the classification between normal and hypernasal speech.

4.3 Classification Between Normal and Hypernasal Speech

The classification between pre-known normal and hypernasal class of high vowel, low vowel, glides, liquids, and voicebar can be done based on a fixed threshold value of PSR in each case. We conducted the classification between normal and

Table 2 Result of classification based on PSR cue, formant-based cue, and combination of two cues

Voiced sound type	Accuracy (%)		
	PSR	Formant-based	Combined
High vowel	70.49	75.41	77.05
Low vowel	78.19	83.46	72.18
Glides	63.15	66.32	77.89
Liquids	60.67	64.04	69.66
Voicebar	67.27	68.48	67.88
Average	67.27	71.54	72.93

hypernasal speech for the same database for which we have plotted the peak to side-lobe ratio. The threshold for each case of voiced speech can be set by looking the median value of PSR in normal or hypernasal speech. Based on the threshold value, the condition for the classification can be set. Table 2 Column 2 shows the result for the classification. The best accuracy for each type of voiced sound is shown in the table. In case of normal and hypernasal high vowel, low vowel, and glides classification, the best accuracy is 70.49%, 78.195%, and 63.15%, respectively. The condition for the classification in all the above cases is if the value for the PSR value is greater than the threshold value, the corresponding voiced sound is classified as the normal sound; otherwise, it is classified as hypernasal sound. Similarly, in case of normal and hypernasal liquids and voicebar, the best accuracy for the classification is 60.67% and 67.27%, respectively. Since the peak to side-lobe ratio for the case of liquids and voicebar is higher in hypernasal speech than the normal speech, the condition for the classification is if the value of PSR is lesser than the threshold value, the corresponding sound is classified as the normal sound; otherwise, it is classified as hypernasal sound. So, the PSR cue classifies the normal and hypernasal speech's highest accuracy of 78.195% for low vowel sounds and the lowest accuracy of 60.67% for liquids with an average accuracy of 67.27%.

To improve the accuracy of the detection, we combined our previous work on the vocal tract response cue with this excitation-based cue [4]. The presence of two formant peaks below 1000 Hz is considered as the cue for hypernasality detection. This is applicable for glides and liquids also, since their characteristics are similar to high vowels. Based on this cue, the sum of the strength of those formants which are below the 1000 Hz is calculated as a feature for hypernasality detection. This sum will be high for hypernasal sound because it contains two formants below 1000 Hz and will be low for normal speech because of only one formant. Table 2 Column 3 shows the threshold-based classification result for each type of voiced sound. It gives the best accuracy of 75.41%, 83.46%, 66.32%, 64.04%, and 68.48% for the high vowel, low vowel, glides, liquids, and voicebar, respectively, with an average accuracy of 71.54%. We combined the excitation source-based cue and vocal tract-based formant cue in equal weight. Table 2 Column 4 shows the threshold-based classification result for each type of voiced sound. The best accuracy of 77.05%, 72.18%, 77.89%, 69.66%, and 67.88% is achieved for the high vowel, low vowel, glides, liquids, and voicebar, respectively, with an average accuracy of 72.93%.

5 Summary and Future Scope

In this work, we analyzed the PSR at each GCIs in HE of LP residual cue for the hyernasality detection in CLP speech. PSR value gets affected in hypernasal speech due to change in intra-oral pressure in the mouth and addition of zeros in the residual of the signal. The analysis shows that PSR value is low in hypernasal speech in the case of high vowel, low vowel, and glides and high for the case of liquids and voicebar. The classification between normal and hypernasal voiced sound gives an average accuracy of 67.27% using PSR value as a feature. To improve the accuracy, we used the formant-based feature, which gives the average accuracy of 71.54%. The combination of two features gives the improvement in the accuracy with an average accuracy of 72.93%. As a future work, we will combine the suprasegmental features to further improve the result. Also, the automatic annotation of vowels, glides, liquids, and voicebar from the words will be done as a future work.

Acknowledgements The authors are very much thankful to Prof. M. Pushpavathi and Prof. Ajish K. Abraham from AIISH Mysore for sharing the hyernasal speech of children with cleft palate.

References

1. Anderson SR, Keating PA, Huffman MK, Krakow RA (2014) Nasals, nasalization, and the velum, vol. 5. Elsevier
2. Cairns D, Hansen JH, Riski JE et al (1996) A noninvasive technique for detecting hypernasal speech using a nonlinear operator. IEEE Trans Biomed Eng 43(1):35–45
3. Dubey AK, Prasanna SM, Dandapat S (2016) Zero time windowing analysis of hypernasality in speech of cleft lip and palate children. In: 2016 twenty second national conference on communication (NCC). IEEE, pp 1–6
4. Dubey AK, Prasanna SM, Dandapat S (2016) Zero time windowing based severity analysis of hypernasal speech. In: Region 10 conference (TENCON), 2016 IEEE, pp 970–974
5. Eshghi M, Alemi MM, Eshghi M (2015) Vowel nasalization might affect the envelop of the vowel signal by reducing the magnitude of the rising and falling slope amplitude. J Acoust Soc Am 137(4):2304
6. He L, Zhang J, Liu Q, Yin H, Lech M (2014) Automatic evaluation of hypernasality and consonant misarticulation in cleft palate speech. Signal Process Lett IEEE 21(10):1298–1301
7. Henningsson G, Kuehn DP, Sell D, Sweeney T, Trost-Cardamone JE, Whitehill TL (2008) Universal parameters for reporting speech outcomes in individuals with cleft palate. Cleft Palate Craniofac J 45(1):1–17
8. Kummer AW, Lee L (1996) Evaluation and treatment of resonance disorders. Lang Speech Hear Serv Sch 27(3):271–281
9. Lee GS, Wang CP, Yang CC, Kuo TB (2006) Voice low tone to high tone ratio: a potential quantitative index for vowel [a:] and its nasalization. IEEE Trans Biomed Eng 53(7):1437–1439

10. Maier A, Hönig F, Bocklet T, Nöth E, Stelzle F, Nkenke E, Schuster M (2009) Automatic detection of articulation disorders in children with cleft lip and palate. J Acoust Soc Am 126(5):2589–2602
11. Medina E, Solorio T (2006) Wavesurfer: a tool for sound analysis
12. Murty KSR, Yegnanarayana B (2008) Epoch extraction from speech signals. IEEE Trans Audio Speech Lang Process 16(8):1602–1613
13. Orozco-Arroyave JR, Rendón SM, Álvarez-Meza AM, Arias-Londoño JD, Delgado-Trejos E, Bonilla JFV, Castellanos-Domínguez CG (2011) Automatic selection of acoustic and non-linear dynamic features in voice signals for hypernasality detection. In: Interspeech. Citeseer, pp 529–532
14. Orozco-Arroyave JR, Arias-Londoño JD, Bonilla JFV, Nöth E (2012) Automatic detection of hypernasal speech signals using nonlinear and entropy measurements. In: INTERSPEECH, pp 2029–2032
15. Rah DK, Ko YI, Lee C, Kim DW (2001) A noninvasive estimation of hypernasality using a linear predictive model. Ann Biomed Eng 29(7):587–594
16. Raykar VC, Yegnanarayana B, Prasanna SM, Duraiswami R (2005) Speaker localization using excitation source information in speech. IEEE Trans Speech Audio Process 13(5):751–761
17. Rendón SM, Arroyave JO, Bonilla JV, Londoño JA, Domínguez CC (2011) Automatic detection of hypernasality in children. In: International work-conference on the interplay between natural and artificial computation. Springer, pp 167–174
18. Sharma B, Prasanna SM (2016) Sonority measurement using system, source and suprasegmental information. IEEE/ACM Trans Audio Speech Lang Process
19. Vijayalakshmi P, Reddy MR, O'Shaughnessy D (2007) Acoustic analysis and detection of hypernasality using a group delay function. IEEE Trans Biomed Eng 54(4):621–629

Estimation in Agile Software Development Using Artificial Intelligence

Prateek Srivastava, Nidhi Srivastava, Rashi Agarwal, and Pawan Singh

Abstract In software development, agile methods are becoming more popular, and in many situations, software development teams are even mandated to use some agile methods in their projects. It is basic to give as exact a gauge as could really be expected. Today, in the data innovation business, for assessment in spry programming advancement, most of the part is dependent on heuristic methodologies like master judgment and arranging poker. It is very hard to gauge coordinated programming advancement without nimble mastery. Various studies have been done throughout the years to evaluate software effort estimating methodologies, but because of the rise of new software development processes, the reviews have not been caught up with them. This article gives an intensive assessment of cost assessment in agile software development, which will help the clients in understanding current expense assessment drifts in ASD. Most agile teams estimate software development effort using expert estimating methodologies, according to a thorough literature analysis and survey. This work includes a thorough literature review that has been updated by examining data from 73 new studies. The majority of the data comes from single-company databases; however, cross-company data is extremely popular. Estimates of effort and cost are typically based on the findings of a study using models or historical data applied to size, activities, and other planning characteristics.

P. Srivastava (✉) · N. Srivastava
Amity Institute of Information Technology, Amity University Uttar Pradesh, Lucknow Campus, Lucknow, India

N. Srivastava
e-mail: nsrivastava2@lko.amity.edu

R. Agarwal
Department of Information Technology, University Institute of Engineering and Technology, Chhatrapati Shahu Ji Maharaj University, Kanpur, India

P. Singh
Amity School of Engineering and Technology, Amity University Uttar Pradesh, Lucknow Campus, Lucknow, India
e-mail: psingh10@lko.amity.edu

M. S. Kaiser et al. (eds.), *Proceedings of Trends in Electronics and Health Informatics*, Lecture Notes in Networks and Systems 376,
https://doi.org/10.1007/978-981-16-8826-3_8

Keywords Agile software development · Cost · Effort · Estimation · Artificial intelligence · Machine learning

1 Introduction

Planning is done iteratively in agile software development (ASD), and project scope is constantly modified and prioritized. In ASD, the most critical considerations to prioritize needs and features are effort and cost. The absolute most popular advancement techniques in ASD are scrum, extreme programming, feature-driven development, lean software development, adaptive software development, crystal methodologies, and the dynamic systems. Development method is probably the most notable improvement procedures in ASD. Exertion assessment assumes a significant and basic part in any product advancement project. Exertion assessment can be as the cycle by which exertion can be assessed, and the assessment is completed as far as the measure of assets needed to end project action to convey an item or administration that meets the given useful and non-practical prerequisites to a client [1].

Cost assessment for ASD strategies is a difficult undertaking. It is so in light of the fact that the dexterous strategy depends on eccentric ideas that are not appropriate for any of the conventional assessment techniques. The utilization of such assessment techniques to nimble advancement instruments brings about significant mistakes, because of the shortfall of basic components like well-qualified assessment and recorded information. Since the coordinated interaction is a lot less difficult and requires quicker work alongside more client inclusion, this adjustment of approach additionally requires an adjustment of the expense assessment measure. Thus, ongoing examination has zeroed in on creating assessment strategies (ETs) that are viable with nimble techniques [2].

Prior to the adoption of agile approaches, lightweight methodologies were used to describe small collocated teams producing software in an iterative, incremental fashion. Agile methodology, on the other hand, may be used for massive projects with the right modeling techniques. Iterative development with changing requirements is the core of agile software development processes [3]. They build on that base with a lighter, more people-centric perspective that mainly relies on users' tacit knowledge. Agile procedures are less document-oriented, with a smaller amount of documentation for a specific task being the norm.

Software engineering is a broad term that refers to the standard practices that apply to all areas of software development, from conception to post-release maintenance. These guidelines ensure that a project is completed in a timely and efficient manner while keeping the greatest level of quality. Certain advantages should be provided by an effective cost estimation process. To begin with, it should support the investigation and reuse of stockroom information to abbreviate assessing time. Second, it is ought to be not difficult to utilize and grasp for end clients. It ought to likewise represent insufficient and vague information. At last, it should list the numerous angles that decide the task's last expense [4].

Estimating software expenses is tough by nature, and humans are notoriously lousy at predicting absolute outcomes. In contrast to traditional acquisition projects, estimating costs in an agile setting demands a more iterative, integrated, and collaborative approach. Cost estimation is a vital activity in agile programs, contrary to popular belief that agile is an undisciplined methodology that ignores cost considerations [5, 6]. There is a widespread misperception that agile software development entails the absence of a long-term strategy. Long-term planning is required in agile development, and cost estimation is a vital task in agile programs. It necessitates early, upfront analysis that indicates a high-level comprehension of the program, as well as the costs and benefits connected with it.

Consistency, broad arranging, systematized measures, and thorough reuse are key components for the proficient advancement of programming. Lithe software development (ASD) is frequently introduced as an option in contrast to more conventional methodologies, like cascade, gradual, or transformative, in which consistency, broad arranging, systematized measures, and thorough reuse are key components for the effective advancement of programming [1]. In any product advancement project, exertion assessment is pivotal and basic. Exertion assessment might be characterized as the method involved with assessing exertion and assessing the measure of assets needed to finish project action to convey an item or administration to a customer that meets the given practical and non-utilitarian necessities [2]. One of the main parts of programming project on the board is assessing exertion. Wrong advancement exertion assessments have brought about significant issues. It is crucial for programming firms to fabricate great items inside spending plan and timetable limitations in the present serious business scene.

Organizations have utilized nimble programming advancement (ASD) strategies [7] in internationally disseminated tasks to lighten a portion of the issues related with creating programming all around the world; light-footed techniques are viewed as being more appropriate to manage projects that present muddled and questionable necessities. Estimating the cost of ASD techniques is a difficult undertaking. Because agile is founded on unorthodox principles that are not compatible with standard estimation methodologies. Due to the absence of crucial components such as expert opinion and historical data, the application of such estimating approaches to agile development procedures results in significant mistakes.

2 Literature Review

The goal of the exact review was to find sensible works that presented methods and estimations answers for deft programming improvement frameworks to recognize: Common undertaking estimation and control rehearses; size measurements utilized; agile advancement research patterns; and open inquiries and examination subjects identified with further developing light-footed improvement project gauges. Research method used in the review is shown in Fig. 1.

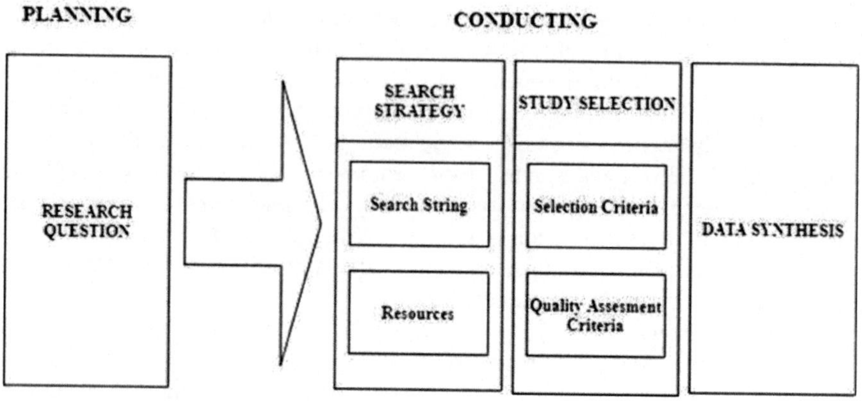

Fig. 1 Research method in systematic literature review

The research incorporates a precise writing survey that was completed by specific standards to gather and handle information from numerous sources. The following are the guidelines, which are based on some standard current research on the subject.

2.1 *Planning Phase*

Proper planning is essential for the effective implementation of a systematic literature review. The research questions are derived from the planning phase of the systematic literature review. A systematic review's most important step is to confirm the research questions.

2.2 *Research Issues*

1. In ASD, what methods were utilized to estimate effort?
2. What are the appropriate situations in which different estimating approaches can be used, and what issues can arise when using different estimation techniques?

3 Conducting Phase

3.1 *Search Strategy*

Three tasks make up the conducting phase: search strategy, study selection, and data synthesis. Unlike independent data synthesis, the search strategy and study selection

Table 1 Search string-based data gathering

S. No.	Search string	Paper from journals	Paper from conference
1	Software cost estimation in agile software development	[8–11]	[12, 13]
2	Framework based for effort estimation in agile software development	[14–17]	[18, 5, 6, 18–21]
3	Effort estimation in agile software development: case study	[22]	[23]

Data sources Springer link, IEEE explore, ACM digital library, Elsevier science direct, and research gate were the digital databases utilized to search for keywords

Table 2 List of resources

S. No.	Source name	URL
1	IEEE explore	www.ieeeexplore.org
2	ACM digital library	http://dl.acm.org/
3	Google Scholar	Scholar.google.com
4	Science direct	www.sciencedirect.com
5	Springer	www.springerlink

are both created by two separate operations. Search strings are a term that is used in search strategy. This phase also identifies the resources that will be used to conduct the search. After the search strings and resources have been determined, this method can be carried out. Search string and list of resources are shown in Table 1 and Table 2.

3.2 *Criteria for Inclusion and Exclusion*

The current study comprised a number of studies, the majority of which focused on cost estimation utilizing ASD. There are a couple of extra investigations that are arranged with exertion and cost assessment using elective advancement approaches, with a definitive objective of quicker and more precise assessment. The examination considers an assortment of distributions from different diaries and meetings. We did not analyze papers that did not serve the expressed point or did not depend on real and exact proof. Criteria for inclusion and exclusion is shown in Table 3.

Table 3 Criteria for inclusion and exclusion

	Criteria	Rationale
Inclusion	The article must address agile and software development in the domain of software engineering and information system	The study focused cost and estimation of agile and software development
Exclusion	Other than English language	Paper in English language
	Article must in the form of keywords, abstract, short paper or thesis	The study does not give sensible measure of data to a target choice
	The article discuss only agile and software development	The study integrates cost and effort estimation of agile and software development

4 Cost Estimation Method

Software cost estimating is a difficult assignment since it necessitates the estimator's precise cost prediction throughout the project's planning phase. Over time, certain software cost estimation methodologies have been presented. [24] To improve the estimation of the software project effort, machine learning techniques were utilized [25]. The historical data set of ninety-three projects was subjected to Naive Bayes, logistic regression, and random forests approaches. It was put up against the constructive cost model (COCOMO). COCOMO drivers and multipliers can be improved to produce more accurate results in the effort estimating process.

The agile software development process is extensively utilized. Agile cost projections are based on a number of project factors, such as prior project data or expert opinion. Principal component analysis (PCA) was used to create a new model. One of the problems for software professionals is to optimize software cost estimation (SCE) with accuracy. To improve SCE, a hybrid technique combining a genetic algorithm and a Tabu search algorithm was devised. As input data, the NASA project data set was used. Summary of cost estimation method and comparative study are shown in Table 4 and Table 5 [24].

Table 4 Summary of cost estimation method

Paper	Limitation
PCA-based cost estimation model for agile software development projects	To generalize the proposed approach, it is suggested that it can be used for a variety of agile software development projects
Predicting software effort estimation using machine learning techniques	Improving the COCOMO drivers and multipliers can help the estimating effort process produce more accurate results
A learning-based adjustment model with genetic algorithm of function point estimation	Alternative strategies for selecting KIFs require more research

Table 5 Comparative study of various papers

S. No.	Title of the paper	Techniques implemented	Dataset	Experimental results	Limitations
1	A method to estimate software strategic indicators in software development: an industrial application	Product readiness SSI estimation model	Normal dataset	More flexibility and adaptive	Some post-deployment part
2	A hybrid software processes management support model	AGOPLAN method	Normal dataset	Model for little and medium-size mixture projects	Developing a bunch of strategies supporting the administration of crossover IT projects
3	Better late than never: Bias and its alleviation in efficient	Mixed-effects logistic regression model	Normal dataset	Time-saving bias	Inaccurate project management
4	A systematic review on software cost estimation in agile software development	Neural network, expert judgment, planning poker, disaggregation, use case point, modified use case point	Normal dataset	Computation of the genuine expense of a project	Did not play out any test to assess the between rater understanding and commentators in the audit action
5	Agile capabilities as necessary conditions for maximizing sustainable supply chain performance: an empirical investigation	Agile approaches	Normal dataset	Critical connection between supportable store network rehearses and coordinated practices	Less accuracy
6	Time pressure in software engineering: a systematic review	Inclusion and exclusion criteria	Normal dataset	Quality reduction becomes effective	Combining different data sources less
7	Risk management in the software life cycle: a systematic literature review	SLR	Normal dataset	Widely used in the field of risk	Harmonization of numerous models of hazard the board
8	DECIDE: an Agile event-and-data-driven design methodology for decisional big data projects	Decisional big data methodology	Normal dataset	A flexible and adaptable methodology for governing, managing and applying data	Designed for big data systems with Big Data technologies

(continued)

Table 5 (continued)

S. No.	Title of the paper	Techniques implemented	Dataset	Experimental results	Limitations
9	Agile supply chain management: where did it come from and where will it go in the era of digital transformation	Co-citation network	Normal dataset	Better integrated in the measurement and metrics of ASC	Less performance

5 Results and Discussions

5.1 *Answers to the Research Questions*

The results produced from the data retrieved from the essential examinations are introduced in this part. These discoveries empowered us to react to the examination's exploration questions (RQ). Information extraction was done by similar gathering of specialists who utilized similar way to deal with and distinguish the essential investigations.

1. **In ASD, what methods were utilized to estimate effort?**

   For assessing the most important work is to potentially the measure of the product to be created, ASD project administrators that favor strategies which permit coordinated effort and agreement. Other than the aforementioned commonly used estimating methods, several regression strategies have been identified in studies. Algorithmic approaches, in addition to regressions, are employed in studies. The distribution of papers in diaries and gathering is shown in Fig. 2.

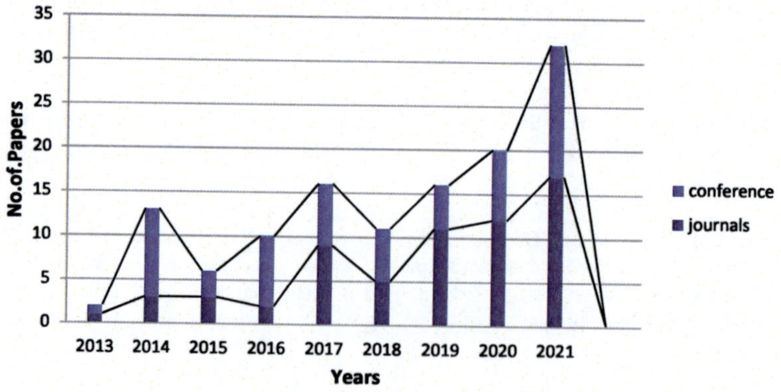

Fig. 2 Number of paper distributed in diaries and gathering each year

Table 6 Comparison table of the existing works

S. No.	Title	Paper and year	Method
1	Effort estimation of agile development using fuzzy logic	IEEE 2018	Fuzzy logic
2	A review on software cost and effort estimation techniques for agile development process	Journal paper 2018	Machine learning
3	Effort, duration and cost estimation in agile software development	IEEE 2016	Simple logarithmic estimation method
4	Support vector regression based on grid-search method for agile software effort prediction	IEEE 2018	Grid-based SVR
5	An ensemble-based model for predicting agile software development effort	Springer 2018	Ensemble-based model
6	Effort estimation in agile software development an updated review	International journal 2018	Artificial intelligence
7	An enhanced framework for effort estimation of agile projects	Research gate 2018	Constructive cost model

2. **What are the appropriate situations in which different estimating approaches can be used, and what issues can arise when using different estimation techniques?**

   For getting an ideal scope of exactness, certain conditions are most appropriate for a particular gauge method. In addition, researchers encounter some challenges when dealing with such circumstances. The comparison table of the existing works is shown in Table 6.

6 Conclusion

This paper presents a purposeful study of programming effort and cost evaluation in quick programming improvement. It shows that light-footed programming improvement has become one of the oftentimes utilized programming advancement devices, which is generally embraced by various analysts just as programming improvement associations. Precise assessment of cost and exertion for a product project assumes a significant part in the accomplishment of that undertaking. The level of programming improvement projects that depend on deft methodologies are quickly expanding. As a result, it is critical to investigate additional methodologies for estimating such model-based projects. A huge expansion in the achievement pace of the various kinds of programming projects are accomplished by the progress in the exactness of the assessment climate. Until this point in time, very little work is done in the field of cost and exertion assessment for nimble programming improvement. As far as future work, the scientists intend to investigate extra late related examinations and give them as a definite review.

References

1. Fernández-Diego M, Méndez ER, González-Ladrón-De-Guevara F, Abrahão S, Insfran E (2020) An update on effort estimation in agile software development: a systematic literature review. IEEE Access 8:166768–166800
2. Trendowicz A, Jeffery R (2014) Software project effort estimation: foundations and best practice guidelines for success. Springer, Berlin, Germany
3. Garg S, Gupta D (2015) PCA based cost estimation model for agile software development projects. In: 2015 International conference on industrial engineering and operations management (IEOM). IEEE, pp 1–7
4. Bilgaiyan S, Sagnika S, Mishra S, Das M (2017) A systematic review on software cost estimation in agile software development. J Eng Sci Technol Rev 10(4)
5. Yadav A, Sharma A (2018) Function point based estimation of effort and cost in agile software development. In: Proceedings of 3rd international conference on internet of things and connected technologies (ICIoTCT), pp 26–27
6. Saini A, Ahuja L, Khatri SK (2018) Effort estimation of agile development using fuzzy logic. In: 2018 7th international conference on reliability, Infocom technologies and optimization (trends and future directions)(ICRITO). IEEE, pp 779–783
7. Usman M, Britto R (2016) Effort estimation in co-located and globally distributed agile software development: a comparative study. In: 2016 joint conference of the international workshop on software measurement and the international conference on software process and product measurement (IWSM-MENSURA). IEEE, pp 219–224
8. Usman M, Börstler J, Petersen K (2017) An effort estimation taxonomy for agile software development. Int J Software Eng Knowl Eng 27(04):641–674
9. Vyas M, Bohra A, Lamba CS, Vyas A (2018) A review on software cost and effort estimation techniques for agile development process. Int J Recent Res Aspects 5(1):1–5
10. Anooja A, Rajawat S (2017) Comparative analysis of software cost-effort estimation and agile in perspective of software development. Int J Adv Res Comput Sci 8(8)
11. Osman HH, Musa ME (2016) A survey of agile software estimation methods. Int J Comput Sci Telecommun 7(3):38–42
12. Owais M, Ramakishore R (2016) Effort, duration and cost estimation in agile software development. In: 2016 Ninth international conference on contemporary computing (IC3). IEEE, pp 1–5
13. Usman M, Mendes E, Börstler J (2015) Effort estimation in agile software development: a survey on the state of the practice. In: Proceedings of the 19th international conference on evaluation and assessment in software engineering, pp 1–10
14. Dragicevic S, Celar S, Turic M (2017) Bayesian network model for task effort estimation in agile software development. J Syst Softw 127:109–119
15. Raslan AT, Darwish NR, Hefny HA (2015) Towards a fuzzy based framework for effort estimation in agile software development. Int J Comput Sci Inf Secur 13(1):37
16. Satapathy SM, Rath SK (2017) Empirical assessment of machine learning models for agile software development effort estimation using story points. Innov Syst Softw Eng 13(2):191–200

17. Raslan AT, Darwish NR (2018) An enhanced framework for effort estimation of agile projects. Int J Intell Engi Syst 11(3):205–214
18. Bilgaiyan S, Mishra S, Das M (2016) A review of software cost estimation in agile software development using soft computing techniques. In: 2016 2nd international conference on computational intelligence and networks (CINE). IEEE, pp 112–117
19. Britto R, Mendes E, Börstler J (2015) An empirical investigation on effort estimation in agile global software development. In: 2015 IEEE 10th international conference on global software engineering. IEEE, pp 38–45
20. Tanveer B (2016) Hybrid effort estimation of changes in agile software development. In: International conference on agile software development. Springer, Cham, pp 316–320
21. Moharreri K, Sapre AV, Ramanathan J, Ramnath R (2016) Cost-effective supervised learning models for software effort estimation in agile environments. In: 2016 IEEE 40th Annual computer software and applications conference (COMPSAC), vol 2. IEEE, pp 135–140
22. Tanveer B, Guzmán L, Engel UM (2017) Effort estimation in agile software development: case study and improvement framework. J Softw: Evol Process 29(11): e1862
23. Tanveer B, Guzmán L, Engel UM (2016) Understanding and improving effort estimation in agile software development: an industrial case study. In: Proceedings of the international conference on software and systems process, pp 41–50
24. Liu J, Du Q, Xu J (2018) A learning-based adjustment model with genetic algorithm of function point estimation. In: 2018 IEEE 20th International conference on high performance computing and communications; IEEE 16th International conference on smart city; IEEE 4th International conference on data science and systems (HPCC/SmartCity/DSS). IEEE, pp 51–58
25. BaniMustafa A (2018) Predicting software effort estimation using machine learning techniques. In: 2018 8th International conference on computer science and information technology (CSIT). IEEE, pp 249–256

Human Fall Detection Analysis with Image Recognition Using Convolutional Neural Network Approach

Kuldeep Chouhan, Ashish Kumar, Ashish Kumar Chakraverti, and Ravindra Raman Cholla

Abstract Human falling may cause injuries and sometimes may lead to deadly conditions. Therefore, in recent decade, the systems used for monitoring of human falling and non-falling are receiving attention among research community for its diversified features and social benefits. These systems solve the problem of falling and gets activated to avert the likely incident with an alarm message, and uses fall recognition classifiers. System helps to identify the human in the intended regions, and classifiers are trained using the information available in the images. The lack of massive scale datasets and human errors limits the generalization of models in terms of robustness and efficiency to invisible regions. In the proposed work, an automatic fall detection using deep learning is modeled using dataset of falling and non-falling images. The sensitive information available in the original images is kept secure and private to maintain the safety and protection by the presented work. The experiments were conducted using real-world fall datasets having both types of human images, i.e., falling and non-falling, and the results obtained clearly indicate system enhancement for falling and non-falling image recognition using convolutional neural network (CNN) algorithm and achieving higher accuracy and reduced loss with a trained dataset which finds the optimal performance from real-time environments.

Keywords Convolutional neural network (CNN) · Deep learning algorithm · Human fall detection · Image recognition

---

K. Chouhan (✉) · A. Kumar
Department of Computer Science and Engineering, I.T.S Engineering College, Greater Noida, India

A. K. Chakraverti
Department of Computer Science and Engineering, Pranveer Singh Institute of Technology, Kanpur, India

R. R. Cholla
Department of Computer Science and Engineering, Bapatla Engineering College, Guntur, India

M. S. Kaiser et al. (eds.), *Proceedings of Trends in Electronics and Health Informatics*, Lecture Notes in Networks and Systems 376,
https://doi.org/10.1007/978-981-16-8826-3_9

1 Introduction

In recent years, the detection of human falls has been a significant global worry for severe injuries which limit comfort and self-sufficiency [1]. The protection of the elderly from injuries is essential and is increasing in current times. The frequency of fall injuries is a significant issue and must be dealt with. In this scenario, an intelligent fall detection and prevention system may assist. For object identification tasks, deep learning models are employed [2]. The model comprises many layers that convert data received from the earlier layer and provide output for the following layer. Many fall detection systems were suggested in the literature, depending on the working techniques, performance, efficiency, and restriction [3]. Different methods are also utilized to enhance the accuracy, sensitivity, specificity, and reaction time [4]. Four generalized stages are followed by fall detection systems: sensing, data processing, fall identification, and alarm system (see Fig. 1).

1.1 Deep Learning Based Fall Detection

The CNN-based fall detection devices reflect fall-related data in the picture dataset collected through sensors. In fall detection systems, CNN architectures identify patterns and forms in a particular picture collection that use different CNN-based image detection architectures. Some have employed a mix of LSTM and CNN to reduce image vision problems [6]. LSTM and CNN are supervised techniques of learning; however, unattended approaches, such as autoencoders, exist that identify data irregularities [7, 8].

1.2 Human Fall Detection

The human fall detection attracts more attention due to its wide range of applications that uses surveillance video or image with low resolution [9]. The majority of scenes

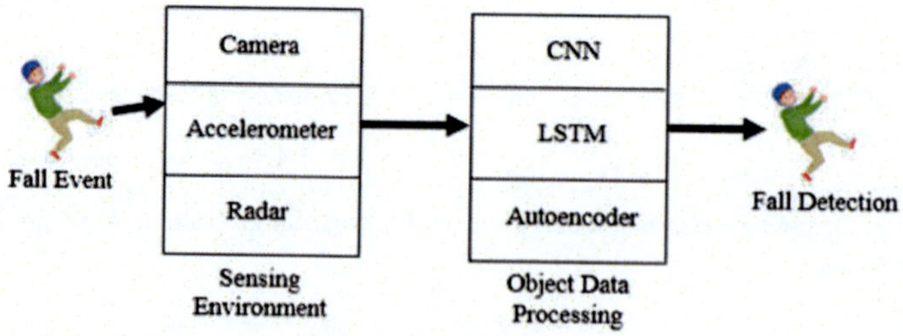

Fig. 1 Generalized view of fall detection systems [5]

taken by a static camera have negligible background alterations. For detecting specific behaviors in a real-time video scene, any item in outdoor surveillance relies on human observers. However, the human capacity to watch several events in surveillance screens has limitations [10]. For accurate object classification and tracking for high-level analysis, an intelligent system recognizes and collects gesture information of moving targets. The aim of this research is on detecting persons without taking into account picture recognition of their complicated actions. From the standpoint of machine vision, human detection is a tough problem since it is influenced by a vast variety of possible appearances; yet prior information may help to improve it. Usually, detection process includes the following steps [11, 12, 29, 30]:

(i) The object detection method uses a pixel-by-pixel filtering procedure to detect moving objects between the current frame and a background frame, resulting in the best possible performance.
(ii) The optical flow-based object detection technique [13] detects an image sequence by analyzing the flow vectors of moving objects [14].
(iii) The spatiotemporal filter approaches that characterize the data volume spanned by the moving person in an image sequence are used to detect movable images [7].

2 Related Work

Ming and Yang [15] have developed a new indoor video surveillance system that can detect human falls and assess the posture of people using the frame ratio and the picture height displacement. Adhikari et al. [16] developed a method of fall detection based on video pictures utilizing the dataset acquired by recording activities of individual populations in various settings. Li et al. [14] presented and developed a method for an individual scenario using CNN for fall detection on each frame picture in the video surveillance environment. H. Yhdego [6] created a pretrained kinematics-based ML method in annotated accelerometry datasets converted into pictures using continuous wavelet transformation and trained deep CNNs. To generalize resource optimization constraints, Tasoulis et al. [17] have developed a CNN method and an efficient algorithm for detecting changes. Zhang and Zhu [18] have shown the gadget used to detect human actions in real time and define deep CNNs for raw data streams. E. Casilari et al. [19] have developed a method of CNN fall detection that utilizes a multi-modal fall detection dataset and a vision and several cameras. Arifa Sultana et al. [20] suggested architecture to differentiate between falls by collecting frames from video records and other indoor natural human activity. Tsai and Hsu [21] presented a one-dimensional CNN technique to convert depth image information into skeleton information and extract feature points through a skeleton extraction algorithm. Illuri and Satyanarayana [2] have an emotional recognition system and is utilized for a CNN-classified video-based recognition system. Min et al. [22] introduced vision-based and deep learning algorithms to train when the system runs smoothly. Ma et al. [23] introduced a fall prevention system predicting fall by utilizing the posture and physical analysis of a person likely to fall and prevented by notifying the person concerned. Wang et al. [24] introduced the CNN algorithm that needs different parameters to deploy facials so as to prevent unpredictability in real-time systems. Seredin et al. [25] suggested a reduction in the description of the skeleton based on the human body's anthropometric features Reddy and Kalaiselvi [4] suggested that the system increases the awareness of fall recognition and obtains a high F-score by carrying out a high-precision fall detection. Zhang et al. [7] have developed a vision-based fall detection method in which visual input is collected and supplied to a fall identification ML classifier. Harrow et al. [26] focus on identifying and classifying falls based on changes in human shape, which remain reliable in fall detection. According to Shu and Shu [9], when left unreported and untreated, human falls are the primary cause of accidental injury and fatality.

3 Methodology of Human Fall Detection

An example falls detection system with picture or video extraction and analysis that includes input data and acquired data using fall detection algorithms and predicts that the data obtained will be taken into consideration. This procedure is illustrated (see Fig. 2), where the fall detection system, i.e., the video analysis and the categorization of human objects, is suggested.

There are environmental changes and adequate sensitivity in a human fall detection picture, and this utilizes medium and mean to define all pixels in the image and is categorized from the video. Kalman filters help eliminate the noise that may

Fig. 2 General process of fall detection system

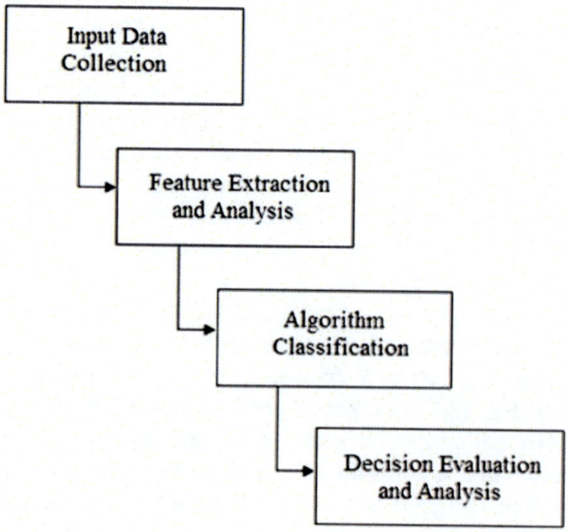

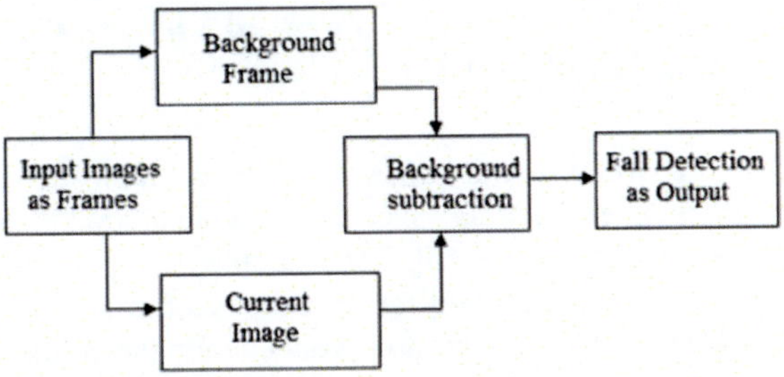

Fig. 3 Human fall detection process used by the algorithm

analyze the video (frame to frame) and identify events produced (see Fig. 3) for better concentrate on the picture.

3.1 Detection of Human and Activities

DL-based architecture uses images to detect a fall and integrates numerous human identifications to correct pose and segmentation errors in the image. It uses various techniques to find and detect a human such as:

(i) To identify a human region using background removal techniques with a low true-positive rate.
(ii) The visual representations protect people's privacy and are unaffected by changes in look.
(iii) Allow the framework to generalize unobserved real-world situations with more effectiveness than approaches for detecting drops using appearance data.
(iv) Significant changes in picture appearance attributes have only a shaky generality.

3.2 Convolutional Neural Network Approach

CNN can extract key features from images to differentiate between one object and another by applying learning weights and biases [27]. For a pixel convolution to produce a convoluted picture, a low-level preprocessing includes an input layer, an output layer, and hidden layers with a stack of coevolutionary layers. The activation function is using a rectified linear unit (ReLU) layer with pooling layers and fully connected layers [5]. CNN uses a series of coevolutionary layers, followed by various pooling layers, a flattening layer, and a fully connected layer, to extract information from images where each layer utilizes several functions for activation [28].

4 Implementation of Human Fall Detection Analysis and Identification

Initialize weights of the nodes in the network model consisting of weights initialized in the next embedding layer for the convolutions layer, which has a null-average Gaussian distribution [2]. For example, in 20 periods, the trained coevolutionary layer and embedding layers are transferred from one end to the next (there are just a few epochs to be shown in work), while the learning rate is set to 0.01, and total weights and amendments are modified. The experimented work is as follows:

INFO: tensorflow: Retraining the models…

Model: "sequential".

Layer (type)	Output Shape	Param #
hub_keras_layer_v1v2 (HubKer	(None, 1280)	2257984
dropout (Dropout)	(None, 1280)	0
dense (Dense)	(None, 2)	2562

Total params: 2,260,546
Trainable params: 2,226,434
Non-trainable params: 34,112

None
Epoch 1/5
99/99 [==============================] - 940s 9s/step - loss: 0.5008 - accuracy: 0.8681
Epoch 2/5
99/99 [==============================] - 1656s 17s/step - loss: 0.3032 - accuracy: 0.9958
Epoch 3/5
99/99 [==============================] - 941s 10s/step - loss: 0.2924 - accuracy: 0.9995
Epoch 4/5
99/99 [==============================] - 925s 9s/step - loss: 0.2892 - accuracy: 0.9995
Epoch 5/5
99/99 [==============================] - 1036s 10s/step - loss: 0.2868 - accuracy: 1.0000
loss, accuracy = model. evaluate(test_data)
12/12 [==============================] - 19s 909ms/step - loss: 0.2848 - accuracy: 1.0000

The model prediction accuracy values are calculated based on the learning rate and run number of epochs that measured or simulated the appropriate accuracy and loss as shown below.

[0.9469696879386902,
0.9968434572219849,
0.9996843338012695,
0.9996843338012695,
1.0] ← Model accuracy values

[0.3905821442604065,
0.30057528614997864,
0.29170241951942444,
0.28913652896881104,
0.2868884205818176] ← Model loss values

5 Results and Discussion

5.1 Datasets

The dataset contains fall and non-falling photos for analytical purposes, and the proposed data samples include diverse activities such as walking, sitting, squatting, and fall images of forward, backward, and sideways motion. The following activities must be taken in order to establish fall detection training and testing are as follow:

(i) Human detection and extraction are carried out, as well as
(ii) Extracted pictures are reframed and scaled to a size of 64 × 64 pixels.

It normally contains varying performances where each performance is acquired via variety of perceptions, and some instances use the reallocation of some objects (Table 1).

We have performed a number of tests utilizing the falling and non-falling picture datasets to verify our fall detection system. We have given particular attention to four kinds of experiments that includes:

(i) Analysis of network design with the goal of determining the best configuration for the problem;
(ii) Compare techniques to state-of-the-art fall detection approaches;

Table 1 Number of frames of each dataset, distribution of frames (falling and non-falling)

Dataset	Total images	Falling images	Non-falling images	Unpredictable images
Fall images dataset	6580	2247	3253	1080
Multiple cameras with images dataset	11,544	3753	5650	2141

(iii) Evaluate the system under various illumination situations; and
(iv) Demonstrate the system's universality by merging all datasets.

5.2 Experimental Results

The experiment setup is done based on the basis of experimental images for the frequency of the falling images and predicted the falling image. The findings are shown based on falling and unsuccessful human pictures, which provide the prediction system output displayed in different epochs in Jupyter along with learning rate of 0.01 accuracy assessed (see Fig. 4).

The human falling and non-falling detection study (see Fig. 5) gives a result shown in different epochs and 0.01 learning rates measuring the loss prevision.

Fig. 4 Optimal accuracy prediction with learning rate using several epochs

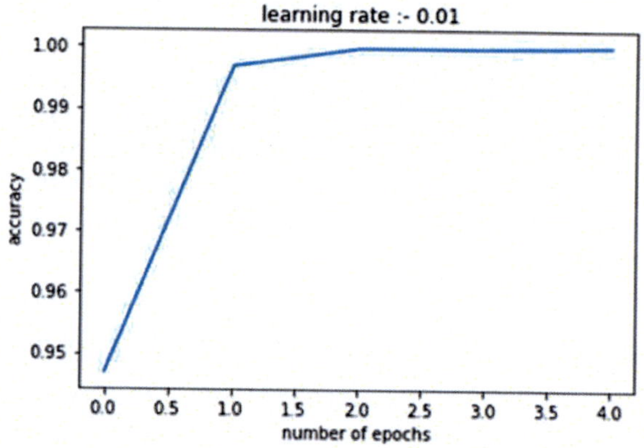

Fig. 5 Loss prediction with learning rate using several epochs

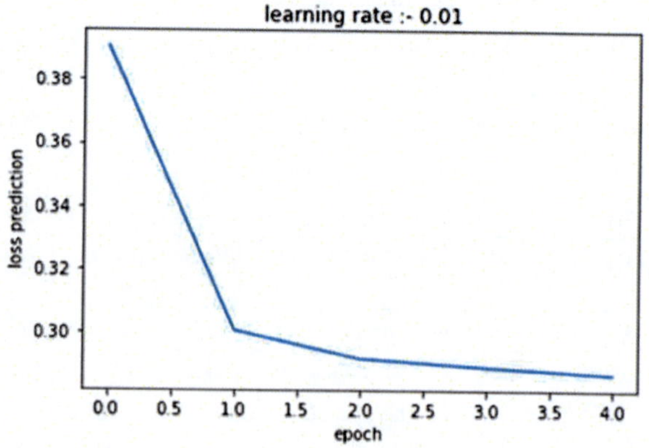

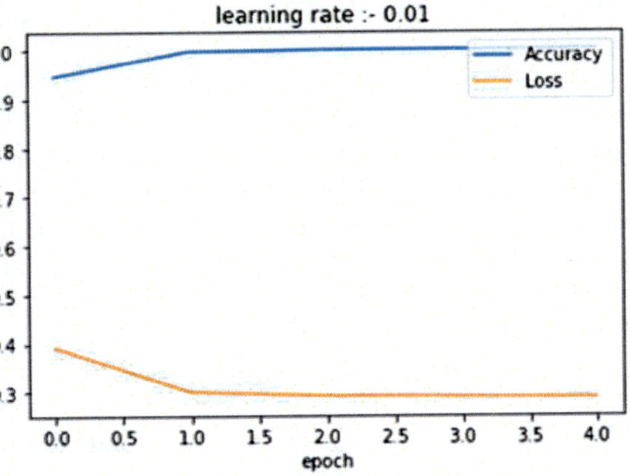

Fig. 6 Total accuracy and loss prediction

Figure 6 represents the accuracy, and loss shows an optimal performance, and there is no overfitting in prediction because accuracy is very close to 1.0; parallel, loss is also measured in stable circumstances till completion of all epochs.

As earlier supposed, we carried out the standardization and the normalization of the data process in this experimental model to promote quicker convergence during falling and non-falling dataset training to assess performance using standardized and un-normalized information as given in Table 2.

The effects of batch normalization for performance measurement are shown in generated error bars (see Fig. 7), used number of epochs along with learning rates (see Fig. 4 and Fig. 5), where losses signify errors only. The error bars represent

Table 2 Effects of batch normalization for performance measurement

	Training accuracy (%)	Validation accuracy (%)	Test accuracy (%)
Normalized data	99.85	99.32	99
Un-normalized data	93.68	84.33	82

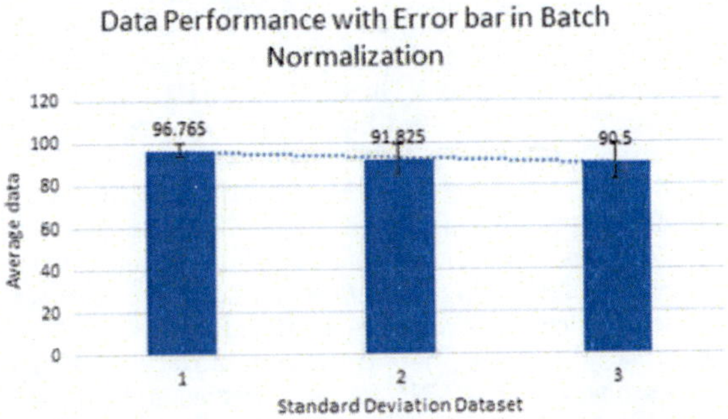

Fig. 7 Error bar generated with normalization data

the graphical representations of the variability of data that indicates the errors or uncertainty in measured data.

It depicts that normalized data achieve a high accuracy rate and reduced error bars within a lower number of epochs than un-normalized data which is experimented with Python code and found that a greater number of data frames can achieve optimal accuracy and less during training and validation of accuracy procedure and reduction in loss due to large number of learning and retested models.

6 Conclusion

This research work presents a human fall dataset consisting of synthetically created human posture and segmentation data under multiple camera perspectives using a CNN model with highly discriminative embedding characteristics for fall identification. In this research work, detecting human beings accurately in a surveillance image or video is a major research work in the area of computer vision despite the challenges to process low-resolution images. This work uses object detection techniques which are categorized according to data shape-based, motion-based, and image texture-based methods that benchmark human detection datasets. In the future study, leveraging a multi-view approach and adopting better models based on restricted sections of the picture will be discussed as ways to improve the human detection process in surveillance photos. The experimental work represents an optimal accuracy and loss prediction that analyses the output, which is demonstrated along with learning rate using several epochs in falling and non-falling images and also eliminate overfitting issues and measure stability in data objects.

References

1. Nasution AH, Emmanuel S (2007) Intelligent video surveillance for monitoring elderly in home environments. In: Proceedings of the IEEE 9th International workshop on multimedia signal processing. Crete, Greece, pp 203–206
2. Sreenidhi I, Satyanarayana P (2020) Real-time human fall detection and emotion recognition using embedded device and deep learning. Int J Emerg Trends Eng Res 8(3):780–786
3. Zhang S, McCullagh P, Nugent C, Zheng H (2009) A theoretic algorithm for fall and motionless detection. In: IEEE 3rd International conference on pervasive computing technologies for healthcare. IEEE Publishing, Piscataway, pp 1–6
4. Reddy GP, Kalaiselvi Geetha M (2020) Video based fall detection using deep convolutional neural network. Eur J Mol Clin Med 7(11):739–748
5. Ghoneim S (2021) Accuracy, recall, precision, f-score and specificity, which to optimize on? Available online: https://towardsdatascience.com/accuracy-recall-precision-f-score-specificity-which-to-optimize-on-867d3f11124
6. Yhdego H (2019) Towards musculoskeletal simulation-aware fall injury mitigation: transfer learning with deep CNN for fall detection. In: Spring simulation conference, pp 1–12
7. Zhang J, Cheng Wu, Wang Y (2020) Human fall detection based on body posture spatio-temporal evolution. Sensors 20(946):1–21

8. Banik A, Shrivastava A, Manohar Potdar R et al. (2021) Design, modelling, and analysis of novel solar PV system using MATLAB. Mater Today Proc. https://doi.org/10.1016/j.matpr.2021.06.226
9. Shu F, Shu J (2021) An eight-camera fall detection system using human fall pattern recognition via machine learning by a low-cost android box. Sci Rep 11:2471
10. Paul M, Haque SME, Chakraborty S (2013) Human detection in surveillance videos and its applications—a review. EURASIP J Adv Signal Process 176:1–16
11. Lorca LA, Sacomori C, Balague-Avila VP, Pino-Marquez LP, Quiroz-Vidal FA, Ortega L (2019) Incidence and risk of falls in patients treated for hematologic malignancies in the intensive Hematology unit. Rev Latino-Americana Enfermagem 27:e3145
12. Islam MdM, Tayan O, Islam MdR, Islam MdS, Nooruddin S, Kabir MN, Islam MdR (2017) Deep learning based systems developed for fall detection: a review. IEEE Access. https://doi.org/10.1109/ACCESS.2020.3021943
13. Das TK, Banik A, Chattopadhyay S, Das A (2021) Energy-efficient cooling scheme of power transformer: an innovative approach using solar and waste heat energy technology. In: Ghosh SK, Ghosh K, Das S, Dan PK, Kundu A (eds) Advances in thermal engineering, manufacturing, and production management. ICTEMA 2020. Lecture notes in mechanical engineering. Springer, Singapore. https://doi.org/10.1007/978-981-16-2347-9_17
14. Li X, Pang T, Liu W, Wang T (2018) Fall detection for elderly person care using convolutional neural networks. In: Proceedings of 10th International congress on image and signal processing, biomedical engineering and informatics, pp 1–6
15. Chen M-C, Liu Y-M (2013) An indoor video surveillance system with intelligent fall detection capability. Math Probl Eng 2013:1–8
16. Adhikari K, Bouchachia H, Nait-Charif H (2017) Activity recognition for indoor fall detection using convolutional neural network. In: Proceedings of the 15th IAPR international conference on machine vision applications, pp 81–84
17. Tasoulis SK, Mallis GI, Georgakopoulos SV, Vrahatis AG, Plagianakos VP, Maglogiannis IG (2019) Deep learning and change detection for fall recognition. Commun Comput Inf Sci 1000:262–273
18. Zhang Q, Zhu S (2018) Real-time activity and fall risk detection for aging population using deep learning. In: 9th IEEE Annual ubiquitous computing, electronics and mobile communication conference, pp 1055–1059
19. Casilari E, Lora-Rivera R, García-Lagos F (2020) A study on the application of convolutional neural networks to fall detection evaluated with multiple public datasets. Sensors 20(5):1466
20. Sultana A, Deb K, Dhar PK, Koshiba T (2021) Classification of indoor human fall events using deep learning. Entropy 23(328):1–20
21. Tsai TH, Hsu CW (2019) Implementation of fall detection system based on 3D skeleton for deep learning technique. IEEE Access 7
22. Min W, Cui H, Rao H, Li Z, Yao L (2018) Detection of human falls on furniture using scene analysis based on deep learning and activity characteristics. IEEE Access 6:9324–9335
23. Ma X, Wang H, Xue B, Zhou M, Ji B, Li Y (2014) Depth based human fall detection via shape features and improved extreme learning machine. IEEE J Biomed Health Inform 18(6):1915–1922
24. Wang S, Wang X, Chen R, Liu Y, Huang S (2019) Real-time detection of facial expression based on improved residual convolutional neural network. In: IEEE International conference on signal processing, communications and computing. Dalian, China, pp 1–4
25. Seredin OS, Kopylov AV, Surkov EE (2020) The study of skeleton description reduction in the human fall-detection task. Comput Opt 44(6):951–958
26. Harrou F, Zerrouki N, Sun Y, Houacine A (2017) Vision-based fall detection system for improving safety of elderly people. IEEE Instrum Meas Mag 49–55
27. Du Y, Wang W, Wang L (2015) Hierarchical recurrent neural network for skeleton based action recognition. In: Proceedings of IEEE computer society conference on computer and visual pattern recognition, pp 1110–1118

28. Ozcan K, Mahabalagiri AK, Casares M, Velipasalar S (2013) Automatic fall detection and activity classification by a wearable embedded smart camera. IEEE J Emerg Sel Top Circ Syst 3(2):125–136
29. Redmon J, Farhadi (2020) YOLO: real-time object detection. https://pjreddie.com/darknet/yolo/
30. http://fenix.univ.rzeszow.pl/~mkepski/ds/uf.html

A Method for Detecting Epileptic Seizure in Pediatrics Patients Based on EEG Signals

Satarupa Chakrabarti, Aleena Swetapadma, and Prasant Kumar Pattnaik

Abstract Epilepsy the disorder of the central nervous system has its worldwide presence in roughly 50 million people as estimated by WHO. The most common non-invasive tool for studying the brain activity of epileptic patient is the electroencephalogram (EEG). Determining the onset of seizures accurately is still elusive, and over the years, developing effective techniques to monitor epilepsy is progressive. In this work, pediatric patients with history of intractable epilepsy have been studied. The EEG signals used here belong to the scalp EEG database of Children's Hospital Boston-Massachusetts Institute of Technology (CHB-MIT). For determining between seizure and non-seizure signals, discrete Fourier transform (DFT) has been used as the feature extraction techniques. The features extracted are then given to the artificial neural network (ANN) to identify the presence of epileptic behavior in the signals. After designing the epileptic seizure detector, a setup has been developed using MATALB/Simulink for real-time applications that recorded an accuracy of 98.6% with specificity and sensitivity of 98.1% and 99.2%, respectively. In this work, an improved method is proposed to provide better solution and enhance the quality of living of the pediatric epilepsy patients.

Keywords Epilepsy · Seizure · Pediatric · Signal processing · DFT · ANN

1 Introduction

Machine learning, in the recent few decades, has become one of the most widely used and sought-after tools for the purpose of prediction and analysis in the medical domain. Researchers all over the world are working to build efficient and cost-effective systems that can single handedly diagnose as well as predict disease. Among the wide array of tools and techniques in machine learning, neural network and its application in the field of neuroscience have been highly benefited with its use and implementation [1]. To understand the underlying brain activities during epilepsy,

S. Chakrabarti · A. Swetapadma (✉) · P. K. Pattnaik
School of Computer Engineering, KIIT University, Bhubaneswar, India

M. S. Kaiser et al. (eds.), *Proceedings of Trends in Electronics and Health Informatics*, Lecture Notes in Networks and Systems 376,
https://doi.org/10.1007/978-981-16-8826-3_10

the reliable way is by using electroencephalogram (EEG) that captures the electrical activity of the brain using electrodes over a certain period of time. As EEG provides huge amount of data about the brain, this information needs pre-processing so that relevant and useful features can be extracted for classification. For automatic detection of epileptic seizure and its prediction, signal processing and machine learning play the pivotal role.

In the recent years, various promising signal processing techniques for EEG signals as well as feature extraction methods useful for detection of seizures have been proposed by researchers [2]. It is generally seen, because of the complex nature of EEG signals, application of any single method for studying its characteristics and features is not very effective. The other most common issue with EEG signals for epileptic patients is the adaptability. From patient to patient, the neuronal activity varies. Therefore, automatic detection mechanism of EEG signals should be able to adapt and distinguish between the different conditions and handle them according to their pre-requisite. Adaptive algorithm that would be capable of learning different subtle features and conditions irrespective of patients is required. Finally, the main issue which needs to be addressed is compliance with long and continuous EEG data rather than recordings comprising of few minutes. The paper is organized as follows. Section 2 addresses the literature review. Section 3 describes the methods used along with the proposed methodology. Results are discussed in Sect. 4, followed by discussion in Sect. 5, and finally conclusion in the last section.

2 Literature Review

Researchers have and are still working on EEG recordings to present newer processes that would help in providing better understanding of brain activity and its antics with respect to epilepsy. Arun Kumar et al. [3] described a novel method using moving window approximate entropy (ApEn) to recognize seizure onset automatically. The average delay recorded was 0.2 s over 200 segments of EEG recordings. Lin [4] presented his work on multivariate analysis for the detection of significant patterns and was based on the combination of principal component analysis—support vector machine for a multisensory system. Ibrahim and Majzoub [5] in their research work used discrete wavelet transform (DWT) along with Shannon's entropy and standard deviation for developing an adaptive seizure detection method from EEG records. Feng et al. [6] brought forward an on-chip portable seizure detection system. An automated seizure detection system [7] would pave way for easier and faster diagnosis of seizure events with minimal misjudgment and error. Although a study dedicated to providing critical facets of preictal duration [8] and its morphology still lacks substantial evidence, yet advancement in developing seizure detection systems would transform patient treatment and management. Devising detection strategies are a challenging task as seizures are patient-specific with distinct characteristic features of each seizure [9].

The onset of an epileptic seizure attack is a widespread manifestation of abnormal electrical activity and spike as well as slow waveforms mark these changes and is considered as the trademark signature of epileptic seizure [10]. Hameed et al. [11] tried to classify and bring distinction between ictal and inter ictal stages with the help of new indices (diagnostic). They implemented the Ggobal PDM or principal dynamic modes for studying the functional activity and connections between the different lobes of the brain. Ke et al. [12] spoke at length about the problem of seizure detection following a shallow-dense network approach. They used maximal information coefficient (MIC) to bring parity among the channels and data. The interesting factor about global MIC was all the coefficients got organized depending on the sequence of time and the way in which the pattern evolved. Thodoroff et al. [13] explored the use of deep neural networks in order to utilize them to learn the different significant characteristics of an EEG recording such that it would be able to distinguish and detect seizure activity from normal condition.

After studying all the above-mentioned techniques and applications, to improve the performance of seizure detection unit and raising an alarm during an epileptic seizure, discrete Fourier transformation has been used. This helped in analyzing the spectral content of the EEG signal and changes in frequency during a seizure attack. As presence of any distortion in signal is best understood in the frequency domain, hence, in this work, discrete Fourier transform to find appropriate features from raw EEG signals. The features are then given to classifier for detecting the epileptic period. The proposed system is implemented so that it can be used in real situations. The performance of the designed system is analyzed in terms of accuracy, sensitivity, and specificity which seem convincing to be implemented in hospitals.

3 Material and Methods

3.1 Dataset Details

The dataset used in this particular work is taken from pediatric database belonging to Children's Hospital Boston (CHB) [14], Massachusetts. The database contained EEG recordings (scalp) of patients with history of intractable seizure and the age group is between 1.5 and 15 years (pediatric). The recordings obtained have specific annotations based on the seizure onset and the duration of the seizure. The number of seizures varied for different patients from minimum of one to a maximum of four seizures. The electrode placement is at par to 10–20 international system and the data are sampled at 256 Hz with 16-bit resolution. There was presence of artifacts such as head, body, and eye movements.

3.2 Methods

Signal processing is done using discrete Fourier transform in this work and the supervised classifier used for classifying the epileptic seizures is ANN. The details have been mentioned in the following subsections.

Discrete Fourier Transform (DFT) The family of Fourier transform and analysis comprises of mathematical procedures whose main principle is centered on signal decomposition into sinusoids. Fourier analysis is one of the most suitable method for analysis of data as this helps in breaking down any signal into its components of various frequencies [15]. DFT or discrete Fourier transform is capable of changing an input signal with N points to output signal with $N/2 + 1$ points. Usually, the input signal is considered to be in the time domain as most of the signals in DFT are in a particular time interval. If the frequency domain is known, then from that the time domain calculation is possible. DFT coefficient (kth) of a sequence $\{x(n)\}$ of length N can be defined as in Eq. (1)

$$X(k) = \sum_{n=0}^{N-1} x(n) W_N^{kn}, k = 0, \ldots, N-1 \tag{1}$$

where

$$W_N = e^{-j2\pi/N} = \cos\left(\frac{2\pi}{N}\right) - j\sin\left(\frac{2\pi}{N}\right)$$

is known as principal root of unity (N-th) since W_N^{nk} is taken as the function of k that has N period and the coefficients obtained from DFT have periodic in accordance to N period. The original sequence $\{x(n)\}$ can be reclaimed back again using the inverse DFT or inverse discrete Fourier transform (IDFT).

$$x(n) = \frac{1}{N} \sum_{k=0}^{N-1} X(k) W_N^{-kn}, n = 0, \ldots, N-1 \tag{2}$$

This can be verified for the principal N-th root of unity W_N

$$\sum_{n=0}^{N-1} W_N^{nk} = N \cdot \delta(k), k = 0, \ldots, N-1 \tag{3}$$

where $\delta(k)$ is known as the Kronecker delta function.

Artificial Neural Network Artificial neural network is a representation of a model that closely resembles the human nervous system but stands on the foundation of mathematical equations and derivations. The key element in the neural network architecture is the neurons or specifically the artificial neurons, sometimes called

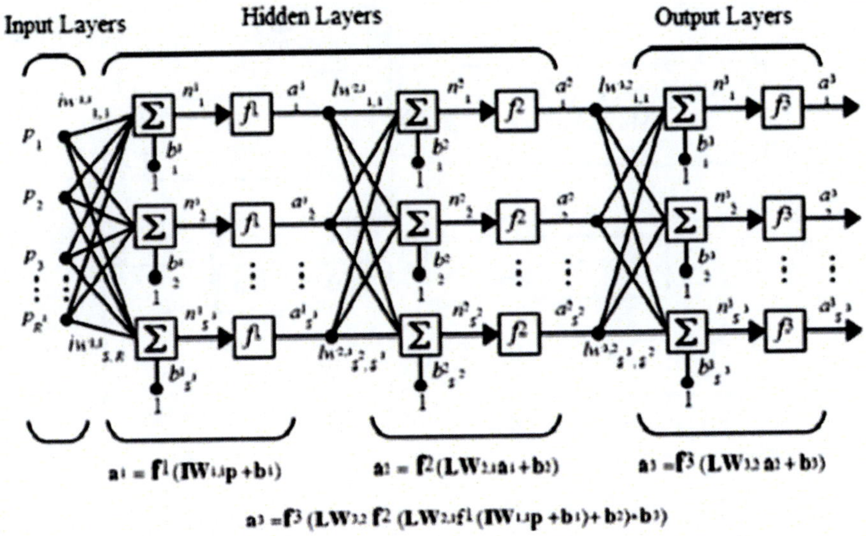

Fig. 1 Feedforward neural network

nodes. The synapses present in the actual nervous system is represented as effect of the different input signals with connection weights, transfer function presents the non-linear features of the neurons [16]. The impulse of the neuron is calculated as the sum of input (weighted) that gets modified with the help of the transfer function. The effectiveness of the learning of neurons is reached by changing and modifying the weights in accordance to the specific learning algorithm that is selected. In Fig. 1, a feedforward multilayer perceptron neural network has been shown. In this work, a neural network has been used as classifier to detect the presence of seizure during epileptic attack.

3.3 Proposed Methodology

The proposed method includes different steps associated with seizure detection as shown in Fig. 2. The elementary step consists of EEG signal collection which is here related to pediatric patients with history of intractable epilepsy. This is followed by the subsequent stage of feature extraction with discrete Fourier transform using an overlapping moving window of 1 s. The extracted features are then given to the artificial neural network for classification. The trained module is tested and validated with data other than the trained data in order to analyze the performance and accuracy.

Multichannel EEG Signals The dataset considered contained EEG signals collected from 23 multiple channels to study the pediatric epileptic seizure. Figure 3

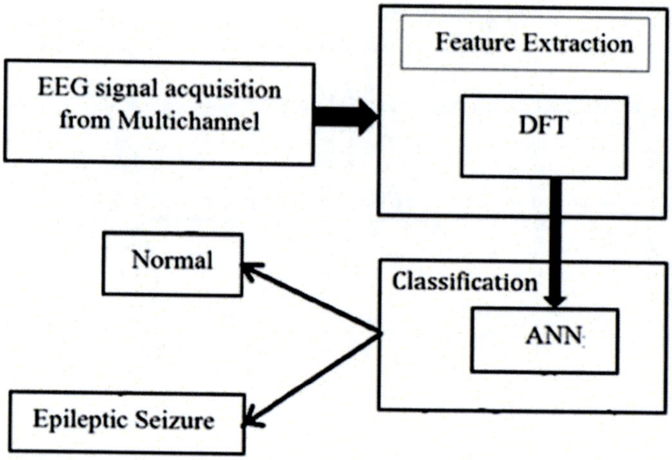

Fig. 2 Flowchart of the proposed methodology

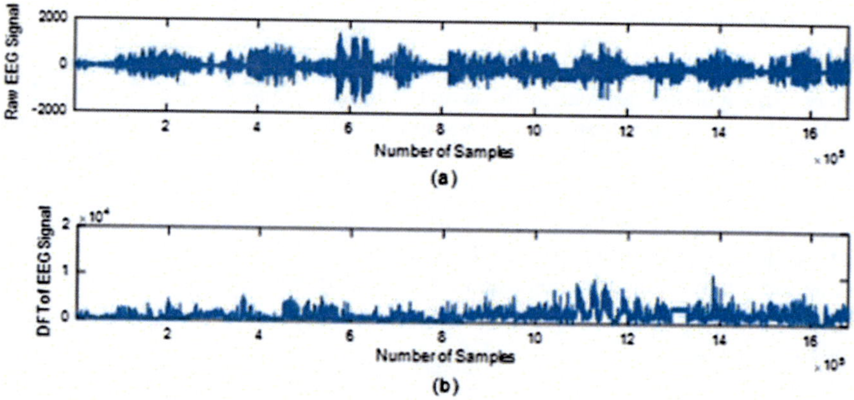

Fig. 3 Signal processing and feature extraction

shows the EEG signals obtained from a patient from 23 channels. The first 80,000 samples are of normal EEG signals and next 80,000 samples of epileptic EEG signals. It can be observed that the amplitude of signals during epilepsy is more than during normal condition. These raw EEG signals are used in signal processing to obtain appropriate features.

Feature Extraction from EEG Signals In this work, DFT has been used as the signal processing technique for extracting appropriate features. Figure 4 shows the feature extraction from EEG signal using DFT in moving window of 256 samples. The first 256 samples of the signal are of zero magnitude as it takes 256 samples to generate one sample. The 257th sample has amplitude which is generated by taking

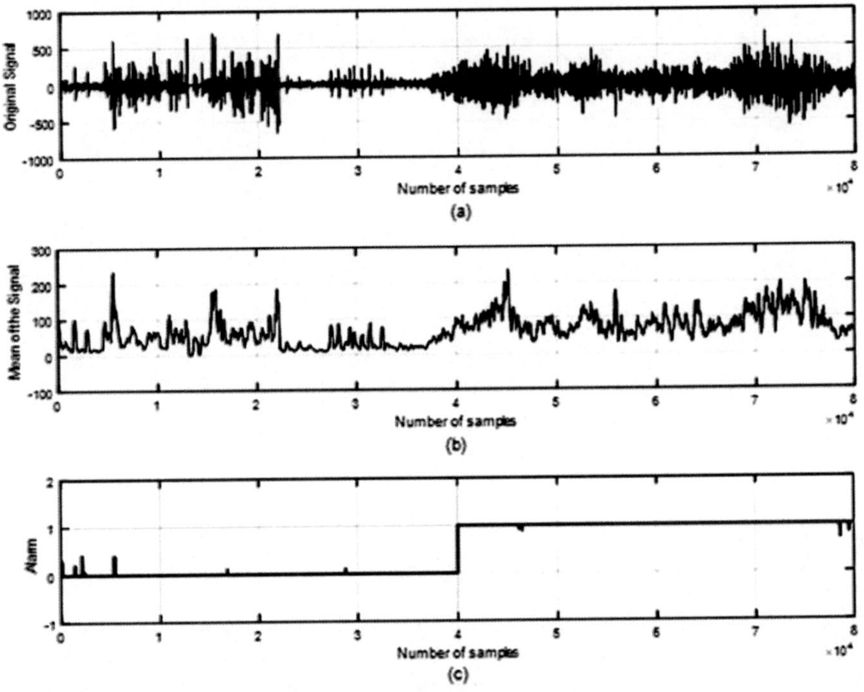

Fig. 4 **a** Original EEG signal of one channel, **b** DFT of the EEG signal, **c** output of the proposed method

the moving window of 1–256 samples. The 258th sample has amplitude which is generated by taking the moving window of 2–257 samples. And the 259th sample has amplitude which is generated by taking the moving window of 3–258 samples. The moving window slides over the length of the signal, and the rest of the designated features are obtained from each window. Figure 3 shows the features obtained from EEG signal used various feature extraction techniques. Figure 3a shows the original signal from one EEG channel. Figure 3b shows the features obtained using DFT from the raw signals.

ANN Classifier Modules In this work, an ANN module has been designed for epileptic seizure detection. Output of the module is set to "0" for normal and "1" for epileptic seizure. Various trials are carried out by changing number of neurons, layers, transfer function, error goal, etc., and after many trials and errors, optimal ANN configuration is chosen for the training module. Table 1 shows the performance of the ANN module. The optimal network architecture obtained is a 3-layered structure with 20 neurons in the hidden layer and having tan-sig as the transfer function. After designing of the ANN module, it is tested and realized using MATLAB/Simulink for easy monitoring of epileptic patients.

Table 1 Performance of patient-specific signal using DFT

Patient	Neural network architecture	Transfer function	Error goal	Accuracy (%)	Specificity (%)	Sensitivity (%)
1	10-10-1	Tan-sig	0.01	99.9	100.0	99.8
2				100.0	100.0	100.0
3				100.0	99.9	100.0
4				99.8	99.9	99.7
5				100.0	100.0	100.0
6				100.0	99.9	100.0
7				99.8	99.7	99.8
8				99.8	99.7	99.9
9				99.9	99.7	100.0
10				99.1	98.4	99.8

4 Results

The proposed method is trained and tested on pediatric patients, and the performance is based on the features that are extracted after transformation. tenfold cross validation has been used to quantity the accuracy, specificity, and sensitivity of the proposed method. In this work, 10 pediatric patients are considered, and using moving window, the features are extracted. Based on features extracted using DFT, the results have been studied for individual subject as well as for the combined dataset of 10 patients. The results in Tables 1 and 2 present the performance of EEG signals after using DFT. Table 1 shows detailed results of each patient while Table 2 shows the different measures for the combined dataset. The highest overall accuracy achieved in DFT is 98.6% (20-20-1). The sensitivity and specificity for the complete dataset are seen to be 99.2% and 98.1%, respectively. In individual patient, the sensitivity is recorded between 98 and 100% while the classifier achieved specificity above 99%. Hence, it can be ascertained that DFT can be used as signal processing tool for effective extraction of features for pediatric epileptic seizure detection.

One of the test results of proposed method using DFT as signal processing has been shown in Fig. 4. Figure 4a shows the original EEG signals of one channel out of 23 channels. The first 40,000 samples are taken from normal condition, and next 40,000 samples are for epileptic condition. Figure 4b shows the DFT value obtained

Table 2 Performance of overall signal using DFT

Neural network architecture	Transfer function	Error goal	Accuracy (%)	Specificity (%)	Sensitivity (%)
10-10-1	Tan-sig	0.01	95.6	94.0	97.3
20-20-1		0.001	98.6	98.1	99.2

from the original EEG signals. Figure 4c represents the output of the proposed method for the samples taken for analysis. It can be observed that the output is "0" for up to 40,000 samples which show there is no requirement for raising an alarm. After that the output becomes "1" denoting presence of seizure and hence, there will be generation of an alarm.

5 Discussion

The performance of the proposed work has been enhanced using the feature extraction techniques which included discrete Fourier transform. Signal processing technique has been used to study the EEG signals in the frequency domain using DFT. The sole reason of using DFT even though knowing that the signals are analyzed in one domain was to have a more elaborate understanding of the different changes in the signals in the frequency domain. DFT provides better frequency resolution and fast Fourier transformation helped in reducing the noise present in the signals, no other filters were used for processing the signals. In order to extract features from the signals, the standard deviation was used to study the variation among the signals using the frequency components. It was seen from the results that for DFT, the classifier has given the highest accuracy of 98.6% with the least number of misclassified data which is necessary for designing a module for accurate detection of epileptic seizures.

Different literatures bring forward works of authors and researchers related to the domain of detection and prediction of epilepsy. A vast array of methods and techniques has been applied ranging from wavelet decomposition to empirical mode decomposition. Some authors have used shallow networks and maximal information coefficients while others have applied deep neural networks and hybrid [17] methods. The choice of classifiers also varied from k nearest neighbor to support vector machine, artificial neural networks, and many more. Table 3 presents a comparative study exclusively based on the works of different authors on the dataset of CHB-MIT using different techniques. Figure 5 shows the comparison of accuracy of some of the methods suggested for detection of pediatric epilepsy. It can be observed that the proposed method works better and is easy and robust.

Table 3 A comparison of few existing studies with the proposed method

Authors	Dataset used	Methods	Accuracy (%)
Ibrahim et al. [5]	CHB-MIT	DWT, Shannon's entropy	94.5
Hameed et al. [11]	CHB-MIT	Global principal dynamic mode	95.0
Ke et al. [12]	CHB-MIT	Shallow dense network, MIC	97.2
Thodoroff et al. [13]	CHB-MIT	Convolutional neural network	85.0
Proposed method	CHB-MIT	Discrete Fourier transform and ANN	98.6

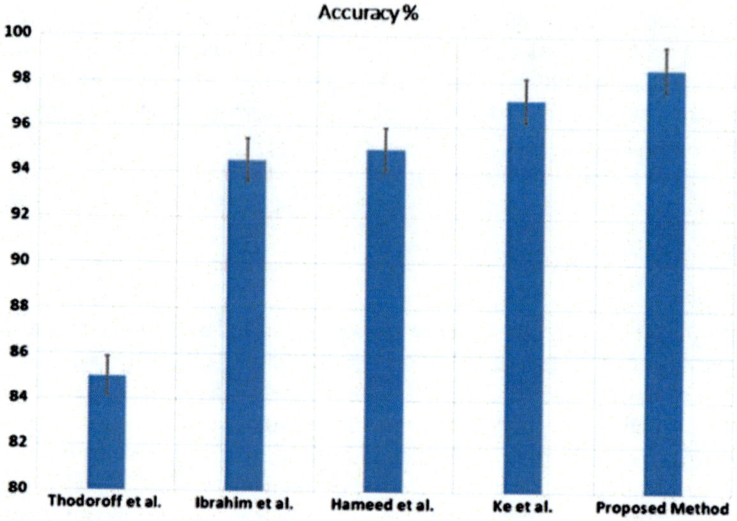

Fig. 5 Comparison study of various methods

6 Conclusion

Over the years, different works have brought forth a clear picture regarding pediatric epilepsy seizure detection and prediction and the drawbacks associated with it. In this work, an improved method has been suggested to distinguish between pediatric seizure and non-seizure EEG signals for patient-specific approach as well as for overall analysis. Various signal processing techniques have been used, and different features extracted are used in the classifier for accurate determination of pediatric seizure. The highlights of the proposed method and the future work can be outlined as follows:

- The accuracy achieved for pediatric epileptic seizure detection is found to be 98.6% which seems promising for monitoring of patients.
- The proposed method is not patient-specific hence can be used for monitoring of any pediatric epileptic seizure patient.
- Better results have been achieved when compared with respect to sensitivity and accuracy.
- There is no requirement of parameter optimization or temporal feature extraction.
- When DFT is used for feature extraction, the number of computations required is reduced.

The future scope of work is to minimize false detection that can be implemented in hospitals for accurate determination of seizure and providing a chance for patients to a better life.

References

1. Koohestani A, Abdar M, Khosravi A, Nahavandi S, Koohestani M (2019) Integration of ensemble and evolutionary machine learning algorithms for monitoring diver behavior using physiological signals. IEEE Access 7:98971–98992
2. Beheshti I, Sone D, Maikusa N, Kimura Y, Shigemoto Y, Sato N, Matsuda H (2020) Pattern analysis of glucose metabolic brain data for lateralization of MRI-negative temporal lobe epilepsy. Epilepsy Res 167:106474
3. Arunkumar N, Ramkumar K, Venkataraman V (2018) A moving window approximate entropy in wavelet framework for automatic detection of the onset of epileptic seizures. Biomed Res 29:161–170
4. Lin T (2018) PCA/SVM-based method for pattern detection in a multisensor system. Math Probl Eng 2018
5. Ibrahim SW, Majzoub S (2017) EEG-based epileptic seizures detection with adaptive learning capability. Int J Electr Eng Inf 9(4):813–824
6. Feng L, Li Z, Wang Y (2018) VLSI design of SVM-based seizure detection system with on-chip learning capability. IEEE Trans Biomed Circuits Syst 12(1):171–181
7. Chakrabarti S, Swetapadma A, Ranjan A, Pattnaik PK (2020) Time domain implementation of pediatric epileptic seizure detection system for enhancing the performance of detection and easy monitoring of pediatric patients. Biomed Signal Process Control 59:101930
8. Medvedev AV, Agoureeva GI, Murro AM (2019) A long short-term memory neural network for the detection of epileptiform spikes and high frequency oscillations. Sci Rep 9(1):1–10
9. Hassan AR, Subasi A, Zhang Y (2020) Epilepsy seizure detection using complete ensemble empirical mode decomposition with adaptive noise. Knowl-Based Syst 191:105333
10. Wang G, Wang D, Du C, Li K, Zhang J, Liu Z, Tao Y, Wang M, Cao Z, Yan X (2020) Seizure prediction using directed transfer function and convolution neural network on intracranial EEG. IEEE Trans Neural Syst Rehabil Eng
11. Hameed Z, Saleem S, Mirza J, Mustafa MS, Qamar-ul-Islam (2018) Characterisation of ictal and interictal states of epilepsy: a system dynamic approach of principal dynamic modes analysis. PLoS ONE, 13(1):1–21
12. Ke H, Chen S, Zhang H, Tang Y, Liu Y, Chen D, Li X (2018) A shallow-dense network approach to synchronization pattern classification of multivariate epileptic EEG. Lect Notes Electr Eng 459:553–563
13. Thodoroff P, Pineau J, Lim A (2016) Learning robust features using deep learning for automatic seizure detection. In: Machine learning for healthcare conference, pp 178–190
14. Physionet CHB-MIT Scalp EEG Database Boston. https://www.physionet.org/pn6/chbmit
15. Engelberg S, Chalom E (2010) Measuring the spectral content of a signal: an introduction. IEEE Instrum Meas Mag 13(6):34–38
16. Kriesel D (2005) A brief introduction to neural networks, p 244. Retrieved August. https://doi.org/10.1016/0893-6080(94)90051-5
17. Zomorodi-Moghadam M, Abdar M, Davarzani Z, Zhou X, Pławiak P, Acharya UR (2021) Hybrid particle swarm optimization for rule discovery in the diagnosis of coronary artery disease. Expert Syst 38(1):e12485

Detection of Brain Tumors in MRI Images Through Deep Learning

Roshan Jahan and Manish Madhav Tripathi

Abstract Brain tumors are abnormal cells that grow within the brain, some of which can cause malignant growth. The standard method for distinguishing between cancer and the mind is magnetic resonance imaging (MRI). Magnetic resonance imaging data enables the identification of the development of strange tissues in the brain. In a variety of review papers, the localization of mind cancer is complemented by the application of machine learning and in-depth learning calculations. After applying these calculations to MRI images, brain tumor prediction is abnormally fast and higher accuracy helps treat patients. The predictions also allow radiologists to make quick choices. In this paper, a combination of artificial neural networks (ANN) and convolutional neural networks (CNN) is proposed and applied to identify the presence of brain tumors.

Keywords Brain tumor · Machine learning · Algorithms · Convolution neural network

1 Introduction

The brain is the major organ of the human organism. It controls the full use of the various organs and assists in making choices. It mainly controls the focal point of the focal sensory system and is responsible for deliberate and mandatory exercises in the human body day after day [1]. Cancer is a tight network of undesirable tissues in our brain that develops and multiplies uncontrollably. In that year, about 3540 children were analyzed at the age of 15 [2], and their minds grew. A correct understanding of

Supported by Integral University, Lucknow (MCN: IU/R&D/2021-MCN0001229).

R. Jahan (✉) · M. M. Tripathi
Integral University Lucknow, Lucknow, India
e-mail: roshan@iul.ac.in

M. M. Tripathi
e-mail: mmt@iul.ac.in

M. S. Kaiser et al. (eds.), *Proceedings of Trends in Electronics and Health Informatics*, Lecture Notes in Networks and Systems 376,
https://doi.org/10.1007/978-981-16-8826-3_11

mental cancer and its staging method is an important task of preventing and supplementing disease rehabilitation methods. As a result, radiologists make extensive use of reverberation imaging (MRI) to dissect brain tumors [1].

In this article, ANN and CNN are used to aggregate typical brains and cancers [3]. Artificial neural network (ANN) operates as a sensory system in the human brain. Under this premise, advanced PCs are associated with a large number of measurements of interconnection and system management. This allows neuron tissues to prepare using basic operating units that are applied to the entire preparation and to store empirical information. There are different layers of neurons related to each other. Neural tissue can obtain information by Nalbalwar et al. [4] using the information index applied to the learning metric. There will be a layer of information and output, and there may be many hidden layers. In the training system, weights and inclination angles are added to the neurons in each layer according to the information highlights and the front layer (for the cover layer and the yield layer). Based on the release work, apply it to the information highlights and build a On the model and secret layer, more learning finally achieved normal performance.

Since ANN works with fully linked layers, it really understands the operation, and in this document, the image is used as the information for its additional focus on CNN applications [3]. In convolution neural network (CNN), convolution is the name of the correct digital activity. Each CNN layer reduces image elements without having to prepare enough data. Unique processing such as convolution, [1] maxpooling, dropout, smooth, and thick are applied to make patterns. The present paper focuses on the self-representation of the engineering of the ANN and CNN models. Finally, ANN and CNN submissions are analyzed when applied to the mental cancer MR dataset.

2 Literature Review

In that paper, ANN was used to develop a system for the detection and classification of brain cancer [4]. When it stands out from various classifiers, the proposed method of using ANN as the classifier of mental image scheme provides good query ability. In addition, it also improves allocability, identity, and accuracy. The proposed method is computer efficient and has incredible results.

In [5], a convolutive neural network (CNN) was performed. For the independent identification of meningiomas, gliomas, and malignant pituitary tumors, the overall accuracy rate was 91.3%, and the survey rates were 88%, 81% and respectively nearly 100%. The important learning configuration for the development of various types of frontal cortex from MRI image slices is represented by the use of 2D convolutional neural associations. In this paper, methods such as data collection, preprocessing data, pre-model data, model smoothing, and adjustment beyond limits are applied. Additionally, 10-layer cross-pricing was performed on the performance dataset to verify that the model was generalizable.

The interaction utilized in this paper depends on Hough's projection of a study [6] structure, a system that mirrors the completely customized counteraction and sharing of plans of presence of interest. It has additionally utilized learning techniques dependent on the divisional framework that is liberal, multi-territorial, flexible and can be effectively altered relying upon various modalities. An unmistakable extent of preparation information and an alternate dimensionality of information (2D, 2.5D and 3D) are applied to foresee unavoidable results. Convolutional neural organizations, [5] Hough projecting an example structure with CNN, voxel-wise solicitations, and efficient fix able assessment by CNN are utilized to dismantle the picture.

The cerebrum is a fundamental organ of the human body that controls a lot the capacities performed by various pieces of the body [1]. It is basically the combination designated spot of the focal touchscreen outline and is liable for carrying out cognizant and required bit by bit exercises in the human body. The illness is a tacky cross-over section of troubled tissue improvement inside our mind that fills in a tranquil way. To counter and fix threat, appealing reverberation imaging (MRI) is utilized comprehensively by radiologists to isolate formative periods from the cerebrum. The deferred result of this evaluation shows that mental health is available.

3 Collection of MR Images

The dataset commences from the GitHub site. This informational collection incorporates MR pictures of mental development. There are two coordinators; one tends to the common mental picture and different addresses the pictures of development. There are, obviously, 2065 photographs in those two envelopes. Figure 1 presents an illustration of normal and mental malignant growth. Completely 1085 growing photos and 980 no cancer are taken. The images have different forms (e.g., 225 $\times$ 225, 630 $\times$ 630,), and these images are resized to 256 $\times$ 256. Total 1672 photos for planning, 171 photos for testing, and 219 photos for analysis are taken. Out of 1672 planning images, 900 images are the image of illness and 772 images are the image without development—a total of 92 malignant photos and 94 free development photos from 186 supported photos and of the 207 screening photos, 116 malignant growth photos, and 91 nonenhancement photos.

4 Implementation

Both ANN and CNN techniques are applied to the psychological development dataset and their openness to image association is analyzed [7–10]. The ways used to apply NA to the collection of information about psychological diseases are.

1. Import the fundamental packs.
2. Import the instructive coordinator.

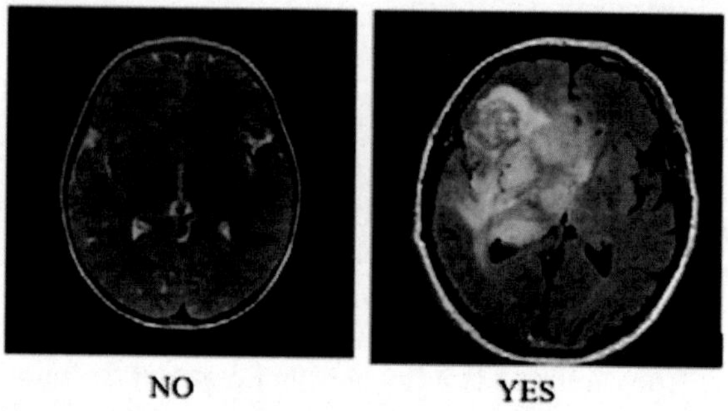

Fig. 1 Natural brain and brain with tumor

3. Look at the pictures, name the picture. (Set the picture with a mind cancer as 1 and the picture without mental development as 0) and store it in the information outline.
4. Edit the picture size as 256 × 256 by filtering the pictures separately.
5. Normalize the table.
6. Divide the instructive file into train, homologation and test congregations.
7. Make the layout.
8. Build the example.
9. Apply the example onto the train.
10. Assess the model utilizing the test set.

There are seven layers in the ANN model utilized here. The primary layer is the smooth layer that changes from 256 × 256 × 3 pictures to a solitary dimensional bunch. The following five coats are the thick coats with the beginning of the work. The level of neurons per layer is 128, 256, 512, 256, and 128 exclusively. These five layers work like mysterious layers, and the last thick layer with the beginning of the work is sigmoid which is the exposure layer with 1 neuron tending to the two classes.

The model is tabulated with the adam progression system and the double-bunking of the cross-entropy incident. The format is done and ready by handing out the planning and underwriting photos. Whenever the format is ready, an effort is made to use the set of test images. Next, the dataset comparing to the CNN system is provided. The steady progress in the use of CNN on the psychological development dataset is:

1. Import the vital groups.
2. Import Information Package (Yes/No)
3. Define class names for pictures (1 for cerebral growth and 0 for cerebral cancer no)
4. Convert Images to Format (256 × 256)
5. Standardization of the picture.
6. Divide the pictures into the Train, Approval and Testbed pictures.
7. Create the significant model.
8. Compile a layout.
9. Apply it to the train dataset (utilize the endorsement set to assess the presentation of the planning).

10. Evaluation of the model utilizing the test pictures.
11. Trace the graph by taking a gander at the readiness and exactness of the endorsement.
12. Compare real and determined execution.

The CNN format back to back is realized using a few layers. The data frame is reconstructed in 256 × 256. The convolve layer is applied to the dataimage with a replay.

Because the beginning works in all cases, the calibration that suggests image execution appears. As if the data picture and channel measurement are 32, 32, 64, 128, 256 for different layers convolve. The largest seam applied with 2 × 2 windows and dropout work is called with 20% dropout. A familiar method is used to turn pieces into a single-dimensional opening. The completely related layer is completed by calling the thickness procedure with the units measure as 256 and replay as activation work. The output layer has one unit to deal with both classes and the sigmoid as an imperious work. The design of the CNN model can be seen in Fig. 2. Performance is limited by using Python and runs in Google Colab. The provision is applied at 200 ages with the readiness and approval data set. The genuine decoration of the display is saved and outlined to understand the models delivered.

5 Review of Results

The information shown is appended to a variable that is considered standard type information. Image class labels are also produced and classified under the variable data target which is additionally a ndarray. As of this time, the images are added to the database. The information index of the image is separated into preparation, approval, and test information. Figure 3 shows the accuracy and misfortune of having applied ANN to the preparation and approval dataset. When the CNN is applied to the preparation of information for 50 deadlines, the accuracy of the acquired preparation is 97.13% and the accuracy of the approval is 71.51%. A similar one when applied to the test information provides 80.77% accuracy.

The highest approval accuracy achieved when the template is applied to the 200-age readiness dataset is 94.00%. The diagram in Fig. 4 demonstrates the relationship between assertion accuracy and accuracy approval and misfortune and loss of preparedness approval.

The model is assessed through the application of the test image layout. The confusion network for the expected result is identified as in the attached Fig. 5. Here are the implications of trial speculation and approval.

Figure 6 illustrates the precision, recall, and f1 rating of the two models.

The CNN model is 89% accurate in terms of test data usage. Have accuracy, callback, and f1 score nearby and by watching the ANN and CNN exposure by distinguishing the presence of brain growth. CNN ends up being the best method of help since it has the highest esteem of accuracy.

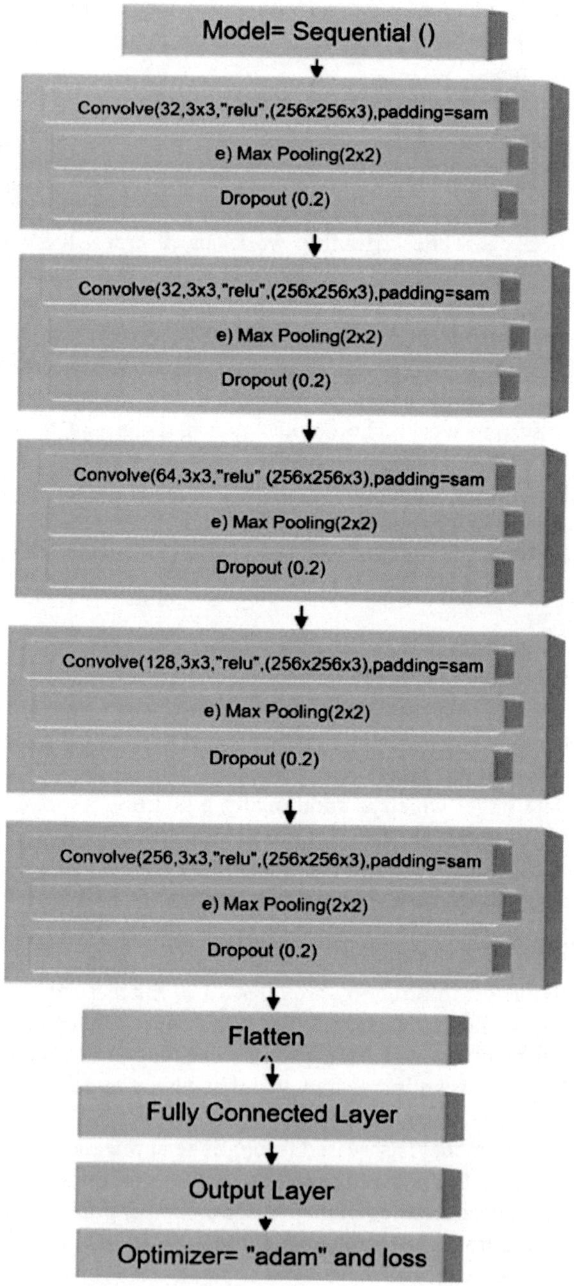

Fig. 2 Design of the CNN model

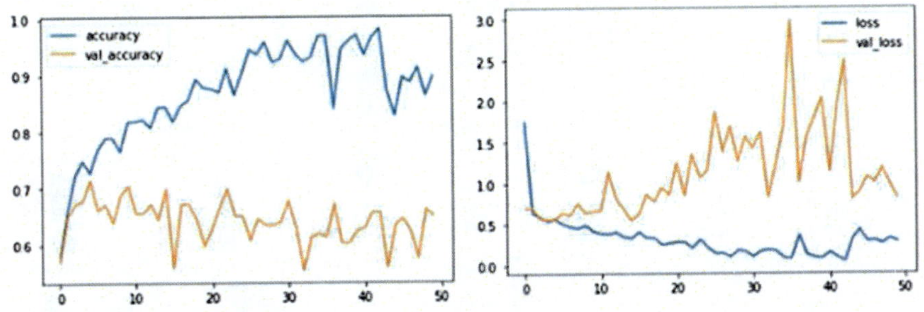

Fig. 3 Compare the precision of training and validation and the loss of the ANN model

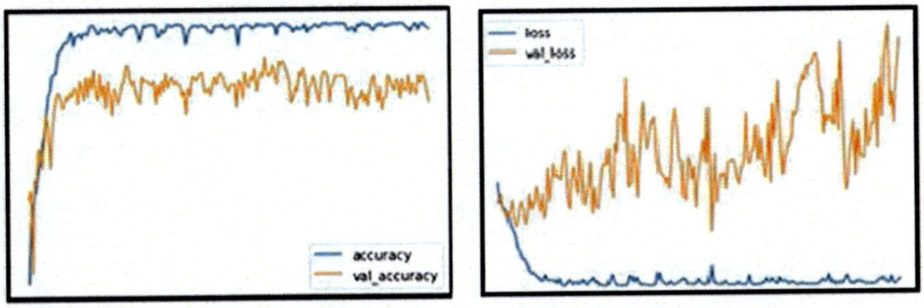

Fig. 4 Compare the precision of the training and validation and the loss of the CNN model

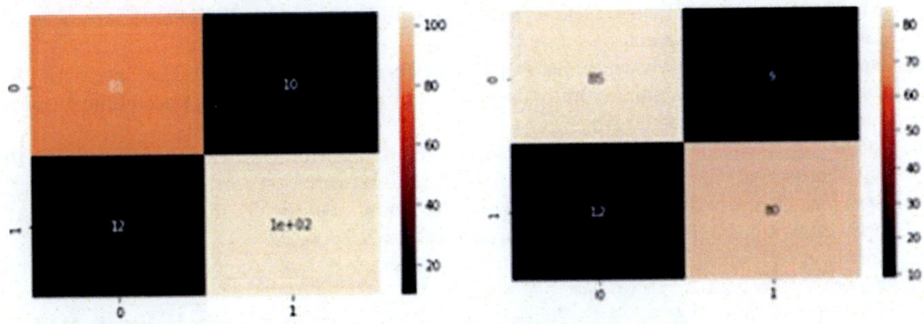

Fig. 5 Training and testing confusion matrix using the CNN

6 Conclusion

CNN is considered unprecedented in relation to the different methods of analyzing the informational index of the image. The CNN predicts by reducing the image size without losing important information for hypothesizing. The ANN model produces 65.21% test accuracy here, and this can be extended by supplying more image data. The comparable should be conceivable using picture development methodologies and the thinking of the ANN and CNN show should be conceivable. The template

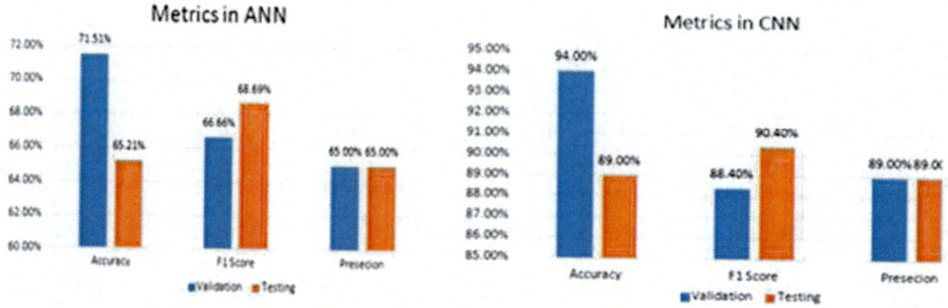

Fig. 6 Metrics

developed here is based on the focus and strategy of the gaffe. In the future, enhancement strategies can be used to determine how many layers and guidelines can be used in a model. In the future, and in the foreseeable future for the given dataset, NA is the best strategy for predicting the presence of frontal cortex development.

References

1. Hashemzehi R, Mahdavi SJS, Kheirabadi M, Kamel SR (2020) Detection of brain tumors from MRI images base on deep learning using hybrid model CNN and NADE. Elsevier B.V. on behalf of Nalecz Institute of Biocybernetics and Biomedical Engineering of the Polish Academy of Sciences Online Publication
2. Cancer data https://www.cancer.net/cancer-types/brain-tumor/statistics. Last accessed 10 Aug 21 https://braintumor.org/brain-tumor-information/treatment-options/clinical-trials/ (Feb2020). Last accessed 10 Aug 21
3. Google Sites https://en.wikipedia.org/wiki/Convolutional-neural-network Last accessed 10 Aug 21 https://en.wikipedia.org/wiki/Artificial-neural-network Last accessed 12 Aug 21 https://www.geeksforgeeks.org/introduction-convolution-neural-network/ Last accessed 11 Aug 21 https://en.wikipedia.org/wiki/Brain-tumor Last accessed 9 Aug 21
4. Nalbalwar R, Majhi U, Patil R, Gonge S (2014) Detection of brain tumor by using ANN. Int J Res Advent Technol 2
5. Milletari F, Ahmadi SA, Kroll C, Plate A, Rozanski V, Maiostre J, Levin J, Dietrich O, Ertl-Wagner B, Bötzel K, Navab N (2016) Hough-CNN: deep learning for segmentation of deep brain regions in MRI and ultrasound. Elsevier Inc., 164, 92-3-102
6. Özyurt F, Sert E, Avci E, Dogantekin E (2019) Brain tumor detection based on convolutional neural network with neutrosophic expert maximum fuzzy sure entropy. Elsevier Ltd., 147
7. Amin J, Sharif M, Raza M, Yasmin M (2018) Detection of brain tumor based on features fusion and machine learning. J Amb Intell Humanized Comput Online Publ
8. George DN, Jehlol HB, Oleiwi ASA (2015) Brain tumor detection using shape features and machine learning algorithms. Int J Sci Eng Res 6(12):454–459
9. Sobhangi K, Avinash S, Sabyasachi K, Satyabrata C, Jong-Seong A, Hee-Cheol S (2020) A CNN based Approach for the detection of brain tumor using MRI Scans. Test Eng Manage 83:16580–16586
10. Sharma K, Kaur A, Gujral S (2014) Brain tumor detection based on machine learning algorithms. Int J Comput Appl 103:7–11

Healthcare Informatics

Machine Learning Algorithm for Detecting Lung Cancer: A Review

Shweta Mallick and Surya Prakash Mishra

Abstract Nowadays, due to a flawed air quality index, many people are suffering from lung disease. These minor diseases could turn into lung cancer. This disease creates problems not only for any specific gender but also causes problems for both genders. So, it is essential to take particular caution before it become dangerous. In our review, we have done a comparative study of early detection of lung cancer. Many methods have been developed in lung cancer diagnosis. Some use x-ray images, and others use CT scan images. Furthermore, to identify lung cancer from the image dataset, multiple classification methods are combined with various segmentation algorithms in this study. We have found that CT scan images over x-ray images have more accuracy. That is why CT scan images are considered for lung cancer detection. Additionally, comparing with other technique, marker-controlled watershed segmentation has a more accurate output. This technique has higher accuracy using the deep learning technique as compared to traditional machine learning algorithms.

Keywords Lung cancer detection · Machine learning · CNN

1 Introduction

Due to lung cancer disease, lots of people lost their life. Therefore, it is necessary to identify lung cancer in the early stage to reduce the deaths of patients. So, detecting and diagnosing lung cancer in the early stage is a great challenge for researchers and doc- tors. To detect lung cancer, the use of medical images like MRI scans, x-rays, and CT scans is considered. Furthermore, ML algorithms identify the primary attributes of heterogeneous lungs datasets. A computer-aided diagnosis (CAD) was introduced in 1980 to analyze medical images that reduce the mortality rate and enhances a patient's survival. This review has also discussed the strategies related

S. Mallick (✉)
Department of Computer Science and Information Technology, WCTM, Gurgaon, Haryana, India

S. P. Mishra
Department of Computer Science and Information Technology, SHIATS, Allahabad, India

M. S. Kaiser et al. (eds.), *Proceedings of Trends in Electronics and Health Informatics*, Lecture Notes in Networks and Systems 376,
https://doi.org/10.1007/978-981-16-8826-3_12

to deep learning, procedures, and designs for different cancer detection, diagnoses, and predictions. The transcendent goal survey aims to introduce a short goal of presenting various disease growths and forecasting lung primary lung cancer in the lungs forecast using deep learning and AI models. Detection is sorted dependent on the area and size of the tumor [1]. However, few algorithms of machine learning that have an intense result on patient health are linear regression, random forest, SVM, and so on. During the beginning phases, it is hard to examine and recognize as this would not cause any ache. However, patients with lung cancer may suffer from shortness of breath, cough, wheezing, chest pain, cough, coughing up blood, shoulder pain, hoarseness, weight loss, fatigue, and weakness (Fig. 1).

90% of it is instigated because of smoking. Passive smoking causes lung cancer. Lung cancer is also hereditary. Factory gases, vehicle smoke, and the ingestion of harmful gases are causing the mortality rate of lung cancer. A gas name Radon is a noble gas and hazardous and causes lung cancer and leads to death. Table 1 shows some of the components which cause lung cancers and the death rate.

Doctors distinguish the presence and phase of disease by inciting different tests, for example, CT scan, bone scan, MRI outputs, x-ray, and PET sweeps.

Depending upon seriousness, NSCLC is split into four stages: In stage 1, this disease is restricted to lungs. In stage 2, it reaches to chest. Then in stage 3, it

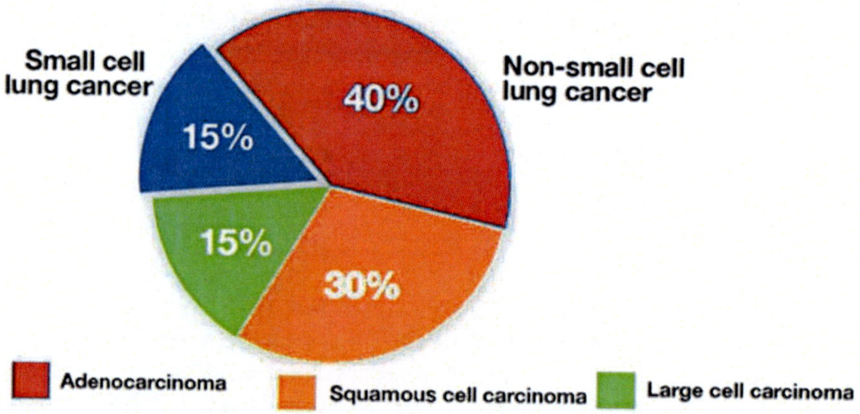

Fig. 1 Lung cancer type

Table 1 Lung cancer factors and its mortality rates [2]

Lung cancer causes	Mortality rate (%)
Smoking	90
Radon	12
Hazardous chemicals	30
Particle pollution	30
Genes	12

Table 2 Death due to lung cancer worldwide [4]

Continent	Deaths (%)
Africa	7.3
America	14.4
Asia	57.3
Europe	20.3

Table 3 Cases of lung cancer and mortality rate in India [4]

Lung Cancer	Deaths (%)
Both cases	21.0
Men	66
Women	23.4

bounded to the chest anyway amid more extensive and significant assertive tumors. Stage 4: developed in different parts of the body. The two-layered model controls SCLC type drug [3]. Table 2 shows the cause of lung cancer globally.

Due to lung cancer, the mortality rate of India is rising, and Table 3 shows the list.

2 Algorithms of Machine Learning

It is seen that the most accurate and effective image-based analysis in machine learning algorithms is support vector machine, k-nearest neighbor, and decision tree etc. [5].

i. **ANN:** ANN is a technique of data processing that is interconnected through components knows as neurons. Typically the neurons are arranged in layer or vector, with the output of one layer serving as an input to the next layer and possibly other layers. A neuron maybe connected to all or a subset of the neurons in the subsequent layers, with these connection simulating the synaptic connects of the brain. There are two steps to do it; first is training, and second is testing. The first step is the training step, and in the training step, it is used to classify the user inputs. The second step is the testing step, in which it analyzes the user input and scans its neurons and generates the output. The ANN approach is beneficial in the healthcare sector. This approach helps detect and predict lung, breast cancer, and other ontology predictions, like medications and symptomatic systems.

ii. **Support Vector Machine:** it is the most suitable method in terms of regression, classification, and forecasting. It draws a boundary based on the classified dataset into two parts which are called a hyperplane. The great resource of SVM is that it is an information determined methodology and without a practical and theoretical plan that creates a precise characterization, especially when the example size is limited. Support vector machines are extensively used to

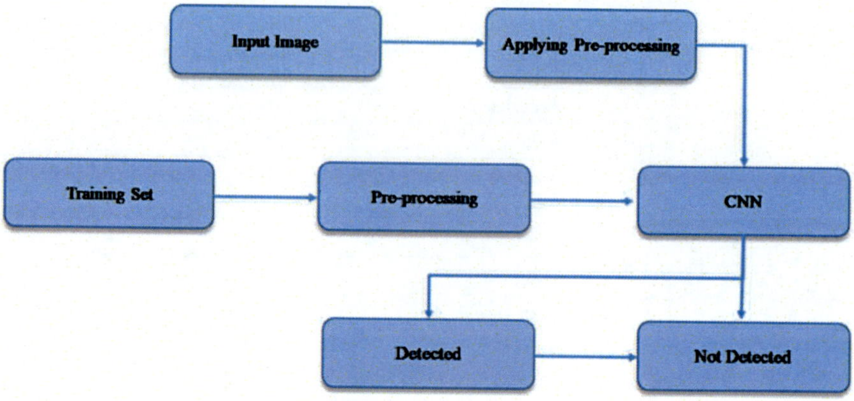

Fig. 2 Flow of CNN

detect and anticipate cancer growth cardiac arrest and neurological issues by for classifying the healthcare datasets.

iii. **Convolutional Neural Network:** The preprocessing needed in a ConvNet is a lot deeper when contrasted with various grouping predictions. CNN is a deep learning prediction that can take in an info picture, allocate significance (learnable loads and proneness) to different perspectives/objects in the image, and separate one from the other. While channels are manually trained, ConvNets can gain proficiency with these channels/attributes with enough preparation (Fig. 2).

iv. **Recurrent Neural Network (RNN):** RNN uses a similar approach for a sequence of components, and the results depend upon the former output. Therefore, the data of the last year is used to analyze which was stored in the memory. It is a development model of the neural network that provides the output network to re-input the network. The RNN architecture uses an Elman-based network with a feedback link from the hidden layer of the input layer.

3 Review of Literature

Janee et al. [6] state that this algorithm was developed in MATLAB and employ gray level cooccurrences method (GLCM) that enhance, segment, detect, and extract the feature of images. For classification purposes, SVM is applied. Converting from gray scale to black and white is called binarization, and this approach is used to make the forecast. They used 600 non-infected and 600 infected CT scan images which are taken from the UCI ML website. The proposed plan identified 126 photos as tainted out of 130 and anticipated 87 views as destructive total of hundred once indicated pictures. The testing result has an accuracy of 97% that recognizable proof and 87% for forecast. Gomathi et al. [7] characterized "A Computer-Aided Diagnosis System for Detection of Lung Cancer Nodules utilizing Extreme Learning Machine." To detect malignancy in CT images, this paper created a CAD model. The necessary period of CAD is to distinguish the district of interest in input CT scan pictures.

Firstly, the lung region segmentation is done; after that, region of the lung is extracted. To detect the cancer nodules, an FPCM clustering algorithm is applied. To formulate the diagnostic rules, a maximum draw able circle intensity value is used. After this step, extreme learning machine (ELM) accompanying with the previous rule is used to train. A most extreme draw able circle force esteem is utilized for defining the analytic guidelines. Then, at that point, these standards are carried out to learn alongside the help of the extreme learning machine (ELM). Takeda et al. [8] suggested a model for detecting lumps in lungs within the chest layer; this is called the CAD layer. The CAD model presented in this paper involves a picture worker and EpiSight/XR programming. This strategy is completed in four essential advances:

- The central collection programmed structure is decreased to deliver various pictures.
- Multiple gray level thresholding methods are used to identify nodule candidates.
- To extract the features, different images are used which distinguish the exact nodules and false positive nodules from chosen images.

Earlier, to reduce the rate of false positive, feature extraction is used. For this purpose, ANN and rule-based analysis are applied. For testing the developed model, the database of 274 radiographs and 323 lung nodules were analyzed. A total of 315 images were considered in which 235(75%) of images are detected as false positive as a normal automatic structure, and pulmonary vessels are detected as 155(49%).

Metin et al. [9] suggested "Lung nodule detection on thoracic computed tomography images: Preliminary evaluation of a computer-aided diagnosis system." The suggested strategy is done in five stages; the first step is to use k-means clustering for segmentation. The suspicious areas are segmented, which causes gaps in the lung areas that generate binarization images, Flood—the filled algorithm—is utilized to filling this gap as nodule candidate is considering as complex instances. The technique may contain a common domain and bud of lungs, containing vessels of blood. Rule-based classifiers using 2D and 3D elements are used to differentiate the buds. Finally, LDA has helped to identify the false positive items. The proposed strategy was broken down on a dataset containing 1454CT pictures accumulated from 34 determined patients to have 63 lung knobs.

Awai et al. [10] depicted a framework for assessing the computer-aided diagnosis impact on radiologist's aspiratory knobs identification. A projected strategy utilized picture preparing methods for intrapulmonary and lung design division dim level limit, 3D naming strategies, and numerical morphological procedures for lung division. For the division of intrapulmonary designs, the top-cap change technique is utilized on an info picture to recognize the smoothed picture. A sifter channel is utilized to recognize essential possible knobs, then, at that point, highlights of these aspiratory knobs are removed to separate genuine knobs from that of bogus positive knobs; ANN is adjusted to choose the likelihood of locale of premium dependent on a picture include. Adaption of this framework improved pneumonic knob occupant's discovery of computed tomography examines. Cheran et al. [11] suggested "PC helped conclusion for lung CT utilizing counterfeit life models." This CAD model is created by sending different calculations. In the first place, the ribcage area is dictated by utilizing a 3D part developing calculation. Then, at that point, the dynamic shape method is executed to make a particular region for the moving toward insects, which are reallocated to foster a specific and exact modifying of the vascular tree and pleura. To recover the bronchial and the vascular trees, fake life models are utilized. By using dynamic shape models, it is resolved whether the recently built branches contain knobs and identify whether the knobs are associated with the pleura. Utilizing calculations like snakes and dab upgrade cleaner calculation is delivered to bind the nodules.

4 Comparison of CT Scan and X-Rays in Lung Detection

4.1 X-Ray

For the detection and identification of medical-related problems, an x-ray is widely used. The widely used x-ray is electromagnetic radiation that helps form images of body parts like lungs, blood vessels, heart, spine, chest, and airways. Generally, x-ray images generate photographic films that need to process before viewing. A digital x-ray is used to solve this issue. In Fig. 3, we show the various examples of chest x-ray which have different lung conditions, collected from other data sources [12].

4.2 CT Scan

It is a type of radiography that creates sectional images through computer processing. Sectional images consist of patient's body images with various angles and can display the parts of images individually.

The images can also be merged to generate 3D images. The 3D pictures can show the skeleton, tissues, and organs of patients that reveal the anomalies. It is seen that CT scan images reveal detailed information compared to X-rays. CT scan images have been taken from various datasets, which is shown in Fig. 4. It is seen that CT scan is widely used in lung disease detection.

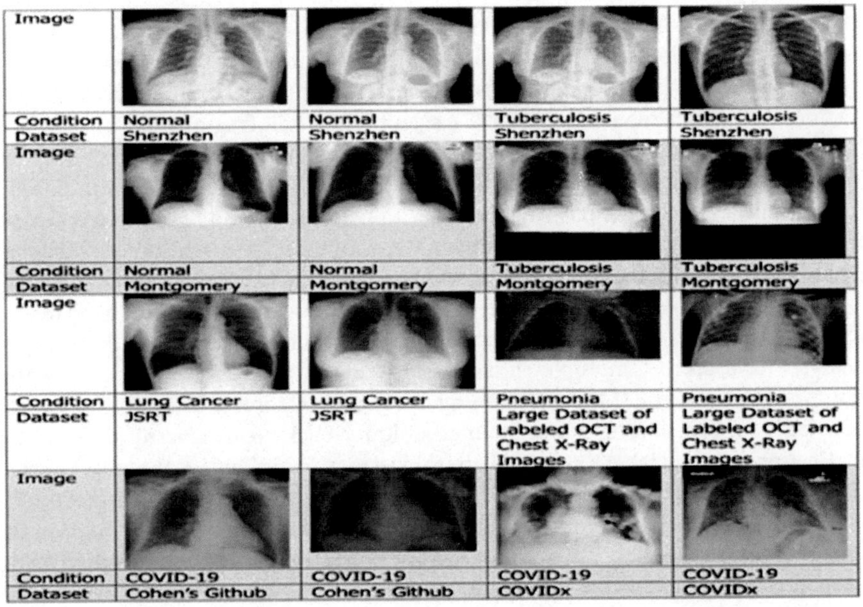

Fig. 3 Chest x-ray images instance

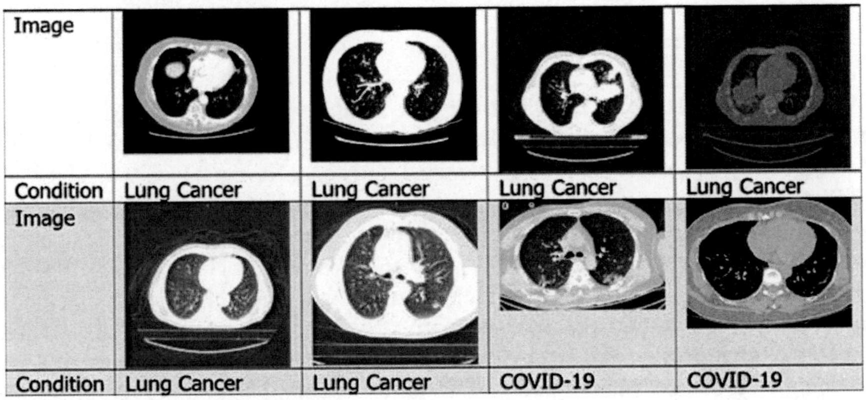

Fig. 4 CT scan images dataset

5 Discussion and Analysis

This approach focuses on lungs classification-based AI strategies to detect lung cancer. Most of the results investigated in writing depended on CT scan pictures, and some utilized x-rays images. Furthermore, in the two cases, the cellular breakdown in the lungs identification system applies through the accompanying stages.

Preprocessing: This is the primary stage where images such as CT scan and the x-ray is considered. Then, at that point, we will apply a few procedures of picture processing, for example, thresholding, denoising, binarization, and standardization. After that, segmentation of CT scan picture will fragment the similar and different areas. For instance, numerous division strategies, marker-controlled watershed, marker-controlled watershed with masking, and area stretching, have utilized in the literature. The watersheds with the concealing technique got higher outcomes are shown in Table 1. At last, it can separate the highlights to be ready for the following stage, addressed by characterization.

Classification: In this stage, the removed highlights are taken care of to the predetermined classifier to order them as ordinary and threatening as needs are. The analysts have utilized multiple classifiers in writing, for example, neural network, multi-facet perceptron (MLP), Naïve Bayes, support vector machine, KNN, gradient boosted tree, decision tree, multinomial arbitrary backwoods classifier, stochastic inclination plunge, Naive Bayes, and group classifier. From Table 1, the most remarkable accuracy output was about 97% acquired by Alam et al. [6] utilizing a multi-class SVM classifier and embracing marker-controlled watershed-based division for picture division. Then again, every one of the works that have been executed using deep learning techniques has the highest accuracy of 99%, where the most meaningful outcome was about by Li et al. [] using various-goal fix CNN.

6 Conclusion

When failure of lungs is examined early, it would be valuable because the drug will then, at that point, be started to keep the illness from having an unsafe outcome. Subsequently, this paper sums up an itemized study on different AI ways to deal with arrange lung malignancies utilizing either CT examine pictures or x-beam pictures. Additionally, scientists have been used multiple classifiers in writing, like neural network, support vector machine, MLP, gradient boosted tree, Naïve Bayes, decision tree, k-nearest neighbors, stochastic inclination plunge, multinomial arbitrary woods classifier, and group classifier. Subsequently, the work has been accomplished and given the broad review; it tends to be presumed that the strategies which used deep learning methods got higher outcomes as far as exactness than other old styles AI procedures, where the most elevated effect was about 99% utilizing multi-goal fix-based CNN.

References

1. Demyanov S, Chakravorty R, Abedini M, Halpern A, Garnavi R (2016) Classification of dermoscopy patterns using deep convolutional neural networks. In: IEEE 13th International symposium on biomedical imaging (ISBI), 2016 IEEE2016, pp 364–368

2. ICMR-National Institute of Cancer Prevention & Research (ICMRNICPR).
3. Lung cancer symptoms, types, causes, treatment & diagnosis. https://www.medicinenet.com/lung_cancer/article.htm
4. The International Agency for Research on Cancer (IARC). Latest global cancer data.
5. Lakshmanaprabu SKG, Mohanty SN, Shankar K, Arunkumar N, Ramirez G (2018) Optimal deep learning model for classification of lung cancer on CT images. Future Gener Comput Syst
6. Janee Alam S, Hossan A (2018) Multi-stage lung cancer detection and prediction using multi-class SVM classifier. In: 2018 International conference on computer, communication, chemical, material and electronic engineering (IC4ME2)
7. Gomathi M, Thangaraj P (2010) A computer-aided diagnosis system for detection of lung cancer nodules using extreme learning machine. Int J Eng Sci Technol 2(10): 5770–5779
8. Kakeda S, Moriya J, Sato H, Aoki T, Watanabe H, Nakata DK (2004) Improved detection of lung nodules on chest radiographs using a commercial computer-aided diagnosis system. Am J Roentgenlogy 182(2):505–510. https://doi.org/10.2214/ajr.182.2.1820505
9. Gurcan MN, Sahiner B, Petrick N, Chan H-P, Kazerooni EA, Cascade PN, Hadjiiski L (2002) Lung nodule detection on thoracic computed tomography images: preliminary evaluation of a computer aided diagnosis system. Med Phys 29(11):2552–2558. https://doi.org/10.1118/1.1515762
10. Awai K, Murao K, Ozawa A, Komi M, Hayakawa H, Hori S, Nishimura Y (2004) Pulmonary nodules at chest CT: effect of computer- aided diagnosis on radiologists' detection performance. Radiology 230(2):347352. https://doi.org/10.1148/radiol.2302030049
11. Cheran SC, Gargano G (2005) Computer-aided diagnosis for lung CT using artificial life models. In: Seventh international symposium on symbolic and numeric algorithms for scientific computing (SYNASC'05). https://doi.org/10.1109/synasc.2005.28
12. Kieu STH, Bade A, Hijazi MHA, Kolivand H. A survey of deep learning for lung disease detection on medical images: state-of-the-art, taxonomy, issues and future directions
13. Nasr-Esfahani E, Samavi S, Karimi N, Soroushmehr SMR, Jafari MH, Ward K, Najarian K (2016) Melanoma detection by analysis of clinical images using convolutional neural network. In: 2016 IEEE 38th Annual international conference of the engineering in medicine and biology society (EMBC), IEEE2016, pp 1373–1376

Toward Machine Learning-Based Psychological Assessment of Autism Spectrum Disorders in School and Community

Sabbir Ahmed, Md. Farhad Hossain, Silvia Binte Nur, M. Shamim Kaiser, and Mufti Mahmud

Abstract The sensory processing system of the human body is capable of collecting, developing, and integrating information through sensory organs. Sensory impairment has been discovered in children with autism spectrum disorder (ASD). People with ASD are susceptible to hyper/hypo-sensitivity that might cause changes in information management, affect cognitive impairment, and social reactions to everyday events. This article proposed a questionnaire based on ASD symptoms found in previous studies with 82 questions. Following that, a dataset is created by conducting a survey using the questionnaire. Several machine learning models that can identify ASD and its types are also compared. Among the machine learning models, the artificial neural network achieved an accuracy of 89.8%. Implicit measurements and ecologically sound settings have shown excellent precision in predicting outcomes and the correct classification of populations into categories.

Keywords Autism spectrum disorder (ASD) · Questionnaire · Support vector machine (SVM) · k-nearest neighbors (KNN) · Random forest (RF) · Artificial neural network (ANN)

1 Introduction

According to the Centers for Disease Control and Prevention, 17 % of children aged three to seventeen were diagnosed with a developmental disability between 2009 and 2017 [1]. Autism spectrum disorder (ASD) is a group of complicated develop-

S. Ahmed (✉) · Md. F. Hossain · S. B. Nur · M. Shamim Kaiser
Institute of Information Technology, Jahangirnagar University, Savar, Dhaka 1342, Bangladesh
e-mail: mskaiser@juniv.edu

M. Shamim Kaiser
Applied Intelligence and Informatics (AII), Wazed Miah Science Research Centre (WMSRC), Jahangirnagar University, Savar, Dhaka 1342, Bangladesh

M. Mahmud
Department of Computer Science, Nottingham Trent University, Nottingham NG1 4FQ, UK

M. S. Kaiser et al. (eds.), *Proceedings of Trends in Electronics and Health Informatics*, Lecture Notes in Networks and Systems 376,
https://doi.org/10.1007/978-981-16-8826-3_13

ment in social contact, speech, and non-verbal expression, and restricted/repetitive behavior that entails ongoing difficulties [2]. In each person, the causes of ASD and the seriousness of the symptoms vary. ASD has been diagnosed in every 1 in 270 people in the world [3]. In the United States of America alone, 1 out of every 54 children has been diagnosed with ASD. Hence, early detection of ASD creates awareness both in the family and socially, enables better care and less negligence for diagnosed individuals, and results in overall better psychological growth. Even though there may be few visible physical impairments, people with ASD suffer from significant psychological sickness. Since there are no physical attributes quantifiable in lab tests, ASD diagnosis has been quite difficult until now. Doctors analyze communication, social, and behavioral development data to make a decision. The Diagnostic and Statistical Manual of Mental Disorders (DSM-5) [2] and Autism Diagnostic Observation Schedule (ADOS) [4], the two most often used manuals, have made a difference in detecting ASD. DSM-5 defined two key domains of ASD in order to assess impairment: (1) communication and social interaction and (2) restricted interests and repetitive behaviors. On the other hand, ADOS evaluation utilizes planned social circumstances to generate target responses and interpersonal interactions divided into four modules. These modules are suited to people depending on their language and stage of development to guarantee that a varied range of behavioral events are covered. Nonetheless, the psychometric features of each method are restricted, dependent on outdated diagnostic standards, various behaviors, restrictions on present operation, and age.

Complex characteristics and symptoms of developmental and cognitive disorders add complications to classifying in clinical decision making as well as deterministic computational methods. Machine learning (ML) algorithms have been utilized broadly to solve developmental disorders, specifically ASD [5, 6]. Hyde et al. [7] addressed the effectiveness of utilizing ML for autism identification and reviewed several detection methods. These methods include detection of behavioral and neuroimaging data, behavioral and developmental data, genetic data, and electronic health records. Reviewed methods include classifiers like support vector machine (SVM), alternating decision tree (AD Tree), neural networks (NN), random forest (RF), logistic regression (LR), decision tree (DT), random tree (RT), Bayesian network (BN), naive Bayes (NB), and more. Our contribution is this paper is given below:

- We have prepared a questionnaire based on ASD symptoms found in previous studies with 82 questions;
- We have conducted a survey in schools and communities leveraging the questionnaire and prepared a dataset;
- We have found the most salient signs that distinguish ASD children from non-ASD children;
- On the created dataset, we compared various machine learning classifiers.

The remainder of the paper is structured as follows: The Sect. 2 reviews the literature; the Sect. 3 discusses the proposed methodology. Section 4 contains the experimental analysis, and Sect. 5 concludes the work.

2 Literature Review

Ample research has been conducted related to ASD, its types, symptoms, and detection. Faras et al. [8] classified autism as a pervasive developmental disorder (PDD) and categorized ASD as autistic disorders (AD), Asperger's syndrome (AS), childhood disintegrative disorder (CDD), pervasive developmental disorder-not otherwise specified (PDD-NOS) and Rett syndrome (RS). Biomarkers related to cognitive, behavioral, visual, and structural connectivity have demonstrated promise in several clinical screening and diagnostic procedures, like ADOS, DSM-5, Autism Diagnostic Interview-Revised (ADI-R), Developmental, Dimensional and Diagnostic Interview (3di), and Social Responsiveness Scale (SRS, SRS-2) [9]. Clinical standards, however, usually require the involvement of multidisciplinary teams in ASD diagnosis, and these processes need substantial amounts of time. Berument et al. [10] developed an autism screening questionnaire (ASQ) with 40 different ASD symptoms and tested a total of 200 individuals. In ASQ, though, there was less distinction between autism from other PDD kinds. Sadek et al. [11] investigated different categories for autism identification and analyzed various types of detection systems that use machine learning, computer vision, and neural networks. Rahman et al. [12] recommended several ways to accelerate the execution of data processing for detecting ASD using ML. They have also looked into several techniques for identifying and processing imbalanced data in these detection techniques. Raj and Masood [13] combined three publicly available datasets and performed a performance comparison of LR, SVM, NN, NB, and convolutional neural network (CNN) with the highest accuracy of 99.53%. Rule-based ML can also be used in autism screening, which further provides understanding to clinical professionals. Thabtah and Peebles [14] proposed such methods and tested them on adult, adolescent, and toddler datasets. Omar et al. [15] combined random forest-CART and random forest-ID3, evaluated it on a similar dataset, and then deployed the trained model in a mobile app. In more recent literature, Hossain et al. [16] tested 25 machine learning classifiers in a collected ASD dataset and concluded that SVM based on sequential minimal optimization (SMO) performs better in their experimental scenario. All aspects of the physiological and psychological activities are hard to be cataloged by health professionals [17]. Hence, a physiological outcome monitoring system that records continuous communication and behavioral changes produce intuition of the patient's well-being [18]. Again these systems assess health professionals to monitor the growth in different contexts [19].

3 Methodology

Symptoms: Seltzer et al. [20] discovered that patients with ASD show a tendency to query inappropriately, spontaneously imitate, lack interest in people, difficulty sharing meals, and repetitive use of objects. Faras et al. [8] explored red flags indicating

ASD in participants and described delays in speaking, repetitive play with toys, and communication difficulties. In addition, there was a lack of facial expression, pretend play, imagination, interest in playing near peers on purpose, ability to comprehend sarcasm, and awareness of personal space. According to Baskin et al. [21], individuals with Asperger syndrome manifest an inflexible adherence to specific nonfunctional routines, schizophrenia, repetitive and stereotyped motor mannerisms, and limited fields of interest. Mirkovic and Gérardin [22] discovered that people engage with others who share similar interests, struggle to maintain and develop acceptable peer relationships, and prefer social isolation. Karabekiroglu et al. researched PDD-NOS symptoms and discovered that the participants exhibit unusual non-verbal movement, lack of eye contact while interacting, hyperactivity and hostility, and inappropriate laughter [23]. Snow and Lecavalier [24] identified a concern with rule-breaking and aggressive conduct, as well as anxiety and depression among PDD-NOS patients. Mehra et al. examined symptoms of childhood disintegrative disorder and discovered that the participants exhibited limited interest, lack of imagination, sleep problems, and decreased motor abilities [25]. Elia et al. observed that the diagnosis of autistic disorder can be based on the first REM delay, muscle twitches density, and rapid eye movement density [26]. Repetitive behaviors may not be significant characteristics of autistic disorder; nevertheless, Militerni et al. [27] discovered that younger subjects demonstrated repetitive motor and sensory behaviors, whereas older youngsters with higher IQ scores demonstrated complex repetitive behaviors. Hagberg et al. [28] discovered that the key clinical features of Rett syndrome are severe progressive dementia and unusual hand movements. Kyle et al. [29] investigated the four stages of Rett syndrome: slow head circumference growth, microcephaly, scoliosis, and wheelchair dependency.

Questionnaire: Previous similar checklists such as Mchat [8] are primarily focused on specific age groups. On the other hand, though DSM-5 [2] gave an overview of symptoms in ASD, the direct questionnaire has not been provided. Again, a straightforward question by asking whether any of the symptoms are present or not in individuals may carry a certain level of human error. The severity of these issues may remain unclear. As a result, a scenario-based severity scaled question was also required. Thus, the creation of a question set for determining ASD and its types was necessary. A questionnaire derived from the symptoms mentioned above has been listed in detail in Fig. 1 with relevant ASD types, which allows measuring across the whole spectrum of autism. The questionnaire consists of 24 questions, with 82 fields representing options for these questions. These questions enable discrimination of the three major components of autism. Each of these options was then graded on a five-point scale. Age, gender, ASD types, and other miscellaneous questions also have been added to the survey.

Participation and procedure: The collection of data from various people of various ages with clinically diagnosed ASD has been the survey's main focus. The scenario of each question has been portrayed in such a way that it can be relatable with all kinds of individuals: toddlers, children, adolescents, and adults. A Google Form has been prepared with multiple-choice options from the questionnaire. The form was sent to

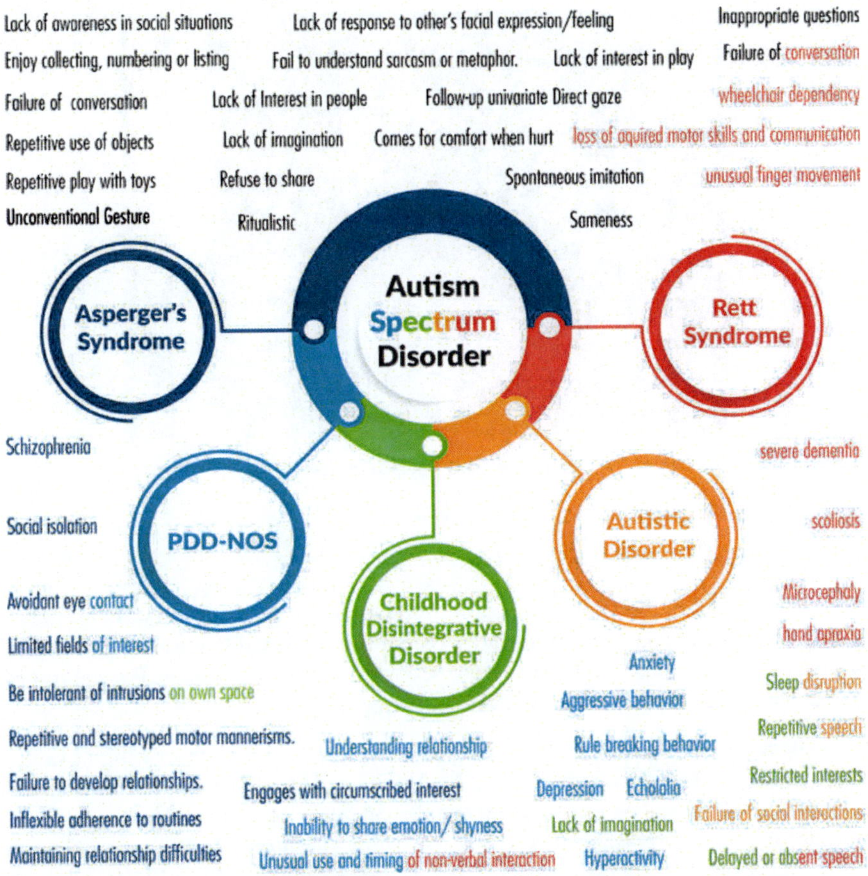

Fig. 1 Symptoms of ASD and types differentiated by color

an autism specialized school, doctors, and students for completion. Filled results have been checked respectively to find out the anomaly. A separate form with the same questionnaire has been sent to ordinary educational institutions. Only form responses correspond to participants who had no prior disorders and were subsequently labeled as neurotypical.

Dataset details and data distribution: There are 71 data instances in the collection; all acquired from the same number of people. The participants were split into two groups: 42 men and 29 women. The ages of the participants ranged from four to twenty-seven, with an average of 18.8 years. The participants filled out 38 forms, family members filled out 32 forms, and a health professional filled out one. Thirty-nine participants were neurotypical, while 32 were clinically diagnosed with ASD, including 16 AD, 4 AS, 4 CDD, 4 RS, and 4 PDD-NOS patients. Figure 2 represents the relationship of responses with the particular question, whereas color represents

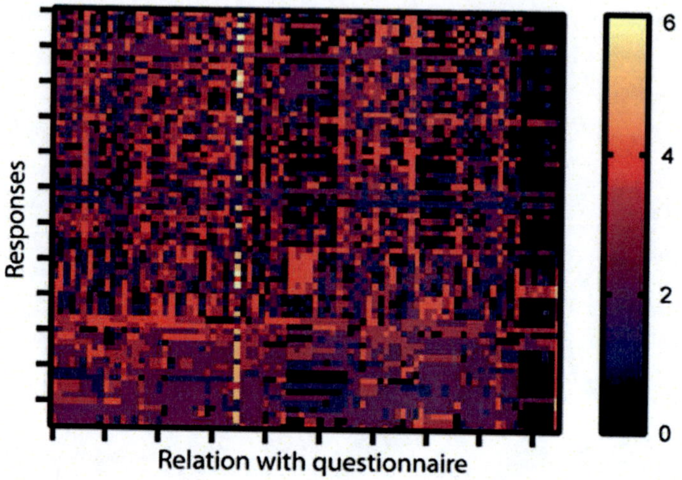

Fig. 2 Values of responses corresponds to questionnaire

the value of each field. The last few questions in the proposed questionnaire delineate physical impairment, which is nonexistent for most ASD cases except for Rett syndrome. Hence, those fields have been occupied with lower values. For the rest of the questionnaire, the values were evenly distributed.

ASD Detection Using ML: Four machine learning techniques, namely support vector machine(SVM), k-nearest neighbors (KNN), random forest(RF), and artificial neural network(ANN), have been utilized for the classification of ASD and its types. SVM assumes data points as support vectors and uses hyperplanes to separate data into classes. One vs. one has been selected as a decision function shape in SVM, which calculates a hyperplane for two classes at a time. Radial basis function (RBF) has been utilized as the kernel. On the other hand, KNN groups together data points based on similarities or distance. The number of neighbors for ASD classification is selected as 20. RF is an ensemble classifier consisting of multiple decision trees, where each tree predicts the output, and the final prediction is given on the majority vote. In the experiment, the number of estimators is set as 20 with two random states and a max depth of 15. SVM, KNN, and SVM have been implemented using the Scikit-learn library. The proposed ANN consists of one input layer, three fully connected hidden layers, two batch normalization layers, two dropout layers, and an output layer. The number of neurons in hidden layers is 32, 256, and 64, respectively. The first two hidden layers utilize rectified linear unit (ReLU) as the activation function, whereas a sigmoid is used in the last hidden layer and the output layer. For loss function, categorical cross-entropy has been used with adam optimizer. All of the ML classifiers have been executed for 100 epochs.

4 Experimental Analysis

Correlation analysis assesses the extent and orientation of the relationship between input and output variables; in this case, values of each question and ASD categories. Figure 3 shows the top 18 symptoms with the highest correlation value, where blue represents negative correlation and red represents positive correlation.

The severity of the dataset has been transformed into numerical values ranging from 0 to 4. The occurrence of any specific value was then determined using the mean value of the symptoms in ASD and neurotypical individuals. Figure 5 depicts the seven symptoms with the highest association between ASD types and neurotypical traits. To determine the most common symptoms among ASD categories, the correlation between ASD types and questionnaires was evaluated individually. In Fig. 6, the symptoms with the highest correlation have been depicted with a mean value. As a result of principal component analysis (PCA), datasets become more interpretable while avoiding performance degradation. It accomplishes this by generating new negatively correlated parameters that sequentially optimize variance–principal component analysis of two components in the ASD dataset depicted in Fig. 7. The dataset has been split into 20% data for testing and 80% data for training. Four

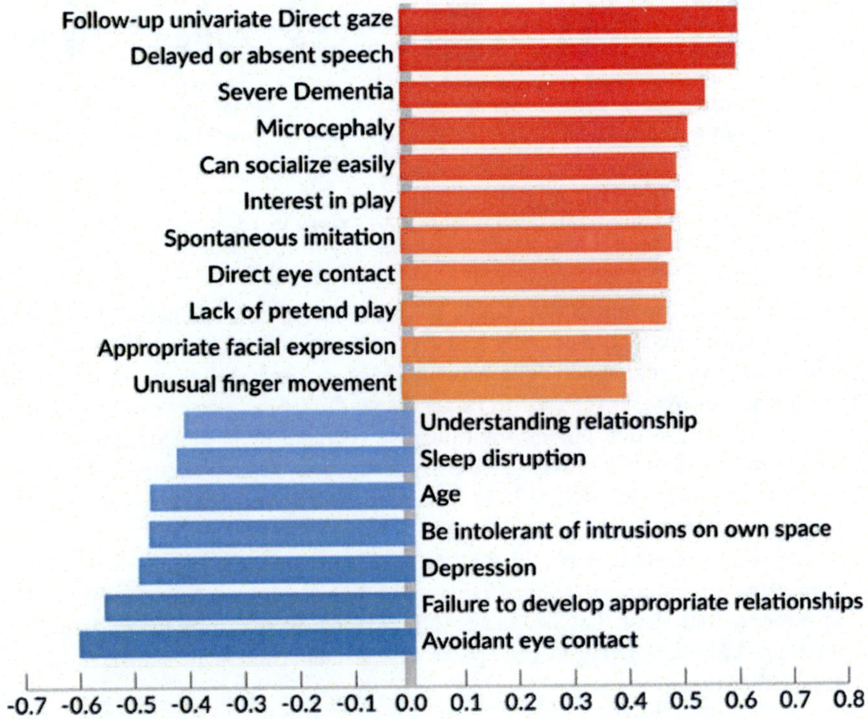

Fig. 3 ASD symptoms with most correlation in dataset

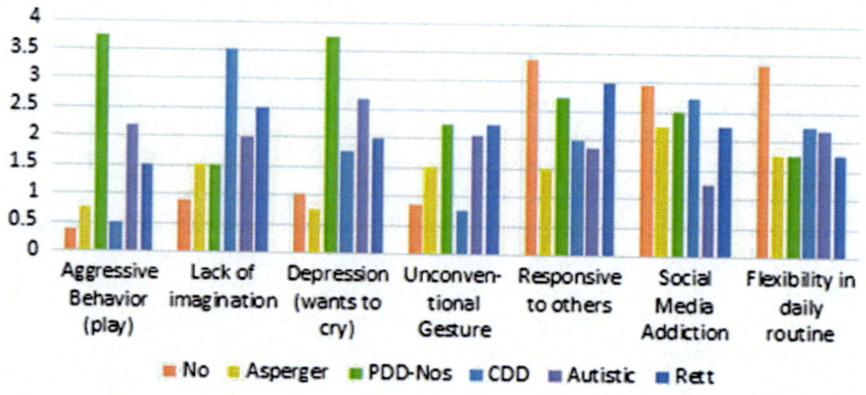

Fig. 4 Comparison of performance metrics in testing data among ML classifiers

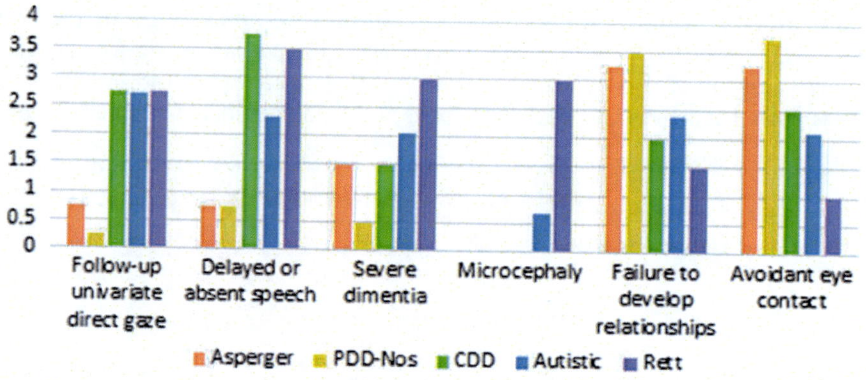

Fig. 5 Mean value of symptoms relevant to ASD types and neurotypical

machine learning models (SVM, KNN, RF, ANN) have been trained and tested on the accumulated dataset. Accuracy and $F1$-Score have been calculated for model performance and comparison. The percentage of correctly predicted classes, both positive and negative, is referred to as accuracy. $F1$-score is the weighted average of accurate classification among total positive predictions and valid classification among correct positive and false negative predictions. Testing accuracy for SVM, KNN, RF, and ANN was 89%, 78%, 83%, and 89.8%, respectively, with training accuracy near 100% for all classifiers. The achieved $F1$-Score of SVM, KNN, RF, and ANN in testing data is 86, 73, 83, and 85% subsequently. Figure 4 depicts the comparison of accuracy, recall, precision and $F1$-Score among ML classifiers. The evaluation metrics show that SVM and ANN perform significantly better than KNN and RF for ASD classification. The epoch-wise test and train AUC and loss of ANN is depicted at Fig. 8.

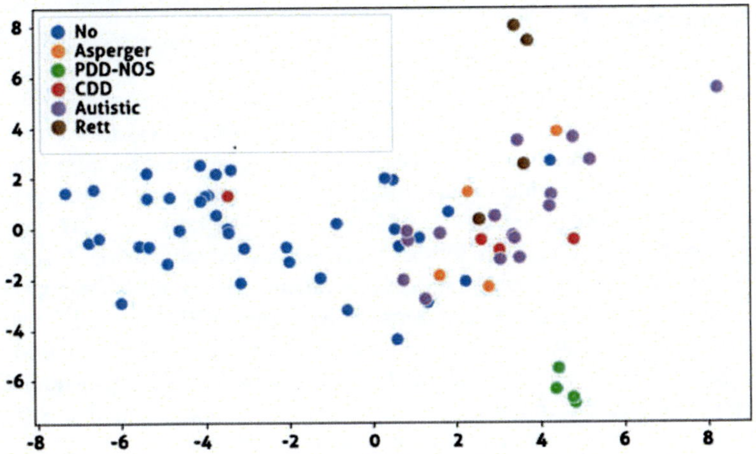

Fig. 6 Mean value of symptoms relevant to ASD types

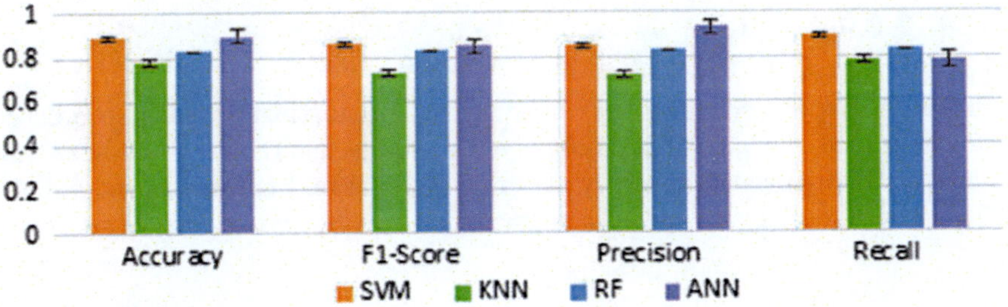

Fig. 7 PCA analysis of dataset

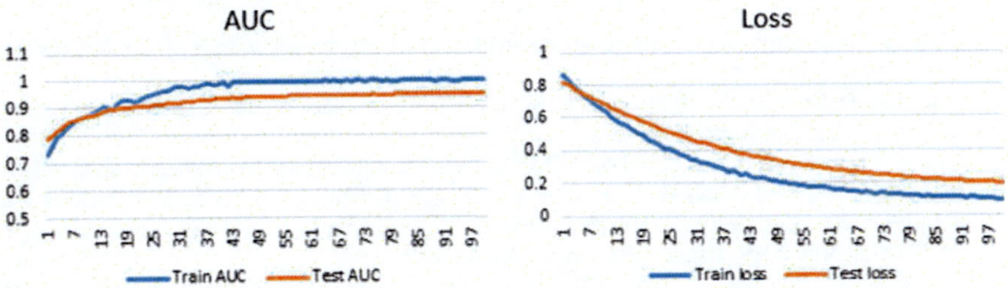

Fig. 8 Epochwise Area Under Curve (AUC) and Categorical Cross-entropy loss of ANN

5 Conclusion

The early and quick diagnostic method of ASD allows early intervention and medical treatment, which reduces the risk significantly. ASD refers to a broad range of psychological deficits that differ in each individual. Hence, detecting autism has been complicated by considering all possible physical and psychological problems. In this article, we have accumulated and analyzed a wide range of ASD symptoms, then converted these symptoms into a scenario-based questionnaire. A survey has been conducted to collect data using a questionnaire. Then, correlation analysis and PCA are used to find out the most prominent symptoms. SVM, KNN, RF, and ANN classifiers have been trained and tested for the classification task. Though ML classifiers achieved good performance, the limited dataset size is a major limitation of this study. In the future, input such as video, voice, and image data that correspond to symptoms can be collected with an open-source platform.

Ethical Approval

All procedures performed in studies involving human participants were in accordance with the ethical standards of the Biosafety, Biosecurity, and Ethical Clearance Committee of Jahangirnagar University, Savar, 1342 - Dhaka, Bangladesh and with the 1964 Helsinki declaration and its later amendments or comparable ethical standards.

References

1. Data & statistics on autism spectrum disorder (2020). https://www.cdc.gov/ncbddd/autism/data.html
2. Association AP et al (2012) Diagnostic and statistical manual of mental disorders (DSM-5®). American Psychiatric Publications
3. Vos T, Lim SS, Abbafati C, Abbas KM, Abbasi M, Abbasifard M, Abbasi-Kangevari M, Abbastabar H, Abd-Allah F, Abdelalim A et al (2020) Global burden of 369 diseases and injuries in 204 countries and territories, 1990–2019: a systematic analysis for the global burden of disease study 2019. Lancet 396(10258):1204–1222
4. Lord C, Risi S, Lambrecht L, Cook EH, Leventhal BL, DiLavore PC, Pickles A, Rutter M (2000) The autism diagnostic observation schedule-generic: a standard measure of social and communication deficits associated with the spectrum of autism. J Autism Dev Disorders 30(3):205–223
5. Biswas M, Kaiser MS, Mahmud M, Al Mamun S, Hossain M, Rahman MA et al (2021) An XAI based autism detection: The context behind the detection. In: International conference on brain informatics. Springer, pp 448–459
6. Ghosh T, Al Banna MH, Rahman MS, Kaiser MS, Mahmud M, Hosen AS, Cho GH (2021) Artificial intelligence and internet of things in screening and management of autism spectrum disorder. Sustain Cities Soc 74:103189
7. Hyde KK, Novack MN, LaHaye N, Parlett-Pelleriti C, Anden R, Dixon DR, Linstead E (2019) Applications of supervised machine learning in autism spectrum disorder research: a review. Rev J Autism Dev Disorders 6(2):128–146

8. Faras H, Al Ateeqi N, Tidmarsh L (2010) Autism spectrum disorders. Ann Saudi Med 30(4):295–300
9. Zwaigenbaum L, Penner M (2018) Autism spectrum disorder: advances in diagnosis and evaluation. BMJ 361
10. Berument SK, Rutter M, Lord C, Pickles A, Bailey A (1999) Autism screening questionnaire: diagnostic validity. Br J Psychiatry 175(5):444–451
11. Sadek ET, AbdElSabour Seada NA, Ghoniemy S (2020) Computer vision techniques for autism symptoms detection and recognition: a survey. Int J Intell Comput Inf Sci 20(2):89–111
12. Rahman M, Usman OL, Muniyandi RC, Sahran S, Mohamed S, Razak RA et al (2020) A review of machine learning methods of feature selection and classification for autism spectrum disorder. Brain Sci 10(12):949
13. Raj S, Masood S (2020) Analysis and detection of autism spectrum disorder using machine learning techniques. Procedia Comput Sci 167:994–1004
14. Thabtah F, Peebles D (2020) A new machine learning model based on induction of rules for autism detection. Health Inf J 26(1):264–286
15. Omar KS, Mondal P, Khan NS, Rizvi MRK, Islam MN (2019) A machine learning approach to predict autism spectrum disorder. In: 2019 International conference on electrical, computer and communication engineering (ECCE). IEEE, pp 1–6
16. Hossain MD, Kabir MA, Anwar A, Islam MZ (2021) Detecting autism spectrum disorder using machine learning techniques. Health Inf Sci Syst 9(1):1–13
17. Alam ME, Kaiser MS, Hossain MS, Andersson K (2018) An IoT-belief rule base smart system to assess autism. In: 2018 4th International conference on electrical engineering and information & communication technology (iCEEiCT). IEEE, pp 672–676
18. Al Banna MH, Ghosh T, Taher KA, Kaiser MS, Mahmud M (2020) A monitoring system for patients of autism spectrum disorder using artificial intelligence. In: International conference on brain informatics. Springer, pp 251–262
19. Sumi AI, Zohora MF, Mahjabeen M, Faria TJ, Mahmud M, Kaiser MS (2018) fASSERT: A fuzzy assistive system for children with autism using internet of things. In: International conference on brain informatics. Springer, pp 403–412
20. Seltzer MM, Krauss MW, Shattuck PT, Orsmond G, Swe A, Lord C (2003) The symptoms of autism spectrum disorders in adolescence and adulthood. J Autism Dev Disorders 33(6):565–581
21. Baskin JH, Sperber M, Price BH (2006) Asperger syndrome revisited. Rev Neurol Dis 3(1):1–7
22. Mirkovic B, Gérardin P (2019) Asperger's syndrome: what to consider? L'encephale 45(2):169–174
23. Karabekiroglu K (2011) Pervasive developmental disorder-not otherwise specified: specifying and differentiating. In: Autism spectrum disorders: the role of genetics in diagnosis and treatment p. 17
24. Snow AV, Lecavalier L (2011) Comparing autism, PDD-NOS, and other developmental disabilities on parent-reported behavior problems: little evidence for ASD subtype validity. J Autism Dev Disorders 41(3):302–310
25. Mehra C, Sil A, Hedderly T, Kyriakopoulos M, Lim M, Turnbull J, Happe F, Baird G, Absoud M (2019) Childhood disintegrative disorder and autism spectrum disorder: a systematic review. Dev Med Child Neurol 61(5):523–534
26. Elia M, Ferri R, Musumeci SA, Del Gracco S, Bottitta M, Scuderi C, Miano G, Panerai S, Bertrand T, Grubar JC (2000) Sleep in subjects with autistic disorder: a neurophysiological and psychological study. Brain Dev 22(2):88–92
27. Militerni R, Bravaccio C, Falco C, Fico C, Palermo MT (2002) Repetitive behaviors in autistic disorder. Eur Child Adolescent Psychiatry 11(5):210–218
28. Hagberg B, Goutières F, Hanefeld F, Rett A, Wilson J (1985) Rett syndrome: criteria for inclusion and exclusion. Brain Dev 7(3):372–373
29. Kyle SM, Vashi N, Justice MJ (2018) Rett syndrome: a neurological disorder with metabolic components. Open Biol 8(2):170216

Design of an Intelligent Diabetes Prediction Model in Big Data Environment

Shampa Sengupta and Kumud Ranjan Pal

Abstract Diabetes is the root cause of various chronic diseases. Developing an intelligent diabetes prediction model can handle the disease efficiently. Disease data is big as it is generated from the patient details with their diagnosis reports. Disease dataset contains the disease features/attributes (symptoms) values of the patient objects. Designing of an efficient prediction model to handle the big data, feature selection is necessary. Sometimes classification result varies with different algorithms for the same dataset. In that case, an ensemble classification approach is the solution. Thus, two modules, such as feature selection and classification, are important to design an efficient prediction model. The paper proposes a diabetes prediction model to handle big data by using genetic algorithm and machine learning techniques in MapReduce framework implementation. In the first phase, genetic algorithm is used to select the optimized feature subset, and in the second phase, ensemble classification system is developed from this reduced subsystem by using classification algorithms Naïve Bayes, random forest, and KNN with majority voting technique. The proposed prediction model can identify the label of the test patient objects correctly. Diabetes dataset is collected from UCI repository to test the model.

Keywords Data mining · Big data · Genetic algorithm · Ensemble classification · Diabetes prediction

1 Introduction

At present, the change of life style are actually affecting people's food habits and physical activities. As a result, various types of chronic disease grow with the time. One of them is diabetes, the root cause for many people's death in the world.

S. Sengupta (✉)
Department of Information Technology, MCKV Institute of Engineering, Liluah, Howrah, West Bengal 711204, India

K. Ranjan Pal
Seharabazar C. K. Institution, Seharabazar, Bardhaman, West Bengal 713423, India

M. S. Kaiser et al. (eds.), *Proceedings of Trends in Electronics and Health Informatics*, Lecture Notes in Networks and Systems 376,
https://doi.org/10.1007/978-981-16-8826-3_14

According to WHO [1], 422 million people are suffering from diabetes worldwide. The number of cases of diabetes is increasing day by day. Diabetes can lead to many difficulties. Normally after consuming food, our body breaks down it into glucose and reach to cell for energy through the bloodstream. Diabetes is three types—Type 1, Type 2, and Type 3. Type 1 diabetes is known as insulin-dependent diabetes mellitus (IDDM) because this type of diabetic patient required insulin injection. Type 2 diabetes continues a shortage of insulin, which may also increase. This type of diabetes is recognized as non-insulin-dependent diabetes mellitus (NIDDM). Type 3 diabetes is known as gestational diabetes which is caused by hormonal changes during pregnancy. The chronic diagnosis depends on the information in the medical data collected by different healthcare industries. Data size is also increasing day by day over a lot of different sources like business processes, social media, etc., and remains both in the form of structured and unstructured.

The proposed prediction model in MapReduce framework is shown in Fig. 1. In the map phase, the whole training data is divided into a number of decision subsystems and assigned in different slave node. Each slave node is performing the feature selection and individual classification job by three existing base classifiers, namely Naïve Bayes, KNN, and random forest. Then, in the reduce phase, all the classification rules are combined with majority voting concept and generate the final classification rules for classification of the disease.

The primary contribution of the work is:

- How to process big data in healthcare domain for the better disease prediction result in MapReduce framework

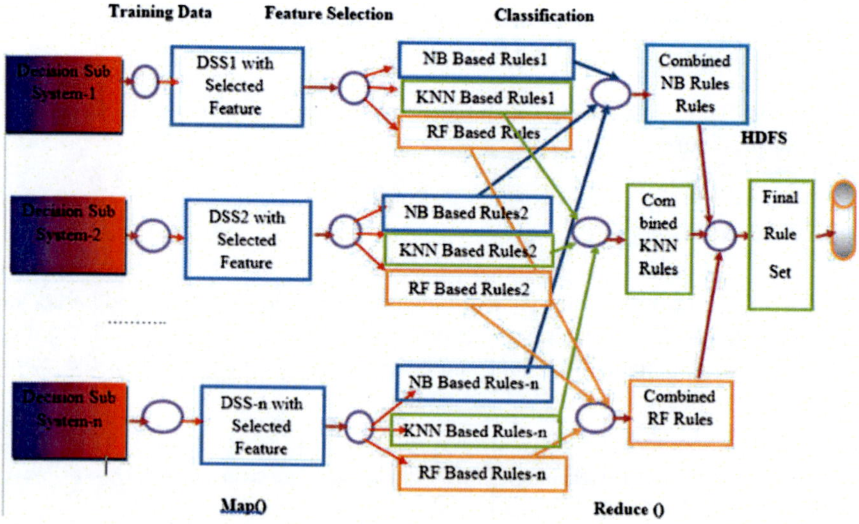

Fig. 1 Proposed diabetes prediction model in big data environment

- Optimal feature subset selection from the feature pool for the big datasets for efficient classification using genetic algorithm
- Development of an efficient ensemble classification System for improved disease prediction results using machine learning techniques in big data environment.

In the paper, Sect. 2 describes the big data in prediction of diabetes, where Sect. 3 describes the working of the prediction model in big data environment. Section 4 shows the experimental results. Section 5 presents the salient features of the method with the conclusion and future scope.

2 Big Data in Diabetes Prediction

Big data [2, 3] describes the huge volume of data that is growing exponentially with time. Big data processing includes data storage, data analysis, data sharing and data mining. Data can be the combination of structured, unstructured and semi-structured data collected from various sources. The characteristic of big data can be expressed by the 5 V's. "Volume" is the huge size of data. This is the amount of generated data. A particular data can be really considered as big data or not dependent on the volume of data. The term "velocity" represents the speed at which data is generated. "Variety" defines the nature and heterogeneous sources of data that can be categorized into structured, unstructured, and semi-structured. "Value" represents the usefulness of data that we can extract. "Veracity" refers to the accuracy of data. Big data is defined as high-velocity, high-veracity, and high-volume data that demands innovative methods to get the knowledge from the data. Big data processing can be applied in various disciplines like science, engineering, business, and as well as health care. The aim of big data processing is to get the insights of the data to help in decision-making job by reducing the processing time. To extract the resultant data from the big data, various tools, models, and technologies have been proposed by the different researchers. Hadoop [4, 5] is one of the popular tools that allow for massively parallel computing used in big data processing.

To manage the healthcare data efficiently for data mining and pattern recognition [6] purpose, the dimensionality of the data is required to be reduced for getting the efficient prediction model. Feature selection [7] and reduct computation [7–10], a term of rough set theory [8–10] is frequently used as a preprocessing step for knowledge discovery [11, 12]. Important and relevant features are selected from the feature space based on certain evaluation criterion, which actually increases the efficiency of the data analysis task like clustering [13] and classification [14, 15]. So feature selection is necessary in the big data environment too for developing the prediction model.

2.1 Review on Feature Selection and Machine Learning Algorithms

In this section, a short literature review on the different feature selection techniques and learning algorithms are presented. Feature selection [7] is an important preprocessing step in machine learning, which is used to reduce the number of input variables/dimensions/features/attributes during the development of predictive model. This process is playing an important role to enhance the performance of the model by reducing the computational cost in terms of space and time. In healthcare field, huge amount of data is generated through the patients' data and reports. A decision system can represent this data in a structured form where row indicates patient objects and column indicates the disease symptoms or the features containing the conditional as well as decision features. Selection of the important features from the feature pool is very important to diagnose a disease. Features those do not contribute to take the decision on disease prediction are required to discard to build up the prediction model efficiently by reducing time and space complexity. So feature selection leads to develop an efficient and accurate prediction model. Three types of feature selection approaches exist, namely *filter* [7], *wrapper* [7], and the *embedded* method [7]. In filter approach [7], no learning algorithms are associated with the approach, whereas in wrapper approach, the feature selection job is associated with the learning algorithm. *Embedded* method [7] takes advantage of its own variable selection method and performs feature selection and classification at the same time.

Learning algorithms [16, 17] play an important role in the development of an automated disease prediction system. Machine learning automates analytical model building task through data analysis method. Machine learning algorithms are traditionally divided into three categories: supervised learning [16], unsupervised learning, [17] and reinforcement learning [17]. Predictive models are developed using supervised learning algorithms. This type of learning algorithms build a realistic model using set of input and output training data to make the predictions for the response to new data. Supervised learning algorithms includes artificial neural network (ANN) [16], Bayesian method [17], decision tree [17], ensemble method [18, 19], random forest [20], KNN [21], etc. Unsupervised learning algorithms are used to develop descriptive models. This type of algorithm uses a known set of input data to analyze and discover pattern within, but output is not known. Semi-supervised learning [16, 17] falls between supervised learning and unsupervised learning. Classification and regression techniques [14, 15] are similar to semi-supervised learning.

Classification analysis [14, 15] serves better understanding of the underlying data. Recently, the structure of the different dataset is so difficult to understand directly, so it is necessary to apply many machine learning tools for classification of the dataset [14, 15]. These methods include the k-nearest neighbors [21], Bayesian approaches [17], SVM [17], ANN [16], and decision trees [17]. Prediction of single classifier depends on the training capability of the classifier on the data itself. Ensemble classification [14, 15] is also a standard approach for improving the classification performance in machine learning by considering the output of more than one classifier decision by a suitable decision combination technique like majority voting, averaging, etc.

2.2 Previous Works on Diabetes Prediction

Many researchers are working in this healthcare analytics domain for predicting the diabetes disease [22] to save people from this deadly disease. Galetsi et al. [23] present a study on a theoretical framework, techniques, and prospects on big data analytics in the health sector to determine the way big data analytics has managed to improve the different decision making job in the healthcare domain. Yuvaraj et al. [24] investigated different machine learning algorithms like decision trees, Naive Bayes, and random forest in Hadoop environment to select best features from the diabetes data using information gain as a parameter for selection of the suitable feature. The generated results were measured by different classification parameter. Finally, it is been concluded that Hadoop cluster-based random forest algorithm performs much better compared to the other two machine learning algorithms in terms of all the different performance measures. Mujumdar et al. [25] developed a classification model with some external factors like BMI, age, glucose, insulin, etc. Their model has five different modules—dataset collection, data preprocessing, clustering, build model, and evaluation. Dataset collection phase is responsible for data collection and understanding the patterns and trends of the data, which helps in prediction and evaluating the results. Data preprocessing phase cleans the raw data to increase efficiency of the model. In the clustering phase, K-means clustering is applied to classify a patient into either a diabetic or a non-diabetes category. Model building is the fourth phase of diabetes prediction model, which is most important. In this phase, authors have implemented various machine learning algorithms for diabetes prediction. The final phase of prediction model is evaluation. In this phase, the authors evaluate the prediction result with the help of different evaluation metrics like confusion matrix, classification accuracy, and f1-score. Ramsingh et al. [26] proposed MapReduce-based hybrid NBC-TFIDF algorithm to diagnose the disease by analyzing these sentiments of the people. This model analyzes the correlation of diabetic risk factors, food habits, and physical activity of Indian people through social media data analysis. The results show that the MapReduce-based model is working extremely efficiently. About 60% of social media data shows the high glycemic index about food items, which is the cause of type 2 diabetes. Ramani et al. [27] proposed a modified artificial neural network (ANN) classifier technique to detect the diabetic chronic disease through MapReduce-based big data framework. This representation exhibits improved accuracy and speed on chronic disease dataset. It also increases the throughput and redundancy of retrieving the huge amount of data. The performance evolution of the proposed artificial neural network with MapReduce structure compared to other existing deep neural network approach. Hadoop MapReduce is a framework for processing a huge amount of data in a cluster of machines, which is reliable. Runtime of the job plays a crucial role for being better management in a platform. In the paper [28], the authors designed an automatic glucose-level prediction model to predict type 1 diabetes mellitus through the wearable processor by investigating minimum data variety, volume, and velocity. They used three standard machine learning algorithms, namely ARIMA, random forest [20], and SVM [17] to measure the performance of the prediction models for execution within a wearable processor. Random forest method given the best performance among all the three used machine learning techniques, but the method is also associated with some cost due to the wearable processor.

Our method is not associated with any cost but generates an intelligent, accurate, and efficient prediction results through feature selection and ensemble classification approach in big data environment.

3 Design of Diabetes Prediction Model

The aim of the proposed work is to development of an integrated big data-enabled diabetes prediction model to predict the diabetes disease efficiently.

Most of the healthcare data is unstructured and huge, so to process this kind of data needs an intelligent big data environment where the tasks can be divided between the nodes to save the processing time of the data. As we know the classification or prediction of the test data is dependent upon the number of input features of a dataset, so finding important and relevant feature subset selection is an important aspect of designing of an efficient prediction model. At the same time, it has been seen that single classifier do not give always best results rather combining the output of the different base classifiers gives improved results. So ensemble classification approach in big data environment is a good solution for better prediction results in healthcare domain.

In the work, a diabetes prediction model in Hadoop platform with MapReduce implementation is proposed to predict the diabetes. The model has two main functionalities such as feature selection and ensemble classification. Feature selection is done through GA [29], and in classification phase, three state-of-the-art classification algorithms such as Naïve Bayes [17], random forest [20], and KNN [21] are used as the base classifiers, and majority voting technique is used to combine the decisions of the base classifiers to develop the efficient prediction model. In the subsequent sections, the detail of the processes and MapReduce implementation of the work is discussed.

3.1 Feature Selection and Classification

Feature selection and classification is the main task of the developing model in MapReduce framework to predict the disease.

3.1.1 Feature Selection

In GA [29], a population is comprised of chromosomes, and the size of the chromosome is the number of features present in the dataset. Each chromosome in the initial population represents the combinations of some features randomly selected. Here in the method, a single objective GA [29] is proposed where fitness function of the GA is defined in the Eq. (1). Positive region overlap (PRO) [29], a concept of rough set theory (RST) [9] is used to design the fitness function. PRO came from the concept of positive region in RST [9]. It finds out the number of objects correctly classified by both the targeted feature subset and the original feature subset of the dataset. So greater the value of PRO, better the fitness value and chance of target feature subset becomes high to be the final feature subset. Then, this feature subset will be considered as the result of the feature selection module.

For a decision system, $DSS = (U, \mathrm{FS}, D)$ where $|U|$= no of objects in the decision system, FS = no of original feature set, and D is decision feature. If the positive region of DSS based on original feature set FS is $\mathrm{POS}_{\mathrm{FS}}(D)$ and the same with target feature subset FS_1 is $\mathrm{POS}_{\mathrm{FS}_1}(D)$, then overlapping positive region is $P_F(D) = \mathrm{POS}_{\mathrm{FS}}(D) \cap \mathrm{POS}_{\mathrm{FS}_1}(D)$ [29]. Fitness function $f(\mathrm{cr})$ for a chromosome cr is defined in Eq. (1) to find out the feature subset R of the system DSS.

$$f(\mathrm{cr}) = \left(\frac{P_{\mathrm{F}}(D)}{|U|}\right) \tag{1}$$

The overall process in feature selection module as follows:

Inputs: Decision subsystem DSS = (U, FS, D).
Outputs: Feature subset A of DSS.
Step I: Compute $POS_{FS}(D)$ of DSS with the feature set FS according to the Eq. (1).
Step II: Initialize GA population with population size = P and chromosome length = |original feature in DSS|.
Step III: Calculate the fitness value of each chromosome cr in the population using $f(cr)$ defined in Eq. (1).
Step IV: Select chromosomes for mating pool using rank selection technique based on the fitness value.
Step V: Crossover and mutation operation on chromosomes using uniform crossover probability $\mathrm{crossp}_{\mathrm{cr}}$ and mutation rate, $\mathrm{mr}_{\mathrm{cr}}$.
Step VI: Choose next-generation chromosomes with some percentage of replacement of the parent population.
Step VII: Repeat Step III to Step VI until GA converges.
Step VIII: Select the best chromosome as the final feature subset A of the entire system DSS.

3.1.2 Ensemble Classification Module

The output from the feature selection module is the reduced training dataset with the selected feature set. Now after applying all the considered three base classification algorithms such as NB [17], KNN [21], and random Forest [20] individually, all classification rule sets are generated, and after that by applying the majority voting concept, the combined final rule sets are generated. The detail implementation of the algorithm in MapReduce framework is described in the next section.

3.2 MapReduce Implementation

For efficient classification, we have implemented the GA [29] and ML algorithms [17, 20, 21] in the MapReduce model of computation [4]. Initial data from HDFS [5] is collected. The work is done on the following directions: Select best-optimized feature subset for each of the data subsystems. Classification rule generation for each of the reduced data using base classifiers applies majority voting to predict the class label of the data.

The work is done through three phases such as map phase, combine phase, and reduce phase.

A. **Map Phase**—In this phase, map function applies feature selection algorithm and computes the best feature subset for the data and then applies the classification algorithms to generate classification rules based on reduced data, and then, output of this phase is send to the Combiner function.
B. **Combine Phase**—In this phase, the combiner function accepts all the output from the previous map phase and arranges the data belonging same class. Next, grouping of the data based on same class labels is done. It keeps record of the number of the objects in the same class label and results of the clusters that are send to the Reducer function.
C. **Reduce Phase**—In this phase, the reduce function accepts the output of the combiner function. Then, ensemble classification rules are generated based on majority voting technique, and the final rule sets are stored in HDFS.

4 Experimental Results

The experiment has been done on the Indian Pima Dataset [30] in the following environment: Intel i5 CPU with 16 GB RAM; using Python language. The accuracy of the method has been compared with existing different single and ensemble classifier and achieves a good accuracy value to prove the efficiency of the method. The method has been compared with existing ensemble model available in Weka [31]. The comparative result based on selected feature is given in Tables 1 and 2. Tenfold cross-validation method is used to build the model.

Table 1 Classification accuracy for diabetes dataset for the proposed and existing ensemble method

Dataset	Classification methods	Accuracy (%)
PIDD(8)	Proposed method	99.02
	Bagging	92.52
	LogitBoost	100

Table 2 Comparative classification results analysis for diabetes dataset

Dataset	Classification methods	Classifiers parameters		
		Precision	Recall	F-measure
PIDD(8)	Proposed method	0.99	0.99	0.99
	Bagging	0.92	0.93	0.93
	LogitBoost	1	1	1

For GA, in every single fold, 20 independent runs are performed and it terminates when no fitness value changes after 2 successive iterations. Other selection of parameter values like crossover probability = 0.9, mutation probability = 0.001.

Classifier performance evaluation [32] is the final step of judging a prediction model. The performance of the classification algorithms is evaluated by the series of experiments. The most commonly used performance metrics are mentioned below.

4.1 Confusion Matrix

The prediction model is judged by the output of the confusion matrix, where TP, FP, FN, TN are four cases depicted in the matrix. True positive (TP) depicts positive objects classified as positive. False positive (FP) depicts positive objects classified as negative. False negative (FN) depicts negative objects classified as positive. True negative (TN) depicts negative objects classified as negative. Followings are the description of the different performance measuring parameters of the classifiers.

Accuracy

$$\text{Accuracy} = \frac{\text{TN} + \text{TP}}{\text{TP} + \text{TN} + \text{FP} + \text{FN}}$$

Recall

$$\text{Recall} = \frac{\text{TP}}{\text{TP} + \text{FN}}$$

Precision

$$\text{Precision} = \frac{\text{TP}}{\text{TP} + \text{FP}}$$

F-Measure

F-measure is the best if there is some kind of balance between precision and recall.

$$\text{F - Measure} = 2 * \frac{1}{\frac{1}{\text{precision}} + \frac{1}{\text{Recall}}}$$

The proposed methodology is evaluated on "Indian Pima Dataset" collected from UCI Repository [30]. This dataset contains 768 instances with eight numeric attributes/features where class "0" represents negative diabetes and class "1" represents positive diabetes. After applying the proposed method on the PIDD data [30], detail classification results of the proposed method and existing methods through Weka tool [31] are given below in Tables 1 and 2. Since accuracy [32] is not only the evaluation metric to judge the classifier performance, so precision [32], recall [32], F-measure [32], and Fall_out [32] are also calculated and presented in Table 2 along with the classification accuracy. The proposed method is compared with two standard ensemble classification method, and results are given in Table 1. Table 2 presents other performance metric values.

Other benchmark disease related datasets also collected from the UCI repository [30] to prove the effectiveness of the method. Tables 3 and 4 provide the detail results of the experiment. The results show that the performance of the proposed method is better comparative to other state-of-the-art methods in all respect to judge a classifier.

The result shows that the proposed method is comparable and efficient with the other mentioned methods with respect to all the performance evaluation metrics of the classifiers. Hence, we can say that the proposed method selects the most important features with a novel ensemble classification approach in the big data environment which provides better performance without losing too much information with good prediction results.

Table 3 Comparative classification accuracy results analysis for other datasets

Dataset (#original attribute)	Bagging (%)	LogitBoost (%)	Proposed method (%)
Breast Cancer (9)	94.43	95.74	95.73
Heart (12)	82.25	82.97	83.21
Dermatology (33)	96.01	96.26	98.99

Table 4 Comparative classification results analysis for other datasets

Dataset (#original attribute)	Classification methods	Classifiers parameters		
		Precision	Recall	F-measure
Breast Cancer (9)	Proposed method	0.96	0.96	0.96
	Bagging	0.95	0.95	0.95
	LogitBoost	0.96	0.96	0.96
Heart (12)	Proposed method	0.83	0.82	0.83
	Bagging	0.82	0.82	0.82
	LogitBoost	0.83	0.83	0.83
Dermatology (33)	Proposed method	0.99	0.99	0.99
	Bagging	0.96	0.96	0.96
	LogitBoost	0.96	0.96	0.96

5 Conclusion

In the work, a diabetes prediction model has been developed by integrating two important data mining tasks such as feature selection and ensemble classification. The model has been implemented in MapReduce framework to handle big healthcare datasets. In MapReduce process, in each node, at first genetic algorithm-based feature selection technique has been used to select the important features, then considered base classifiers are applied to generate the classification rules and after that output from all the node combined with majority voting technique and ensemble classification technique evolved to classify the disease efficiently. As we know, GA is a time-consuming technique for the bigger dataset, so applying GA for feature selection is a matter of concern. Since here, the MapReduce approach has been used, so efficiency will not be the issue at all because data is divided between the nodes. Classification model provides the accuracy level of about 99.02% for the diabetes dataset. The proposed method is a generalized prediction method and can be used for the prediction purposes for other datasets too. In spite of the above benefits, some more experiments to be conducted for the bigger datasets to check the efficiency with different machine learning approaches in big data environment.

References

1. World Health Organization (2021) Diabetes statistics reports for the world. http://www.who.int/diabetes/en/
2. Shafqat S, Kishwer S, Rasool RU, Qadir J, Amjad T, Ahmed HF (2018) Big data analytics enhanced healthcare system: a review. LLC, part of Springer Nature
3. Mehta T, Mangla N, Gurgaon G (2016) A survey paper on big data analytics using map reduce and hive on Hadoop framework. Int J Recent Adv Eng Technol 4(2):112–118

4. Ramini R, Devi KV, Soundar KR (2020) MapReduce-based big data framework using modified artificial neural network classifier for diabetic chronic disease prediction. Soft Comput. https://doi.org/10.1007/s00500-020-04943-3
5. Nishadi Thanuja AS (2019) Healthcare big data analysis using Hadoop MapReduce. Int J Sci Res Publ 9(3)
6. Bishop C (2010) Pattern recognition and machine learning, 1st edn. Springer, New York, NY, USA
7. Jain A, Zongker D (1997) Feature selection: evaluation, application, and small sample performance. IEEE Trans Pattern Anal Mach Intell. https://doi.org/10.1109/34.574797
8. Das AK, Paul A, Sil J (2009) Generation and analysis of classifiers using reducts and support vector machines. In: International conference on intelligent systems and networks. India, pp 159–164
9. Zhang Q, Xie Q, Wang G (2016) A survey on rough set theory and its applications. CAAI Trans Intell Technol 1(2016):323–333
10. Pawlak Z (1998) Rough set theory and its applications to data analysis. Cybern Syst 29:661–688
11. Alasadi SA, Bhaya WS (2017) Review of data preprocessing techniques in data mining. J Eng Appl Sci 12(16):4102–4107
12. Marban O, Marisal G, Segovia J (2009) A data mining & knowledge discovery process model, data mining & knowledge discovery in real life applications. ISBN 978-3-902613-53-0, p 438
13. Eick CF, Zeidat N, Zhao Z (2004) Supervised clustering-algorithms and benefits. In: 16th IEEE international conference on tools with artificial intelligence, pp 774–776
14. Choubey DK, Paul S, Kumar S (2017) Classifications of PIMA Indian diabetes dataset using Naïve Bayes with genetic algorithm as an attribute selection. In: Prasad et al. (eds) Communication and computing systems
15. Maniruzzaman Md, Rahman Md J, Ahammed B, Abedin Md M (2020) Classification and prediction of diabetes disease using machine learning paradigm. In: Health information science and systems. Springer Nature Switzerland AG.
16. Otchere DA, Ganat TOA, Gholami R, Ridha S (2020) Application of supervised machine learning paradigms in the prediction of petroleum reservoir properties: comparative analysis of ANN and SVM models. J Petrol Sci Eng 108182:2020
17. Hasan MdK, Alam MdA, Das D, Hossain E, Hasan M (2020) Diabetes prediction using ensembling of different machine learning classifiers. IEEE Access 8:76516–76531
18. Dvornik N, Schmid C, Mairal J (2019) Diversity with cooperation: Ensemble methods for few-shot classification. In: IEEE/CVF International conference on computer vision, pp 3723–3731
19. Zhou ZH (2019) Ensemble methods: foundations and algorithms. Chapman and Hall/CRC
20. Azar AT, Elshazly HI, Hassanien AE, Mohamed A (2014) A random forest classifier for lymph diseases. Comput Methods Programs Biomed 113(2):465–473
21. Gaur S (2017) Comparative analysis between GA, KNN and hybrid algorithm to optimize the classification of fuzzy KNN. In: 46th ISTE annual national convention and national conference 2017. International journal of advance research and innovation (ISSN 2347-3258)
22. Fiarni C, Sipayung EM, Maemunah S (2019) Analysis and prediction of diabetes complication disease using data mining algorithm. In The fifth information systems international conference
23. Galetsi P, Katsaliaki K, Kumar S (2020) Big data analytics in health sector: theoretical framework, techniques and prospects. Int J Inf Manage 50:206–216
24. Yuvaraj N, SriPreethaa KR (2019) Diabetes prediction in healthcare systems using machine learning algorithms on Hadoop cluster. Clust Comput 22:S1–S9
25. Mujumdar A, Vaidehi V (2019) Diabetes prediction using machine learning algorithms. In: International conference on recent trends in advanced computing ICRTC 2019
26. Ramsingh J, Bhuvaneswari V (2020) An efficient map reduce-based hybrid NBC-TFIDF algorithm to mine the public sentiment on diabetes mellitus—a big data approach. J King Saud Univ Comput Inf Sci
27. Peyravi N, Moeini A (2020), Estimating runtime of a job in Hadoop MapReduce. J Big Data

28. Rodríguez-Rodríguez I, Chatzigiannakis I, Rodríguez JV, Maranghi M, Gentili M, Zamora-Izquierdo M-Á (2019) Utility of big data in predicting short-term blood glucose levels in type 1 diabetes mellitus through machine learning techniques. Sensors 19:4482. https://doi.org/10.3390/s19204482
29. Das A, Sengupta S, Bhattacharyya S (2018) A group incremental feature selection for classification using rough set theory based genetic algorithm. Appl Soft Comput 65. https://doi.org/10.1016/j.asoc.2018.01.040
30. Murphy P, Aha W (1996) UCI repository of machine learning databases. http://www.ics.uci.edu/mlearn/MLRepository.html
31. WEKA. Machine Learning Software. https://www.cs.waikato.ac.nz/
32. Yahyaoui A, Jamil A, Rasheed J, Yesiltepe M (2019) A decision support system for diabetes prediction using machine learning and deep learning techniques. In: 1st International informatics and software engineering conference (UBMYK), pp 1–4

Secure Data Sharing of Electronic Health Record (EHR) on the Cloud Using Blockchain in Covid-19 Scenario

Deepak Kumar Verma, Rajesh Kumar Tyagi, and Ashish Kumar Chakraverti

Abstract In the current scenario of Covid-19, health data are stored in a centralized server at hospitals and medical institutions, which is susceptible to diverse extortions, such as malicious tinkering, patient data loss, and natural disasters. The advent of blockchain expertise fetches a new-fangled notion to decipher the abovementioned security issues due to its features of immutability, verifiability, and decentralization. This technology was initially invented for money-associated exchanges and financial transactions using centralized authorities. Nowadays, the popularity of blockchain technology is increasing enormously in the field of healthcare. Healthcare devices having a great utilization in the field of healthcare, but they pose several privacy and security threats to the sensitive data of a patient. To overcome these issues, we have proposed a novel hybrid system that combines the merits of centralized and decentralized blockchain for the secure sharing of health data between health devices and hospitals. The proposed system will be useful in the context of protected, interoperable, and effectual admittance to health registers by patients, hospitals, and third revelries while maintaining the privacy of patients' penetrating data. Also, we used smart contracts in an Ethereum-based blockchain for access control. Ethereum is a programmable blockchain platform that utilizes the strong environment of solidity (a state-based scripting language). By using both centralized and decentralized properties of blockchain together, we can effectively secure the patient's sensitive data. The data of a patient generated by heterogeneous devices would be shared in a secured manner. We have analyzed that the proposed system is better than the existing systems in terms of scalability, data ownership, and interoperability. The deployment cost of

D. K. Verma (✉)
Department of CSE, Greater Noida Institute of Technology, Greater Noida, Uttar Pradesh 201310, India

R. K. Tyagi
Department of CSE, Amity School of Engineering and Technology, Amity University Haryana, Manesar, Gurgaon, India

A. K. Chakraverti
Department of Information Technology, Pranveer Singh Institute of Technology, Kanpur, UP, India

M. S. Kaiser et al. (eds.), *Proceedings of Trends in Electronics and Health Informatics*, Lecture Notes in Networks and Systems 376,
https://doi.org/10.1007/978-981-16-8826-3_15

the proposed hybrid model may be the limitation. In the forthcoming, we would implement the suggested hybrid exemplary to advance the security of health data.

Keywords Blockchain · Smart contract · Ethereum · Privacy · Security · Healthcare

1 Introduction

Now a days, cloud computing technology is in trend, offers Internet-based resources at a quick release with minimal organizational efforts. The technology implementation is by the data center hardware situated at a distant location from users. Security of the cloud data is one of the major issues, which has been improved continuously in the past decade. The growth of medical data from hospitals and wearable health devices is becoming more useful to analyze. It is becoming more important to secure that data.

In the era of the digital globe, many organizations are generating a huge quantity of insightful data from various domains such as healthcare, education, finance, and research institutions. The volume of such data is increasing enormously. Most of the organizations have availed the facility of cloud computing for the storage and maintenance of sensitive data. Nowadays, cloud computing is becoming popular due to its potential computing capacity and large data storage. The organizations transfer their burden of handling the enormous amount of sensitive data to the cloud service provider due to its characteristics such as on-demand access, scalability, and security in an economical manner (Verma and Tyagi [18]). A large number of organizations have a barrier in adopting cloud computing technology due to privacy and security issues of data (Bollineni and Neupane [15]). The term "cloud computing" was, first, coined by John McCarthy in the 1960s. He stated that "computation may someday be organized as a public utility" (Joshua and Francisca [16]). Verma et al. [37] optimized the setup phase cost in the cloud storage using multithreading architecture. Gupta et al. [38] presented an improved RSA algorithm for data security in the cloud.

With the dawn of healthcare digitization, the trend of data distribution of patients and hospitals on the cloud has seen massive expansion. It was predicted that a huge escalation in the number of healthcare devices that will be linked to the Internet by 2030. An electronic health record is a way of storing health records in an electronic format. It has various advantages like ease of storing, searching for a specific disease, and appending details to previous records. Several privacy and security issues arise with the increasing use of digital devices in healthcare data sharing such as patient data ownership, interoperability, access control, and scalability. Data owners are worried about their sensitive data which is stored in the cloud as the control of their data is out of their hands. Blockchain has become a prominent technology to overcome the abovementioned security and privacy issues in electronic health records (Ali et al. [1]). Health data integration is a big problem in health professional organizations. After the innovation of smart contracts in blockchain technology for storing patients' health data, any legitimate user can access their data securely. This novel technology gives the right to the patients for accessing and sharing sensitive data with health professionals and institutions. Blockchain technology enables accessibility at a large scale, provides data privacy, incurring costs, and also provides an untrusted information system. Blockchain technology is increasing in popularity due to its usage in cryptocurrency like Bitcoin, it is used to implement various types of decentralized applications. Blockchain technology is based on the notion of a distributed ledger that acts as a database that consists of historical data of transactions that become occupied agents (Gordon and Catalini [5], Vazirani et al. [11]). Li et al. [10] proposed a tamper-proof electronic health system based on blockchain and cloud to secure the outsourced data of EHRs from any tempering in integrity.

They have been found that the existing systems are not able to guarantee the exactness and integrity of outsourced EHRs when the nasty doctor colludes among the cloud server to alter outsourced EHRs. Mor et al. [36] reviewed the literature on blockchain for its applications in data security. In the current state of interoperability, interoperability may be defined as "the ability of different information technology systems and software applications to communicate, exchange data and use the information that has been exchanged." Interoperability has various benefits such as improving operational efficiency and also improving clinical care. However, interoperability is an essential part of cost-effective, comprehensive clinical care. To simplify the diagnosis and healing procedure, healthcare professional players are currently taking on IoT-enabled wearable devices (Zhang and Ji [13]). On the other hand, these technologies cause severe privacy and security risks concerning the data transmission of a patient. Fan et al. [4] used blockchain for securing patients' health data in the hospital. The security of data in a blockchain is based on a Proof of Work (PoW) model, in which a contract is only measured legitimate once the system gets proof of computational exertion by authorizing nodes. The miners (accountable for generating blocks) continually try to resolve Proof of Work (PoW) in the figure of hash computation. A hash is used to identify every block in the header of the chain. The hash is exceptional and generated by SHA-256. The failure to delete or modify data from blocks makes the blockchain a preeminent suitable tool for the healthcare scheme (Zheng et al. [14], Han et al. [7]).

Bhuiyan et al. [2] proposed a blockchain-based scheme for achieving security, interoperability, and proficient access to patients' health data. They used smart contracts on the Ethereum platform for sensitive data obfuscation and access control of the data by employing cryptographic schemes for additional security. Zheng et al. [14] and Kaur et al. [9] designed a system for secure storage and managing personal health records using blockchain technology. In the existing environment, mostly, health data management systems are governed by health service providers that mean there is no control of the patient on their data. This leads to the loss of the reliability and integrity of patient health records due to centralized storage.

Blockchain technology is becoming popular for storing healthcare data as a supply chain in which each process might be verified, answerable, and immutable. Such intrinsic uniqueness makes it a latent way out for healthcare records.

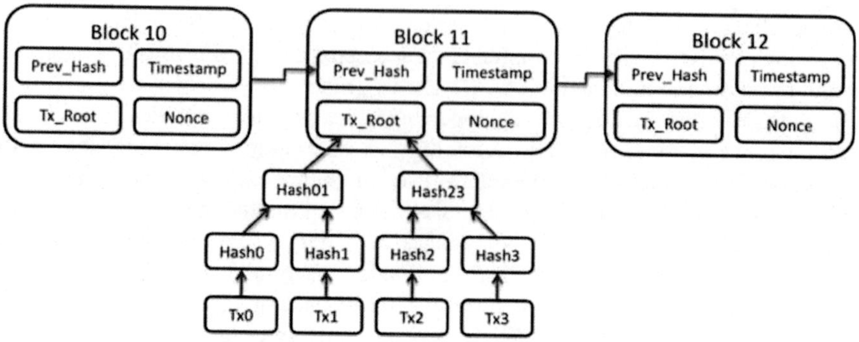

Fig. 1 Schematics of blockchain

Figure 1 represents the schematics of blockchain. A blockchain contains the following components.

- **Timestamp**: It is the time of block foundation.
- **Reference to Parent (Prev_Hash)**: It is the hash of the preceding block header which associates every block to its parent. This sequence of references is the eponymy notion for the blockchain.
- **Merkle Root (Tx_Root)**: It is a set of confirmed transactions in a block. At least one transaction must be executed by a block such as Coinbase. The Coinbase is a unique transaction uses to generate new bitcoins and collects the transactions fees.
- **Target**: Target supports the default in finding a new block. The target corresponds to the difficulty of finding a new block. When a default comes, it updates it after every 2016 block.
- **Nonce**: A random number is used to add entropy to a block header easily without reconstructing the Merkle tree.
- **The block's hash**: All the above items of the header accept the transaction data being hashed into the block hash. It has been confirmed that no other parts of the header altered.

2 Related Work

Due to the growing development of cloud computing in every field, several privacy and security concerns have arisen that are obstacles in the wide acceptance of cloud services. Confidentiality, integrity, and availability are the three main pillars of security in cloud computing (Sumter [17], Feng et al. [27] and Lombardi et al. [19]). The explosion in cloud computing has given several privacy and security challenges for the clients (Bleikertz et al. [20] and Lu et al. [21]). Many researchers explored the privacy and security issues with their distinct solutions (see, for instance, Altman [22], Bayardo and Srikant [23], Bertino et al. [24], Brodkin [25], Vimercati et al.

[26], Feng et al. [27], Jadeja and Modi [28], Verma et al. [35]). Verma et al. [34] proposed a novel scheme for securing data by improving Baptista's cryptosystem.

An electronic health record (EHR) consists of a patient's health data such as prescription, X-ray, diagnosis report, and ultrasound report. An EHR is useful for sharing the patient's data with other doctors or hospitals for their better diagnosis (Achampong [29]). The security of the patient's sensitive data is a constant issue. To conquer this issue, Wang et al. [30] and Kahani et al. [31] provided a secured mechanism for sharing and accessing the health data of a patient. The rise of cloud computing explores a new section for the healthcare industry. In e-healthcare, cloud computing lowers the cost of health care and increases system availability (Deshmukh [32], Indhumati and Prakasham [33]).

Kaur et al. [9] proposed a scheme for quick access to patient records, electronic health records that are being adopted by many hospitals. To handle data efficiently, one of the most suited technology is blockchain. This serves multiple applications such as patient record management and pharmacies. Interoperability of the system is being enhanced by moving entire data electronically and then to a distributed decentralized network.

Han et al. [7] stated that there is a problem of data isolation as maximum hospitals and medical institutions are storing their healthcare data on their platforms. Also, secure data storage, privacy protection, and data sharing in synergetic phenomena are troublesome tasks. To handle these tasks, a novel technology, blockchain has been used for securing health data. To fulfill the security measures, healthcare data are being encrypted by asymmetric encryption technique.

Katuwal et al. [8] explored the challenges of blockchain in the healthcare industry. They found that this technology helps in solving problems of data exchanging, secure repository and integrity preservation, monitorability, and answerability of data. The proposed applications include data provenance, counterfeit drugs identification, and consent management. Zhang and Ji [13] found that interoperability is one of the major problems with healthcare record systems. Da et al. [3] also found that interoperability is a major issue in electronic health records. To improve electronic health records, blockchain and smart contracts can be applied. This solution can permit huge-scale accessibility, facts privacy, decreasing medical treatment expenses, and providing trust in the information system.

Fan et al. [4] suggested a blockchain primarily based information management system named 'Medblock'. It illustrates superior information security combining altered access control protocols and symmetric cryptography. Vazirani et al. [11] performed a methodical survey to analyze the potentiality of blockchain, and found that blockchain should grow interoperability while retaining the privateness and safety of EHR information saved at the cloud. The outcome of the studies and independent assessment shows that blockchain could determine the efficient management of EHR data. Gordon et al. [5] discovered that transferring of organization pushed interoperability to user-pushed interoperability is a famous trend in healthcare that has altered ways of clinical data exchange and ownerships. Authors show that the patient-centric model is more useful which is shared among many stakeholders.

Wang and Song [12] and Guo et al. [6] proposed an attribute-based signature mechanism with multiple authorities, wherein the affected person allows a message consistent with the attribute and prevents disclosing the facts which are not signed by the patient. There are multiple authorities to distribute the public or private keys to users in this system which helps to eliminate the escrow problem as well as comply with distributed data storage in the blockchain. The EHR system having multiple authority and blockchain has been introduced into the attribute-based signature (ABS) scheme for preserving patient privacy which has been improved as multiple authority attribute-based signature (MA-ABS) scheme. This system reaches all the requirements of blockchain. The comparison analysis shows the linearly increasing cost and performance with the number of authority and patient attributes. Table 1 represented the detailed analysis of the methodologies proposed by researchers.

3 Proposed Solution

The proposed scheme implements a hybrid blockchain on the Ethereum platform to enhance the interoperability of the systems by using tracking all activities that take place to the information in the databases. Smart contracts are applied for including particular items in records to the blockchain for tracking. In the proposed system, one may keep less sensitive information on a centralized server by interlinking it with data stored on the blockchain. We can store it in an encrypted and anonymous way. The less sensitive information can be anonymously stored details about hospitals, doctors, and encrypted documents (Fig. 2).

On the other side, a blockchain has been used to store highly sensitive information of patients securely. A smart contract is itself be ownership free that is the ownership of the smart contract will be destroyed once it is uploaded on the blockchain (Table 2).

4 Conclusion

Blockchain plays an essential role in securing the health data of a patient in a healthcare repository. In the pandemic of Covid-19, a lot of health data has been generated in the healthcare market. This data contain the confidential information of a patient that has to be secure from any breaches. Blockchain is the best tool for the same. One huge benefit of the usage of blockchain in the healthcare industry is that it can reform the interoperability of healthcare databases. We proposed a hybrid blockchain scheme for improving the performance of the system. Our proposed scheme will take care of patient data ownership and interoperability. In the future, we shall implement the proposed hybrid blockchain scheme for improving the security of health data in the repository.

Table 1 Critical analysis of literature on blockchain-based EHR

Reference	Title	Pros	Cons
[1]	Blockchains in the Internet of Things	Develop a fast and secure system for IoT applications	Implementation of the proposed work has not been done
[2]	Blockchain and big data to transform healthcare	Proposed a model for health data management for an individual patient using a distributed ledger	No concrete results have been presented
[3]	Electronic health records using blockchain technology	Design and implement an information architecture to admittance EHRs using smart contracts	Only data privacy and accessibility issues have been discussed
[4]	Medblock: Efficient and secure medical data sharing via blockchain	In the proposed scheme, distributed ledger has been used to allow electronic medical records admittance and recovery	MedBlock may be used for securing sensitive information of the patient
[5]	Blockchain technology for healthcare: facilitating the transition to patient-driven interoperability	In the proposed system, the researchers worked on the following concepts 1. Digital access rules 2. Data aggregation 3. Data liquidity	The proposed system was patient-centric only
[6]	Secure attribute-based signature scheme with multiple authorities for blockchain in electronic health records systems	Proposed an attribute-based signature scheme with multiple authorities to provide better security and privacy under random oracle model	Empirical comparison with the existing methods has not been done
[7]	The architecture of a secure health information storage system based on blockchain technology	The proposed scheme united consortium blockchain and fully private blockchain as a hybrid blockchain to improve the delay of data validation	No critical analysis has been done related to the proposed scheme
[8]	Applications of blockchain in healthcare: current landscape and challenges	Discussed the issues related to practical, monitoring, and business defies to the acceptance of blockchain in the healthcare diligence	A theoretical study has been discussed

(continued)

Table 1 (continued)

Reference	Title	Pros	Cons
[9]	A proposed solution and future direction for blockchain-based heterogeneous medicare data in a cloud environment	A blockchain-based system has been proposed in the cloud environment	No privacy and security issues have been discussed
[10]	Using blockchain for data auditing in cloud storage	Proposed a security mechanism for cloud data auditing based on blockchain	No batch auditing
[11]	Implementing blockchain for efficient healthcare: systematic review	An empirical review has been discussed based on the use of blockchain in the healthcare industry	No implementation was done

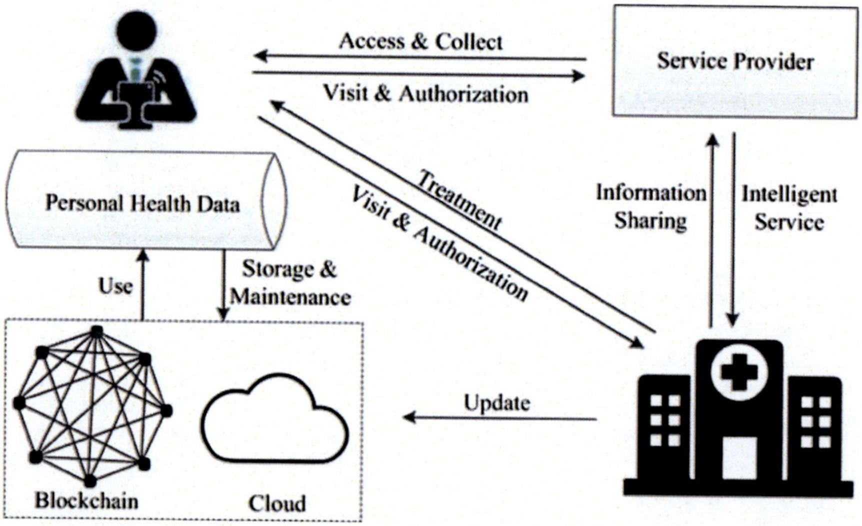

Fig. 2 Proposed framework

Table 2 Comparison between a centralized, decentralized system with the proposed system

Factor	Centralized system	Decentralized system	Proposed hybrid system
Authentication	Easy	Not easy	Easy
Security	Low	High	High
Scalability	High	Low	High
Storage cost	Low	High	Low
Interoperability	No	Yes	Yes
Setup	Easy	Not easy	Easy
Patient data ownership	No	Yes	Yes

References

1. Ali MS, Vecchio M, Pincheira M, Dolui K, Antonelli F, Rehmani MH (2018) Applications of blockchains in the Internet of Things: A comprehensive survey. IEEE Commun Surveys Tutorials 21(2):1676–1717
2. Bhuiyan MZA, Zaman A, Wang T, Wang G, Tao H, Hassan MM (May 2018) Blockchain and big data to transform healthcare. In Proceedings of the international conference on data processing and applications, ACM, pp 62–68
3. da Conceição AF, da Silva FSC, Rocha V, Locoro A, Barguil JM (2018) Electronic health records using blockchain technology. arXiv preprint arXiv:1804.10078
4. Fan K, Wang S, Ren Y, Li H, Yang Y (2018) Medblock: efficient and secure medical data sharing via blockchain. J Med Syst 42(8):136
5. Gordon WJ, Catalini C (2018) Blockchain technology for healthcare: facilitating the transition to patient-driven interoperability. Comput Struct Biotechnol J 16:224–230
6. Guo R, Shi H, Zhao Q, Zheng D (2018) Secure attribute-based signature scheme with multiple authorities for blockchain in electronic health records systems. IEEE Access 6:11676–11686
7. Han H, Huang M, Zhang Y, Bhatti UA (Jun 2018) An architecture of a secure health information storage system based on blockchain technology. In International conference on cloud computing and security. Springer, Cham, pp 578–588
8. Katuwal GJ, Pandey S, Hennessey M, Lamichhane B (2018) Applications of Blockchain in healthcare: current landscape and challenges. arXiv preprint arXiv:1812.02776
9. Kaur H, Alam MA, Jameel R, Mourya AK, Chang V (2018) A proposed solution and future direction for blockchain-based heterogeneous medicare data in a cloud environment. J Med Syst 42(8):156
10. Li C, Hu J, Zhou K, Wang Y, Deng H (Jun 2018) Using blockchain for data auditing in cloud storage. In International conference on cloud computing and security. Springer, Cham, pp 335–345
11. Vazirani AA, O'Donoghue O, Brindley D, Meinert E (2019) Implementing blockchains for efficient health care: systematic review. J Med Internet Res 21(2):e12439
12. Wang H, Song Y (2018) Secure cloud-based EHR system using attribute-based cryptosystem and blockchain. J Med Syst 42(8):152
13. Zhang M, Ji Y (2018) Blockchain for healthcare records: a data perspective. PeerJ PrePrints 6:e26942v1
14. Zheng X, Mukkamala RR, Vatrapu R, Ordieres-Mere J (Sept 2018) Blockchain-based personal health data sharing system using cloud storage. In 2018 IEEE 20th international conference on e-health networking, applications and services (Healthcom). IEEE, pp 1–6

15. Bollineni PK, Neupane K (2011) Implications for adopting cloud computing in e-Health, Blekinge Institute of Technology SE—371 79 Karlskrona Sweden.
16. Joshua A, Ogwueleka F (2013) Cloud computing with related enabling technologies. Int J Cloud Comput Services Sci 2(1):40
17. Sumter R, La'Quata (2010) "Cloud computing: security risk classification." In ACMSE
18. Verma DK, Tyagi RK (2015) A new era of computing: cloud computing. Int J Comput Electron Eng (IRJCEE) 3(1):1–4
19. Lombardi F, Di Pietro R (Mar 2010) Transparent security for the cloud. In Proceedings of the 2010 ACM symposium on applied computing, pp 414–415
20. Bleikertz S, Schunter M, Probst CW, Pendarakis D, Eriksson K (Oct 2010) Security audits of multi-tier virtual infrastructures in public infrastructure clouds. In Proceedings of the 2010 ACM workshop on Cloud computing security workshop, pp 93–102
21. Lu R, Lin X, Liang X, Shen X (Apr 2010) Secure provenance: the essential bread and butter of data forensics in cloud computing. In Proceedings of the 5th ACM symposium on information, computer and communications security, pp 282–292
22. Altman I (1977) Privacy regulation: culturally universal or culturally specific. J Soc Issues 33(3):66–84
23. Bayardo RJ, Srikant R (2003) Technological solutions for protecting privacy. Computer 36(9):115–118
24. Bertino E, Paci F, Ferrini R, Shang N (2009) Privacy-preserving digital identity management for cloud computing. IEEE Data Eng Bull 32(1):21–27
25. Brodkin J (2008) Gartner: seven cloud-computing security risks. InfoWorld 2008:1–3
26. Di Vimercati SDC, Foresti S, Jajodia S, Paraboschi S, Samarati P (Sept 2007) Over-encryption: management of access control evolution on outsourced data. In Proceedings of the 33rd international conference on Very large databases, pp 123–134
27. Feng DG, Zhang M, Zhang Y, Xu Z (2011) Study on cloud computing security. J Softw 22(1):71–83
28. Jadeja Y, Modi K (Mar 2012) Cloud computing-concepts, architecture and challenges. In 2012 International conference on computing, electronics and electrical technologies (ICCEET). IEEE, pp 877–880
29. Achampong EK (2013) Electronic health record (EHR) and cloud security: the current issues. International Journal of Cloud Computing and Services Science 2(6):417–420
30. Kumar PS, Subramanian R, Selvam DT (Oct 2010) Ensuring data storage security in cloud computing using Sobol Sequence. In 2010 first international conference on parallel, distributed and grid computing (PDGC 2010), IEEE, pp pp217–222
31. Liu J, Xiao Y, Chen CP (Jun 2012) Authentication and access control in the internet of things. In 2012 32nd international conference on distributed computing systems workshops. IEEE, pp 588–592
32. Deshmukh P (2017) Design of cloud security in the EHR for Indian healthcare services. J King Saud Univ-Comput Inf Sci 29(3):281–287
33. Indhumathi V, Prakasham V (Mar 2015) On-demand security for Personal Health Records in cloud computing. In 2015 International conference on innovations in information, embedded and communication systems (ICIIECS). IEEE, pp 1–5
34. Verma DK, Rani M, Tyagi RK, Sagar BB (2019) Baptista chaotic cryptosystem based on an alternate superior dynamic lookup table. J Discrete Math Sci Cryptography 22(8):1383–1392
35. Verma DK, Tyagi RK, Chaudhury V (2019) Enhanced security of public integrity auditing for outsourced data in cloud storage. Int J Adv Sci Technol 27:187–209
36. Mor P, Tyagi RK, Jain C, Verma DK (2021) "A systematic review and analysis of blockchain technology for corporate remittance and settlement process", in 4th Int. conf. on computational intelligence and communication technologies (CCICT) organized by B.M. institute of engineering and technology, Sonipat, Haryana on July 03, 2021, pp 121–128, IEEE. https://doi.org/10.1109/CICT53244.2021.00034

37. Verma DK, Gupta P, Tyagi RK (2019) Cloud storage–optimization of initial phase for privacy-preserving public auditing. In Ambient communications and computer systems. Springer, Singapore, pp 353–365
38. Gupta P, Verma DK, Singh AK (Jan 2018) Improving RSA algorithm using multi-threading model for outsourced data security in cloud storage. In 2018 8th International conference on cloud computing, data science and engineering (Confluence). IEEE, pp 14–15

A Study Towards Recent Trends, Issues and Research Challenges of Intelligent IoT Healthcare Techniques: IoMT and CIoMT

Garima Verma, Aditya Pratap Shahi, and Shiva Prakash

Abstract Present scenario deals with lots of complexities and drawbacks of healthcare systems. These systems help in transforming and providing various solutions to replace the use of traditional monitoring systems. The advanced healthcare monitoring systems are dealing with the reduced cutting cost and also they are improving the treatment methodologies of the patients. These systems gives the opportunities to the patients for online tracking of their health related data without moving to the doctor's clinic and one can easily check the related data by just sitting online. A framework is required for the combination of verification convention with a vitality proficient access control instrument. In the wake of experiencing the philosophy for validation convention and for a proficient access control system, a consolidated procedure is proposed to be received to pool the hole. This paper shows an exhaustive literature review and describing the related work done by the existing authors based on the Wireless Body Area Networks (WBANs) and the latest technologies used in connected health like CIoMT and IoMT. Through this paper; various comparisons between several parameters and techniques are being done. The new researchers will be able to get more ideas about the past researches and the emerging trends in the healthcare field based on IoT.

Keywords Internet of Things (IoT) · Internet of Medical Things (IoMT) · Internet of Healthcare Things (IoHT) · Cognitive Internet of Medical Things (CIoMT) · Comparative Study of Parameters

G. Verma (✉)
Department of Computer Science, Pranveer Singh Institute of Technology, Kanpur, India

A. P. Shahi
Department of Mechanical Engineering, B. N. College of Engineering and Technology, Lucknow, India

S. Prakash
Department of Information Technology and Computer Application, Madan Mohan Malaviya University of Technology, Gorakhpur, India

M. S. Kaiser et al. (eds.), *Proceedings of Trends in Electronics and Health Informatics*, Lecture Notes in Networks and Systems 376,
https://doi.org/10.1007/978-981-16-8826-3_16

1 Introduction

Internet of Things plays a very important role in providing various applications and benefits to the clients and consumers. In the current scenario, more than 1 billion users are there which are interconnected and communicate with each other. There are a lot of devices which are electronically and mechanically connected with each other for providing a better aspect of communication to the users. Internet is a technology that has somehow incorporated various devices and their technical solutions as per the needs of the users [1]. IoT has revolutionized the world with the ability to identify and track all other devices as per the requirements [2]. But at present, IoT healthcare is emerging as one of the recent challenge for the researches since it is providing new scopes and research domains for the IoT developers [3]. As predicted by the Cisco Systems, it has been told that in the upcoming years, the IoT is enlarging itself into so many other domains. But there are many drawbacks also which are considered for IoT devices like cybercrimes and hackers which harm the security of the data. More the devices which are available online, more number of chances of hacking the data. There are various types of medical devices that are available for the users like smart diagnostic tools, smart healthcare devices etc. which are providing great applications for the mobile health users all over the world [4]. From hand bracelets to home automation systems, all the frameworks need a tight security for protected data. According to the researchers, IoT threats are being increasing day by day potentially in all the domains. One of the basic issues is privacy of data. In [5], the author has given a systematic approach for the healthcare technologies using the fog network for designing devices that can be used in Internet of Medical Things. The security of the accumulated data is the main concern that the data privacy should not get loss or the individual's information should not be misused. There are several devices which are operated on this layer and various networking protocols are being used. Some of the devices are repeaters, Network Interface Cards (NICs) etc. In fact, has given the facility to extend the current IPv4, expands the current IPv4 protocol from 32 to 128 bits for every IP address which offers great flexibility for IoT world. IPv6 supports dynamic objectives of networking to achieve flexibility and reliability in a system. A comprehensive study of IoT in medical things of healthcare has been discussed [6]. Well-ordered guidelines to approve the healthcare devices are similarly a critical research zone. Usually, confirmation is cultivated through various methods, for instance, ID/mystery word, pre-shared special bits of knowledge are some examples. There are various software platforms used for the implementation of IoT devices such as Raspberry Pi [7], Arduino Uno. Figure 1 shows the various architectural frameworks of IoT Domain.

The IoT has the empowering capability to change the whole world where we are living today. The architectural work goes for planning and actualizing an IoT-mindful Smart Hospital System (SHS) having, as principle characteristic, the capacity to promptly join extraordinary, yet corresponding, advancements empowering novel functionalities. Essentially, the framework we imagine ought to have the capacity to

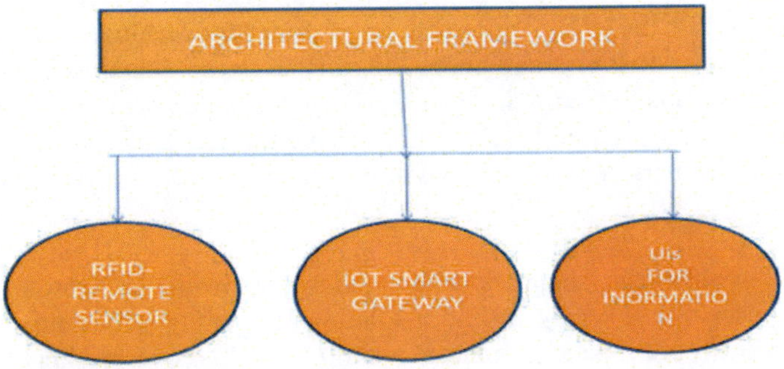

Fig. 1 Components of Healthcare Frameworks

gather, progressively, both natural conditions and patients' physiological parameters and convey them to a control focus. IoT has been a promising field since many years.

IoT presently utilizes various gadgets, administrations and conventions to accomplish a shared objective. In any case, for better coordinating of any system it should be required to use the architecture standards. In any case, the security necessities for IoT can't be accomplished by essentially putting explicit arrangements from every layer together. Indeed, it is important to consider IoT framework, overall framework and security is one of the major factor that should be considered in the IoT structure. In this manner, to improve IoT security, we additionally need some participation between various layers by planning security answers for cross layers use beating heterogeneous combination issues. This component of extraction was basically combined with the hashing techniques to avoid several assaults. The exhibited model explains the versatility and adaptability which are the highlighting concepts of this model. A lot of detailed work on diabetes diagnosis and detection using IoMT has been discussed [8].

- **IoT and related background referring to COVID-19**

Talking about the Internet of Things (IoT), it can be simply defined as the network of interconnected devices which can be incorporated in any communication network using various hardware, software, RFIDs (Radio Frequency Identification Devices) etc. or any other required components. In the current pandemic situation, whole world is fighting with this corona virus and researchers are in race of trying to develop a successful vaccine but still the vaccine is in the development phase. Doctors and researchers are still looking for a feasible solution to develop a vaccine that could somehow reduce the infection rate of this dangerous corona virus. Researchers involved in various departments like computer science, physical engineering etc. are in a continuous attempt to develop new approaches, theories, study problems for giving a successful solution to this COVID 19 pandemic. IoT is an innovative approach of implementing several kinds of healthcare systems that can easily reduce the work load of the doctors and also help in developing cost-effective methodologies for patients. At this point of time, there is a great need of such scenario where one can easily integrate the technologies with new theories for developing best solutions for this pandemic. Talking more about IoT, it is a concept which is incorporating many other domains like artificial intelligence, machine learning, data science etc. It also helps in implementing such sort of techniques which will help in complete integration of the person who is in need of the services and the service providers.

- **Research focus**

In such problematic situation, where the whole world is fighting with the pandemic, everyone is trying to find a solution for getting out of this. On daily basis, the records of the patients infected with COVID-19 are increasing day by day. Every day, a new record of data is set breaking all other records. There is a great need of utilizing the existing facilities and technologies integrating with the Internet of Things (IoT). Moreover, IoT has already been implemented in several domains in different forms and is serving great roles in helping people with different aspects like Internet of Healthcare Things (IoHT) and Internet of Medical Things (IoMT). By using different tools and techniques of IoHT and IoMT, the number of cases can be reduced up to certain level. For example, there should be proper monitoring systems in every room of the quarantined patients so that proper care can be taken of those patients. Along with all this, various body sensors like temperature sensors, BP sensors etc. can be used for regular updates of the patients so that if some other diseases are there, they can be easily cured and timely treatment can be given to the patients.

2 Literature Review

The concept of fog computing and edge computing has somehow affected the overall technology in IoT as it has given a new approach for the researchers to work in this area. Along with this, the data generated from the healthcare industry carries major sensitive data that requires critical care and security. There are lot of developments being made on daily basis regarding the healthcare platforms for better optimization of technologies. Home care monitoring systems have emerged as one of the very helpful technological frameworks in IoT [9].

One of the recent studies [10], a framework developed using AI based technology to battle with the novel corona virus has been developed using the smartphones is discussed in this paper. A novel study [11] has discussed the design and implementation of Remote Monitoring Systems for Low Cost devices for Limb health. In [12], authors has done a detailed survey in the usability of AI in the field of IoT using Embedded NN-Techniques for developing smart mobiles devices for better computing. Further, a study discussed the pruning convolution networks for the healthcare systems in [13]. Monteiro [14] has discussed a lot of tele-treatment methods for the healthcare domains using different fog computing devices for the treatment of patients on several nodes of parameters. The healthcare systems that are being developed today are of great benefits for the patients but there are still various loopholes on which, the researchers are working today for better design and development of such devices.

Further, G. Muhammad [15] has done the study on different smart health solutions by integrating various domains but mainly IoT and cloud computing along with a case study on it. There are numerous solutions possible for the technological advancement of healthcare problems by integrating different domains into one. In [16], a detailed discussion for developing a smart healthcare framework has been discussed using the concept of Artificial Intelligence and Edge Computing that can be implemented in the smart cities for progressive developments of areas. In [17], a smart framework has been developed for persons with voice disorder and their treatments using edge computing with cloud framework. In [18], various frameworks for checking the health status using the records of the health conditions can be seen in this work. Further, a recent approach of Body Area Networks has been discussed in which different types of studies has been done incorporating the transmission policies of the networks [19]. Pham et al. [20] have proposed a new technological framework for the designing of smart healthcare solutions using cloud based architectures (CoSHE).

Here, a comparative study has been discussed with various parameters like sensors used, fog/cloud devices, methodology used, their advantages and disadvantages. Various authors have researched on IoT fundamentals given in the Table 1.

3 Research Objective

The COVID-19 is a very challenging situation for everybody and especially for the doctors, healthcare workers, nurse staffs and many medical personnels to deal with patients and offer them services. These people are trying to serve the patients in more impactful and effective way. The paper is a comprehensive study of various tools and techniques of offering the services to the corona patients by the means of IoMT/ IoHT. Patients today are suffering from various problems like visiting the hospitals, corona testing, report monitoring and medicine purchasing. There are further more issues with regards to the COVID-19 which can be resolved more effectively and more efficiently by using the IoT healthcare approaches. These techniques can also be helpful for those patients which are quarantined at a remote place [27].

The main objective of this proposed work is to develop such a framework in which the system will consist of several layers including the physical layer, middleware layer, network layer, transport layer etc. Firstly, on the physical layer, there will be several embedded devices responsible for data collection, data transmission and data controlling. These devices will contain the sensors, transmitters, LowPAN Networks etc. Hence, this layer will perform several processes of data collection and transmission. Further, the next layer is the network layer which plays the role of transmitting the signals [28]. The signals are transmitted from the sensors to the cloudlets or cloud servers. And meanwhile, middleware layer helps in storing and collecting the data and then depositing that data into the cloud. Another function of middleware layer is that it helps in making the data available for the users who

Table 1 Comparative study of different parameters of technologies used

Authors	Contributions	Sensors Used	Fog/cloud devices used	Methodology used	Advantages	Disadvantages
Devarajan et al. [21]	Diagnosis, prediction and controlling the risk of diabetic patients based on real-time framework	BP sensors, Motion sensors, Heart sensors	No fog/ Cloud devices were provided	Used Hybrid Technique neutrosophic VIKOR methods	Efficient technique with smart sensors based operations	Difficulty in handling large samples of data
Oniga [22]	Various parameters recorded by using Arduino Microcontroller	Body specialized sensors	Arduino, System	Data was transferred into PC for further processing	Better monitoring and controlling	Cost Factor
Yakut et al. [23]	Use of ECG signals using Raspberry pi	E-Health sensors	Raspberry Pi	Raspberry Pi records the data for processing in Matlab	Faster Processing of signals	Hardware constraints and cost factors
Dubey et al. [24]	Speech Monitoring Mechanisms using PD and ECG sensors	Microphone	Intel Edison	Dynamic Time Warping (DTW) method is used for processing	Efficient Speech recognition method	Difficulty in speech conversion of data
Monteiro et al. [14]	Worked on tele-treatment techniques of patients	Microphone	Intel Edison	Numerous features was sent to the cloud server	Easy approach for tele-medicine techniques	Cost factors
Mathur et al. [11]	Temperature monitoring of residual limb	Motion sensors, thermistors	Raspberry pi, Arduino	Machine Learning is used for measuring skin temperature	Easy monitoring of sensors	Difficulty in Accessing the Sensor data quickly

(continued)

Table 1 (continued)

Authors	Contributions	Sensors Used	Fog/cloud devices used	Methodology used	Advantages	Disadvantages
Kaur et al. [7]	Worked on measuring pulse rate and temperature	Temperature and pulse rate sensors	Raspberry Pi	PANGEA platform has been used using wifi networks	Provides accurate results	Cost factor and difficult implementation
Satija et al. [25]	ECG measurement using signal quality	ECG sensors	Linux, GPU as hardware	SVM technique in machine learning along with deep learning	Better signal quality results	Design and implantation is difficult
Pham et al. [20]	Collection of Physiological signals and motion	Smartwatch and environmental sensors	arduino mega	Data transmitted from the sensors is processed at home gateway networks	Quick implementation and results	Environmental parameters are difficult to sustain
Queralta et al. [26]	Cardiovascular and diabetes monitoring	ECG, EMG	Raspberry Pi, Gateways are used	LSTM RNN networks were used for data processing	Easy monitoring and controlling	Cost factor is a limitation

are in need of that data at a particular point of instance. And at last, the application layer responsible for the final processing of data by using the data analysis and data diagnosis techniques.

4 Proposed Architecture of IoMT (Internet of Medical Things)

Now-a-days, there are a lot of complex architectures leading to tedious implementations of the recent technologies. Basically, the devices present in the IoMT architecture are connected to the cloud servers and the data is stored in the cloud and then the data is being easily accessed through the clouds [29]. There are a lot of implementations of IoMT architectures like remote monitoring of patients having serious issues related to health and treatment can be given instantly without hectic movement from one place to another. Along with various important services, the IoMT architecture offers numerous other important administrative and medical facilities [30]. Consultation of telemedicine has become easier through such implementations of IoMT architectures. These architectures are very helpful to reduce the cases in COVID-19 pandemic. There are several functions that are carried by the IoMT implementations as given below:

- IoMT architectures help in managing the data of the patients online. The patient does not have to depend on physical movement from one doctor to another.
- IoMT facilities leads to accessing of the data easily like one can use the facility of block chains.
- Helps in measuring the different parameters like robustness, efficiency, productivity etc.
- Easy identification of healthcare issues and problems.
- Patients can be easily traced simultaneously using remote monitoring
- Services will become internet based services.

Since, there are a lot of barriers in the way of accessing the health services due to increase in the number of connected medical devices, a need rises for designing the IoMT devices for various parameters like lowering the costs, efficiencies, improvement in the capabilities of managing devices etc. IoMT services has the ability to easily collect, analyze and transmit the healthcare data where required [31]. Therefore, IoMT techniques and tools are continuously transforming the way of healthcare services delivery. There is connectivity between the medical devices and the sensors being implemented in the IoMT architecture which leads to proper management and improvement in the patient's healthcare services (Figs. 2 and 3).

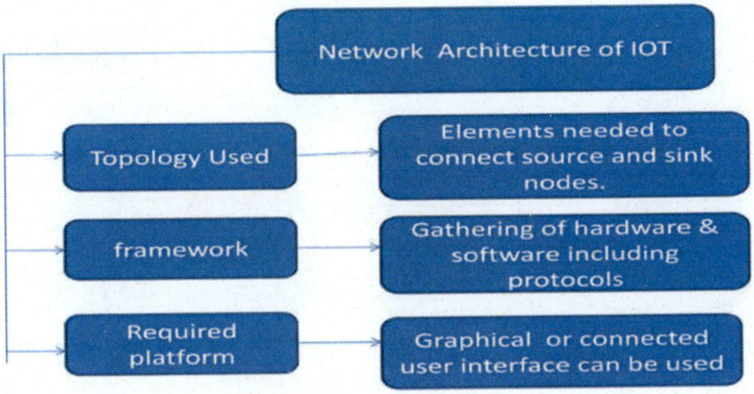

Fig. 2 Flow diagram for healthcare framework

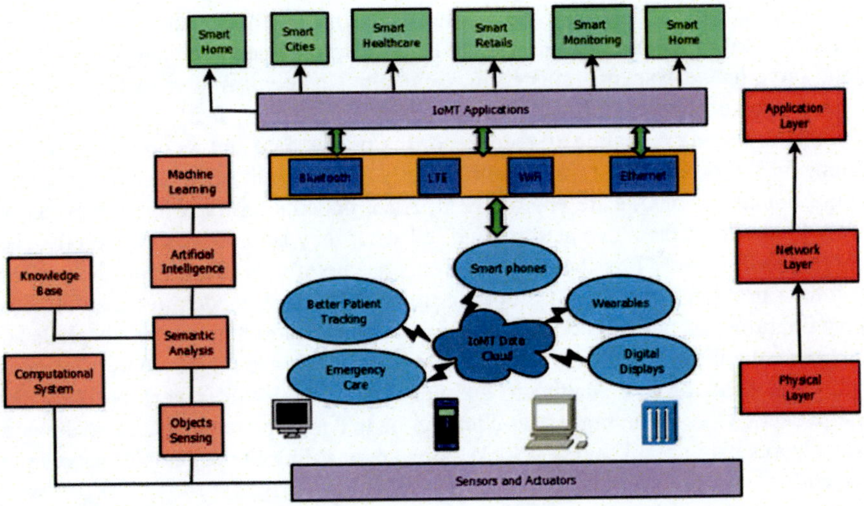

Fig. 3 Architecture of IoMT

5 CIoMT (Cognitive Internet of Medical Things)

Basically, CIoMT is a class of CIoT (Cognitive Internet of Things) made specifically for the medical industry in order to support the recent technologies in smart health-care. The need of such technologies is to track and record the patient's real time data like diabetes check, glucose level, blood pressure level, heart rate, temperature, humidity etc. According to the current scenario of COVID-19, there is a great need of such Cognitive architectures that can tackle with corona cases. With such systems,

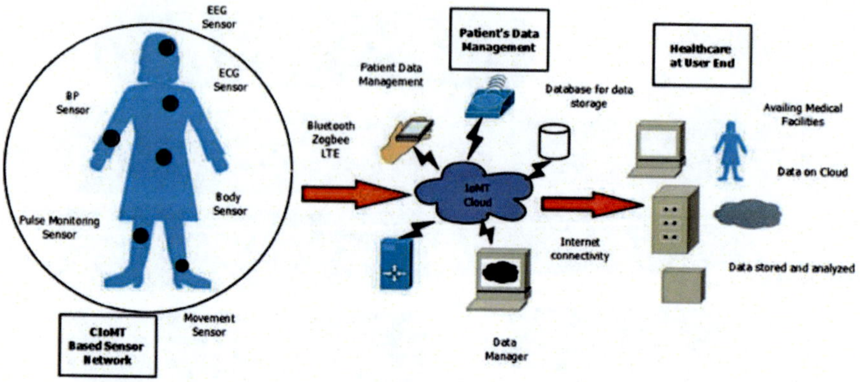

Fig. 4 Architecture of CIoMT

data tracking can become easy and monitoring of the patient can also become effective. The CIoMT technology will lead to better recording and analyzing of real-time data, surveillance, tracking, clustering, prevention and control of virus [32].

A connected medical infrastructure provides with so many features like easy data sharing, accessing o healthcare data, reporting of live data and recording them etc. Along with this, CIoMT systems will enhance the capability and robustness of the entire domain of healthcare environment. Also, patients on track mode can easily record and report their live activity and tell what they actually feel. Currently, the biggest use of CIoMT is that these systems are helpful in diagnosing the patient and their problems easily [33]. Looking upon the current pandemic situation, it is very important to pay attention to the healthcare infrastructure of the hospitals so that better facilities can be provided to the patients. It is the high time to increment and implement the IoT healthcare architectures to deal with severe problems of the patients. One of the biggest application of IoT is implementing the healthcare frameworks using blockchains. Blockchains are enabling the patients to access the patient's data from the cloud and many more facilities (Fig. 4).

It is being expected that the investment on the IoT healthcare solutions will somehow reach to $1 trillion by 2025 and it will be set on the stage for the overall high adaptability, accessibility and durability of the data. This will help in providing on-time healthcare services to the users by using the real-time scenarios of collecting the data, analyzing the data and then storing the data for the future use. Hopefully, by 2026, remote monitoring implementations will create approx. $1.15 trillion in value which will help in improving the healthcare conditions of the patients. These implementation systems will lead to develop better healthcare systems that will help to deal with chronic diseases easily. Internet of Medical Things (IoMT) has covered almost each and every part of the healthcare systems by which the medical facilities has increased up to a certain level.

Talking about the current scenario, there are approx. 3.8 million medical devices which are connected all together in order to give quick response to the healthcare

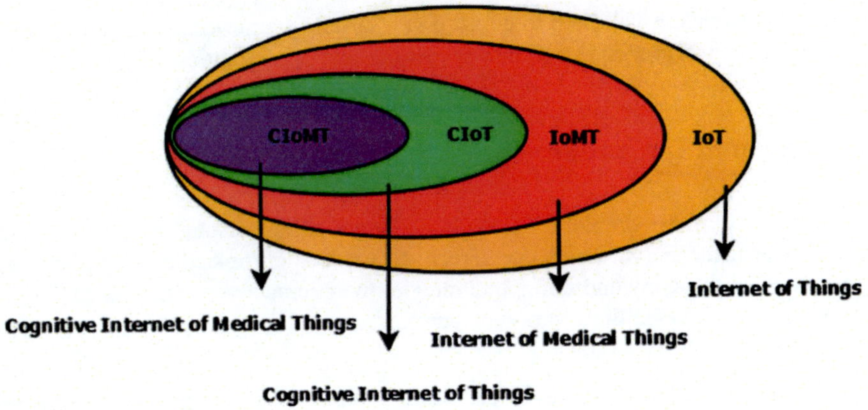

Fig. 5 Subsets of IoT

decisions. Using such cognitive architectures of medical devices, it has become very easy to monitor the activities of the patients and make decisions accordingly. Doctors and scientists are using such medical systems for better healthcare facilities which is making the patient tracking more easier and efficient [34]. CIoMT is a field of cognitive healthcare study which offers preventive care for the patients as it is somehow reducing the paper work and making the healthcare processes digital So, the areas having most critical need can be easily tracked using the IoT deployed systems. Moreover, there are more advanced devices which provide internal surveillance with embedded sensors and chip technologies allowing smart medical services. By using such smart surveillance systems, it is easier to tackle with all such situations of forgery and cheat. These devices were not available before for use but now they are available with most recent advanced embedded sensors (Fig. 5).

6 Proposed Services of IoMT

IoMT and CIoMT are the two most trending concepts for the healthcare infrastructures which are in progress to be implemented for better monitoring and tracking of the patients. There are a lot of services which are being offered by the Internet of Medical Things as discussed below:

- Smart and early diagnosis of diseases in the patients.
- Smart Tracking systems will help in proper monitoring and surveillance of the patients and will help in recording the live activities of the patients.
- It will help in better risk prediction which allows identifying the problems at a very early stage helping the easy diagnosis.
- Smart monitoring systems leads to smart tracking of patients.
- Smart wearable devices can be implemented easily.

- Smart healthcare will help to develop new system frameworks that will revolutionize the world with lots of new inventions and opportunities.

7 Research Limitations

Subsequently, there should be some pre-characterized personality of the board element or center point which can screen the association procedure of gadgets by applying cryptography and different strategies to anticipate wholesale fraud [35]. It may also ensure to facilitate various security issues and helps in better management of the network in IoT model.

- On the basis of the risks evolved, listing should be done and accordingly the devices should be deployed.
- In any IoT communication process, there are various encrypt and decrypt cycles taking place in the mechanism and these cycles are very much vulnerable to attacks and are prone to high security attacks. So, this point should be considered while designing any IoT device.
- There are many security issues which are being rectified using the communication protocols to combine with IoT security in IoT systems and to provide basic level security at each layer in the IoT model [36].

8 Conclusion

This paper basically presents about the various contributions of different authors and their respective works in the field of IoT. This paper will help in making a better comparative study and will help various new authors to develop and create a new scenario for the betterment and development of new healthcare related technologies. The paper consists of various recent concepts of healthcare like IoMT, CIoMT etc. Since, the validation of conventions gives confirmation of the client, while different assaults like secrecy, trustworthiness, revocation, and so forth are not tended to. IoT techniques play a very important role in connected health and also providing various services.

References

1. Niranjana S, Balamurugan A (Dec 2015) "Intelligent e-health gateway based ubiquitous healthcare systems in internet of things". IJSEAS 1(9)
2. Asif-Ur-Rahman M et al (June 2019) Toward a Heterogeneous Mist, Fog, and Cloud-Based Framework for the Internet of Healthcare Things. IEEE Internet Things J 6(3):4049–4062. https://doi.org/10.1109/JIOT.2018.2876088

3. Yehia L, Khedr A, Darwish A (Jul 2015) "Hybrid security techniques for internet of things healthcre applications"
4. Sermakani V (2014) "Transforming healthcare through internet of things". The internet of thingsfor medical devices prospects, challenges and the way forward
5. Ibrahim WN, Selamat A, Krejcar O, Chaudhry J (2018) Recent advances on fog health—a systematic literature review new trends in intelligent software methodologies. Tools Tech, IOS Press
6. Islam SMR, Kwak D, Kabir MH, Hossain M, Kwak KS (2015) The internet of things for health care: a comprehensive survey. IEEE Access, 678–708
7. Kaur A, Jasuja A (2017) Health monitoring based on IoT using raspberry PI. 2017 International conference on computing, communication and automation (ICCCA), Greater Noida, 1335–1340
8. Klonoff DC (2017) Fog computing and edge computing architectures for processing data from diabetes devices connected to the medical internet of things. J Diabetes Sci Technol 11(4):647–652
9. Magana-Espinoza P, Aquino-Santos R, C˜ardenas-Benitez N, Aguilar-Velasco ´J., Buenrostro-Segura C, Edwards-Block A et al (2014) WiSPH: a wireless sensor network-based home care monitoring system. Sensors 14(4):7096–7119
10. Maghdid HS, Ghafoor KZ, Sadiq AS, Curran K, Rabie K (2020) A novel ai-enabled framework to diagnose coronavirus covid-19 using smartphone embedded sensors: design study arXiv preprint arXiv:2003.07434
11. Mathur N, Paul G, Irvine J, Abuhelala M, Buis A, Glesk I (2016) A practical design and implementation of a low cost platform for remote monitoring of lower limb health of amputees in the developing world. IEEE Access 7440–7451
12. Poniszewska-Maranda A, Kaczmarek D, Kryvinska N, Xhafa F (2019) Studying usability of AI in the IoT systems/paradigm through embedding NN techniques into mobile smart service system. Computing 101(11):1661–1685
13. Meola A (2016) Internet of things in healthcare: information technology in health. Business Insider
14. Monteiro A, Dubey H, Mahler L, Yang Q, Mankodiya K (May 2016) Fit: a fog computing device for speech tele-treatments In 2016 IEEE international conference on smart computing (SMARTCOMP), pp 1–3. IEEE
15. Muhammad G, Rahman SMM, Alelaiwi A, Alamri A (2017) Smart healthsolution integrating iot and cloud: a case study of voice pathology monitoring. IEEE Commun Magazine 55(1):69–73
16. Muhammed T, Mehmood R, Albeshri A, Katib I (2018) UbeHealth: a personalized ubiquitous cloud and edge-enabled networked healthcare system for smart cities. IEEE Access 6:32258–32285
17. Muhammad G, Alhamid MF, Alsulaiman M, Gupta B (2018) Edge computing with cloud for voice disorder assessment and treatment. IEEE Commun Mag 56(4):60–65
18. Numenta Community (2018) Introduction to HTM, https://numenta.org IoanOrha, Stefan Oniga, Automated system for evaluating health status. Design and technology in Electronic Packaging (SIITME), 2013, IEEE 19th international symposium for, pp 219–222
19. Park J, Samarakoon S, Bennis M, Debbah M (2019) Wireless network intelligence at the edge. Proc IEEE 107(11):2204–2239
20. Peng Y, Peng L (2016) A cooperative transmission strategy for body-area networks in healthcare systems. IEEE Access 9155–9162
21. Pham M, Mengistu Y, Do H, Sheng W (2018) Delivering home healthcare through a cloud-based smart home environment (CoSHE). Future Gener Comput Syst 81:129–140
22. Devarajan M, Subramaniyaswamy V, Vijayakumar V, Ravi L (2019) "Fog-assisted personalized Healthcare-support system for remote patients with diabetes. J Ambient Intell Humaniz Comput 22:1–14
23. Orha I, Oniga S (2013) "Automated System for evaluating health status, "Design and Technology in electronic Packaging (SIITME). IEEE 19th International symposium 219–222

24. Yakut O, Solak S, Dogru E (2014) Bolat measuring ECG signal using e-health sensor platform. Int Conf Chem Biomed Environ Eng (ICCBEE'14), 65–69
25. Dubey H, Yang J, Constant N, Amiri AM, Yang Q, Makodiya K (2015) "Fogdata: enhancing telehealth big data through fog computing. In Proceedings of the ASE bigdata and social informatics, ACM, 1–14
26. Satija U, Ramkumar B, Sabarimalai Manikandan M (2017) Real-time signal qulity-aware ecg telemetry system for iot-based healthcare monitoring. IEEE Internet of Things J 4(3):815–823
27. Queralta JP, Gja TN, Tenhunen H, Westerlund T (2019) "Edge-AI in LoRa-based health Monitoring: fall detection system with fog computing and lstm recurrent neural networks. 42nd International conference on telecommunications and signal processing (TSP), 601–604
28. Abdel-Basset M, Manogaran G, Gamal A, Chang V (2019) "A novel intelligent medical decision support model based on soft computing and iot
29. Prakash S, Rajput A (Sep 2nd–3rd, 2017) "Hybrid cryptography for secure data communication in wireless sensor networking". Proceeding of Springer, International conference on recent advancement in computer, communication and computational sciences (RACCCS-2017), at Aryabhatta College of Engineering and Research Center, Ajmer, Paper id-82, pp 589–599
30. Verma G, Prakash S (2020) Design and implementation of modified unicode strategy for data security in IoT. Int J Adv Sci Technol (IJAST) 29(06):6271–6294
31. Garima Verma, Shiva Prakash, "Pneumonia Classification using Deep Learning in Healthcare", International Journal of Innovative Technology and Exploring Engineering (IJITEE), Volume 9, Issue 4, ISSN: 2278–3075, Feb 2, 2020, pp. 1715–1723.
32. Verma G, Prakash S (Nov 21–22, 2019) "A study towards current trends, issues and challenges in internet of things (IoT) based system for intelligent energy management". 4th International conference on information systems and computer systems (ISCON 2019), Venue- IEEE Conference Record Number: #47742, GLA University, Mathura, Uttar Pradesh, India, 297
33. Verma G, Prakash S (Jun 4–05, 2020) "A Comparative Study based on different energy saving mechanisms based on green internet of things (GIoT)". IEEE 8th International conference on reliability, infocom technology and optimization (ICRITO-2020), IEEE Conference Record Number 48877, Amity University, Noida, India, 631
34. Shahi A.P., Dwivedi V., Garima Verma, "A Review on Latest Trends on Different Research Domains of Composite Materials", In: Agrawal R., Jain J.K., Yadav V.S., Manupati V.K., Varela L. (eds) Recent Advances in Smart Manufacturing and Materials. Lecture Notes in Mechanical Engineering. Springer, Singapore. https://doi.org/10.1007/978-981-16-3033-0_8, (2021).
35. Hegde C, Suresha PB, Zelko J, Jiang Z, Kamaleswaran R, Reyna MA, Clifford GD (2020) "autotriage-an open source edge computing raspberry pi-based clinical screening system"
36. Verma G, Prakash S (2021) "Emerging security threats, countermeasures, issues, and future aspects on the internet of things (IoT): a systematic literature review". In Kumar N, Tibor S, Sindhwani R, Lee J, Srivastava P (eds) Advances in interdisciplinary engineering. Lecture notes in mechanical engineering. Springer, Singapore. https://doi.org/10.1007/978-981-15-9956-9_6

Digitalization of Healthcare System in India—A Perspective and PESTLE Analysis

Chandrahash Patel and Kunal Sinha

Abstract In the time of emergency, where there is an urgent need for healthcare services, the digitalization of health care ensures active delivery of the services to their consumers and citizens. Telecommunication, especially Internet-based technologies, plays a vital role in collecting health-based data to deliver and employ people. The healthcare sector is directly responsible for human well-being and health and needs continuous political, economic, social, technological, legal, and environmental up-gradation and development that only improves the system but also its effectiveness and efficacy. E-health services have a tremendous blow worldwide and have positively prepared us with more knowledge, healthcare accessibility and reduce the distance and divide in demand between patients and healthcare providers. This paper attempts to address the Indian perspective on healthcare system digitalization and the different components based on secondary sources.

Keywords Healthcare · Digital healthcare · Digitalization · Digital technology · NDHM BluePrint · PESTLE

1 Introduction

Indian healthcare sector is the largest in India in terms of size and growth. With a growing population of over a billion individuals and changing disease patterns, the healthcare sector will become a USD 400 billion markets by 2024. The World Health Organization (WHO) recommends a doctor to patient ratio of 1:1000, whereas in India, as of 2020, this ratio is 0.95:1000. Furthermore, India accounts for nearly 22% of the global disease burden, putting more pressure on the existing healthcare

C. Patel (✉)
Research Scholar, Centre for Studies in Science Technology and Innovation Policy (CSSTIP), School of Social Sciences (SSS), Central University of Gujarat, Gandhinagar 382030, India

K. Sinha
Assistant Professor, Centre for Studies in Science Technology and Innovation Policy (CSSTIP), School of Social Sciences (SSS), Central University of Gujarat, Gandhinagar 382030, India

M. S. Kaiser et al. (eds.), *Proceedings of Trends in Electronics and Health Informatics*, Lecture Notes in Networks and Systems 376,
https://doi.org/10.1007/978-981-16-8826-3_17

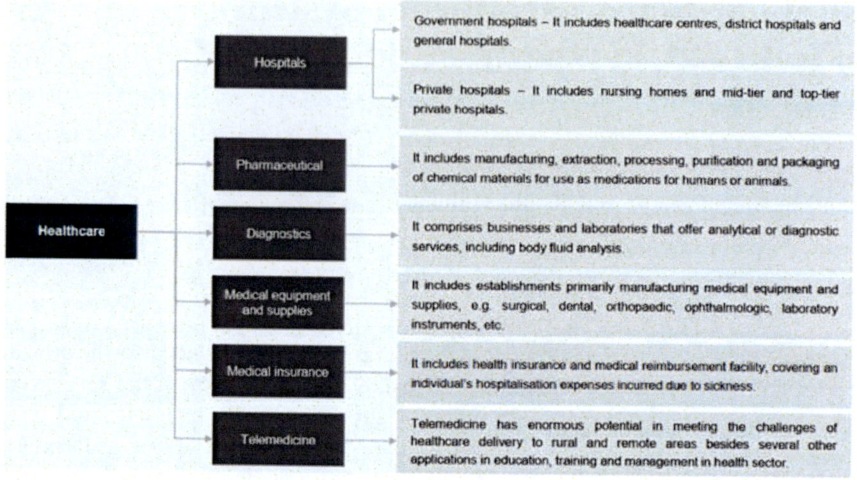

Fig. 1 Classified view of Indian healthcare [3]

delivery model. Approximately 65% of the Indian population lives in rural regions, with less than 30% healthcare infrastructure [1].

The Indian healthcare sector is the sector that needs upgradation and development in the infrastructure and technologies, services, human resources, etc. The Healthcare sector here means hospitals, hospitals beds, pharmaceuticals, medical insurance, medical equipment, supplies, diagnostics, and telemedicine. However, with the series of IPOs and private equity over the past few years, innovative processes, and more prominent players, the Indian healthcare sector is presently the most adored investment destination by the investing community. Most of the revenue of this sector comes from hospitals. Like other sectors, this sector also has two forms, public and private [2]. Figure 1 gives you a classified view of this sector market structure having different blocks.

The Indian healthcare system structure is not as simple as it seems to be but comprises various segments (refer Fig. 2), where many stakeholders are involved and are interconnected [4]. In this, patient care is mainly given through primary/community healthcare center (PHC/CHC), secondary healthcare center (District hospital), and tertiary healthcare center (National level) (refer Fig. 3). Currently, 4833 CHCs, 24 049 PHCs, 148 366 SCs, and 722 district hospitals are based on the distributional pyramid. These are functioning under the egis of the state and central governments [5].

In our dynamic digital era, the convergence of science and technology has resulted in innovative digital health devices that allow accurate and easy characterization of health and disease. In the current context, healthcare system is at the nib of a digital transformation. Digitalization aims to provide universal, affordable, equitable, and quality care to all citizens, leveraging digital technologies. However, looking at the country demographics and complexity, this would be a challenging journey.

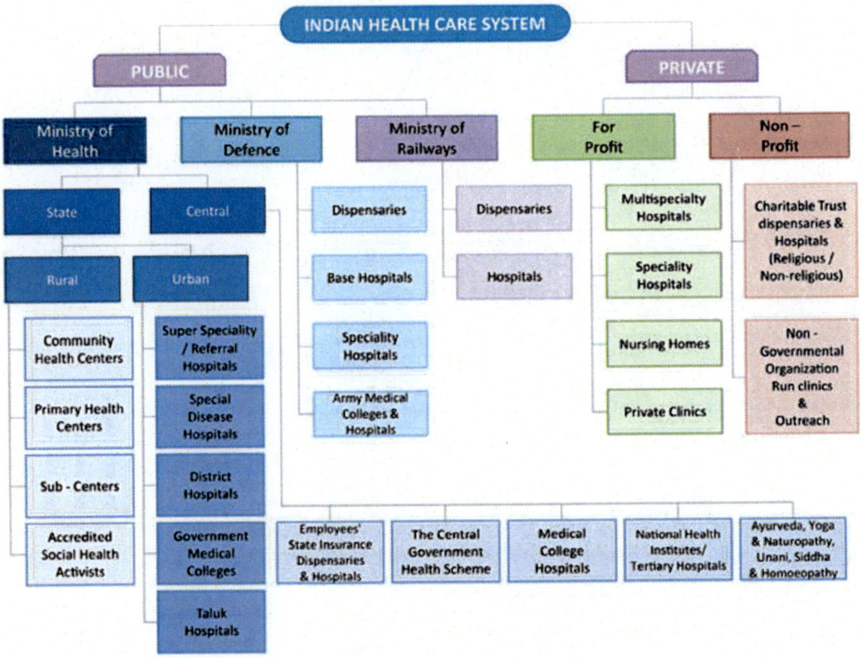

Fig. 2 Indian healthcare system [4]

Therefore, there is a need for such an ecosystem where all stakeholders (individuals, public, private, and government) will need to collaborate closely to make this happen.

Henceforth, the paper analyses the perspective of the Indian government on the digitalization of the Indian healthcare system considering the political, economic, social, technological, legal, and environmental (PESTLE) factors. As it is a long-term process, so there is a need to understand these associated elements, so that the planning that has been done can be achieved successfully. The structure of the paper is as follows, it starts with the introduction (Sect. 1), followed by background discussion on the Indian perspective (Sect. 2), that the methodology section discusses the way and the method used for the study (Sect. 3), then the discussion (Sect. 4), and lastly the conclusion part (Sect. 5).

2 Digitalization of Healthcare System: A Background

One of the journals Health Policy and Technology 9 (2020) has an issue on the "Digital transformation in healthcare: New value for a new movement," where a discussion is made on the three revolutions in aspect to the healthcare information technology. The first movement of healthcare IT includes telehealth and telemedicine,

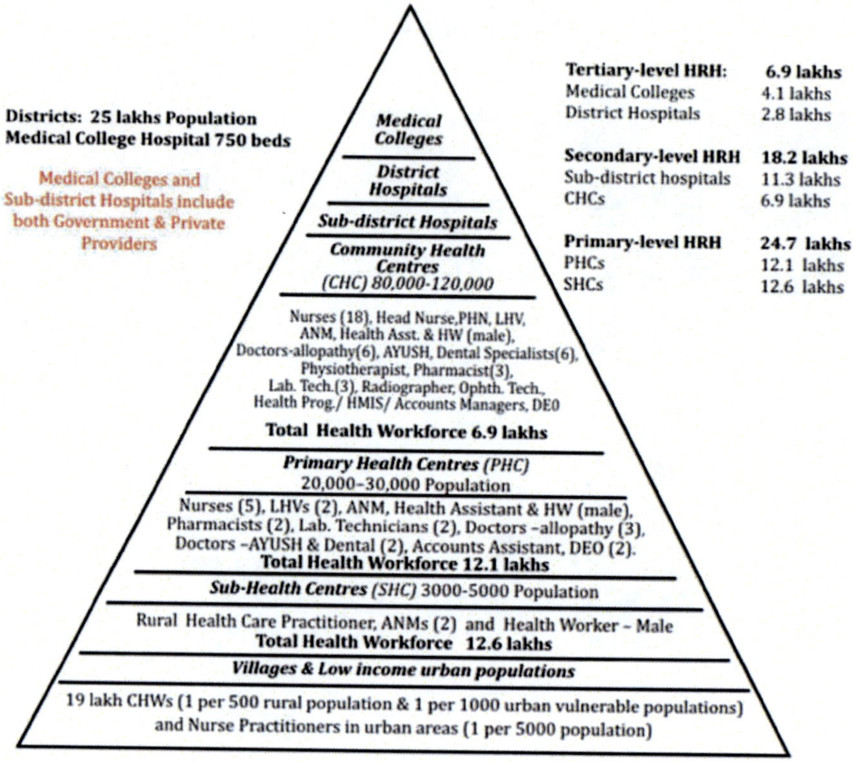

Fig. 3 Norms at primary, secondary, and tertiary levels [5]

where under this, research centered on using information communication technology (ICTS) to connect providers with patients or patients with providers and both over a geographic distance. The second movement of healthcare IT can be characterized by the movement to evaluate the technology's ability to benefit outcomes that are critical to healthcare that is enterprise resource planning (ERP) which includes picture archiving and communications systems (PACS), electronic medical records (EMRs), electronic personal health records (ePHRs), and a multitude of Web and mobile app-based innovations meant for physicians, nurses, patients, and other stakeholders; and the third movement in healthcare IT is the digital transformation in healthcare (DTHC) that emerges as distinct movement has attracted interest from both researchers and practitioners focusing on digital technologies [6].

Digitalization was used in conjunction with computers somewhere in the mid-1950s and referred to as "an organization, company, or a country embracing or using digital or computing technologies." Innovation in that aspect is moving in the Indian healthcare sector in the future of sophisticated, practical, and linked technologies. E-heath is one of the rising areas connected to community health, medical informatics, and industry, with concern to health services and facts provided or improved through the Internet and its related technologies. E-health is described by the European Commission as "the use of new communication and information technology to address the needs of people, patients, healthcare practitioners, healthcare providers, and decision-makers."

Digitalization here refers to various medical facilities focusing on digital health (refer Fig. 4) accessible to the citizen. The WHO defines the term digital health as "a broad umbrella term encompassing eHealth, as well as emerging areas, such as the use of advanced computing sciences in 'big data, genomics, and artificial intelligence'" that means using tools and services that use ICTs to improve the accuracy of monitoring and diagnosis of chronic diseases and improve patient treatment outcomes [7].

There are various forms of digital technologies used in the healthcare sector. Still, the service delivery through telemedicine, mHealth, EHR/EMR systems, healthcare analytics, and robot-assisted surgery has been gaining popularity in recent years (refer to Fig. 5). But the traces of digital health can be found from the year 2000 in telemedicine, but the least used digital services despite almost two decades of pilot

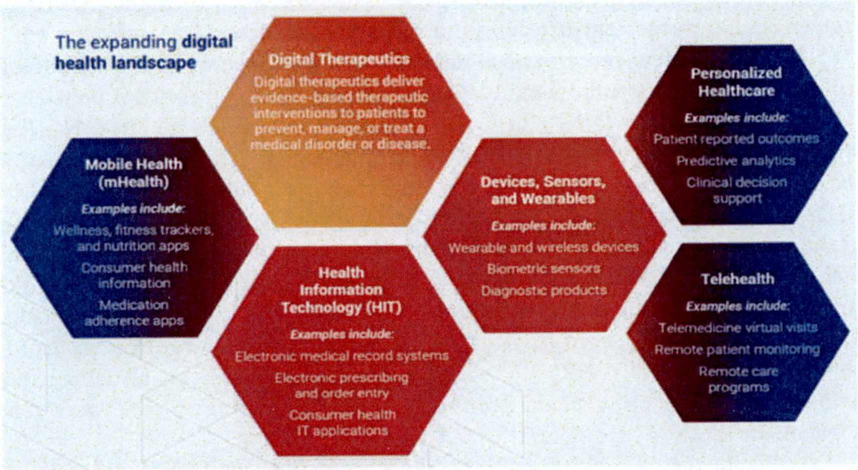

Fig. 4 Six categories of digital health [7]

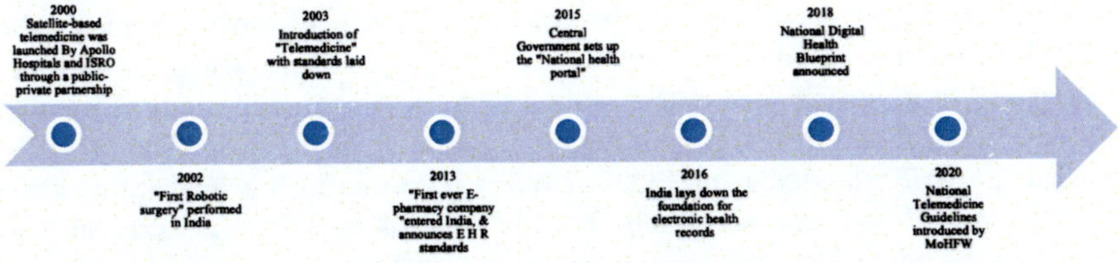

Fig. 5 Evolution of digital Healthcare in India (Adopted from [1])

studies and planning. Satellite-based telemedicine in 2000 was launched by Apollo Hospitals and the Indian Space Research Organization (ISRO) through a public–private partnership (PPP) [8–10]. In addition, a national telemedicine task force was established as early as 2005. However, a practical model could not be produced due to the lack of technological constraints such as low Internet speed. But teleradiology as notable success can be seen due to the need for less infrastructure and natural digital workflow.

Since 2002, GOI has released plans every five years, highlighting the progress in health care, including inputs and actions needed in digital health care. In the last two decades, India has continuously achieved a significant milestone. From 2015 onward, with the launch of the Digital India initiative and the last six years shows a societal transformation due to the digital revolution, directed efforts toward health care have increased significantly.

Various researchers, scholars, and practitioners, newspapers articles activists related to this sector in their blogs, articles, and research work have shown the changing scenario, challenges, and the availing opportunities arising due to the digitalization of the healthcare system as Aggarwal (2020) has tried to picturize the stages of digital health evolution taking place in Indian context when the COVID-19 pandemic has emerged and accelerated the need for health services (refer Fig. 6).

Talking of last few years, various steps taken by the Government of India (GoI) to promote and support the digital health journey by framing national policies as National Health Policy (NHP) 2017, National Health Stack (NHS) 2018, National Digital Health Blueprint (NDHB) 2019, and National Digital Health Mission (NDHM) launched in 2020 intending to create an "open digital health ecosystem" (ODE) featuring the required parameters and the ecosystem. In the "open digital health ecosystem," there would be digital infrastructure shared and to be used by both stakeholders (public and private) to deploy and build new innovative health solutions. The proposed digital infrastructure will comprise of two building blocks, first electronic health record (EHR) (patient digital medical record) and second is personal health record (PHR) (controlled by the patient and holds all HER data), with the adoption of open standards and a national health information network to be deployed by 2025.

Broadly, the digital health in India is seen through five significant categories, viz MHealth (Medical and public health practice is endorsed by mobile devices such as personal digital assistants (PDAs), other wireless devices, patient monitoring devices, and mobile phones. This also includes monitoring devices and services, followed by diagnosis, treatment, and healthcare practitioner support); Telemedicine (means the use of ICT to deliver healthcare services. It encompasses the exchange of information related to diagnosis, preventive and curative treatment, and medical training and development at a distance or in remote locations.); EHR/EMR (The MoHFW notified the EHR standards for India. It refers to capturing medical information about an individual concerning their current diagnosis as well as a focus on their longitudinal health); Healthcare analytics (an umbrella term that includes offering insights regarding patient records, costs, diagnoses, pharmaceutics, and medical research data, among others, by leveraging technologies such as big data, science and

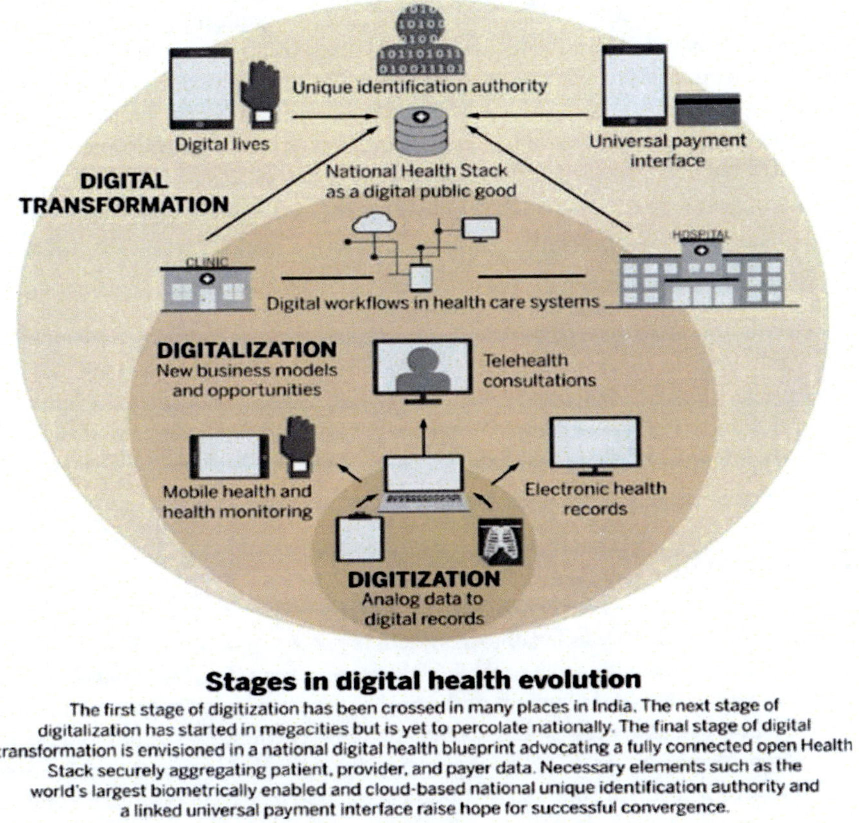

Fig. 6 Stages in digital health evolution in India [8]

analytics, and artificial intelligence); Robot-assisted surgery (method of executing surgery using minimal tools attached to robotic arm. The surgeon sits and instructs a robot's movements at the computers station through devices connected to the robot's arms).

In addition, there are various schemes launched by GoI that is helping in the transformation of the Indian healthcare ecosystem, that includes National AIDS and STD Control Programme; Pradhan Mantri Swasthya Suraksha Yojana; National Pharmacovigilance Programme; National Organ Transplantation Programme, Family Welfare Schemes; Swachhta Action Plan (SAP); and Impacting Research Innovation and Technology (IMPRINT) scheme covered under central. Furthermore, programs such as the National Rural Health Mission (NRHM), the National Health Mission (NHM), and the National Urban Health Mission (NUHM) as centrally supported schemes covering other sub-scheme [11–23].

The Indian perspective on healthcare system digitalization is evident and focuses on "reaching services to citizens" and "citizen empowerment through information dissemination" to improve public healthcare delivery significantly. And the success of this government-led transformation is crucial for the future economic growth of the country and directly or indirectly would benefit all the stakeholders, including individuals, government, payers, private health providers, healthcare technology companies, and startups in to achieve universal healthcare goal and provide every Indian citizen the choice of access to personalized quality care.

3 Methodology

The paper's objective is to explain the Indian perspectives on the healthcare system digitalization and the opportunities of the present Indian healthcare system. For analysis purpose, the researchers have used the PESTLE analysis. The researcher relied on secondary sources like journals, Web sites, editorials, and published reports.

4 Discussion

Digitalization of the Indian healthcare system is not a simple task. However, India is among the few countries that, over the few years, emerged as the fastest-growing digital economy due to the growth of the digital adoption index between 2014 and 2017. To improve accessibility and quality, the Indian healthcare sector has adopted digital transformation. By 2024, the digital healthcare market is expected to increase at a CAGR of 27.41% to US$ 485.43 billion compared to 2018, US$ 116.61 billion. Capital investment has been fueled due to the increasing importance of digital health and technologies. In 2019, 53% of angel investments were made in healthcare. Some of the notable deals Iora Health Inc. (US$ 126 million) were Curefit (US$ 111.5 million) and HealthCare Global Enterprise Ltd. ($119.7 million) [24].

However, compared to the BRICS Peers and Developed countries like the United Kingdom, New Zealand, Finland, Netherlands, and Australia spend 9% of total GDP, whereas Japan, Germany, France, Canada, and Switzerland spends 10%. While the United States over 17% of its GDP, adjacent countries like Bangladesh and Pakistan spend on the public healthcare system around 3% of GDP. The country's expenditure on health is far below, which is approximately 1.3% of GDP. Thus, government expenditure by 2025 on health to be increased to 2.5% of GDP was recommended by the National Health Policy of 2017, but that seems to be a far-off vision as to reach the target set, for that the country needs by 0.35% each from now. On the contrary, there has just been a mere increase of 0.02% in the health budget in India between 2015 16 and 2020–21 [25–26].

The growth in the digital adoption index of India has motivated the Indian government to focus on the digitalization of the Indian healthcare system. Within healthcare digitization, digital health is based on six pillars (refer to Fig. 7) interlocked with

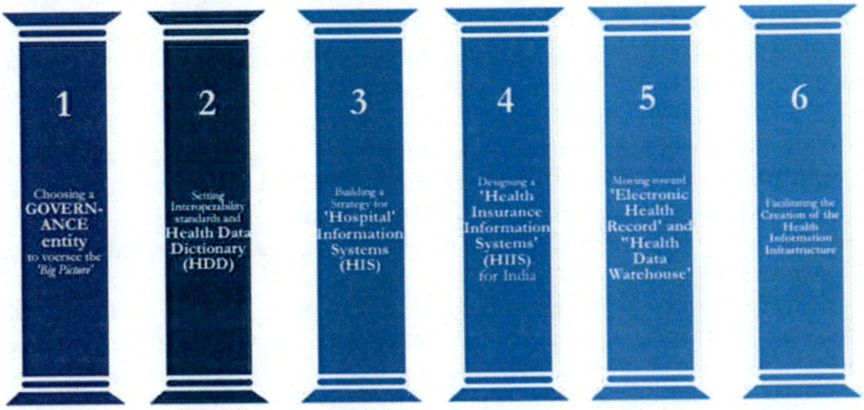

Fig. 7 Six pillars of digital health world [27]

each other. Each pillar has its purpose, communicates, interacts, and adds strengths and synergy to others.

Pillar One: Governance includes both technical and non-technical elements within itself. Technical as hardware, software, cloud technology, standards, network control center, road map implementation, certified skills, maintenance desk, etc. At the same time, non-technical includes creating innovative culture and environment, encouraging healthcare information technology (HIT) vendors to maintain records and resolve complaints.

Pillar Two: Health Data Dictionary (HDD) and Master Registries is an assemblage of standards that collectively define this common language in two ways, first in technical terms, nurtures "interoperability," and other in the non-technical term, becomes a way to communicate digitally with one another for all stakeholders. The HDD process includes a universal coding syntax, a unique patient identifier, and the semantics of each used medical reference with eDischarge and eClaims formats briefings.

Pillar Three: Building a strategy for Hospital Information Systems (HIS) for ALL facilities, both public and private, has various purposes: Their primary and first task is to aid in efficiently handling the facility administratively, financially, and clinically; They collate and assemble outputs which will eventually form the basis of the personal health record [PHR] and electronic health record [EHR] that includes diagnostic results, clinical reports, eDischarge summary objects, etc.; and so. That is, they maintain all the records from finance to the health information of patients and payers.

Pillar Four: Health Insurance Information Systems [HIIS] for health payers helps maintain the eClaims and has a few essential functions 1. Beneficiary enrollment and roaring; 2. Contribution fund and management; 3. Claim processing and payment; and 4. Utilization and quality management.

Pillar Five: Anywhere, anytime records for clinicians (Electronic Health.

Records [EHR]) and for patients (Personal Health Records [PHR]) are primarily a compilation of information gathered from other digital sources. The digital diagnostic results, physician orders positioned using the Hospital Information System (HIS), and the digital outputs from those similar systems.

Pillar Six: Facilitating the creation of the health information infrastructure: the 2–5 Pillars, of course, require considerable computer power amount, human expertise, and network connectivity on which to operate. This pillar mainly focuses on the technical infrastructure and the human capacity needed to maintain and run this digital healthcare system [27].

Digitalization of any system is based on five domains **Customers** (harnessing the networking among them), **Competition** (building platform, not just products), **Data** (as health data stored as PHI, and its privacy and use), **Innovation** (building something new by rapid experimentation) and **Value** (in the form of market value, demand–supply chain, and so). Each of them is very important and interlinked. As each digital technology are redefining, many of the underlying principles of strategy and changing rules decide the success of any company operating in this domain. This is what is needed to look at healthcare digitalization [28].

In addition to the above discussion, the crucial factors that also play a vital role in the digital healthcare transformation are the political, economic, social, technological, legal, and environmental factors that upgrade and impact the system's efficacy.

Political includes government industry-related policies, laws and regulations, trade restrictions, tax policies, tariffs, etc. This can be seen in the five-year plans and the initiative taken in the form of policies, schemes, Yojnas as acts, and rules. Some of them are defined above, which are laying the foundation of digital health.

Economic, include economic growth, interest rates, exchange rates, inflation rates, etc. The last five years shows the rapid growth of the country's healthcare sector, particularly since 2016, with a compound annual growth rate (CAGR) of approximately 22%. In terms of revenue and employment, health care has become one of the most significant sectors of Indian economy. KPMG and FICCI reports show that the healthcare sector in 2015, employing directly 4.7 million people. The NSDC estimates that by 2022, the sector will directly employ around 7.5 million people, adding up approximately 2.7 million more jobs between 2017 to 2022. In health, FDI has been focused on pharmaceuticals, comprising about two-thirds of the entire health sector. The healthcare sector has received keen interest from investors (venture capital and private equity) over the previous few years, with an increase from 94 Million USD (2011) to 1275 Million USD (2016) transaction value.

Social, this looks at cultural aspects that are sociocultural. It includes an increase in the aging population and life expectancy. In India, the fraction of the population aged 65 years and over is also on the rise. Others are based on demographic disease profiles, trends, and lifestyle diseases—cancer, cardiovascular diseases, and asthma have become the most vital segments, and in-patient expenditure and the healthcare market depend.

After that, the higher population and literacy display a massive opportunity for the health sector in their sheer volume. Also, there is a vast rural–urban shift in

India, offering an opportunity for this to have a roadmap on the digitalization of the Indian healthcare system. Rising literacy also improves health awareness about lifestyle-related diseases (tend to be more costly to treat than infections).

Technological, this is related to the application of new inventions, new technology (digital), R&D activity, automation, the rate of technological change, and technology incentives. This focuses on quality service and offers cost-competitive medical treatment and cardiology technological advances, orthopedic surgery, cosmetics, eye care, precautionary health checkups, and dentistry. Technology for healthcare includes machinery/equipment/ devices or methods for therapeutics and diagnostics that may be used to provide healthcare services.

Legal is related to the context of patient health information sharing, stored in the digital health apps, telemedicine that benefits both the providers and patients. In addition to protected health information (PHI), essential aspects are data use, data sharing, intellectual property (Patents, Copyrights, Trademarks, and Designs), commercial agreements, offenses, and penalties.

Environmental, the studies related to this focuses on whether the industry is working environment friendly and ethics are followed or not [29–37].

If the healthcare digitalization ensures efficient services delivery to their citizens of the nation, and consumers, thus can appreciates in a true sense of the Digital Nation India. Overall, the entire digital health ecosystem of technologies is represented in Fig. 8, focusing on quality care, improved access, better information management, better patient outcomes, and patient engagement. The six pillars and the essential key elements that are needed to understand has been discussed above. In addition, there is a blueprint prepared by the Indian Government, defining all the prospects but still has challenges and based on that the future possible opportunities.

While studying, particular challenges were found as implementing digital health across India is one of the major challenges, as health is a state-subject matter, where the states have to take responsibility, whereas the policies are centrally directed. The others are as lack of infrastructure (hospitals (private and public), beds, medical equipment, and devices, staff, and so) and the implementation capacity due to the absence of good leadership and management capability. This is followed by the shortage of human resources for health and their inequitable geographical distribution, noncompliance to standards, limited interoperability, and lack of data governance frameworks, thus drawing attention to the need for dedicated personnel to manage health and health information. As stated above, the ethical challenges of health data in digital formats is around data privacy and security and to counter that, to counter that the Draft Personal Data Protection Bill, 2018, was tabled and which when passed offers to set up National Data Protection Authority to regulate access to those who collect data, thereby ensuring privacy protection. However, challenges discussed above, besides difficulties, also provide an opportunity in the form of investments, employment generation, capacity building program, frameworks for clinical and operational data collection, evidence-informed development of policies, collation and governance to facilitate research and development, healthcare startups, for the adoption of EHRs need of a nation-wide framework, sustaining efficacy and quality of the digital healthcare system [38–47].

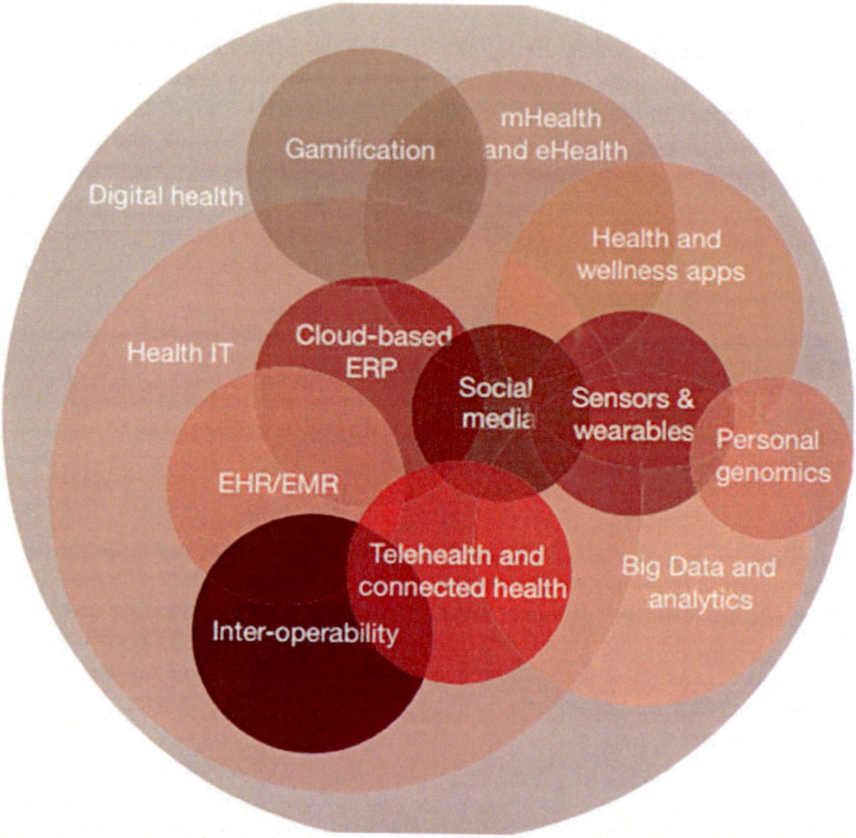

Fig. 8 Digital health ecosystem and its components [38]

5 Conclusion

In today's interconnected and interlinked world, health is not an internal matter but has its influence on the world, as in the case of a pandemic. Digital health or digitalization of healthcare is the emerging trend and has impacted the geopolitical and socioeconomic realities in the present and future. That is also the case in India too. The article focuses on the issue of healthcare digitalization, there are several essential parameters: innovative care, care anywhere, empowered care and intelligent healthcare enterprise, and the intelligent ecosystem where all players can work under one umbrella. And the government various initiatives and the associated political, economic, social, technological, legal, and environmental factors pointed to the need for digital health. Followed by India's current status, challenges, future prospects, and National Digital Health Blueprint would also help India better prepare to achieve sustainable development goals inclusively with the regulatory framework and ecosystem and to face unwanted circumstances such as the ongoing COVID-19. The article is expected to help researchers, analysts, strategists, policymakers, and scientists to develop the policies and intangible designs and models to enhance and sustain the stability for health reforms in the present and future.

References

1. Swiss Business Hub India. (2020) Digital healthcare industry in India. https://www.s-ge.com/en/publication/industry-report/20211-c3-medtech-india-digital-healthcare. Last accessed 23 Aug 2021
2. Kiran Kumar KV A sector that's all in the pink of health. https://www.isme.in/a-sector-thats-all-in-pink-of-hea/. Last accessed 23 Aug 2021
3. IBEF. Indian healthcare industry report. https://www.ibef.org/download/Healthcare-May-2021.pdf. Last accessed 23 Aug 2021
4. DRISHTIIAS (May 2020) Public health system in India. https://www.drishtiias.com/daily-updates/daily-news-editorials/public-health-system-in-india. Last accessed 23 Aug 2021
5. UHC-India. Chapter 4 human resources for health, http://uhc-india.org/reports/hleg_report_chapter_4.pdf. Last accessed 23 Aug 2021
6. Dohan M, Califf C, Ghosh K, Tan J (2020) Digital transformation in healthcare: new value for a new movement. Health Policy Technol 9. https://doi.org/10.1016/j.hlpt.2020.04.003
7. RUNWAY. Digital health: categories and trends [2020 Research]. https://runway.is/blog/digital-health-trends/. Last accessed 23 Aug 2021
8. Kumar A, Verma AK, Bharti J (2020) Aspects of digitalization of healthcare in India. 7:404
9. Anurag A (2020) Bridging digital health divides COVID-19 is accelerating digital transformation in the Indian health sector. Science, 1050–1052
10. Thyagaraja CM, Lakshmi S (2021) Telemedicine in India—perspective and SWOT analysis. IJCRT 9(1):1325–1330
11. Chokshi M, Patil B, Khanna R, Sharma J, Paul VK, Zodpey S (2016) Health system in India. J Perinatol 36:S9–S12
12. Ivančić L, Glavan ML, Vesna V (2020) A literature review of digital transformation in healthcare. https://doi.org/10.23919/MIPRO48935.2020.9245259
13. Kumar S (2018) Digitization of hospital services and operations: a conceptual framework. Int J Healthcare Educ Med Inf 05:1–5. https://doi.org/10.24321/2455.9199.201801
14. Nilaish N (2017) A review of Indian healthcare sector. SSRN Electron J. https://doi.org/10.2139/ssrn.2952286
15. Kraus S, Schiavone F, Pluzhnikova A, Invernizzi A (2020) Digital transformation in healthcare: analyzing the current state-of-research. J Bus Res, 123. https://doi.org/10.1016/j.jbusres.2020.10.030
16. Sarbadhikari S (2019) Digital health in India—as envisaged by the national health policy (2017). BLDE Univ J Health Sci 4(1). https://doi.org/10.4103/bjhs.bjhs_8_19; Roy M (2020) Digital health evolution and propagation in rural healthcare in India: a review
17. CIVILSDAILY (Sept 2020) Rolling-out of national digital health mission. https://www.civilsdaily.com/burning-issue-rolling-out-of-national-digital-health-mission/. Last accessed 23 Aug 2021
18. Srinivisan R Health care in India—visio 2020 issues and prospects. https://niti.gov.in/planningcommission.gov.in/docs/reports/genrep/bkpap2020/26_bg2020.pdf. Last accessed 23 Aug 2021
19. Olayan N, Morisaki S, Yamamoto S (2019) ARM analysis case study: digital Indian health care system business model and review. Acta Sci Med Sci 3(9):77–85

20. Prasad S (Mar 2021) Demystifying the digital healthcare transformation in India. https://www.cxotoday.com/big-data/demystifying-the-digital-healthcare-transformation-in-india/. Last accessed 23 Aug 2021
21. Hermes S, Riasanow T, Clemons EK et al (2020) The digital transformation of the healthcare industry: exploring the rise of emerging platform ecosystems and their influence on the role of patients. Bus Res 13:1033–1069. https://doi.org/10.1007/s40685-020-00125-x
22. FICCI-BCG-HEAL-2020-REPORT (2020) Leapfrogging to a digital healthcare system re-imagining healthcare for every Indian
23. IBEF, Knowledge Centre (Nov 2020) Digital healthcare to witness exponential growth In India, https://www.ibef.org/blogs/digital-healthcare-to-witness-exponential-growth-in-india. Last accessed 23 Aug 2021
24. Shob K (Jan 2021) "Will the upcoming budget address the needs of India's ailing health-care sector?" https://www.dailyrounds.org/blog/will-the-upcoming-budget-address-the-needs-of-indias-ailing-healthcare-sector/. Last accessed 23 Aug 2021
25. Mondal D (Jan 2021) "India spends just 1.26% of GDP on public healthcare". https://www.sundayguardianlive.com/news/india-spends-just-1-26-gdp-public-healthcare
26. NITIAyog (2019) Health system for new India: building blocks potential pathways to reform. https://www.slideshare.net/PankajGupta9/reimagining-indias-digital-health-landscape-wiring-the-indian-health-sector. Last accessed 23 Aug 2021
27. Rogers DL (2016) e digital transformation playbook; rethink your business for the digital age, Columbia University Press, New York
28. Pai RR, Alathur S (Ph.D.) (2019) Mobile health system framework in India. In Proceedings of dg.o 2019: 20th Annual International Conference on Digital Government Research (dg.o 2019), Dubai, United Arab Emirates. ACM, New York, NY, USA, p 10. https://doi.org/10.1145/3325112.3325235
29. NITIAyog (2021) Investment opportunities in India's healthcare sector. https://www.niti.gov.in/sites/default/files/2021-03/InvestmentOpportunities_HealthcareSector_0.pdf. Last accessed 23 Aug 2021
30. Nitish Desai Associates (2020) Digital health in India legal, regulatory and tax overview. https://www.nishithdesai.com/fileadmin/user_upload/pdfs/Research_Papers/Digital_Health_in_India.pdf. Last accessed 23 Aug 2021
31. Ranganathan S (2020) Towards a holistic digital health ecosystem in India. ORF Issue Brief No. 351, Observer Research Foundation. https://www.orfonline.org/research/towards-a-holistic-digital-health-ecosystem-in-india-63993/. Last accessed 23 Aug 2021
32. ACCENTURE. Digital Health Technology Vision2020. https://www.accenture.com/_acnmedia/PDF-130/Accenture-Health-Tech-Vision-2020.pdf. Last accessed 23 Aug 2021
33. Mitchell M, Kan L (2019) Digital technology and the future of health systems. Health Syst Reform 5. https://doi.org/10.1080/23288604.2019.1583040
34. Sehgal DR (2020) A legal study of digital healthcare in India. https://blog.ipleaders.in/legal-study-digital-healthcare-india/. Last accessed 23 Aug 2021
35. MoHFW (2019) Report on national digital health blueprint. https://www.nhp.gov.in/NHPfiles/National_Digital_Health_Blueprint_Report_comments_invited.pdf. Last accessed 23 Aug 2021
36. FXB CHH. India digital health net. https://fxb.harvard.edu/fxb-intersect/idhn/. Last accessed 23 Aug 2021
37. India Health (2020) Digital healthcare in India "healthcare of the future", https://www.indiahealth-exhibition.com/content/dam/Informa/indiahealth-exhibition/en/downloads/Digital%20health%20report%202020.pdf. Last accessed 23 Aug 2021
38. PWC. Indian Healthcare on the cusp of a digital transformation. https://www.pwc.in/publications/2016/indian-healthcare-on-the-cusp-of-a-digital-transformation.html. Last accessed 23 Aug 2021
39. Kumar R (2015) Lack of social or political demand for good health care in India: impact on unfolding universal health coverage. J Fam Med Primary Care 4(1):1–2. https://doi.org/10.4103/2249-4863.152234

40. Gudi N, Lakiang T, Pattanshett S, Sarbadhikari SN, John O (2021) Challenges and prospects in India's digital health journey. Indian J Public Health 65:209–212
41. Ministry of Health and Family Welfare Government of India (Apr 2019) National digital health blueprint. https://www.nhp.gov.in/NHPfiles/National_Digital_Health_Blueprint_Report_comments_invited.pdf. Last accessed 23 Aug 2021
42. Prasad MD, Menon CS (2020) The personal data protection bill, 2018: India's regulatory journey towards a comprehensive data protection law. Int J Law Inform Technol 28:1–9
43. Guo C, Ashrafian H, Ghafur S, Fontana G, Gardner C, Prime M (2020) Challenges for the evaluation of digital health solutions—a call for innovative evidence generation approaches. NPJ Digital Med 3:110. https://doi.org/10.1038/s41746-020-00314-2
44. Dr. Abidi FA (2020) "Does India need a digital health mission?". https://science.thewire.in/health/does-india-need-a-digital-health-mission/. Last accessed 23 Aug 2021
45. PBNS (Aug 2021) "The rise of India's healthcare: upgraded digital response ready for next big challenge", https://newsonair.com/2021/08/14/the-rise-of-indias-healthcare-upgraded-digital-response-ready-for-next-big-challenge/?__cf_chl_managed_tk__=pmd_D9ivDqO03ixdNLB33SFIdmAZoHsTFdyMs_ldzyTy5dI-1633930515-0-gqNtZGzNA1CjcnBszRQ9. Last accessed 23 Sep 2021
46. Tewari V (Jul 2021) "India's journey towards a digital healthcare ecosystem: taking the leap of faith" https://www.financialexpress.com/lifestyle/health/indias-journey-towards-a-digital-healthcare-ecosystem-taking-the-leap-of-faith/2281853/. Last accessed 23 Sep 2021
47. Ashvini Danigod (May 2021) 5 reasons why India's healthcare system is struggling https://www.thehindubusinessline.com/news/national/5-reasons-why-indias-healthcare-system-is-struggling/article34665535.ece. Last accessed 23 Sep 2021

A De-Speckling Framework for Optical Coherence Tomography Images

Pradeep K. Gupta and Farooq Husain

Abstract OCT is a very promising method to diagnose the diseases related to eyes. But in image acquisition process, a special noise known as speckle noise also present in the image. Due to present of this noise, diagnosis will be difficult. This paper proposed a framework that helps to reduce the noise. This framework apply curvelet transform to reduce the noise along with SRAD Filter and Huber variant of TV regularization. Firstly, noisy image passed through SRAD filter then curvelet transform is apply, and finally, we got de-noised image by applying Huber variant of TV regularization. Developed framework experimented on OCT images. Results concluded that this framework gives better performance along with better edge preservation capability.

Keywords SRAD · Curvelet transform · Huber variant · OCT

1 Introduction

Enhancement of OCT images is always prime concern for the accurate diagnosis of retinal diseases. At present, OCT widely used in ophthalmology for the detection of glaucoma, cataract disease [1, 2, 3]. OCT imaging technique used the detection of coherence source for the formation of image; therefore, OCT images have inherent feature of speckle noise; therefore, the image analysis of OCT images is a very difficult task [4]. It is a locally correlated and multiplicative in nature noise. Therefore, preprocessing is a necessary step in OCT image analysis. A number of de-speckling filters already have been proposed for de-speckling the OCT images.

In the literature, different types of spatial and non-linear filters [5, 6] are used to de-speckling the OCT images. These filters are trade-off between noise reduction and edge preservation. Linear filters also admit blur into the images and therefore degrade

---

P. K. Gupta (✉)
Pranveer Singh Institute of Technology Kanpur, Kanpur, U.P., India

F. Husain
SSITM Aligarh, Aligarh, U.P., India

M. S. Kaiser et al. (eds.), *Proceedings of Trends in Electronics and Health Informatics*, Lecture Notes in Networks and Systems 376,
https://doi.org/10.1007/978-981-16-8826-3_18

the contrast of the image [7]. Partial diffusion equation is also used to proposed a filter [8]. The noise reduction capability of these filters depends on different variables. Adaptive filters like hybrid median filter [9, 10] used the local neighborhood concept to calculate the de-noised pixel value. The structural information of image is restored by bilateral filter [11] and trilateral filter [11]. The drawback of these type filters is that the performance of these filters is noise dependent. To deal with the correlated noise, wavelet-based filters are proposed. Multi-scale resolutions are used to decompose the image in these filters. Out of different variants of wavelet transform, shift invariant wavelet give better results [12]. Recently, curvelet transform [13] and dual tree complex wavelet [14] are also used to remove the noise from the OCT images. These transforms give better result in comparison to conventional wavelets. The speckle noise from the OCT images can also be reduced by sparse and redundant representation of image along with K-SVD algorithm [15]. Discrete wavelet transform with Bayesian threshold is also used for speckle noise removal from OCT images [16].

Recently, a number of combinational techniques are also used to de-noising the images. These techniques exploited properties of different filters to achieve the better performance. In hybrid techniques, one or two filters are used serially. A number of hybrid techniques are being proposed in literature. Combination of discrete wavelet transform and anisotropic diffusion filter has been used to improve the de-speckling capability of the filter. This technique also has the capability of edge preservation [17]. SRAD filter, wavelet soft thresholding along with guided filter is also used to design a hybrid technique [18–20]. In hybrid technique, there is a trade-off between de-speckling capability and edge preservation ability of the filter. This paper also applies two different filters for noise reduction along with edge preservation capability.

The proposed framework used a preprocessing filter, curvelet transform along with post-processing filter. The remaining sections of this paper are: Sect. 2 explains the modeling of speckle noise and Sect. 3 about the proposed framework. Sections 4 tells about the materials and methods used in this paper. Sections 5 discuss about the results, and Sects. 6 concludes the outcome of the proposed framework.

2 Speckle Noise Modeling

The nature of the speckle noise present in the OCT image is multiplicative; therefore, mathematically it is represented as

$$I_o = \mathrm{IN}_m + N_a \tag{1}$$

I represent noiseless image, I_o represent the output image corresponding to input image I, N_m represent the multiplicative part of speckle noise, and N_a represent the additive part of the speckle noise [21].

3 Proposed Framework

The proposed de-speckling framework is a type of hybrid approach. This approach is a three-step approach. In first step, preprocessing filtering is performed by using SRAD filter. SRAD filter gives better result for lower noise variance in comparison to conventional methods [18]. In second step, the proposed framework used curvelet transform. It is the extension of wavelet transform. In this. transform image is decomposed at specified scales, locations and orientations. The curvelet transform is helpful to preserve the structure of the image [22]. The last step of proposed framework used a post-processing filter. This step used a variant of total variation. Last step of the proposed framework is used for edge preservation [23]. The procedural steps of our proposed framework are:

Step 1: Apply SRAD filtering on noisy OCT image using Eq. (2).
Step 2: Apply curvelet transform de-noising on output of step 1.
Step 3: Apply Huber variant of TV regularization on the output of step 2 to get the de-noised image (Fig. 1).

3.1 SRAD Filter

OCT image de-speckling can be perform by SRAD filter. SRAD filter is a partial differential equation (PDE)-based speckle reducing filter. SRAD filter is used to preserves the edge details of image along with reducing the speckle noise. Let $I_0(x, y)$ is given gray level image, corresponding to this $I_o(x, y; t)$ is the output image as per the following equation

$$\begin{cases} \frac{\partial(x,y;t)}{\partial t} = \mathrm{div}[c(q)\nabla I(x, y; t)] \\ I_o(x, y; 0) = I_o(x, y), \left.\frac{\partial I(x,y;t)}{\partial \vec{n}}\right|_{\partial B} = 0 \end{cases} \tag{2}$$

here div, ∇ represent divergence and gradient [8].

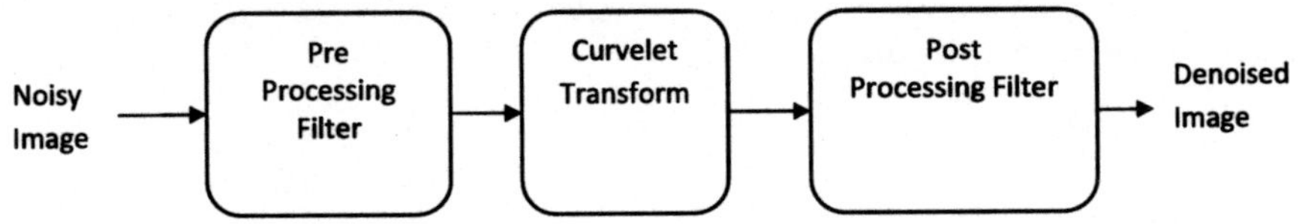

Fig. 1 Block diagram of proposed de-speckling framework

3.2 Curvelet Transform

Curvelet transform is helpful to represent the image at various scale, and orientation is proposed. This transform decomposes the image with the help of basis function. It has time–frequency localization properties of wavelets [22]. The main advantage of curvelet transform is that it has superior performance over local ridgelet transform. Basically, 2D curvelets are 2D extension of wavelets. Scale, orientation, and two translation parameters decide the curvelets. Curvelets used a spatial band-pass filter with multiscale ridgelets to isolate different scales [24]. The following steps are used in curvelet decomposition.

1. Subband decomposition—The object O is decomposed into subbands such that

$$O \leftrightarrow (\Delta_0 O, \Delta_1 O, \Delta_2 O \ldots\ldots\ldots\ldots\ldots\ldots\ldots)$$

2. Smooth partitioning—Each subband is smoothly windowed into sequence of an appropriate scale

$$\Delta_s O \leftrightarrow \left(w_Q \Delta_s O\right)_{Q \in Q_s}$$

3. Renormalization—Output of step 2 is convert into unit scale.

$$g Q = \left(T_Q\right)^{-1}\left(w_Q \Delta_s O\right), \quad Q \in Q_s$$

4. Ridgelet analysis.

3.3 Huber Variant of TV Regularization

In step 3 of this framework, a variant of TV regularization is applied. Last step of the proposed framework is used for preserving the structure with speckle noise reduction. During this post-processing step of proposed framework, it is assumed that speckle is a multiplicative noise and converted into a Gaussian distribution with a square-root transformation [23]. Staircase artifacts due to traditional TV regularization are remove by Huber penalty function.

4 Material

To demonstrate the worthiness of this framework, the results of proposed framework are compared with many filters proposed by different researchers. These filters are speckle reducing anisotropic diffusion (SRAD) [8], hybrid median filter (HMF) [13], weighted guided filter [25], and TGVD filter [26].

4.1 Image Database

Real images of OCT provided by Jinming Duan [26] are used for experiments.

4.2 Quality Matrices

The different quality matrices used in this proposed framework are: Structural residual (SR), peak signal to noise rati(PSNR), structure similarity index (SSIM), and contrast-to-noise ratio (CNR).

4.2.1 Peak Signal to Noise Ratio(PSNR)

Ratio of maximum power to noise power.

$$\mathrm{PSNR(dB)} = 10\log_{10}\left(\frac{I_{\mathrm{MAX}}^2}{\mathrm{MSE}}\right) \tag{3}$$

where I_{MAX} is the maximum power of signal and MSE is mean square error of signal.

4.2.2 Contrast-To-Noise Ratio (CNR)

Calculate the contrast of interested ROI and noisy background of the image and defined as

$$\mathrm{CNR} = \frac{1}{N}\left[\sum_{n=1}^{N}\frac{\mu_n - \mu_b}{\sqrt{(\sigma_n^2 + \sigma_b^2)}}\right] \tag{4}$$

where μ_b, σ_b^2 are mean and variance of the background noise of the image and μ_n,σ_n^2 are the nth ROI of the image.

4.2.3 Structural Similarity Index Metric (SSIM)

It measures the similarity between noisy and noiseless image defined as:

$$\mathrm{SSIM}(I, O) = \frac{(2\mu_I\mu_O + c_1)(2\sigma_{I,O} + c_2)}{(\mu_I^2 + \mu_O^2 + c_1)(\sigma_I^2 + \sigma_O^2 + c_2)} \quad (5)$$

where (μ_I, σ_I^2) and (μ_O, σ_O^2) are the mean and variance, and $\sigma_{I,O}$ is the covariance.

5 Result

The visual and numerical results of this framework are calculated by performing an experiment on real OCT images. The output results are compared with four different filters.

Tables 1, 2 and 3 show PSNR, CNR, and SSIM values comparison for real OCT image 1, 2, and 3. From the numerical values, it is clear that this technique is outperformed in terms of PSNR, CNR,SR, and SSIM in comparison to other compared

Table 1 PSNR, CNR, and SSIM comparison for real OCT image 1

Filter	PSNR	CNR	SSIM
SRAD[8]	30.7539	4.96632	0.60584
HMF[13]	27.9743	3.59154	0.52962
WGF[25]	22.2599	3.10091	0.99996
TGVD[26]	32.2799	5.28452	0.65039
Proposed	**35.9128**	**7.50471**	**0.99997**

Table 2 PSNR, CNR, and SSIM comparison for real OCT image 2

Filter	PSNR	CNR	SSIM
SRAD[8]	29.5751	4.1081	0.61977
HMF[13]	26.5936	6.7111	0.53541
WGF[25]	25.5966	3.7574	0.99996
TGVD[26]	24.9841	2.8149	0.66266
Proposed	**35.5866**	**6.5724**	**0.99996**

Table 3 PSNR, CNR, and SSIM comparison for real OCT image 3

Filter	PSNR	CNR	SSIM
SRAD[8]	29.6477	4.1106	0.5939
HMF[13]	26.2189	6.5147	0.5005
WGF[25]	25.9129	3.1009	0.9999
TGVD[26]	25.0964	4.0207	0.6455
Proposed	**35.9128**	**7.2103**	**0.9999**

filters. Figures 2, 3, and 4 show the visual comparisons of the proposed framework with other state of the art filters. The visual results also support the numerical values. This technique significantly removes the speckle noise along with edge preservation capability.

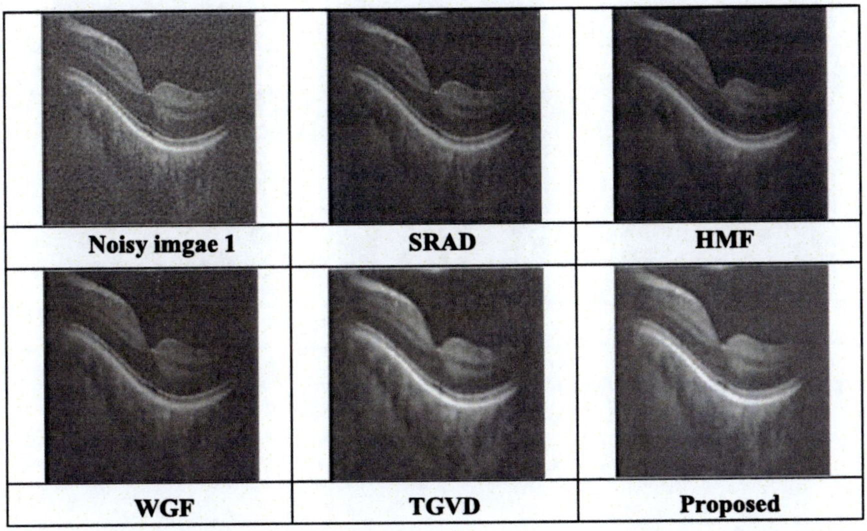

Fig. 2 Visual comparison of real OCT image 1

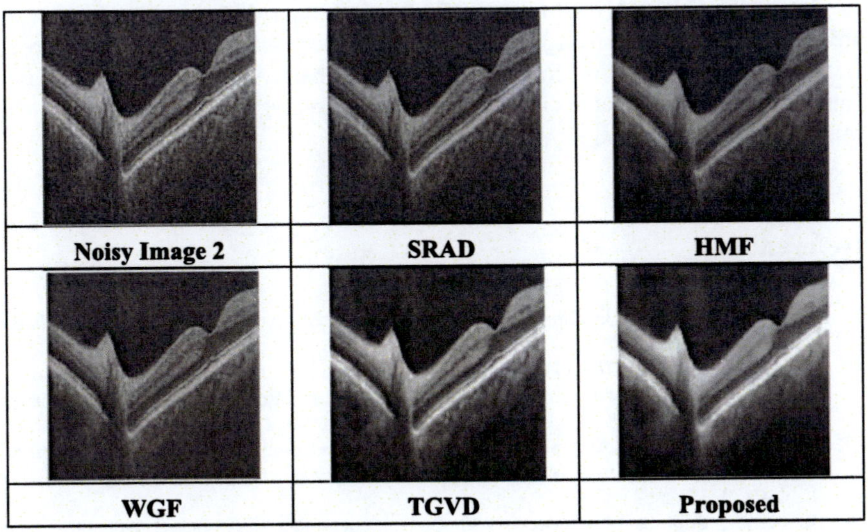

Fig. 3 Visual comparison of real OCT image 2

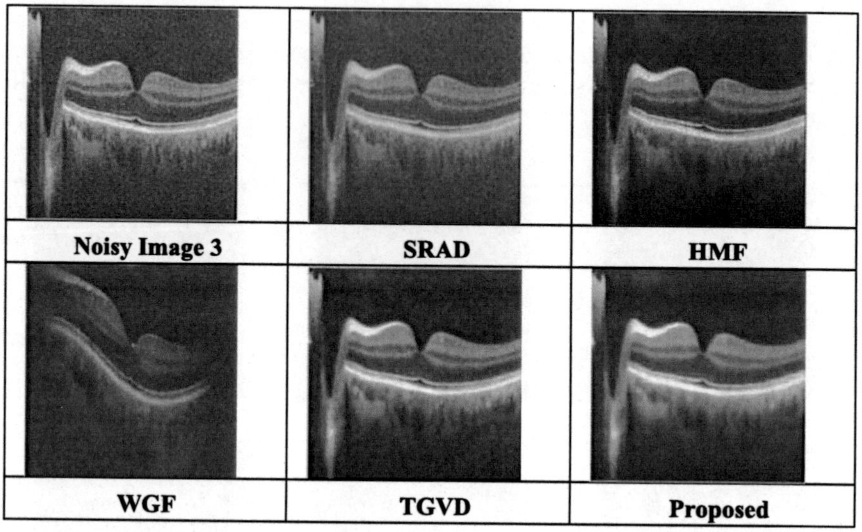

Fig. 4 Visual comparison of real OCT image 3

6 Conclusion

This researcher paper proposed a de-speckling framework for real OCT image. The proposed framework shows the ability of speckle noise reduction with the preservation of fine detail. An experiment has been conducted on real OCT images to find out the PSNR, CNR, and SSIM values. The results obtained for proposed framework are compared with the existing de-speckle filters. The results show that the proposed framework outperforms in comparison to various filters. Visual results of proposed framework also show that the technique is capable to preserve the edges along with original structures of image.

References

1. Drexler W et al (2001) Ultrahigh-resolution ophthalmic optical coherence tomography. Nature Med 7(4):502–507
2. Khaing TT, Aimmanee P (2017) "Optic disk segmentation in retinal images using active contour model based on extended feature projection." 2017 8th international conference of information and communication technology for embedded systems (IC-ICTES). IEEE
3. Zhang L et al (2017) "Automatic cataract detection and grading using deep convolutional neural network." 2017 IEEE 14th international conference on networking, sensing and control (ICNSC). IEEE
4. Drexler W, Fujimoto JG (eds) (2008) Optical coherence tomography: technology and applications. Springer Science and Business Media
5. Serkan M et al (2008) Edge and fine detail preservation in SAR images through speckle reduction with an adaptive mean filter. Int J Remote Sens 29(23):6727–6738

6. Perreault S, Hébert P (2007) Median filtering in constant time. IEEE Trans Image Process 16(9):2389–2394
7. Kato H, Goodman JW (1975) Nonlinear filtering in coherent optical systems through halftone screen processes. Appl Opt 14(8):1813–1824
8. Yu Y, Acton ST (2002) Speckle reducing anisotropic diffusion. IEEE Trans Image Process 11(11):1260–1270
9. Anantrasirichai N et al (2014) Adaptive-weighted bilateral filtering and other pre-processing techniques for optical coherence tomography. Comput Med Imaging Graph 38(6):526–539
10. Xie H, Pierce LE, Ulaby FT (2002) SAR speckle reduction using wavelet denoising and Markov random field modeling. IEEE Trans Geosci Remote Sens 40(10):2196–2212
11. Hao Y, Feng X, Jianlou X (2012) Multiplicative noise removal via sparse and redundant representations over learned dictionaries and total variation. Signal Process 92(6):1536–1549
12. Zeng Z, Cumming I (1998) "Bayesian speckle noise reduction using the discrete wavelet transform." IGARSS'98. Sensing and managing the environment. 1998 IEEE international geoscience and remote sensing. Symposium proceedings. (Cat. No. 98CH36174). vol 1. IEEE
13. Nieminen A, Heinonen P, Neuvo Y (1987) A new class of detail-preserving filters for image processing. IEEE Trans Pattern Anal Mach Intell 1:74–90
14. Chitchian S, Fiddy MA, Fried NM (2009) Denoising during optical coherence tomography of the prostate nerves via wavelet shrinkage using dual-tree complex wavelet transform. J Biomed Optics 14(1):014031
15. Jian Z et al (2010) Three-dimensional speckle suppression in optical coherence tomography based on the curvelet transform. Opt Express 18(2):1024–1032
16. Ozcan A et al (2007) Speckle reduction in optical coherence tomography images using digital filtering. JOSA A 24(7):1901–1910
17. Bhateja V et al (2015) Speckle suppression in SAR images employing modified anisotropic diffusion filtering in wavelet domain for environment monitoring. Measurement 74:246–254
18. Choi H, Jeong J (2018) Despeckling images using a preprocessing filter and discrete wavelet transform-based noise reduction techniques. IEEE Sens J 18(8):3131–3139
19. Fernández DC, Salinas HM, Puliafito CA (2005) Automated detection of retinal layer structures on optical coherence tomography images. Opt Express 13(25):10200–10216
20. Weickert J (1998) Anisotropic diffusion in image processing, vol 1. Teubner, Stuttgart
21. Zadeh LA (1996) "Fuzzy sets." Fuzzy sets, fuzzy logic, and fuzzy systems: selected papers by Lotfi A Zadeh, 394–432
22. Candes E et al (2006) Fast discrete curvelet transforms. Multiscale Model Simul 5(3):861–899
23. Li M et al (2017) Statistical model for OCT image denoising. Biomed Opt Express 8(9):3903–3917
24. CandÃÍs EJ, Donoho DL, Schumaker L (1999) "Curvelets–a surprisingly effective nonadaptive representation for objects with edges." Curve and surfaces. Nashville, TN: Vanderbilt University Press, 105–120
25. Li Z et al (2014) Weighted guided image filtering. IEEE Trans Image Process 24(1):120–129
26. Duan J et al (2016) Denoising optical coherence tomography using second order total generalized variation decomposition. Biomed Signal Process Control 24:120–127

Rotational Opponent Motion Detection Impact in Biological Motion Perception

Khashayar Misaghian, J. Eduardo Lugo, and Jocelyn Faubert

Supported by an NSERC-Essilor Research Chair the NSERC discovery grant And FESP-E´OUM

Abstract Analyzing the underlying mechanisms of biological motion perception in the visual system as a critical feature to survival and social life of human beings has been an interesting study subject for a while. Earlier, a descriptive implementational-level model to characterize the dorsal pathway of an expert observer visual system has been proposed. Moreover, the model has been successfully used to model the behavior (psychometric function) of 35 expert athletes who participated in one previous psychophysics study. Here, rotational optical flow pattern detection feature has been implemented at the evidence-encoding stage of the model mentioned above to investigate further the effect of different visual cues involved in biological motion perception. The increased capacity of the new version of the model to simulate more subjects with more precision and flexibility, as a result, gives valuable insight into the importance of rotational optical flow in the decision-making process and how expert observers could perform on a different level compared to the non-experts.

Keywords Biological motion perception · Rotational optical flow · Descriptive model · Implementational-level model · Psychometric function · Expert observer · Dorsal pathway

K. Misaghian (✉) · J. E. Lugo · J. Faubert
Faubert Lab, School of Optometry, University of Montreal, Montreal, QC 3T 1P1, Canada
e-mail: k.misaghian@umontreal.ca

J. E. Lugo
Facultad de Ciencias Fisico-Matematicas, Benem´Erita Universidad Aut´Onoma de Puebla, Av. San Claudio y Av. 18 sur, Col. San Manuel Ciudad Universitaria, Pue, 72570 Puebla, Mexico

M. S. Kaiser et al. (eds.), *Proceedings of Trends in Electronics and Health Informatics*, Lecture Notes in Networks and Systems 376,
https://doi.org/10.1007/978-981-16-8826-3_19

1 Introduction

One of the most prominent objectives of finding neural correlates of decision making is to ultimately model the behavior beyond research paradigms and closer to real-world situations [18, 19]. One great example of a real-world situation is the motion perceived only from the conjoint movement of a living body's optimum number of key points. This body motion analysis by the brain is called biological motion perception. This trait of the visual system has indeed proven to be critical to the survival of human beings in the wild and society [7]. Modeling biological motion perception as one form of decision making at different levels of analysis, especially representational and implementational level and after that putting one step further and model the human behavior using that model is indubitably in a direction toward a more unified understanding of the brain [10, 12, 16]. One seminal investigation in the field of representational/implementation level of the biological motion perception modeling has been done by Giese and Poggio, suggesting the more significant contribution of the dorsal pathway (motion processing pathway) compared to the ventral pathway (dynamic form processing pathway) in the visual system. Contradicting the earlier speculations from psychophysics study favoring form pathway as the prominent role player [1, 4]. Later, Casile and Giese honed in on the previous idea from the 2003 study above and proposed a model solely based on the dorsal pathway [3]. Furthermore, the thorough review from Blake and Shiffrar proposed a more redundant view indicating that both pathways are synergistically working toward a robust decision based on the situation and conditions [2]. Moreover, Thurman and Lu proposed a computational-level Bayesian template-matching model for biological motion perception. They concluded that the dynamic form pathway processes the motion of a live body in the same way it processes non-biological dynamic form evolution [17]. While the ongoing investigation of the neural correlates of biological motion perception has corroborated the activation of vast cortical areas, including form and motion areas, the causality of these activations is not clear [5, 6, 9]. One fascinating study invited participants with focally compromised ventral visual cortex and demonstrated that they could perceive biological motion almost at the same level as healthy participants [5]. Later, an implementational-level model of the dorsal visual cortex to perceive high complexity biological motion was proposed, and the model successfully simulated the behavior of 35 elite athletes replicating their psychometric functions. Even though most of the athletes' behavior was simulated, few behaviors were not reenacted favorably [11].

Additionally, one study has demonstrated that training with a perceptual-cognitive exercise called "3D Multiple Object Tracking" enhances athletes' ability to make decisions in sports scenarios, where many decisions revolve around biological motion processing. Interestingly, this cognitive task has no sport-related content or information [14]. The mechanics of how "3D Multiple Object Tracking" training contributes to the biological motion perception substrates are yet to be discovered. However, it is apparent that this type of cognitive training would not directly enhance the internal generative models or prototypes. The reason is that the observer receives no context-related (biological motion-related) information that could affect the internal prototypes directly in terms of learning and denoising. However, it is established that the executive functioning would improve by this type of training, and having a better working memory and other factors may correlate to a better inference from internal models. Nevertheless, one question remains: what other context-independent factors in biological motion perception differentiate an expert from a non-expert. One undeniable hypothesis is that the rotations in the scene could be the cues that the non-experts would have a hard time picking up for a better assessment. One way to test such a hypothesis is to examine it with the implementational-level model mentioned above [11]. The second hierarchy level of the original model was only capable of sensing expansion and contraction opponent motions. Now, one could examine how the implementation of local rotation detection in the model would contribute to the betterment of the model and behavior modeling. Therefore, we have implemented the clockwise and counterclockwise rotation sensing neurons in the previously proposed biological motion perception model to investigate how local rotations would contribute to the expert human behavior facing a complex biological motion perception task [11].

2 Methods

A descriptive risk-averse biological motion perception model to simulate human expert behavior in a soccer biological motion task has been proposed and achieved to simulate the behavior (psychometric function) of 35 but not all human expert participants of an earlier psychophysics study [13]. To find out if implementing the rotational motion sensing in the model would enhance the model's performance (or not) and its extent is a matter of the investigation of this study [11]. The model detects the direction of a soccer ball from stimuli adopted from the work of Romeas and Faubert, which is a biological motion of the soccer kick captured by Mixamo studio. Fifteen point-lights characterize the head and 14 major joints of the kicker (no ball marker). The motion capture stimulus is 4.5 s with 90 frames, and to create kicks stimuli with different angles to the right or left, the original motion capture stimulus has been rotated around the Z-axis [13]. Moreover, implementations and data fitting are achieved using MATLAB. This implementational-level decision-making model consists of two levels for the evidence-encoding stage, one level for the integration stage, and finally, one last level for the thresholding stage. The first two consecutive evidence-encoding hierarchical levels are:

Local motion energy detectors: At their small and overlapping receptive fields (approximately 0.4 deg), these detectors sense the basic upward, downward, leftward and rightward motions in different locations of the scene and communicate it to the second level [3, 11].

Opponent-motion sensors: With their wider and again conjoining receptive fields of 4.5 degrees, they sense the vertical and horizontal expansions and contractions at the lower hierarchy level. However, in reality, there exist sensors at this level that sense rotational motions of the lower level which, for the sake of simplicity, have not been implemented in the previous version of the model [3, 11, 15].

For the clockwise (counterclockwise), motion-sensing 20 neurons are implemented to cover the whole local motion detection grid of the previous local motion energy detection level. Each rotation neuron looks at four abutting and overlapping subfields accommodating the neuron to sense the highest localized rotational activity of the scene with max-pooling. For clockwise (counterclockwise), rotation sensing neurons are arranged in a 4×5 grid. Each neuron receives signals from four abutting and overlapping subfields from the lower level. Each subfield is made of a grid of 14X14 local motion detectors to cover the whole rotational activity of the lower level (Fig. 1). To paint a clearer picture of the implementation, consider four neighboring receptive fields of one of the clockwise rotation neurons, the upper-left, the upper-right, the lower-left, and the lower right subfields (Fig. 2). Since local motion detection sensors only pick up on the fundamental rightward, leftward, upward, and downward motions, the clockwise rotation neuron only would get activated under the two conditions illustrated in Fig. 2. The range, 1°–20° of deviation for both left and right sides, has been used for training, testing, and cross-validation purposes. The enhanced model with rotation detection capability has been cross-validated using fivefold cross-validation [8]. Furthermore, the range of 7°–20° was used to train the model. After that, complying with the psychophysics study mentioned above, it has been tested randomly on 2°,4°,8°, and 15° angles to the left or to the right kick stimuli [11, 13]. In the psychophysics study mentioned above, a forced-choice paradigm task has been utilized. In the task, expert athletes and non-athletes were asked to detect

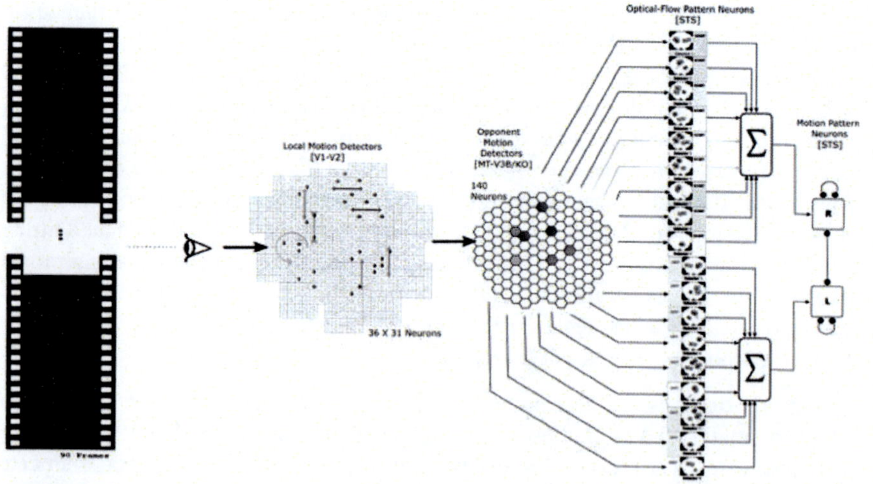

Fig. 1 Four hierarchical levels of biological motion perception with added rotation detection at the second level

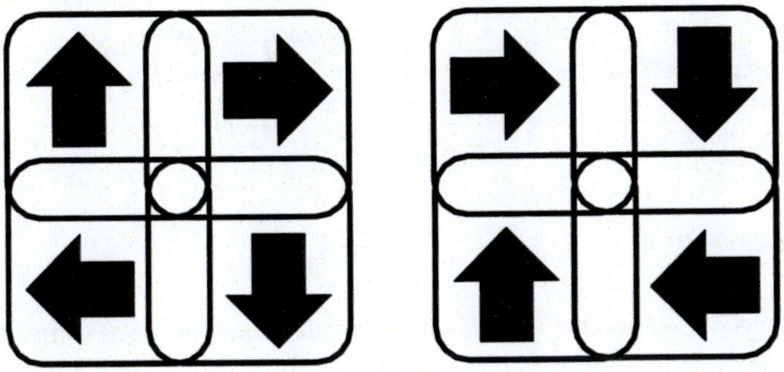

Fig. 2 Subfields in one clockwise rotation receptive field of our model

the direction of the ball as fast as possible from the biological motion stimuli of the soccer kick explained above [13]. A set of 1080 randomized stimuli (of 2°,4°,8° and 15° angles of deviation to the left and right was assigned to each participant as their task (120 times for each angle and side). Subsequently, the acquired data were used to calculate the psychometric function parameters of the participants (angular deviation thresholds and slope) [13]. The same task protocol has been given to the model to replicate the conditions of the psychophysics study. The process has been repeated 30 times (30 times more than the human subject), and the results were used to calculate the simulated psychometric functions parameters (angular deviation thresholds and slope).

3 Results

Similar to the previous work, the expert participants' behaviors (psychometric functions) have been simulated in a grid-search fashion by modifying the model's parameters [11]. The rotation detection neurons at the second hierarchy level were integrated to include the occurrences of local rotations of the scene into the decision process. Unsurprisingly, the rotation features combined with expansion/contraction features lead to more accurate fittings of the behavior in all computed states of the model with no exception. To be more precise, simulating high-performance behaviors of steeper slopes and lower angular thresholds were attainable with this new model. In an impressive turnout, integration of rotation receptive fields resulted in simulating the behavior of the athlete participant B10, which could not be achieved by the previous version of the model [11], leaving us with two participants out of 38 athletes whose behaviors could not be simulated with the proposed model. These findings only corroborate that different visual systems strategize differently in what combination of expansion/contraction and rotation signals they use to perceive the same biological motion stimulus.

Table 1 Subject B10's simulated behavior versus experimental behavior

Subject	Experimental angular threshold	Simulated angular threshold	Experimental slope	Simulated slope
B10	13.160 ± 3.02	13.36312 ± 0.56	0.103 ± 0.015	0.101 ± 0.0027

4 Discussion

The results above imply that knowing how one visual system gives weight to expansion/contraction information versus rotation information, the simulation of the two left-out subjects would be attainable. Subsequently, implementing a mechanism by which the model could give weight to different opponent motion signals sounds like a promising future work. The characterization of the neural hierarchies at each level could generally have different forms due to how different variants of that level are combined. When these diverse levels connect to other diverse hierarchy levels, the number of possible combinations becomes vast, and the proposed model has not indeed explored many of these interesting conditions [10]. Having a better simulation of the behavior by bringing the rotational motion detection feature into the equation was not far from the expectation, given that more information might lead to more accurate decisions. Nevertheless, the valuable finding was the more extensive range of angular threshold to slope ratio, which interpreted into the model's capacity to reproduce a much more extensive range of behaviors. Moreover, to simulate one behavior that could not be reproduced earlier rejects the hypothesis that the expert observer does not leverage from heeding to purported rotational motions of the scene (Table 1).

References

1. Beintema J, Lappe M (2002) Perception of biological motion without local image motion. Proc Natl Acad Sci 99(8):5661–5663
2. Blake R, Shiffrar M (2007) Perception of human motion. Annu Rev Psychol 58:47–73
3. Casile A, Giese MA (2005) Critical features for the recognition of biological motion. J Vis 5(4):6–6
4. Giese MA, Poggio T (2003) Neural mechanisms for the recognition of biological movements. Nat Rev Neurosci 4(3):179–192
5. Gilaie-Dotan S, Saygin AP, Lorenzi LJ, Rees G, Behrmann M (2015) Ventral aspect of the visual form pathway is not critical for the perception of biological motion. Proc Natl Acad Sci 112(4):E361–E370
6. Grosbras MH, Beaton S, Eickhoff SB (2012) Brain regions involved in human movement perception: a quantitative voxel-based meta-analysis. Hum Brain Mapp 33(2):431–454
7. Johansson G (1973) Visual perception of biological motion and a model for its analysis. Percept Psychophys 14(2):201–211
8. Jung Y, Hu J (2015) Ak-fold averaging cross-validation procedure. J Non–parametric Statistics 27(2):167–179
9. Kourtzi Z, Krekelberg B, Van Wezel RJ (2008) Linking form and motion in the primate brain. Trends Cogn Sci 12(6):230–236

10. Kriegeskorte N, Douglas PK (2018) Cognitive computational neuroscience. Nat Neurosci 21(9):1148–1160
11. Misaghian K, Lugo JE, Faubert J (2021) An implementational-level model of the humandorsal pathway for biological motionperception of high complexity
12. Newell A (1994) Unified theories of cognition. Harvard University Press
13. Romeas T, Faubert J (2015) Soccer athletes are superior to non-athletes at perceiving soccer-specific and non-sport specific human biological motion. Front Psychol 6:1343
14. Romeas T, Guldner A, Faubert J (2016) 3d-multiple object tracking training task improves passing decision-making accuracy in soccer players. Psychol Sport Exerc 22:1–9
15. Smith AT, Snowden RJ (1994) Visualdetection of motion. Academic Press
16. Standage D, Blohm G, Dorris MC (2014) On the neural implementation of the speed-accuracy trade-off. Front Neurosci 8:236
17. Thurman SM, Lu H (2014) Bayesian integration of position and orientation cues in perception of biological and non-biological forms. Frontiers human Neuro–Sci 8:91
18. Wang XJ (2008) Decision making in recurrent neuronal circuits. Neuron 60(2):215–234
19. Wang XJ (2012) Neural dynamics and circuit mechanisms of decision-making. Curr Opinion Neurobiol 22(6):1039–1046

Radiation Pressure in Opal-Based Microcavities

M. Toledo-Solano, M. A. Palomino-Ovando, E. Sánchez-Mora, Jocelyn Faubert, and J. Eduardo Lugo

Abstract In this work, we studied theoretically the induction of electromagnetic forces in three-dimensional photonic crystals when light impinges normally onto an assembly of SiO_2 nanospheres known as artificial opals. We investigated the electromagnetic propagation along a high symmetry direction of the crystal, specifically along the [111] crystal axis and the scalar wavelength approximation is used. The studied photonic structure consists of a microcavity-like structure formed of two opals, separated by a variable air gap, and the working wavelength is 630 nm. We show that the radiation pressure can be as high as $3 \times 10^{-5}\ \mathrm{N/m^2}$ and electromagnetic force value of 0.1 nN when the laser optical power is 13 mW with beam size of $3\ \mathrm{mm^2}$.

Keywords Light propagation · Electromagnetic force · Opal · Gap

M. Toledo-Solano (✉)
CONACYT-Facultad de Ciencias Físico-Matemáticas, Benemérita Universidad Autónoma de Puebla, Av. San Claudio y Av. 18 sur, Col. San Manuel Ciudad Universitaria, Puebla Pue. 72570, Mexico
e-mail: mtoledoso@conacyt.mx

M. A. Palomino-Ovando
Facultad de Ciencias Físico-Matemáticas, Benemérita Universidad Autónoma de Puebla, Av. San Claudio y Av. 18 sur, Col. San Manuel Ciudad Universitaria, Puebla Pue. 72570, Mexico

E. Sánchez-Mora
Instituto de Física "Luis Rivera Terrazas", Benemérita Universidad Autónoma de Puebla, Col. San Manuel Ciudad Universitaria, Puebla, Mexico

J. Faubert · J. E. Lugo
Faubert Lab, Ecole d'optométrie, Université de Montréal, Montreal QC H3T1P1, Canada

M. S. Kaiser et al. (eds.), *Proceedings of Trends in Electronics and Health Informatics*, Lecture Notes in Networks and Systems 376,
https://doi.org/10.1007/978-981-16-8826-3_20

1 Introduction

Photonic crystals (PC) are commonly made of periodic dielectric materials [1], and sometimes these dielectrics are nanostructures that alter the propagation of light [2]. It was observed that light with wavelength close to the period of the dielectric lattice will bounce in the bulk of a crystal and reflect back. This phenomenon, known as Bragg diffraction, has been investigated in photonic crystals over the last decade, and it was shown that there exists a range of wavelengths called stop bands, through which electromagnetic waves cannot propagate through the photonic crystal along certain directions. These forbidden bands give rise to different optical phenomena, for example, high reflection omnidirectional mirrors [3], Bloch oscillations [4, 5], sensing [6], negative refraction [7] and mechanical oscillations [8].

Self-assembled PCs are generally three-dimensional structures. For example, self-assembly of silica or polymethylmethacrylate spheres can be used to form uniform layers of compact, stacked spheres exhibiting three-dimensional PC (PC-3D) characteristics [9, 10]. These types of PCs are commonly known as colloidal crystals or artificial opals [11]. The crystal structure of such opal photonic crystals has a face-centered cubic lattice. Many approaches have been employed to prepare PC-3D by self-assembly of colloidal spheres such as evaporation [12, 13], dip coating [14] and free standing [15].

In recent years, porous silicon one-dimensional photonic crystals have been used as mechanical oscillators, forced and auto-oscillators [8]. These oscillators are known as photodynes which are activated with light. The mechanism employed to induce mechanical oscillations is the generation of electromagnetic forces: a particular photonic mode is excited by using a modulated laser light wavelength. The maximum force and amplitude of the oscillations are of the order of 100 nN and 150 microns, respectively.

In what follows, we discuss first the theoretical reflectance and transmittance spectra under the scalar wavelength approximation (SWA). The light wave vector within the proposed photonic structure is obtained, along with the Bragg condition. The theoretical framework outlined here allows to predict the conditions to observed localized modes within the bandgap and also the electrical filed intensity spatial profile. These are key elements to calculate electromagnetic forces and radiation pressure within the photonic structure. Finally, we wrap up this work by giving the radiation pressure order of magnitude for the same experimental conditions already found in the literature.

2 Reflectance and Transmittance Spectra

In Fig. 1, the opal consists of 12 close-packed silica spheres layers, with diameter D and dielectric constant $\varepsilon_s = 1.46^2$, with air in the interstitial regions of dielectric constant $\varepsilon_a = 1$. It is assumed that both the spheres and the air exhibit no absorption.

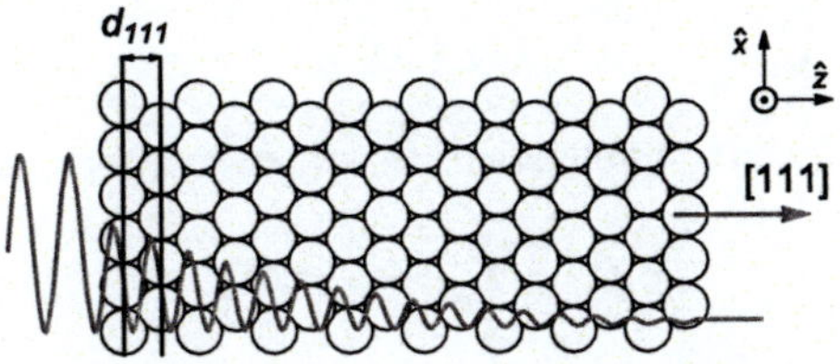

Fig. 1 Schematic of a lateral view of the FCC array of spheres. The parallel straight lines represent the planes (111), whose interplanar distance is d_{111}. The crystal is oriented such that the [111] axis is normal to the planar surfaces. The incident wave traveling in the +z direction is localized within the photonic band gap

Moreover, Fig. 1 shows a electromagnetic (EM) propagation along a high symmetry direction of the crystal, in particular at normal incidence along the [111] crystal axis. In this case, SWA [16–18] is appropriate due to their reasonable agreement with experimental observations [19]. The SWA considers two important assumptions [18]. First, the electric field is treated here as scalar and expanded into Bloch states

$$E(\mathbf{r}) = \sum_{\mathbf{G}} \sum_{\mathbf{k}} C_{\mathbf{k}-\mathbf{G}} e^{i(\mathbf{k}-\mathbf{G})\cdot\mathbf{r}}, \tag{1}$$

where $\sum_k$ is summed over the first Brillouin zone and where G is a reciprocal lattice vector. Second, light scattering is only given by the plane set [111], while the effects of all the other lattice planes are neglected. Thus, only two terms $\mathbf{G} = \mathbf{0}$ and $\mathbf{G} = \mathbf{G}_L$ are considered. $\mathbf{G}_L$ is the shortest reciprocal lattice vector along the L direction and their value is given by $G = 2\pi/d_{111}$, where $d_{111} = 2D\sqrt{2/3}$ is the distance between crystalline planes in the [111] direction. Therefore, the radiation light wave vector inside the photonic crystal [18], $k(\lambda)$, is given by

$$k(\lambda) = 2\pi\sqrt{\epsilon_0}\left[\frac{1}{\lambda_B} \pm \sqrt{\frac{1}{\lambda^2} + \frac{1}{\lambda_B^2} - \sqrt{\frac{U_G^2}{\epsilon_0^2\lambda^4} + \frac{4}{\lambda^2\lambda_B^2}}}\right], \tag{2}$$

where U_G are the Fourier coefficients for a fcc lattice and spheres of radius R_s,

$$U_G = \frac{16\pi}{(GR_s)^3}(\varepsilon_s - \varepsilon_a)\left[\sin(GR_s) - GR_s\cos(GR_s)\right]. \tag{3}$$

λ_B is the wavelength corresponding to the Bragg condition, and is given at normal incidence by

$$\lambda_B = 2d_{111}\sqrt{\varepsilon_0}. \tag{4}$$

Finally, ε_0 is the average dielectric which depends on the volume fraction ($f \approx 0.74$) occupied by the spheres,

$$\varepsilon_0 = f\varepsilon_s + (1-f)\varepsilon_a, \tag{5}$$

Then, the dielectric function of the cristal is written as a constant plus a periodically varying term,

$$\varepsilon_{opal}(z) = \varepsilon_0 + 2U_G\cos(Gz). \tag{6}$$

Consider a N-layers crystal and an incident wave traveling in the +z direction. The wave is described by [16]

$$E(z) = \begin{cases} e^{ik_0z} + r\cdot e^{-ik_0z}, & z<0, \\ C_1\dfrac{e^{ik(z-Nd_{111})} + \Sigma\cdot e^{i(k-G)(z-Nd_{111})}}{1+\Sigma} \\ +C_2\dfrac{e^{-ik(z-Nd_{111})} + \Sigma\cdot e^{-i(k-G)(z-Nd_{111})}}{1+\Sigma}, & 0<z<Nd_{111}, \\ t\cdot e^{ik_0(z-Nd_{111})}, & z>Nd_{111}. \end{cases} \tag{7}$$

k_0 is the free-space wave vector. The parameter Σ is given by

$$\Sigma = \varepsilon_a\frac{2(k-\sqrt{\varepsilon_0}k_0)}{U_G\sqrt{\varepsilon_0}k_0}. \tag{8}$$

The coefficients r and t are determined by the continuity of $E(z)$ and $\mathrm{d}E(z)/\mathrm{d}z$ at the surfaces and can be expressed analytically:

$$r(\lambda) = i\frac{(1-\beta_0^2)\sin(kNd_{111})}{2\beta_0\cos(kNd_{111}) - i(1+\beta_0^2)\sin(kNd_{111})}, \tag{9}$$

$$t(\lambda) = \frac{2\beta_0}{2\beta_0\cos(kNd_{111}) - i(1+\beta_0^2)\sin(kNd_{111})}, \tag{10}$$

where

$$\beta_0 = \frac{k_0(1-\Sigma)}{k(1-\Sigma)+G\Sigma}. \tag{11}$$

Figure 2 shows a series of reflectance (R) and transmittance (T) spectra for a sample composed of N-layers in the case of normal incidence. The wavelength is normalized to the spacing between adjacent (111) lattice planes. As the number of layers increases, the maximum of R that defines the photonic band suffers a red shift until it reaches the value of $2\sqrt{\epsilon_0}$ for $N > 50$. Also, both spectra were obtained using the discrete dipole approximation (DDA) model [20]. The comparison shows that the SWA could be a good option to have an insight about the number of layers of the crystal in less time.

In the case of two films of opals separated by an air gap of width d, the reflectance and transmittance spectra can be analyzed using the SWA and the transfer matrix

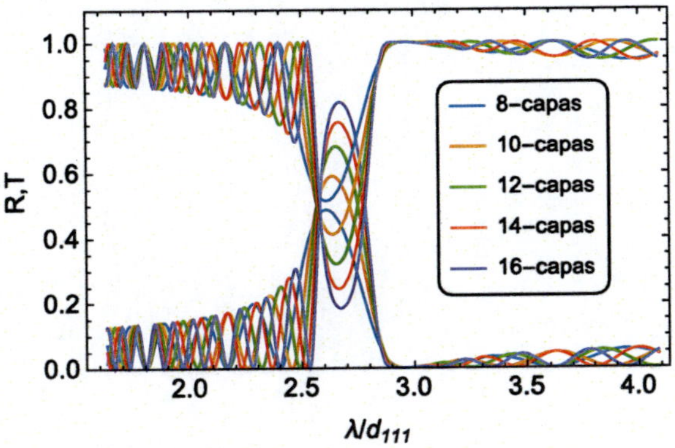

Fig. 2 Reflectance and transmittance of a thin film composed of N-layers of SiO_2 spheres. The incident light comes normal to the surface

method [21]. The last approximation assumes that the individual opals can be characterized by the well-defined reflection and transmission coefficients, which depends on the number of layers. These coefficients can be denoted as as r_1, t_1 and r_2, t_2 for the first and second film, respectively. Then, the reflection and transmission coefficients for the two opals can be written as

$$\mathfrak{r} = \frac{r_1 t_1^* + r_2 t_1 e^{ik_0 d}}{t_1^* + r_1^* r_2 t_1 e^{2ik_0 d}}, \tag{12}$$

$$\mathfrak{t} = \frac{t_1 t_1^* t_2 e^{ik_0 d}}{t_1^* + r_1^* r_2 t_1 e^{2ik_0 d}}. \tag{13}$$

When both opal films have the same number of layers

$$r_1 = r_2 = \sqrt{R_1} e^{i\alpha}, \qquad t_1 = t_2 = \sqrt{T_1} e^{i\delta}. \tag{14}$$

Using Eqs. (12)–(14), the transmittance of the double films can be written in the form

$$\mathfrak{T} = |\mathfrak{t}|^2 = \frac{T_1^2}{1 + R_1^2 + 2R_1 \cos[2(k_0 d + \delta)]}. \tag{15}$$

For some N in the range shown in Fig. 1, expanding the $\cos[2(k_0 d + \delta)]$ about $2n\pi$ and about $(2n-1)\pi$ for $n = 1, 2, \ldots$, it is possible to observe maxima and minima in the reflectance spectrum around $\lambda = 8/3d_{111} \approx 2.66 d_{111}$ when $d = (4n-1)/3d_{111}$ and $d = (4n-3)/3d_{111}$, respectively. However, considering that $\varepsilon_{opal}(Nd_{111}) = \varepsilon_{\text{opal}}(Nd_{11} + d)$, only the values $d = (4m+1)d_{111}$ for $m = 0, 1, \ldots$ and $d = (4m-1)d_{111}$ for $m = 1, 2, \ldots$, are considered correct.

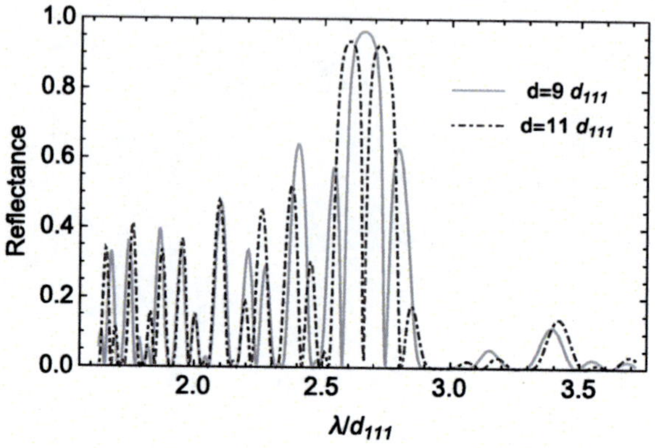

Fig. 3 Reflectance spectra for a double layer of opals with an air gap of 9 and 11 d_{111}

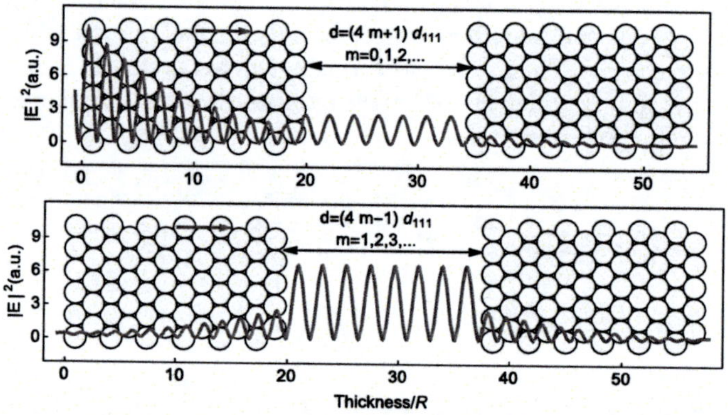

Fig. 4 Shows the distribution of the intensity of the electric field of modes localized at photonic band gap and transmitted modes that are located in an air gap

Figure 3 shows the R spectra when the separation distance of the opals is $d = 9d_{111}$ and $d = 11d_{111}$, respectively. Clearly in the latter case, it can be observed the presence of a localized mode. Figure 4 shows the the electric field intensity spatial distribution of modes localized within the photonic band gap and transmitted modes that are located in the air gap.

3 Force on the Crystal

The force exerted by the EM radiation on the crystal can be known from the direct application of Lorentz force method [22]. At normal incidence, the force on the crystals of N-layers is in the wave propagation direction. The time-averaged Lorentz force volumetric density is written

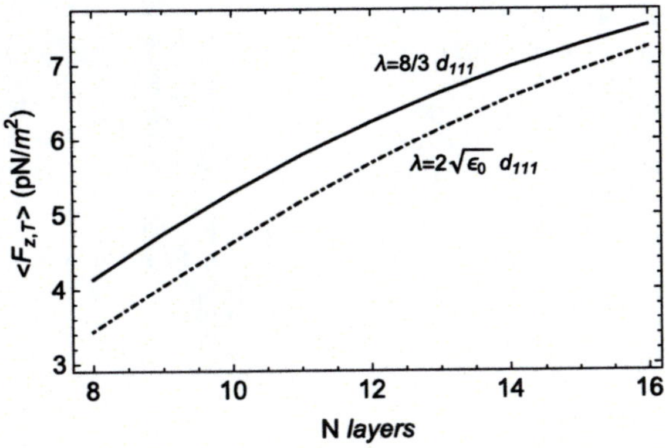

Fig. 5 Force density from normal incident light onto an opal as a function of the number N of layers. The incident electric field has a magnitude of 1 V/m

$$<f_z> = \frac{1}{2}\mathrm{Re}\left[\epsilon_0(\varepsilon_{\mathrm{opal}}(z) - 1)E^*(z)\mathrm{d}E(z)/\mathrm{d}z)\right], \tag{16}$$

where $\epsilon_0 = 8.85 \times 10^{-12}$ F/m is the permittivity of free space. The total pressure is

$$<F_{z,T}> = \int_0^{Nd_{111}} \mathrm{d}z <f_z>. \tag{17}$$

Figure 5 shows the volumetric density force on a opal film composed of layers ranging between 8 and 16, as in Fig. 2. The force is calculated at $\lambda = 8/3d_{111}$ and at $\lambda = 2\sqrt{\varepsilon_0}$, the values corresponding to the maximum in reflectance for 16 layers and the corresponding value to the center of the photonic band gap for a 3D opal.

Using the obtained solution (16), the total pressure on the double opal film can be written as

$$<F_{z,T}> = \int_0^{Nd_{111}} \mathrm{d}z <f_z> + \int_{Nd_{111}+d}^{2Nd_{111}+d} \mathrm{d}z <f_z>. \tag{18}$$

Figure 6 shows the volumetric density force on a double opal film composed by 12 layers as in Fig. 4, around the incident wavelength $\lambda = 8/3d_{111}$. At maximum pressure, 93.7% of the force is exerted on the first opal, while only 6.3% on the second opal as expected for a mode in the gap region. At minimum pressure, the localized mode in the air gap, moves the first opal to the left with a pressure about 19.6 $\mathrm{pN/m^2}$ and in turn, with equal pressure but in the opposite direction to the second opal. Other pressure values are obtained due to the shift of the resonance mode from the chosen wavelength. However, a periodic variation of the radiation pressure is observed as a function of the air thickness. The incident electric field has a magnitude of 1 V/m; however, if we use experimental values already reported in the literature like laser light of 630 nm with 13 mW and beam size of 3 $\mathrm{mm^2}$ then the electric field intensity

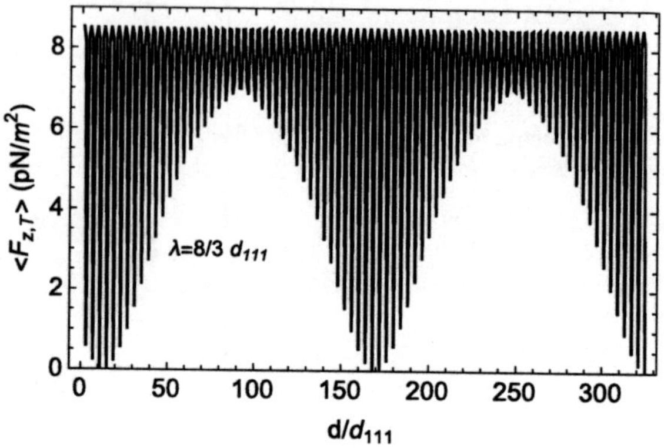

Fig. 6 Force density from normal incident light onto a double layer of opals depending on the thickness of the air gap. The incident electric field has a magnitude of 1 V/m

value is 1808 V/m. The electromagnetic forces scale with the electric field intensity square and the pressure value increases to $3 \times 10^{-5}\ \mathrm{N/m^2}$.

Acknowledgements This work was supported by CONACYT (Cátedras Project No. 3208) and through Grant A1-S-38743.

References

1. Joannopoulos JD, Johnson SG, Winn JN, Meade RD (2008) Photonic crystals molding the flow of light. Princenton University Press, Princeton and Oxford
2. Lugo JE, Lopez HA, Chan S, Fauchet PM (2002) J Appl Phys 91:4966
3. Fink Y, Winn JN, Fan S, Chen C, Michel J, Joannopoulos JD, Thomas EL (1998) Science 282:1679
4. Agarwal V, del Río JA, Malpuech G, Zamfirescu M, Kavokin A, Coquillat D, Scalbert D, Vladimirova M, Gil B (2004) Phys Rev Lett 92:097401
5. Estevez JO, Arriaga JA, Mendez-Blas A, Reyes-Ayona E, Escorcia J, Agarwal V (2012) Nanoscale Res Lett 7:413
6. Rodriguez GA, Lawrie JL, Weiss SM (2014) Porous silicon biosensors for DNA sensing. In: Santos HA (ed) Porous silicon for biomedical applications. Woodhead Publishing Ltd., University of Helsinki, Finland
7. Lugo JE, Doti R, Faubert J (2011) PLoS ONE 6:e17188
8. Lugo JE, Doti R, Sanchez N, de la Mora MB, del Rio JA, Faubert J (2014) Sci Rep 4:3705
9. Romero-Cruz LA, Santos-Gómez A, Palomino Ovando MA, Cristobal H, Orlando S, Mora E, González AL, Toledo Solano M (2018) Superlatt Microstruct 123:71
10. Matamoros-Ambrocio M, Sánchez-Mora E, Gómez-Barojas E, Luna-López (2021) Polymers 13:2171
11. Norris DJ, Arlinghaus EG, Meng L, Heiny R, Scriven LE (2004) Adv Mater 16:1393
12. Fudouzi H, Xia Y (2003) Adv Mater 15:892
13. Huang CK, Chan CH, Chen CY, Tsai YL, Chen CC, Han JL (2007) Nanotechnology 18:265305
14. Ye J, Zentel R, Arpiainen S, Ahopelto J, Jonsson F, Romanov SG, Torres CMS (2006) Langmuir 18:7378
15. Chan CH et al (2005) Nanotechnology 16:1440
16. Shung KW-K, Tsai YC (1993) Phys Rev B 48:11265

17. Tarhan I, Watson GH (1996) Phys Rev B 54:7593
18. Mittleman DM et al (1999) J Chem Phys 111:345
19. Bertone JF, Jiang P, Hwang K, Mittleman DM, Colvin VL (1999) Phys Rev Lett 99:300
20. González AL, Santos A, Toledo M (2019) In: Ghamsari MS, Dhara S (eds) Nanorods and nanocomposites, vol 90313. IntechOpen, pp 1–17. https://doi.org/10.5772/intechopen.90313
21. See, e.g., Yen P (1988) Optical waves in layered media. Wiley
22. Mizrahi A, Schachter L (2006) Phys Rev E 74:036504

An Implementational-Level Model of the Human Dorsal Pathway for Biological Motion Perception of High Complexity

Khashayar Misaghian, J. Eduardo Lugo, and Jocelyn Faubert

Abstract The ability to recover information about a moving living object from a sparse input is known as biological motion perception. Biological motion's importance in various aspects of human lives like survival, social life, and interactive activities is a well-established consensus. So, it is no surprise that determining its mechanisms and affiliated neurobiological substrates have been a subject of interest for quite a while. We proposed a descriptive Bayesian simulation model representing the visual system's dorsal (motion) pathway. Recent studies have inspired this approach questioning the degree of impact of dynamic form cues in biological motion perception and were developed based on earlier neurophysiologically plausible model assumptions. The neurophysiologically plausible, implementational-level model was trained to distinguish the soccer ball's direction (invisible ball) from a set of biological motion soccer kick stimuli used in an earlier psychophysical study of our lab. The athlete subjects' psychometric functions have been simulated with high precision by adjusting the model parameters merely to simulate the behavior of the athlete subjects in the same study. The correlation analysis demonstrates a significant, almost perfect correlation between experimental and simulated data. Even though all available information gets optimally integrated to make a decision by the visual system, the results are in accord with the speculations favoring motion cue importance over dynamic form by testing the limits when biological motion perception only depends on motion information processing.

Keywords Biological motion · Bayesian · Hierarchical simulation model · Dorsal pathway · Supported by an NSERC-Essilor Research Chair · The NSERC discovery grant · FESP-E´OUM

K. Misaghian (✉) · J. E. Lugo · J. Faubert
Faubert Lab, School of Optometry, University of Montreal, Montreal, QC 3T 1P1, Canada
e-mail: k.misaghian@umontreal.ca

J. E. Lugo
Facultad de Ciencias Fisico-Matematicas, Benem´Erita Universidad Aut´Onoma de Puebla, Col. San Manuel Ciudad Universitaria, Av. San Claudio y Av. 18 sur, Puebla, Pue. 72570, Mexico

M. S. Kaiser et al. (eds.), *Proceedings of Trends in Electronics and Health Informatics*, Lecture Notes in Networks and Systems 376,
https://doi.org/10.1007/978-981-16-8826-3_21

1 Introduction

The robustious capacity in the mammalian brain to collect a wide range of information strictly from the movement of a live body is renowned as biological motion perception. For the first time in 1973, Johansson introduced a stimulus that represented biological motion by placing light bulbs [9]. The biological motion perception is integral to humans' physiological and social survival and has received a great deal of attention from many research areas [3, 6].

The result from many psychophysical, neurophysiological, and functional imaging experiments pointed toward the involvement of the dorsal pathway, ventral pathway, and their convergence at the STS area in the human visual system [1, 16]. Consequently, the accumulation of evidence of experimental data would necessitate and provide the means to consolidate a theoretical framework as in characterizing the aforementioned system at different levels of abstraction of modeling [3, 15].

Later, a representational level model of biological motion perception under certain assumptions was proposed [6]. Both form processing stream (ventral pathway) and optic flow processing stream (dorsal pathway) have been implemented to conclude that the local motion analysis by the dorsal pathway outweighs the form processing for the model to detect the biological motion stimuli [3, 5, 6]. These findings were at odds with an earlier prominent psychophysics study on the subject [1]. Later further studies and investigations set the scale by suggesting that the robustness of biological motion hinges on integration of both local motion and dynamic form processing [3].

Moving beyond the notion of regarding motion pathway and form pathway as two separated streams, further investigations of the neural correlates suggest a broader and more interconnected cortical network. Hence, questioning the causal nature of the activation of some of the areas associated with particular visual cues [7, 8, 12].

To follow up on the effectiveness of motion and form cues, in an interesting study, six patients with focal injuries at multiple regions of the ventral visual cortex (form processing stream) have managed to detect the biological stimuli with not significantly different threshold than the control group. While interestingly, they have outperformed the participants with impairment at other regions believed to be critical to biological motion perception significantly, shedding more insight into the role of different visual cues in biological motion perception [7].

The modeling of the biological motion perception falls into the domain of decision-making modeling that could be scrutinized at different levels of abstraction. Also, algorithmic and implementational levels are not being considered discrete but rather spectral classes. Moreover, analytic studies in the domain of decision-making modeling signify that under specific assumptions, the two levels could be formalized interchangeably [4, 14, 20].

Accordingly, it is also crucial to model uncertainty, and consequently, risk as an inseparable aspect stemming from the generative model of the observer and the presence of noise in its input process [2, 11]. A feed-forward hierarchical risk-averse Bayesian model of the visual system dorsal pathway has been proposed, assuming that the prototypical patterns are stored at the STS area in the brain's temporal lobe.

Moreover, a mutual inhibition dynamic has been adopted for the motion pattern neurons that are also believed to reside in the STS area [13].

Detecting the ball's direction from the biological motion of a soccer kick taker has been assigned as a task to the model. The model has been tuned to replicate the existing behavioral data of 35 human athletes [18], demonstrating a significant correlation between simulated and human psychometric function parameters.

2 Model

The presented model shares the main assumptions of the model proposed by Cassile and Giese [5]: Hierarchical nature of dorsal stream like other visual pathways, predominantly feed-forward structure, and storage and utilization of prototypical for perception (Fig. 1).

There are four hierarchical levels to the model:

Local motion energy neurons: At the first stage of evidence collection, neurons are sensitive to basic motion directions at their small receptive fields (approximately 0.4 deg). These neurons are arranged to a 36×31 matrix of detectors sensitive to leftward, rightward, upward, or downward motions. The details of the implementation have been made according to the work of Casile and Giese [5, 19].

Opponent-motion sensors: The first encoding of the evidence, as the second part of the evidence collection stage, occurs at the opponent-motion neuronal level. Six types of neurons sensitive to expansion or contraction in both horizontal and vertical

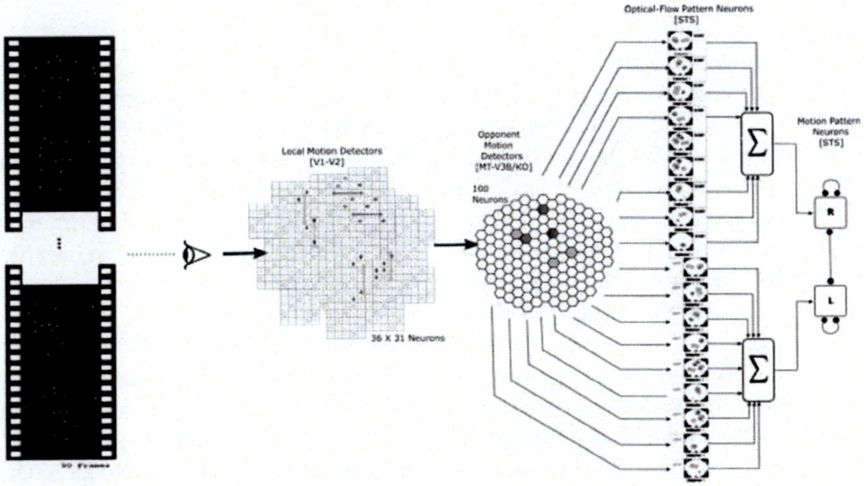

Fig. 1 Four hierarchical levels of biological motion perception

manners and rotations in clockwise or counterclockwise directions are believed to reside at this level, with their respective receptive field of 4.5 degrees. Here, only the contraction/expansion neurons have been organized in four 5×5 arrangements, again, conforming to the work of Casile and Giese [5].

Global optical-flow pattern detectors: Capable of detecting complex global optic flow patterns at the correct, timely instance, this hierarchy constitutes the integration of the evidence level of this decision-making model. Each column neuron is tuned to a specific chronological stage of the optic flow pattern of interest. Neurons of the column are laterally coupled through asymmetrical excitatory or inhibitory connections in a way that the active neuron excites the neurons tuned to the later chronological stages of the activity and inhibits the neurons tuned to the earlier chronological stages compared to what chronological stage the active neuron is tuned to [17].

Complete motion pattern detectors: The last hierarchy of a decision-making model is the thresholding level. At this level, the neurons tuned to different complete motion patterns receive the signals from the thresholding level and interact until only one neuron reaches its activation level, hence the decision-making [20]. There are multiple proposed dynamics for the decision-making neurons interactions; here, we have modified the dynamic proposed in the work of Lugo et al. [13].

The physiological noise in the dorsal pathway has been simulated by assuming the output of the integration level as a Gaussian process, $N H_i\ (t),\ \Delta t\sigma 2$. Where, $H_i\ (t)$ is the activity of the ith optic flow neuron in time, and the Gaussian internal noise is of the variance, $\sigma 2$.

3 Methods

The model implementation, data fitting, and statistical analyses are executed in MATLAB. Since one purpose of the study is to simulate the psychophysics work of Romeas and Faubert [18], we adopted the same biological motion of the soccer kick captured by Mixamo studio from the study above. The head, shoulders, hips, elbows, wrists, knees, and ankles in the stimuli are represented by 15 point-lights. Each stimulus is 4.5 s with 90 frames. Leftward and rightward stimuli of different angles have been created by rotating the original stimulus around the Z-axis, just like in the aforementioned study [18].

Assuming that the visual system of a soccer player is trained within the range of a soccer penalty kick, we have assimilated the shooting range of 1°–20° for training and cross-validation of the proposed dorsal pathway model. First, The model got cross-validated with k-fold cross-validation of $k = 5$ [10]. After cross-validation, the model has been trained with the stimuli of 7°–20° and tested with stimuli of 2°, 4°, 8°, and 15°, to replicate the conditions in the work of [18]. The first two hierarchy levels have been implemented according to the previous works [5, 6].

Given that each biological motion stimulus comprises 90 frames, we decided to assume that each stimulus has nine chronological stages and each stage comprises ten consecutive frames. At the third level, we have implemented 18 neurons. The first nine neurons are tuned to right-side kicks and the other nine neurons are sensitive to the leftward kicks. Moreover, each neuron is sensitive to one and only one chronological stage of their respective kick stimuli. To solve the neuronal system's dynamic at this level, Euler's method has been used.

The neuronal dynamic of the thresholding level has been implemented using the modified mutual inhibition mentioned above and has been solved using the fourth-order Runge–Kutta method.

In an earlier behavioral study, a forced-choice paradigm task has been devised for expert athletes and non-athletes to recognize the ball's direction from the biological motion stimuli mentioned above [18]. A total of 1080 randomized stimulus queue of leftward and rightward kicks of the deviations, 2°,4°,8° and 15° angles have been presented to the subjects (120 times for each angle at each side). Subsequently, psychometric functions for the angular deviation thresholds and slope were calculated [18].

To reproduce behavioral study conditions, for each angle and side, each specific stimulus has been presented to the model 120 times to generate an error percentage quantity. Furthermore, the whole process has been repeated 30 times, and the results were used to calculate corresponding simulated psychometric functions.

4 Results

The proposed model was fivefold cross-validated with 87.5% average success. The behavioral performances of 35 athletes have been simulated by tuning the proposed models' parameters. Results have been subsequently plotted: experimental angular thresholds and their corresponding simulated angular thresholds have been plotted in Fig. 2, and experimental slopes of the subjects' psychometric functions against their corresponding simulated slopes have been plotted in Fig. 3. Correlation analysis demonstrates a positive correlation of significance between experimental and simulated angular threshold values, with the Spearman correlation coefficient $r_s = 0.991$, *p-value* = 7.08*E* 31 (p <0.001). Moreover, simulated and experimental slope values also show a significant positive correlation with Spearman correlation coefficient r_s0.963, *p-value* $= 2.70E - 20$ ($p < 0.001$).

5 Discussion

The proposed model showed notable success in simulating human behavior, while the previously proposed networks failed to detect the biological motion of this complexity. Despite all limiting assumptions, the model managed to reproduce the

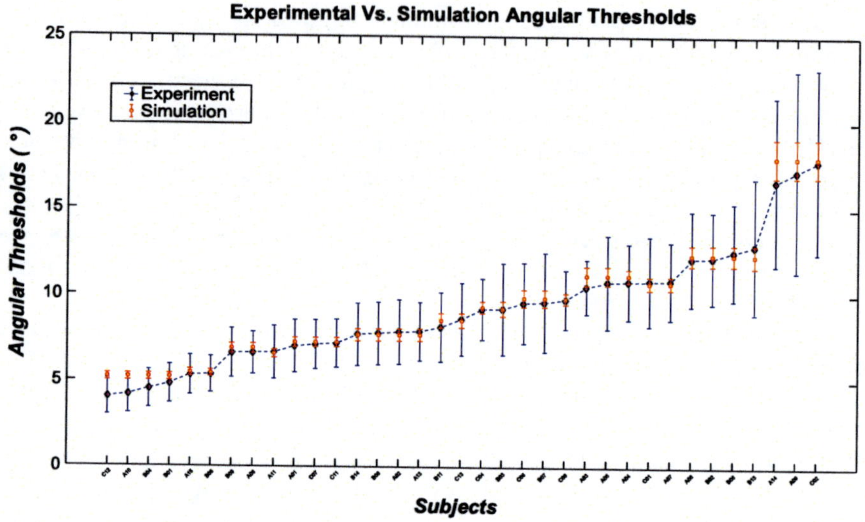

Fig. 2 Diamonds depict the calculated experimental angular thresholds of the subjects and the circles display the simulated angular thresholds

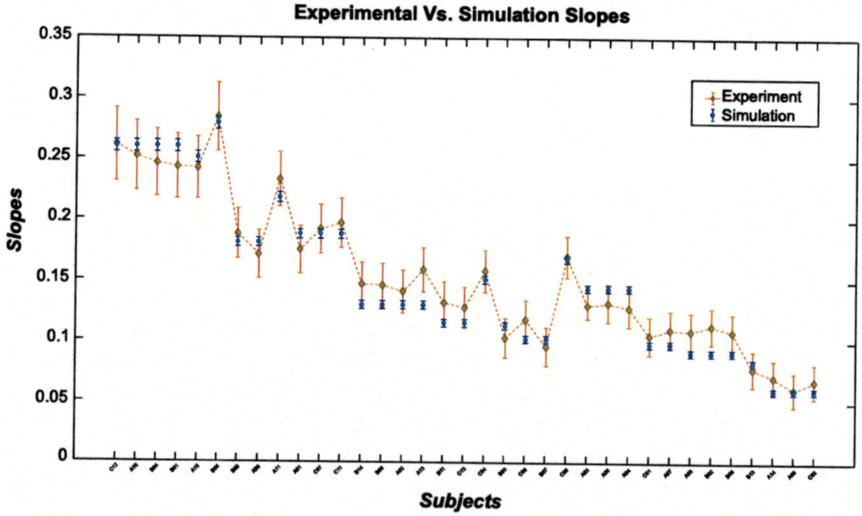

Fig. 3 Diamonds depict the calculated experimental slopes of the subjects and the circles display the simulated slopes

psychometric function of 35 expert athletes. However, a more inclusive model would respond to the stimuli in a measurable reaction time.

It is consensus that the visual system adopts different contingencies to deploy all sources of information like form cues and motion cues for optimal biological motion perception [3]. Here, we have theoretically examined the capacity of the dorsal pathway to perceive a complex manifold of biological motion stimuli. The results fall in line with the suggestions from the work of Gliaie and Dotan, which tests the integrity of the form cues in the biological motion perception and also, the work of Thurman and Lu, indicating that there are no differences in processing the biological and non-biological form cues in the ventral pathway (form pathway) [7, 21]. However, the limitations of the model are to be considered. For example, while in reality there are opponent-motion neurons with receptive fields far from each other, allowing the visual system to detect global expansions, contractions, and rotations, the opponent-motion neurons of the proposed model only regard the adjoining receptive fields. They do not account for rotations altogether [19]. Moreover, for the sake of simplicity, the first two levels are assumed to be noise-free. Also, inference prototypes in the integration level are assumed to be fixed and non-updating, albeit online adaptation mechanisms are at play in reality. All mentioned limitations would clarify the next steps toward a more thorough model and, therefore, a better understanding of this phenomenon.

References

1. Beintema J, Lappe M (2002) Perception of biological motion without local image mo- tion. Proc Natl Acad Sci 99(8):5661–5663
2. Bitzer S, Park H, Blankenburg F, Kiebel SJ (2014) Perceptual decision making: drift-diffusion model is equivalent to a bayesian model. Frontiers in human neu- roscience 8:102
3. Blake R, Shiffrar M (2007) Perception of human motion. Annu Rev Psychol 58:47–73
4. Bogacz R, Brown E, Moehlis J, Holmes P, Cohen JD (2006) The physics of optimal decision making: a formal analysis of models of performance in two- alternative forced-choice tasks. Psychol Rev 113(4):700
5. Casile A, Giese MA (2005) Critical features for the recognition of biological motion. J Vis 5(4):6–6
6. Giese MA, Poggio T (2003) Neural mechanisms for the recognition of biological movements. Nat Rev Neurosci 4(3):179–192
7. Gilaie-Dotan S, Saygin AP, Lorenzi LJ, Rees G, Behrmann M (2015) Ventral aspect of the visual form pathway is not critical for the perception of biological motion. Proc Natl Acad Sci 112(4):E361–E370
8. Grosbras MH, Beaton S, Eickhoff SB (2012) Brain regions involved in human movement perception: a quantitative voxel-based meta-analysis. Hum Brain Mapp 33(2):431–454
9. Johansson G (1973) Visual perception of biological motion and a model for its analysis. Percept Psychophys 14(2):201–211
10. Jung Y, Hu J (2015) Ak-fold averaging cross-validation procedure. J Non-Parametric Statistics 27(2):167–179
11. Kahneman D, Tversky A (2013) Prospect theory: an analysis of decision under risk. In: Handbook of the fundamentals of financial decision making: Part I, pp 99–127, World Scientific

12. Kourtzi Z, Krekelberg B, Van Wezel RJ (2008) Linking form and motion in the primate brain. Trends Cogn Sci 12(6):230–236
13. Lugo J, Mejia-Romero S, Doti R, Ray K, Kothari S, Withers G, Faubert J (2018) A simple dynamic model that accounts for regulation of neuronal polarity. J Integr Neurosci 17(4):323–330
14. Marr D (1982) Vision: a computational investigation into the human representation and processing of visual information, henry holt and co. Inc., New York, NY **2**(4.2)
15. Marr D, Poggio T (1976) From understanding computation to understanding neural circuitry
16. Mather G, Radford K, West S (1992) Low-level visual processing of biological motion. Proceedings of the royal society of London. Series B: Biol Sci 249(1325):149–155
17. Mineiro P, Zipser D (1998) Analysis of direction selectivity arising from recurrent cortical interactions. Neural Comput 10(2):353–371
18. Romeas T, Faubert J (2015) Soccer athletes are superior to non-athletes at perceiving soccer-specific and non-sport specific human biological motion. Front Psychol 6:1343
19. Smith AT, Snowden RJ (1994) Visual detection of motion. Academic Press
20. Standage D, Blohm G, Dorris MC (2014) On the neural implementation of the speed-accuracy trade-off. Front Neurosci 8:236
21. Thurman SM, Lu H (2014) Bayesian integration of position and orientation cues in perception of biological and non-biological forms. Frontiers Human Neuro-Sci 8:91

All Basics that Are Wrong with the Current Concept of Time Crystal: Learning from the Polyatomic Time Crystals of Protein, microtubule, and Neuron

Komal Saxena, Pushpendra Singh, Pathik Sahoo, Subrata Ghosh, Daya Krishnanda, Kanad Ray, Daisuke Fujita, and Anirban Bandyopadhyay

Abstract The time crystal concepts introduced by Winfree in the 1960s and Wilczek in 2012 have identical definitions. If a perturbed system's inherent clock spontaneously runs a new clock before returning to the original clock, then it is assumed that the system breaks time symmetry. If repeated perturbation recurrently generates new clocks, it resembles a crystal, together, its time crystal. One essential part of this definition is that the ratio of frequencies between the original and new clock is an integer, making the existing time crystal concept extremely controversial. By studying protein, microtubule, and neuron, we propose that the ratio of frequencies between original and newly created clocks is not low-value integers as believed for half a century. New clocks are not harmonics of the original clock. Time symmetry is truly broken. We detect the formation of new clocks at a 1000 times lower frequency range than the original clock, harmonics of molecular oscillators cannot exhibit an organized clocking behavior at 1000 times lower frequency than the original. Most importantly, we measure clocks remotely. No physical contact ensures a non-demolition type detection of the time crystal. Finally, we found many fundamental clocks, far from the original clock frequency, so its polyatomic time crystal. Thus,

K. Saxena · D. Krishnanda
Microwave Physics Laboratory, Department of Physics and Computer Science, Dayalbagh Educational Institute, Dayalbagh, Agra, Uttar Pradesh 282005, India

K. Saxena · P. Singh · P. Sahoo · D. Fujita · A. Bandyopadhyay (✉)
International Center for Materials and Nanoarchitectronics (MANA), Research Center for Advanced Measurement and Characterization (RCAMC), NIMS, 1-2-1 Sengen, Tsukuba 3050047, Ibaraki, Japan

P. Singh · K. Ray
Amity School of Applied Science, Amity University Rajasthan, Jaipur Delhi Highway, Kant KalwarJaipur, Rajasthan N11C303007, India

S. Ghosh
Chemical Science & Technology Division, CSIR North East Institute of Science andTechnology, Jorhat, Assam 785006, India

Academy of Scientific and Innovative Research (AcSIR), Ghaziabad, Uttar Pradesh 201002, India

M. S. Kaiser et al. (eds.), *Proceedings of Trends in Electronics and Health Informatics*, Lecture Notes in Networks and Systems 376,
https://doi.org/10.1007/978-981-16-8826-3_22

we not only change the basic definition of a time crystal, but possibly discard existing time crystals as mere harmonics.

Keywords Microtubule · Protein · Electromagnetic resonance · Time crystal

1 Introduction

The research on time crystals has received enormous attention because the transformation of human civilization started when we learned how to break spatial symmetry [1]. The next revolution would come from breaking the time symmetry. It is an old concept of the 1960s [2, 3]. A time crystal is expected to contribute to the understanding of artificial and virtual atoms-based new age materials science, regulating the spatio-temporal dynamics at higher dimensions, information processing, and computing, medical science like modeling brain [4] and intelligence in biomaterials etc. When clocks rotate continuously, hold periodicity, it is said that temporal symmetry is preserved. However, if the periodicity changes, it is believed that time symmetry is broken, time crystal is realized. Since there is no known master clock integrating all systems in the universe, a local system's particular recurrent dynamics is assigned as a clock, and associated time symmetry. Recently there are multiple claims of realizing the time crystal as the advent of a new scientific and industrial revolution. However, they lack the foundation or conceptual understanding of the true configuration space in the time symmetry. Researchers could not formulate beyond the configuration space of spatial symmetry and inherently considered temporal symmetry should have a similar configuration space. Consequently, the whole adventure of time crystal has become a spatial illusion.

The recurring transitions within a set of energy levels may give rise to multiple clocks. However, if all clocking frequencies are integrally related to the fundamental frequency, all clocks belong to a particular time symmetry. The way all current time crystal breakthroughs argue as if switching to different harmonics is breaking time symmetry, then every single matter in the universe being a resonator would produce time crystals. We repeat, when a system resonates, there could be multiple symmetries, wherein each symmetry is associated with a dynamic change; e.g. orbital symmetry, functional symmetry etc. One or a few symmetries could break, switch symmetry and others may remain unchanged. It is not necessary that all symmetries should break at once. To break time symmetry, all clocks associated with a particular symmetry could be made silent and all clocks following a new symmetry could be activated. At this particular point, we make our argument clear that be it classical time crystal [5]; or quantum time crystal [6], the new clocks produced spontaneously by the system should not have half or double the frequency of the original clock. First two or three harmonics could be a simple perturbation of the resonantly vibrating oscillators. By suppressing the fundamental note, drums are often played, switching between different energy levels could be assigned as breaking orbital symmetry but not breaking the temporal symmetry.

To hold entanglement, Quantum clocks would not change periodicity, but the geometric phase of oscillations and that phase would return after a certain time [7]. In other word, the geometric phase instead of its dynamic phase would break time symmetry. Recently, several works on the quantum version of the time crystal were proposed by Wilczeck [8, 9]. However, in all works, at the ground state, if a clock is perturbed, the system changes its clock frequency to one of its harmonics just like a classical resonator [10]. There has been significant criticism of this approach [11]. First of all, if clock frequency changes, the system breaks the quantum ground state forever, and then, even if it returns, it cannot be the same state. The hurriedly made theory of quantum time crystal does not incorporate the situation when the frequency remains unchanged, and it's the network of geometric phases that could break time symmetry and realize the true time crystal. Therefore, we agree with the criticism that so far proposed and realized quantum time crystals are not a quantum entity, as they do not exhibit any exclusive property of a quantum effect, nor are they time crystals of any nature. Consequently, generated experimental evidences and theoretical predictions are exclusive classical properties. Often it is thought quantized electromagnetic energy ($E = h\upsilon$) contains Plank's constant and in the disguise of minimum time uncertainty [12], demonstration of the existence of Plank constant is considered as the reflection of a quantum effect. Primarily, they fit amplitude change [13] during quantum measurement in the Plank scale and assign small-scale energy exchange to be a quantum effect. It is easy to realize due to pure classicality.

However, some quantum researchers understand the problem and raise voices against this culture from time to time. Inherently, the quantum effect happens without exchanging energy. For example, see quantum tunneling; it is not hopping the barrier. The molecular orbitals are quantum systems, but orbital transition measurements from emitted quanta or noticing the existence of Plank constant are not exclusively a quantum effect. We need a metastable state made of a large number of overlapped energy levels within a small energy gap ($\Delta E = h\upsilon \sim k_B T$), so that input states prepared from different sources attain the metastable state, when transit to the common ground state, a stream of pulses with a singular phase and amplitude is emitted. This is the preparation of a quantum state, but still not a quantum effect, until more filtering of coherent states would allow a higher degree of transmission of probability wave. This concept is inverse of classical transmission and constitutes the foundation of Bell's inequality. Therefore, preparing a quantum clock is simply a stream of pulses with identical phases and amplitude moving in a loop. Thus far, all experimental realizations of quantum clocks are fine. The problem begins when they change the period and break the entangled state. This is where classic quantum researchers become a severe critic of breaking the symmetry that the quantum state holds, i.e. current foundation of a time crystal.

1.1 Conceptual Foundation for the Temporal Configuration Space

First of all, we have to realize the temporal configuration space. For the formation of matter-based crystals many singularities occur in space as shown in Fig. 1a, each singularity would depict an atom or real matter. Symmetry of space is broken by singularities; we get crystal made of matters. Matters are singularities in the curved space, similarly, time is a singularity in the curvature produced by clocks, each clock represents a point or a pixel in the configuration space of time. Therefore, unlike infinite spatial coordinates and their symmetry builds spatial configuration space, the clocks build a periodic architecture similar to curved space as shown in Fig. 1b. Then, the system has to create a singularity in the periodicity that could allow another set of clocks to operate for a short period, as shown in Fig. 1c. In the spatial configuration space, we can change spatial ordering, but in the temporal configuration space, it is the unit or constituent clocks of a larger clock that needs to be changed or redefined. These two configurations should not be treated equally.

Therefore, the physical ordering of resonators is not the concern here, they could vibrate in sync to run a clock or set of clocks following one symmetry. It is their

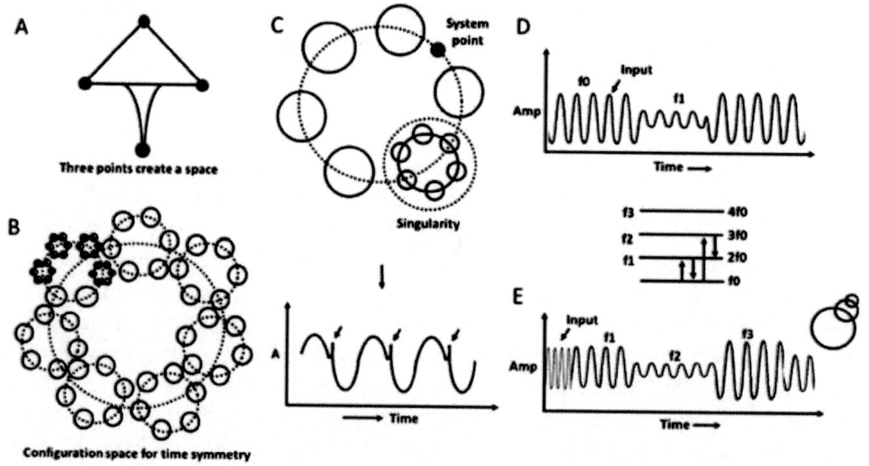

Fig. 1 **A**. A spatial domain requires at least three points or pixel arranged side by side. A spatial configuration space is shown in terms of generalized coordinates. **B.** A temporal domain requires at least three layers of clocks arranged within and above. A temporal configuration space is shown in terms of generalized temporal coordinates (temporal coordinate = clock). **C.** Singularity in the temporal configuration is a guest clock system in the host. The system point of the host traps in the guest. If guest has a similar guest, it would look like panel B and the system would be ready to create a time crystal. **D.** Current concept of a time crystal where input is given as a signal and its harmonics are realized. **E.** Our proposed concept of time crystal where input is given as noise and different composition of clocks is periodically activated and deactivated spontaneously without repeated trigger of noise

temporal ordering that matters. While it's true larger structure resonantly vibrates slowly, our concern is not the speed of vibration, it's the ordering of unit time or unit space. One of the simplest models that could allow a mechanism to switch off a time symmetry and switch on to another time symmetry, then return to the original one, is shown in Fig. 1c. Here we could see that a clock made of many clocks in its perimeter could have one clock replaced by a loop of elementary clocks. Such hierarchical integration of clocks delivers a suitable data structure in breaking time symmetry. The system point running constituent clocks or pixels on its perimeter would trap into the specific clock or pixel with an internal structure. That special clock with an internal structure takes the system point into the loop, which follows a new symmetry, so, the transition from the host clock's symmetry to the guest clock's symmetry is a break in time symmetry. Triplet clocks are historic in time crystal research [14].

Therefore, it's a conceptual paradigm shift in the field of time crystal research. Using a new concept to construct a time crystal, we have challenged the existing culture of defining the time crystal. While curved space could generate mass and the materials science we explore is based on various atoms, or various distinct ways to create singularities in the space. On the other hand, temporal symmetry requires a temporal space made of clocks. Each clock acts as a pixel there, providing an opportunity for us to create a temporal singularity. Without a temporal singularity in the within and above network of clocks it is not possible to construct two distinct time symmetries. Therefore, we cannot imitate the spatial time crystal construction trick to build temporal time crystals. While spatial crystals could form side by side, temporal crystals have to grow within and above, so the spatial and temporal crystals are orthogonal to each other in the configuration space. Another interesting point to note for a within and above network is that the unit clock used to create the guest clock would be several orders lower in time domain than the unit clocks of the host clock. Therefore, the ratio of two units of clocks used to construct two distinct temporal symmetries would not be 2, 3 or ½ or 1/3 etc. [10] Rather, it would be a few thousand, depending on the nature of the oscillators used to build the clock (Fig. 1d for harmonics). Finally, when the time symmetry breaks, the guest clock would be inactive for a moment, yet the amplitude of the output frequencies during that time would remain the same. The only parameter that would change would be the phase of the host clock. The signal from the guest clock would continue with a nearly noisy signal, while an additional signal would generate from the guest clock (Fig. 1e). Still, we cannot say, the guest clock system is the time crystal. When each constituent clock of the guest clock has a loop of clocks inside (guest of guest), we have three nested layers of clocks grown within and above. The central layer of clocks makes the time crystal.

2 Experimental Realization of the New Paradigm of Time Crystal

To practically realize a time crystal, we need a special material with at least two coupled systems of resonators with at least two fundamental frequencies and multiple different clocks belonging to each set of resonators that would hold a distinct temporal symmetry. The system, under external perturbation, would switch from one set of clocks to another or one fundamental frequency to another before returning to the initial frequency.

The first thing that we have shown experimentally to demonstrate a time crystal is that the ac signal generated by the new clock in the middle layer would be independent of input frequency, input signal amplitude. The uppermost and innermost layers of clocks could be tuned and edited but not the central one. Therefore, time symmetry has a configuration space grown within and above and the time crystals could form in any of the nested layers except the innermost and the outermost layer. The upper limit of the innermost clock sets the fastest clock of the time crystal or the central layer (Fig. 1b). The longest clock adopted by the time symmetry is the fastest clock of the upper layer. If at least, three time symmetries are nested one inside another, then, in the central symmetry one could build the true time crystal that we have already reported [15]. Just like three points are required to create a finite space, three layers of clocks are required to create a timeline where time symmetry could be encoded [16].

To observe each temporal atom of a time crystal, we need a distinct trigger, which signifies discrete, isolated temporal atoms. Temporal atoms are not part of a singular crystal. The current idea of conceptualizing a time crystal by repeated perturbation is wrong. One should see multiple distinct temporal atoms spontaneously (Fig. 1e), as a result of only one perturbation. Here we have experimented with single protein molecule, filaments and the hippocampal neuron cells [17, 18], to measure time crystals by sending noise bursts and measuring the emitted optical vortex condensate usingquantum optics [19] (Fig. 2a–c). It means, right after sending one perturbation, the original clock and the new clocks alternately appear and disappear to create a time crystal (Fig. 1e). No repeated trigger should be required if at all we want to realize time crystals. Even if one changes the noise frequency, amplitude, or duration, optical vortex condensate that reads the time crystal using quantum optics remains identical [16, 19]. To us, this is the ultimate proof that time crystal truly exists, which is a standalone system like atoms or crystals made of matter.

At resonance, electric and magnetic fields loop in separate spatial domains on the surface of the resonating material. These loops overlap and exchange energy as they synchronize and create a new loop. Consequently, a set of frequency peaks in a resonance band activate in a loop, we get a temporal clock with a phase and a spatial signature.

When incident photon interacts with the resonating surface-loops and emits photons acquiring the angular momentum, from the rotating photon's polarization state and topological charge we can gather information about the localized resonance

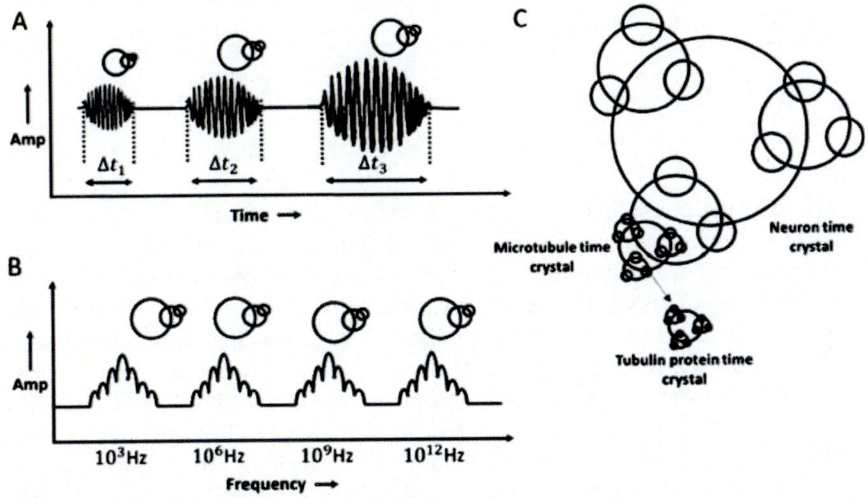

Fig. 2 **A.** Noise burst sent to tubulin protein, microtubule, and neuron for different amplitude and temporal duration creates similar optical vortex condensate (time crystal) for tubulin protein, microtubule, and neuron. **B.** Noise bursts created at different frequency domains generate similar optical vortex condensate (time crystal) for tubulin protein, microtubule and neuron. **C.** Triplet of triplet optical vortex condensate (time crystal) of a tubulin protein is the guest of the optical vortex condensate (time crystal) of a microtubule, and the optical vortex condensate (time crystal) of a microtubule is a guest in the optical vortex condensate (time crystal) for the neuron [15]

of the surface [16, 19]. Localized resonance via evanescent wave is not a singular event. For a molecular complex, several locally derived clocks form a 3D vortex assembly which we read instantly as a time polycrystal. Recently we demonstrated that neuron, microtubule, and protein all biomaterials have distinct signatures of time polycrystal [16, 19] and they follow the fundamental principles of fractal information theory (FIT) we proposed earlier [20, 21]. Our work paves the way to understand the data structure and information processing in biomaterials and build 2D, 3D, and polyatomic time crystals analogous to Mendelive's periodic table for materials crystals.

The phase diagram of the polyatomic time crystal would be different from that proposed thus far. Phase resetting curves are the foundations of time crystal [22], since they determine synchronization, phase locking, and clustering of resonating dielectric oscillators [23, 24]. Pre-thermalization, means we pump the system with a high-frequency signal, it is so fast that the system heats up very slow. Then, how the time crystal would look like we do not know. Not published yet, and people are looking for such a system. Pre-thermalization is the system where we probe the singularity domain, where the phase is discontinued. For the proposed structure of temporal configuration space, we visualize the time crystals with pre-thermalization.

3 Results and Discussion

3.1 *Wide Ranges of Resonant Frequencies of Proteins and SHG Technique*

It was hinted that phase singularity points in a time crystal could act as self-assembling centers for bonding multiple time crystals and create a giant architecture. However, no proposal was made on the possible routes of self-assembly. Here we find that the microtubule's time crystal architecture follows a unique rule of mathematical symmetries while bonding its elementary time crystals. Even pumping resonant frequencies (10^{-9} s) to a local functional group of tubulin protein triggers its giant complex microtubule resonantly vibrating spontaneously & changing polarity of resonance to run a network of clocks all over the time domain (from 10^{-3} s to 10^{-9} s). Clocks memorize and process the geometric shapes, make decisions [16, 19] (Fig. 2c). 10^6 order cascade effect by local tubulin is possible by time crystal engineering of ~50 nested time crystals; it could be replicated in artificial time crystals to build massive machines of the future.

The electromagnetic resonance of proteins is being measured since the 1930s. Since biomaterials are dielectric materials, it is natural to observe resonance frequencies. However, what has been missing is the dispersion relation of resonance frequencies in a biomaterial. For nearly a century now, most of the studies have been limited to only one frequency domain. Large temporal ranges are reported, but the geometry of time was never underpinned. Surprisingly, no other group than us talks about nature's writing of geometric shapes using resonance frequencies. Resonance frequency generates patterns in the dancing matter, but that is not everything. Those frequencies are patterns of primes. Phase part is explicit in the electromagnetic resonance of biomolecules [25]. We use the sum-frequency generation (SHG) technique to find the clocking relationship between several resonance frequencies (online article A). We built a two-frequency laser interferometer to measure small protein's very slow clocks, which are the foundation of the largest clocks we see in the time crystal map [26]. Small harmonics generation (SHG) techniques were used extensively in protein vibration measurement [27] to understand the chirality made modulation of combining two clocks [28]. We exclusively ruled out the wetting effect [29] (Chi Hieu et al.) due to the air–water interface [30] to deconvolute the time crystal contributions of individual components in the neuron i.e. microtubule, actin nanowire, proteins.

Proteins vibrate from milliseconds to the femtoseconds time scale, unfolding its dynamics is a multi-clock process though the structure of time is a mystery [31]. Different structures vibrate in different time scales [32]. Even the protein folding happens in nanoseconds and microseconds time-domain [33]. What begins at nanoseconds reaches a biologically noticeable formation in the microseconds time-domain [34]. Though we are the first group to predict triplet of triplet resonance band for time-correlated energy and information transfer, triplet–triplet energy transfer is evident in proteins in various modes [35]. The origin of protein's noise harvesting clocks (Fig. 2a, b) is the helical symmetry, the nucleation time of α-Helix suggests noise-induced condensation [36], there are various temporal limits, quantized speeds of folding similar to the one suggested here for creating the temporal configuration space [37]. Multi-time scale is the foundation of forming the whole life form starting from a single protein molecule [38]. It was unfortunate that we did not know the structure of time-based on which we could study spatio-temporal events much better than what we do today.

Time crystal was discovered in the 1960s to explain the intelligence of viruses. Finding biological clocks is not a complicated matter. However, the problem is holding the clock under noise (Fig. 2a, b). Whenever a biological clock is perturbed, it should get destroyed, but biological clocks shift to another clock and then return to the original clock. This particular phenomenon haunted scientists in the 1960s, and they suggested assembling newly born clocks in a single line, like a 1D single crystal. In materials science, we find 2D and 3D crystals, polyatomic crystals and polycrystals as a combination of several crystals or superpositions of materials with various symmetries. Significant research interests have enriched the knowledge in recent times on the time crystal. Unless and until we invent 2D and 3D time crystals, most importantly, polyatomic time crystals the true industrial revolution cannot begin. The oldest material detection technique was to measure non-linear changes in its resistance. Over time, dielectric technologies started finding their change in capacitance. We envision a new tool that accounts for the changes in the topology of phase spheres of materials as a time crystal. Our Geometric musical language (GML), as part of fractal information theory (FIT) provides these provisions since it combines the within and above configuration space of the temporal symmetry and at the same time side by side configuration space of the spatial symmetry.

4 Conclusion: Challenging the Exiting Paradigm of the Time Crystal

We have challenged the existing paradigm of constructing a time crystal on three accounts. First, we suggest that both the earliest proposal of time crystal by Arthur Winfree in the 1960s and Frank Wilczek in 2012 do not address the basic requirement to create a configuration space for time symmetry prior to building a time crystal. All subsequent works supporting their concept have theoretically investigated a resonating oscillator with its infinite harmonics series, furthermore consolidating that switching from fundamental frequency to the harmonics is breaking time symmetry and harmonics are time crystal. Though they do not write it explicitly, they follow these premises to realize a time crystal experimentally. The other two accounts assign quantum resonators as quantum time crystals, compromising the quantum essence of time symmetry. Finally, the necessity to externally perturb the inherent clock repeatedly to create what we call atoms for time crystal is contradictory to the basic definition of a crystal. In our experimental verification, we found the three nested time symmetries in a single protein, a protein made filament and neurons, and spontaneous generation of 3D clock assemblies 10^3 orders lower frequency domains than the original clocks. Therefore, the configuration space made of time symmetries that we have conceived outright rejects all existing concepts of time crystals; however, it stands the test of practical realization.

5 Competing Interests

The authors declare that there is no competing interest.

Acknowledgements Authors acknowledge the Asian office of Aerospace R&D (AOARD) a part of United States Air Force (USAF) for the grant no FA2386-16-1-0003 (2016–2019) on electromagnetic resonance-based communication and intelligence of biomaterials.

References

1. Strocchi F (2005)): Symmetry breaking. The lecture notes in physics. Springer, Berlin Heidelberg
2. Winfree AT (1970) Integrated view of resetting a circadian clock. J Theor Biol 28(3):327–374
3. Winfree AT (2001) Biological rhythm research. In The geometry of biological time. 2nd ed, Springer, New York, NY, USA
4. Singh P, Saxena K, Singhania A, Sahoo P, Ghosh S, Chhajed R, Ray K, Fujita D, Bandyopadhyay A (2020) A self-operating time crystal model of the human brain: can we replace entire brain hardware with a 3D fractal architecture of clocks alone? Information 11(5):238
5. Shapere A, Wilczek F (2012) Classical time crystals. Phys Rev Lett 109(16):160402
6. Wilczek F (2012) Quantum time crystals. Phys Rev Lett 109(16):160401
7. Susskind L, Glogower J (1964) Quantum mechanical phase and time operator. Physica 1(1):49–61
8. Zhang J, Hess PW, Kyprianidis A, Becker P, Lee A, Smith J, Pagano G, Potirniche ID, Potter AC, Vishwanath A et al (2017) Observation of a discrete time crystal. Nature 543:217–220
9. Blum R, Rovny J, Barrett S (2019) NMR observations of discrete time crystalline signatures in an ordered crystal of ammonium dihydrogen phosphate. In APS Meeting Abstracts
10. Yao NY, Potter AC, Potirniche ID, Vishwanath A (2017) Discrete time crystals: Rigidity, criticality, and realizations. Phys Rev Lett 118:030401
11. Sacha K, Zakrzewski J (2017) Time crystals: a review. Rep Prog Phys 81(1):016401
12. Faizal M, Khalil MM, Das S (2016) Time crystals from minimum time uncertainty. The European Physical Journal C 76(1):30
13. Han, X., Wei, M., Bi, Q., Kurths, J.: Obtaining amplitude-modulated bursting by multiple-frequency slow parametric modulation. Physical Review E 97, 012202 (2018).
14. Berliner, M.D.: Neurath PW. The rhythms of three clock mutants of Ascobolus immersus. Mycologia 57 (5), 809–17 (1965).
15. Saxena K, Singh P, Sahoo P, Sahu S, Ghosh S, Ray K, Fujita D, Bandyopadhyay A (2020) Fractal, scale free electromagnetic resonance of a single brain extracted microtubule nanowire, a single tubulin protein and a single neuron. Fractal and Fractional 4(2):11
16. Singh P et al (2021) Electrophysiology using coaxial atom probe array: Live imaging reveals hidden circuits of a hippocampal neural network. J Neurophysiol 125(6):2107–2116

17. Ghosh S, Sahu S, Agrawal L, Shiga T, Bandyopadhyay A (2016) Inventing a co-axial atomic resolution patch clamp to study a single resonating protein complex and ultra-low power communication deep inside a living neuron cell. J Integr Neurosci 15:403–433
18. Agrawal L et al (2016) Inventing atomic resolution scanning dielectric microscopy to see a single protein complex operation live at resonance in a neuron without touching or adulterating the cell. J Integr Neurosci 15(04):435–462
19. Singh, P. et al. Sahoo, P., Saxena, K., Manna, J.S., Ray, K., Ghosh, S., Bandyopadhyay, A.: Cytoskeletal Filaments Deep Inside a Neuron Are Not Silent: They Regulate the Precise Timing of Nerve Spikes Using a Pair of Vortices. Symmetry 13, 821 (2021b). https://doi.org/10.3390/sym13050821.
20. Agrawal, L. et al.: Fractal Information Theory (FIT)-Derived Geometric Musical Language (GML) for Brain-Inspired Hypercomputing. In: Pant, M. et al (eds) Soft Computing: Theories and Applications. Advances in Intelligent Systems and Computing, vol 584, pp. 343–372 (2018). https://doi.org/10.1007/978-981-10-5699-4_33
21. Bandyopadhyay, A. et al: Universal Geometric-musical language for big data processing in an assembly of clocking resonators. JP-2017–150171, 8/2/2017: World patent (February 2019), WO 2019/026983; US Patent App. 16/635,900 (2020).
22. Canavier CC, Kazanci FG, Prinz AA (2009) Phase Resetting Curves Allow for Simple and Accurate Prediction of Robust N:1 Phase Locking for Strongly Coupled Neural Oscillators. Biophys J 97(1):59–73
23. Achuthan S, Canavier CC (2009) Phase Resetting Curves Determine Synchronization, Phase-locking, and Clustering in Networks of Neural Oscillators. J Neurosci 29(16):5218–5233
24. Zlotnik A et al (2016) Phase-selective entrainment of nonlinear oscillator ensembles. Nat Commun 7:10788
25. Paliwal, A. et al.: Complex dielectric constant of various biomolecules as a function of wavelength using surface plasmon resonance. J. Appl. Phys. 116, 023109 (2014)
26. Ohtsuka Y, Itoh K (1979) Two-frequency laser interferometer for small displacement measurements in a low frequency range. Appl Opt 18(2):219–224
27. Fu L, Wang Z, Yan ECY (2011) Chiral Vibrational Structures of Proteins at Interfaces Probed by Sum Frequency Generation Spectroscopy. Int J Mol Sci 12(12):9404–9425. https://doi.org/10.3390/ijms12129404
28. Okuno M, Ishibashi T (2014) Chirality Discriminated by Heterodyne-Detected Vibrational Sum Frequency Generation. Physical chemistry letters 5(16):2874–2878. https://doi.org/10.1021/jz501158r
29. Chi Hieu, H.et al: Wetting effect on optical sum frequency generation (SFG) spectra of d-glucose, d-fructose, and sucrose; Spectrochimica Acta Part A: Molecular and Biomolecular Spectroscopy. 138, 834–839 (2015).
30. Engelhardt K, Peukert W, Braunschweig B (2014) Vibrational sum-frequency generation at protein modified air–water interfaces: Effects of molecular structure and surface charging. Curr Opin Colloid Interface Sci 19(3):207–215
31. Levy RM, Dai W, Deng N, Makarov DE (2013) How Long Does It Take to Equilibrate the Unfolded State of a Protein? Protein Sci 22:1459–1465
32. Hamm, P.: Ultrafast peptide and protein dynamics by vibrational spectroscopy. In: Braun, M., Gilch, P., Zinth,W. (eds) Ultrashort laser pulses in biology and medicine. Berlin, pp. 77–94 (2008).
33. Ballew RM, Sabelko J, Gruebele M (1996) Observation of distinct nanosecond and microsecond protein folding events. Nat Struct Biol 3:923–926
34. Duan Y, Kollman PA (1998) Pathways to a Protein Folding Intermediate Observed in a 1-Microsecond Simulation in Aqueous Solution. Science 282:740–744
35. Bieri O, Wirz J, Hellrung B, Schutkowski M, Drewello M, Kiefhaber T (1999) The speed limit for protein folding measured by triplet-triplet energy, transfer. Proc Natl Acad Sci USA 96:9597–9601
36. Serrano AL, Tucker MJ, Gai F (2011) Direct Assessment of the α-Helix Nucleation. Time J. Phys. Chem. B 115:7472–7478

37. Mukherjee S, Chowdhury P, Bunagan MR, Gai F (2008) Folding Kinetics of a Naturally Occurring Helical Peptide: Implication of the Folding Speed Limit of Helical Proteins. J Phys Chem B 112:9146–9150
38. Lü, Z., Zhao, C., Zhang, B., Duan. L.: Multitime Scale Study of Bursting Activities in the Pre-Bötzinger Complex. International Journal of Bifurcation and Chaos 27(11), 1750172 (2017).

Meta-Analysis of fMRI for Emotional and Cognitive States Shows Hierarchical Invariant Optimization in Brain

Anindya Pattanayak, Tanusree Dutta, Piyush Pranjal, Pushpendra Singh, Pathik Sahoo, Soumya Sarkar, and Anirban Bandyopadhyay

Abstract The brain's cognitive operation for emotion and perception is captured by fMRI images, which activates or deactivates different functional regions in synchronization with the human thoughts and expressions of emotional states. These synchronized pairs of emotional states and images of activated brain regions of interest (ROI) are called functional images. These images are not useful until we couple the brain's anatomical map or brain atlases with the ROI images. The coupling of two maps is called normalization, here we used both MNI and Talairach standards. Then, we investigated five ROI domains of behavioral response shifts, e.g., Action, Cognition, Emotion, Interoception, and Perception to find spatial jumps, periodic jumps between spaces, or multiple ROIs to find invariant geometric shapes. Each brain function has a specific set of geometric shapes that remain invariant in a 3D orientation, invariants are subject independent, correlate brain behavior and functions with comparative geometric shapes. Our finding paves the way to integrate spatio-temporal dynamics of hierarchically connected behavioral responses.

Keywords Human brain · Meta-analysis · Region of Interest ROI · Action · Cognition · Perception · fMRI · Human subject

---

A. Pattanayak · T. Dutta
Organizational Behavior and Human Resource Management, Indian Institute of Management, Ranchi 834008, India

P. Singh · P. Sahoo · A. Bandyopadhyay (✉)
International Center for Materials and Nanoarchitectronics (WPI-MANA) and Research Center for Advanced Measurement and Characterization (RCAMC), National Institute for Materials Science (NIMS), 1-2-1 Sengen, Tsukuba, Japan

P. Pranjal
Management Department, O.P. Jindal Global University, Sonipat 131001, India

S. Sarkar
Marketing Management, Indian Institute of Management, Ranchi, 834008, India

M. S. Kaiser et al. (eds.), *Proceedings of Trends in Electronics and Health Informatics*, Lecture Notes in Networks and Systems 376,
https://doi.org/10.1007/978-981-16-8826-3_23

1 Introduction

It is now well established that the brain has two coupled hierarchically organized structures, one anatomical and the other functional. The multi-layered, one above another integration of brain hardware [1], for example, Rich club organization of connectome [2], feedback signal transmission loops in visual cortex [3]. Linking dense network of cortico-cortical axon-paths with human behaviors is the hallmark of neurogenesis, the unfolding of these networks from spatial and topological centrality of the core in the cortex [4] suggest a scale-free energy transmission [5]. Helmholtz suggested that brain minimizes energy to make decisions, later, free energy concept was introduced to mathematically put forth the argument. Free energy minimizes the probability differences between environmental variables and network's configuration-induced arbitrary contributors by changing network geometry [6].

Integrating different energetically active brain parts with their specific behavioral and functional features into a singular correlated hierarchical architecture has been a challenge [7]. Linking active ROI sites in the fMRI, EEG or PET scans required a mathematical model to integrate information from all evaluation and attention systems to generate perceptual cognitions simultaneously using short-term and long-term memory. Causal relationship between active hardware part and behavioral response is difficult to model.

Optical imaging of brain's intrinsic signals (OIS) is used to map the functional topography of human cortex [8]. To model spatial scale hierarchy, the limitations of current models have been outlined by Simon et al., and they have described the recent trend to imagine neurobiological atoms or functional nodes that act as basic units which self-assemble with different multimodal functional features in the brain [9]. Our time crystal-based brain model extends the multimodal approach [10] to 537 modes (one mode = one clock system) in the brain integrating 12 layers of fractal hardware starting from proteins to the entire body's neural network [11]. Imagining hypothetical neurons based on global workspace of cognitive responses [12].

One of the novel ideas that have contributed to the understanding of the emotional structures of the brain is the ordering of phases of the transmitted signals. The distribution of phases across the brain could be ordered and disordered, its entropy could be calculated to estimate the information quantity and quality [13]. Since direction of information flow is decided by the frequency of signal [14], our time crystal-based modeling of the entire human brain, where 537 classes of clocks are integrated to estimate the whole brain's spatio-temporal network holds true [11].

Wide spectrum of cortical functional features originates from structural constraints, which leads to invariants of functional properties [15]. Here in this work, we have made an effort map invariant in the complete integrated emotional and functional maps of the brain [11].

Automated brain image analysis uses keywords for datamining several papers and identifying the complexity of brain signaling by filtering essential information from free large datasets [16]. Emotion and perception-driven thoughts and expressions have been correlated with bright active regions in the fMRI, EEG, and PET scans in wide ranges of high-volume databases. One of the key problems in identifying a particular emotional state with a distinct region of interest (ROI) is that most functional domains largely overlap.

1.1 Software Tools and Online Brain Databases Used for Meta-Analysis

Metadata analysis from "brainmap's" behavioral taxonomy of "axon motor learning" and "neurosynth's" interhemispheric energy transfer:

In this study, we used a meta-analytic approach to the functional MRI studies 81 distinct research described by Yarkoni et al. (http://Neurosynth.org). We downloaded the Neurosynth database that contained interhemispheric transfer details (https://neurosynth.org/analyses/terms/interhemispheric/). We downloaded the files and visualized them in https://socr.umich.edu/HTML5/BrainViewer/ and https://rii-mango.github.io/Papaya/ http://rii.uthscsa.edu/mango/mango.html used behavioral analysis plugin http://rii.uthscsa.edu/mango/plugin_behavioralanalysis.html talairach labels atlas applied on input image before behavior analysis plugin is run in the metadata analysis software http://www.brainmap.org/ale/ 52. Here for action motor learning 27 publications were compiled.

http://www.brainmap.org/taxonomy/behaviors/Action.Motor_Learning.html following tutorials http://rii.uthscsa.edu/mango//videos.html

1.2 Our Background Studies in Neuroscience and Mathematics

We have developed integrated clock architecture by measuring resonant oscillation frequencies of neurons, microtubules, etc. [17, 18], and discovering a fractal network of clocks. There are many hidden circuits in the brain, each in a particular time domain [19, 20]. Based on triplet of triplet fractal scale-free resonant bands connecting the microtubule, protein, and the neuron [21] we have already created a self-operating mathematical universe, SOMU model for understanding the human brain [22, 23]; eventually developing a complete-time crystal model of the human brain [11].

2 Experiment on Human Subject and Invariant Calculation Methods

Declaration on human subjects: The local ethics committee approved the study (Indian Institute of Management, IIM Ranchi). It was performed following the ethical standards in the Declaration of Helsinki (last modified, 2004). All 89 subjects were above 18 years and written informed consent was taken from all of them.

Human Subjects: For the experiment, 20 students aged between a maximum of 23 years and a minimum of 21 years were selected, all of whom were healthy, their body temperatures around 98 deg F, initial pulse rate between 78 to 132, brought down to 80–85; blood pressure 85–130 and the oxygen level in their blood between 95 to 97%. For matching the subjects' circadian rhythm, all experiments were performed in the evening, after the students were done with their classes for the day. Subjects with high fever, neurological disorders, major diseases in the past, or any forms of abnormal responses were rejected.

2.1 EEG Measurements to Compare with the fMRI Hierarchical Network

All subjects were asked to engage in an emotional state while measuring EEG. We tested 30 subjects for the emotional tests, the hierarchical architecture that we obtained from the fMRI-based meta-analysis was compared to the hierarchical invariant structure made from the EEG pattern.

Methods for determining the invariant map: In Fig. 1A we have explained how fMRI data obtained from the brainmap database project has been analyzed. The activated brain regions for different functions are connected by loops, we notice variations in the data as the loop. Note that our data is not dynamic, however, there are several online videos that suggest that dynamic regions are spatial loops. Therefore, we consider the statistical database as various activated loops, these loops are considered clocks and 3D assembly of clocks are created to take into account the phase relations between clocks. Once the clock structures are built we start finding the differential clocks following the protocol described in Fig. 1B. When the differential clocks are considered as a single point, we find elementary 1D, 2D, and 3D geometric shapes are remaining constant for all the papers used to create this brain metadata. Thus, we conclude those shapes are invariants.

2.2 What is Invariant? How Do We Detect It Here?

In Fig. 1C we have shown the typical feature that we observe in the EEG patterns and also in the FMRI images that 1D, 2D, and 3D patterns of exciting regions form differential 3D clocks, which we call 4D. Some of these differential clocks vibrate in a plane, we check the 2D shapes, we call it 5D. Some of these planes follow some lines when they change case to case basis (list of papers used in the database are online), so we get 1D invariants, this database of lines is called 1D invariant. Actually, we read three types of invariants from EEG and fMRI database, and mostly

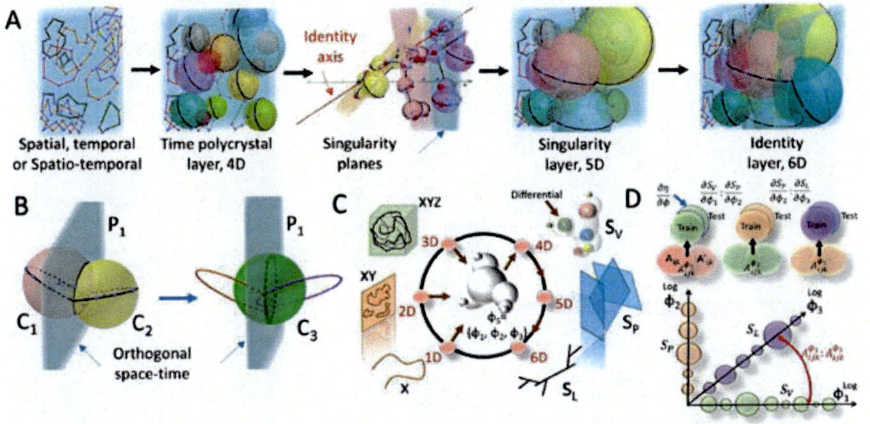

Fig. 1 **A**. Spatio-temporal data obtained from fMRI, EEG, or PET scans are processed step by step following this procedure. The loops of similar values of intensities are connected and a clock is assigned. In the second step, these clocks are integrated based on a concept that clocks synchronized in a plane vibrate together, and planes vibrating along a line are assigned a new clock. The integration of clocks continues until at the highest level, a singular clock is obtained. **B**. Hierarchical integration of clocks is achieved by differential integration of clocks. Two clocks C1 and C2 overlap and the different volumes of clock-holding sphere are assigned a new clock that is invariant. This particular concept is used in developing the hierarchical integration of clocks. **C**. The procedures noted in the captions for panels A and B are summarized. 1D, 2D, and 3D datasets are used to build the invariant network. The information in the brain is invariant network, brain integrates invariants to make decisions. **D**. Mathematical representation of panel C. Here along three orthogonal axes three types of invariants, volumetric, planar, and linear arrangement of differential clocks are placed, the derived invariant pattern is the decision made by the brain

the invariant geometric shapes obtained from the brain surface and inside are identical for a particular brain function.

An invariant is a geometric shape created by the unchanged 1D line, 2D area, and 3D volume arrangement of differential clocks. Once the differential clock-based patterns are ready, we replace clocks using a point to find that geometric shape that does not change. As a result, we get elementary geometric shapes like triangle, square, pentagon, hexagon for all the five mental states that we are investigating here from the large fMRI database.

3 Results and Discussion

In Fig. 2A, three images show that two triangular domains work at a time in two perpendicular planes in the brain (see images 1 and 3). They together govern the energy transfer between left and right hemispheres. Interhemispheric transfer's invariant geometry is shown in the Figure itself. However, this particular meta-analysis does not reveal the energy transfer process. So, we carried out behavioral

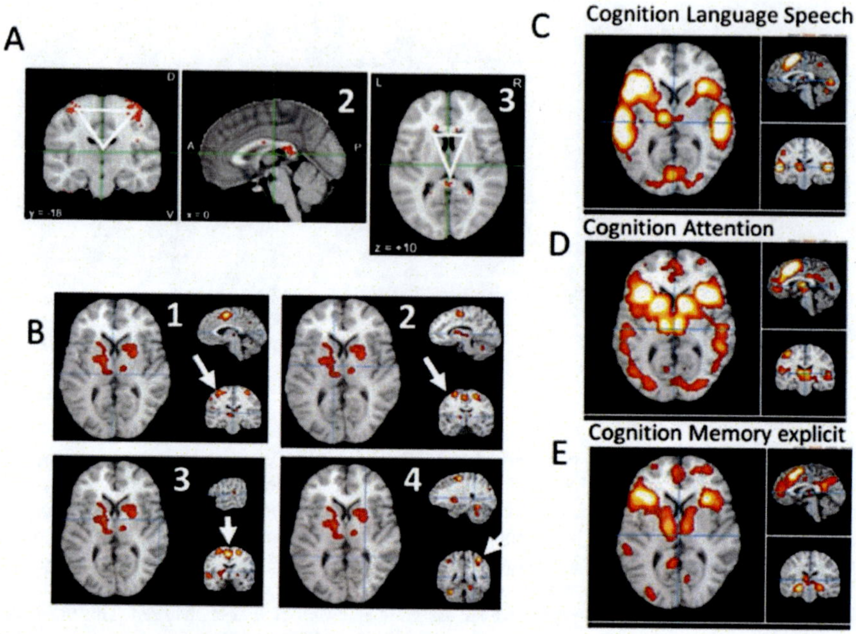

Fig. 2 **A** The load of "interhemispheric" meta-analysis, in 81 papers from Neurosynth brain scan database. "association" function has been applied for generating the metadata (see methods for details). **B** Action motor learning of brainmap database. Here metadata is a compilation of 27 relevant publications; 114 experimental contrasts; 1080 coordinates reported. **C**. Cognition language speech, 228 relevant publications, 1028 experimental contrasts, 8977 coordinates reported. **D**. Cognition attention, 664 relevant publications, 2748 experimental contrasts, 21,797 coordinates reported. **E**. Cognition memory explicit, 262 relevant publications, 1110 experimental contrasts, 8403 coordinates reported

analysis from another brain database called brainmap (see methods). We selected metadata of motor control learning that closely associates to EEG task for five emotional states, sum of 27 associated publications presented in Fig. 2B shows an unprecedented three-point energy transfer (see 3). Three bright spots blink in sequence, two spots are identified in the two lobes of the brain, but the central one is a common energy transfer domain that regulates the laterization process. Both meta-analyses of panels (A) and (B) suggest that energy transfer happens by jumping through space by spending specified time, leading to spatio-temporal quantization of lateralization. We wanted to find whether if such quantization in the hardware-based behavioral analysis has a real effect on the human subject responses.

In Fig. 2C, we have shown three cognition functions, language, speech shows a pentagon, attention shows a circle with a V shape on the top part of its perimeter (Fig. 2D). Explicit memory shows a U shape and an ellipsoid kept on top of it (Fig. 2E). These invariant patterns are visible and understood even without much analysis. Since this is the first work of trying to find invariants in the information processing of brain, we have limited ourselves only within the framework of apparent solution. Another reason is that we believe in hierarchy within and above network of clocks following fractal information theory (FIT) and model brain as a time polycrystal (Singh 2020). However, when the databases are created only the apparent area is noted and contributions of a large number of independently carried out experiments are merged. Therefore, to carry out true analysis to verify our brain model is not possible. Most information captured from the brain ignores how differential loops behave, instead crudely merge. In the future, we would create our own brain signal database to get rid of such problems.

In Fig. 3A–F we have investigated positive and negative emotions to find the invariant geometric shapes. Figure 3A–C are positive emotions while Fig. 3D–F are negative emotions. The invariant geometries for positive emotions are lines in distinct 3D orientations when we see transverse cross-sectional view of the image. In sharp contrast, we see that along the longitudinal cross-section, loops form for negative emotions. For negative emotions, the transverse view shows X for anger, two connected squares for fear, and a line for sadness. Thus, negative emotions build two orthogonal invariant patterns. Activation for happiness is discrete S shape in the transverse cross-section while a semicircular loop in the longitudinal cross-section. Humor is probably a dark emotion state where distantly located discrete activation does not reveal any inherent geometric shape. Valence is the most conservative emotional state and it originates from a tiny looped activation at the frontal lobe of the human brain.

In Fig. 4A–D, we have shown four interceptions, hunger, sexuality, sleep, and thirst, while Fig. 4E–H shows four perceptions, vision for color motion and shape, then somesthesis pain. While hunger is a very local effect in the mid-brain, sexuality is an open-loop visible in the orthogonal cross-section, possibly sexuality is the only brain state that forms an incomplete loop. Sleeping and thirst are very localized effects originating from isolated discrete memory locations. While perception for color is a V shape, for motion, a flower pot like a nearly close necked object is the invariant loop. Shape activation is a hexagon and pain is a dumbbell-shaped activation.

4 Conclusions and Mathematical Model for Cognitive Engineering

We investigated five ROI domains of behavioral response shifts, e.g. Action, Cognition, Emotion, Interoception, and Perception to find spatial jumps, periodic jumps between spaces, or multiple ROIs to find invariant geometric shapes. The above discussion accounts for 19 cognitive states of the brain which could be modeled using dodecanions or 12D tensors (Singh 2021c,d) and applying them in the space–time-topology-prime metric. All 19 brain states have a typical geometric shape of activation in the human brain. Therefore, our geometric language of time crystals could integrate periodic vibrations in different organs occurring at different time

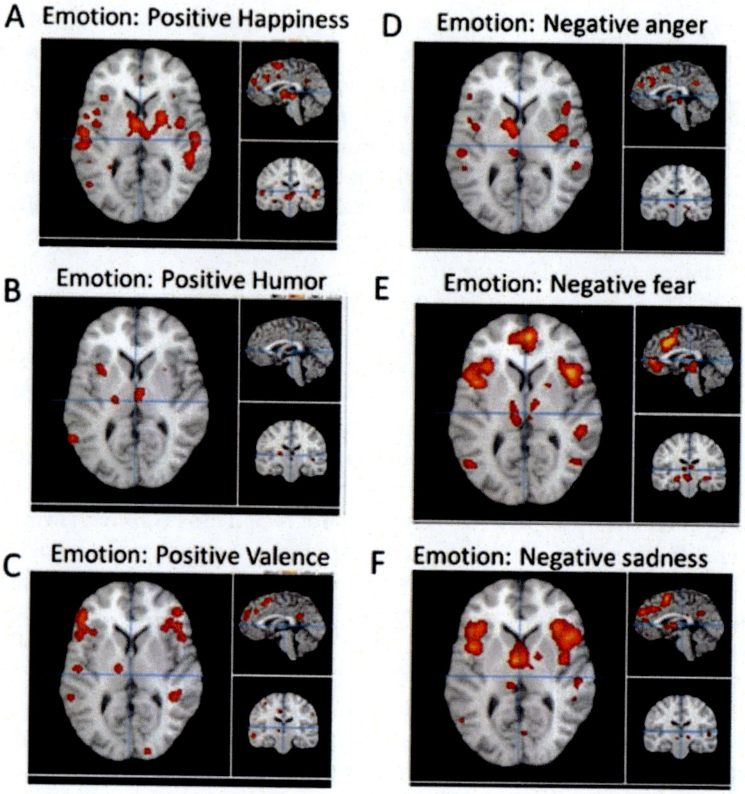

Fig. 3 **A** The load of "emotion" meta-analysis, for emotion positive happiness (117 relevant publications; 411 experimental contrasts; 2458 coordinates reported); **B** For positive emotion humor (7 relevant publications; 34 experimental contrasts; 202 coordinates reported); **C** Emotion, positive valence (intrinsic goodness) 43 relevant publications 150 experimental contrasts 1119 coordinates reported. **D** Emotion negative anger 64 relevant publications, 275 experimental contrasts, 1496 coordinates reported. **E** Emotion negative fear, 133 relevant publications, 531 experimental contrasts, 3089 coordinates reported, **F** Emotion negative sadness, 92 relevant publications, 350 experimental contrasts; 2399 coordinates reported. Collected from Neurosynth brain scan database. "association" function has been applied for generating the metadata (see methods for details)

domains into a unified structure that represents resonant oscillations of the brain components as well as the brain functions, behavioral responses.

5 Contributions

A.B. and T.D. conceptualized the idea, A. P; P. P.; P. Sa., and P. Si. did the experiment, A. B analyzed the data and wrote the paper with A.P. and P. Si. S.S. verified

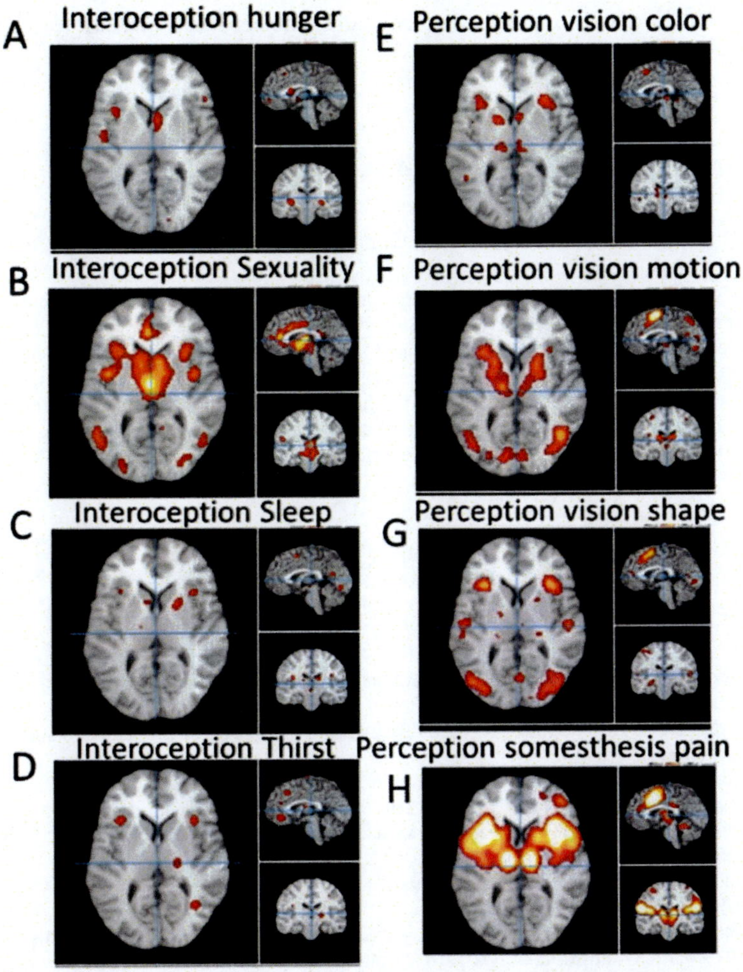

Fig. 4 The load of "emotion" meta-analysis, **A** Interoception hunger; 23 relevant publications, 90 experimental contrasts, 505 coordinates reported. **B** Interoception sexuality, 73 relevant publications, 426 experimental contrasts, 3486 coordinates reported, **C** Interoception sleep, 12 relevant publications, 45 experimental contrasts, 278 coordinates reported. **D** Interoception thirst, 6 relevant publications, 28 experimental contrasts, 246 coordinates reported. **E** Perception vision color, 40 relevant publications, 117 experimental contrasts, 1112 coordinates were reported. **F** Perception vision motion, 94 relevant publications, 318 experimental contrasts, 3038 coordinates reported. **G** Perception vision shape, 165 relevant publications, 606 experimental contrasts, 4483 coordinates reported. **H** Perception somesthesis pain, 147 relevant publications, 553 experimental contrasts, 5354 coordinates reported. Collected from Neurosynth brain scan database. "association" function has been applied for generating the metadata (see methods for details)

experimental protocol and helped in the human subject study, M.K.M. reviewed the validity of the data.

6 Competing Interests Statement

The authors declare that they have no competing financial interests.

Acknowledgements We thank Dave Sonntag and Martin Timms for the independent test and verification of our device as part of patent US9019685B2. Authors acknowledge the Asian office of Aerospace R&D (AOARD), a part of the United States Air Force (USAF), for Grant no. FA2386-16-1-0003 (2016–2019) on the electromagnetic resonance-based communication and intelligence of biomaterials. Authors also acknowledge the financial assistance of Scheme for Promotion of Academic and Research Collaboration (SPARC) an MHRD, Govt of India initiative for the project titled 'Management of Fractal Time in High-level Decision Making' (Govt of India, MHRD; project number P 524; Start date: 15.03. 2019-14.03.2021; Duration:2 years).

References

1. Felleman DJ, Van Essen DC (1991) Distributed hierarchical processing in the primate cerebral cortex. Cereb Cortex 1:1–47
2. van den Heuvel MP, Sporns O (2011) Rich-club organization of the human connectome. J Neurosci 31:15775–15786
3. Markov NT et al (2014) Anatomy of hierarchy: feedforward and feedback pathways in macaque visual cortex. J Comp Neurol 522:225–259
4. Hagmann P et al (2008) Mapping the structural core of human cerebral cortex. PLoS Biol 6:e159
5. Friston KJ, Stephan KE (2007) Free-energy and the brain. Synthese 159(3):417–458. https://doi.org/10.1007/s11229-007-9237-y
6. Friston K, Kilner J, Harrison L (2006) A free energy principle for the brain. J Physiol Paris 100(1–3):70–87. https://doi.org/10.1016/j.jphysparis.2006.10.001 Epub 2006 Nov 13 PMID: 17097864
7. Deco G, Vidaurre D, Kringelbach ML (2021) Revisiting the global workspace orchestrating the hierarchical organization of the human brain. Nat Hum Behav 5:497–511. https://doi.org/10.1038/s41562-020-01003-6)
8. Pouratian N, Sheth SA, Martin NA, Toga AW (2003) Shedding light on brain mapping: advances in human optical imaging. Trends Neurosci 26(5):277–282. https://doi.org/10.1016/S0166-2236(03)00070-5 PMID: 12744845
9. Eickhoff SB, Constable RT, Yeo BTT (2018) Topographic organization of the cerebral cortex and brain cartography. Neuroimage 170:332–347. https://doi.org/10.1016/j.neuroimage.2017.02.018 Epub 2017 Feb 20. PMID: 28219775; PMCID: PMC5563483
10. Glasser MF et al (2016) A multi-modal parcellation of human cerebral cortex. Nature 536:171–178
11. Singh P, Saxena K, Singhania A, Sahoo P, Ghosh S, Chhajed R, Ray K, Fujita D, Bandyopadhyay A (2020) A self-operating time crystal model of the human brain: can we replace entire brain hardware with a 3D fractal architecture of clocks alone? Information 11(5):238
12. Dehaene S, Kerszberg M, Changeux JP (1998) A neuronal model of a global workspace in effortful cognitive tasks. Proc Natl Acad Sci USA 95(24):14529–14534

13. Lobier M, Siebenhuhner F, Palva S, Palva JM (2014) Phase transfer entropy: a novel phase-based measure for directed connectivity in networks coupled by oscillatory interactions. Neuroimage 85:853–872
14. Hillebrand A et al (2016) Direction of information flow in large-scale resting-state networks is frequency-dependent. Proc Natl Acad Sci USA 113:3867–3872
15. Huntenburg JM, Bazin PL, Margulies DS (2018) Large-scale gradients in human cortical organization. Trends Cogn Sci 22:21–31
16. Lancaster JL, Laird AR, Eickhoff SB, Martinez MJ, Fox PM, Fox PT (2012) Automated regional behavioral analysis for human brain images. Front Neuroinform 6:23. https://doi.org/10.3389/fninf.2012.00023
17. Agrawal L et al (2016) Inventing atomic resolution scanning dielectric microscopy to see a single protein complex operation live at resonance in a neuron without touching or adulterating the cell. J Integr Neurosci 15(04):435–462
18. Ghosh S, Sahu S, Agrawal L, Shiga T, Bandyopadhyay A (2016) Inventing a co-axial atomic resolution patch clamp to study a single resonating protein complex and ultra-low power communication deep inside a living neuron cell. J Integr Neurosci 15:403–433
19. Singh P et al (2021) Electrophysiology using coaxial atom probe array: live imaging reveals hidden circuits of a hippocampal neural network. J Neurophysiol 125(6):2107–2116
20. Singh P, Sahoo P, Saxena K, Manna JS, Ray K, Ghosh S, Bandyopadhyay A et al (2021) Cytoskeletal filaments deep inside a neuron are not silent: they regulate the precise timing of nerve spikes using a pair of vortices. Symmetry 13:821. https://doi.org/10.3390/sym13050821
21. Saxena K, Singh P, Sahoo P, Sahu S, Ghosh S, Ray K, Fujita D, Bandyopadhyay A (2020) Fractal, scale free electromagnetic resonance of a single brain extracted microtubule nanowire, a single tubulin protein and a single neuron. Fractal Fractional 4(2):11
22. Singh P et al (2021c) Quaternion, octonion to dodecanion manifold: stereographic projections from infinity lead to a self-operating mathematical universe. In Singh P, Gupta RK, Ray K, Bandyopadhyay A (eds) Proceedings of International conference on trends in computational and cognitive engineering. Adv Intell Syst Comput, Springer, Singapore, vol 1169, pp 55–77
23. Singh P et al (2021d) A space-time-topology-prime, stTS metric for a self-operating mathematical universe uses dodecanion geometric algebra of 2–20 D complex vectors. In Ray K, Roy KC, Toshniwal SK, Sharma H, Bandyopadhyay A (eds) Proceedings of international conference on data science and applications. Lecture notes in networks and systems, Springer, Singapore, vol 148, pp 1–31

IoT and Data Analytics

A Framework of an Obstacle Avoidance Robot for the Visually Impaired People

Sudipto Chaki, Shamim Ahmed, Milon Biswas, and Iffat Tamanna

Abstract Human being precepts its visual information with the help of eyes. But, some people are visually impaired and are incapable to collect visual information. That is why they have to rely on others while walking or moving somewhere. So, we have proposed a framework that can solve this issue effectively and give the blind people a scope to move around freely. Some researchers have already contributed to this issue and proposed some walker-based systems to assist visually impaired people. But, most of the walkers are either heavy or big. Heavyweight restricts them from being user-friendly, and big size makes it impossible to be used in a narrow space. In this regard, we have developed a lightweight robot that can assist blind people to find an obstacle freeway while moving. Our robot is integrated with a Microsoft Kinect camera and to process the captured images, we use the Raspberry Pi as its computational unit. By using the depth sensor of the Kinect device, the robot collects its surroundings images and is sent to the Raspberry Pi unit to analyze them to detect any obstacles coming toward. We accommodate our robot with an obstacle avoidance algorithm so that if any obstacle is detected within a certain range, the robot can automatically move either right or left depending on the intensity values of the images.

Keywords Microsoft kinect · Raspberry pi · Robot · Depth sensor · Object detection

1 Introduction

Navigation without vision is difficult. Navigating in spaces is quite a challenge for the users who are blind as they largely have to rely on their hands and ears for spatial perception. These people suffer from serious visual impairments preventing them from traveling independently. Several technologies have been emerged to help visually impaired people. In this regard, we have built a prototype robot that can

S. Chaki (✉) · S. Ahmed · M. Biswas · I. Tamanna
Bangladesh University of Business and Technology, Dhaka 1216, Bangladesh

M. S. Kaiser et al. (eds.), *Proceedings of Trends in Electronics and Health Informatics*, Lecture Notes in Networks and Systems 376,
https://doi.org/10.1007/978-981-16-8826-3_24

securely guide visually impaired people. The self-driving car concept is now a very popular application area in autonomous vehicle management systems. A laser light reflection-based obstacle avoidance vehicle management is proposed by Baras et al. [1]. The authors have used Raspberry Pi as its processing unit that is integrated with its obstacle avoidance algorithm. But, they have built their systems which are largely dependent on Wi-Fi for navigation purposes which may fail due to the absence of it while moving in a robust environment. Nowadays, infrared light is being used in automatic vehicle management systems [2]. The authors have proposed a prototype-based automatic vehicle for any indoor environment. But, they have failed to deploy their prototype autonomous vehicle in outdoor environments. The future of our transportation will be largely dependent on the autonomous vehicle management system. The key contributions of our proposed framework is highlighted in the following:

- We develop a prototype of obstacle avoidance robot that is capable of providing a safe passage by avoiding obstacles in its way.
- Our prototype robot is integrated with an obstacle avoidance algorithm that performs better with lower time complexity.
- Our proposed framework can be beneficial for the visually impaired people if we integrate our robot with a smart cane.

The rest of the part of this paper is organized in the following manner. Section 2 describes the research background of our proposed work. Section 3 provides the robot based framework of this paper. We show some experimental result analysis in Sect. 4. Finally, we add the conclusion and future works in Sect. 5.

2 Related Research

Some previous researches on collision avoidance technique for a robot are being treated as high-level tasks. But, Takizawa et al. [3] have proposed a novel technique for mobile robots that shows the robot can be controlled in a real-time monitoring system. Microsoft Kinect [4] has a depth sensor and is equipped with an infrared light imaging technique that helps to identify any type of 3D objects from the environment. But, this system is integrated with a tactile device that needs to be held by its user and this may not be user-friendly for visually impaired people. To remove this problem, we have integrated a Kinect device with a robot that is equipped to pave an obstacle freeway without any physical involvement. To process in real-time, we have a Raspberry Pi unit that can process our captured image faster than in [5, 6]. Apart from the Kinect device, the radio frequency identification-based object detection technique [7] is applied for blind people so that they may move freely in the indoor environment by using tags attached to the objects. For identifying obstacles while moving, blind users need to wear a glove to their hands to detect obstacles while touching the objects. A novel approach for the surveillance purpose [8] that integrates with computer vision and neural network techniques is proposed by Budiharto.

A recent advancement for the obstacle avoidance robot is proposed by Naveen et al. [9, 10] where they built a prototype of ultrasonic sensor-based electronic travel aid to avoid obstacles while moving in the environment. But, due to the large size of this prototype device, it is not suitable for lightweight vision-less robots. SICK sensor-based [11] object detection and identification for the ground robots is proposed by Yan Peng et al. To reduce noise from the sensed images, they have applied a filtering technique to improve the performance by reducing noise levels. Over the few years, Raspberry Pi [12, 13] is being used as a very popular computational processing unit especially in miniature robots. In our works, we have used it to process our novel obstacle avoidance algorithm and hence to send signals to the robot to avoid the upcoming obstacles by turning its wheels in a certain direction provided by it.

An experimental autonomous [14, 15] ground vehicle system is used to test a unique obstacle avoidance approach. In comparison to prior techniques, the suggested method provides a novel solution to the problem and has numerous advantages. This innovative method is simple to tweak and takes into account the robot's range of vision as well as non-holistic restrictions. The bug algorithms [16], the potential field techniques, and the vector field histogram approach, all active sensor-based methods [17] are discussed in this article for obstacle avoidance and path planning. Unlike most existing hybrid navigation systems [18], in which deliberative layers play a dominant role and reactive layers are merely simple executors, the proposed architecture focuses on the navigation problems and pursues a more independent reactive layer that can guarantee convergence without the assistance of a deliberative layer. These papers [19, 20] describe a hybrid approach (roaming trails) that combines a prior knowledge of the environment with local perceptions to complete assigned tasks efficiently and safely; that is, by ensuring that the robot never becomes stuck in deadlocks, even when operating in a partially unknown dynamic environment. The obstacle avoidance robot uses sonar range sensors as a sensory element [21]. The authors introduced an improved artificial potential field-based regression search (improved APF-based RS) technique [22] in this work, which can quickly get a global sub-optimal/optimal path with complete known environment information without local minima and oscillations. The use of computer vision and picture sequence algorithms to detect and avoid obstacles for autonomous land vehicle (ALV) [23] navigation in outdoor road conditions is proposed.

In our work, we have used the Microsoft Kinect sensor to obtain the depth information of the scene for obstacle classification. The advantage of our framework with an existing product is its ability to detect obstacles within the specified range in a faster manner because of our obstacle avoidance algorithm. Besides, our robot automatically moves in a direction where no obstacle is present that can lead the user to an obstacle-free path. It will be much cheaper compared to all the other devices currently available in the market. A lower price and its ability to detect obstacles will be greatly helpful for visually impaired individuals.

3 Overview of Our Proposed Framework

We have focused on designing an obstacle avoidance robot which is a lightweight one so that visually impaired people can easily navigate among the obstacles both in the indoor and outdoor environments. The system overview of our proposed framework is shown in Fig. 1.

This device will start up when power will be given to the processor and the Microsoft Kinect camera. After booting up the Raspberry Pi which is used as the processing device, a program inside the Raspberry will automatically run. This task is done by writing a bash script. A bash script is a text file containing a series of commands. The camera will sense the surrounding environment. Based on the position of the obstacle, the processor will send signals to the motor driver. Depending

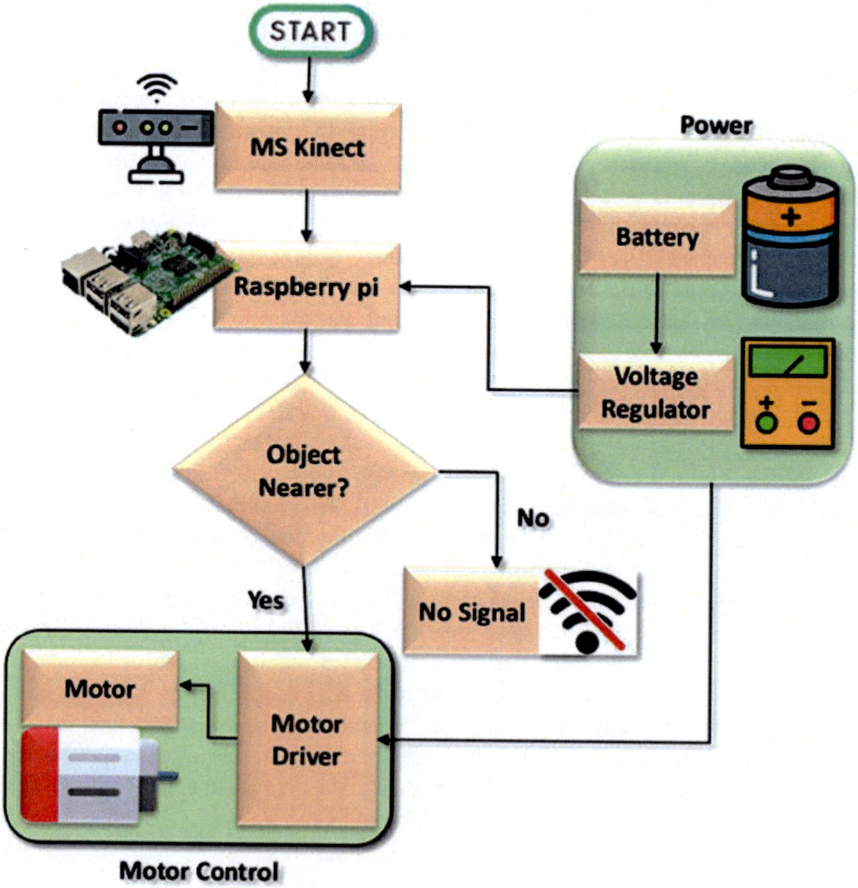

Fig. 1 System overview of our proposed robot framework

on the signal of the motor driver, it will turn the wheels attached to that device. A battery of 12 V is used to supply power to the Raspberry Pi unit and the Microsoft Kinect sensor. The voltage regulator regulates the voltage level. As the Raspberry Pi operates on 5 V, a bug module is used to supply the exact amount of voltage. The Kinect is powered by using a booster module.

Having the position of the obstacle detected, the Raspberry Pi will send signals to the motor drivers. It amplifies the level of current. Two types of polarity are given to the motor driver. Depending on the polarities, the wheels are rotated. To provide a clear understanding of the proposed system, we have subdivided the whole system into mainly two parts, and they are the object detection phase and obstacle avoidance phase.

3.1 Object Detection Phase

In this phase, from the environment, the object is detected as an obstacle. For system debugging purposes, the OpenNI framework is configured with OpenCV that is an open-source computer vision library. Object detection is done mainly by detecting the depth of the image. This depth image is obtained by an infrared projected-matrix bouncing camera over the objects. The infrared camera (IR) captures the beams which contain an intensity variance. This intensity variance helps to compute the distance to every object in the scene. To analyze the depth image, preprocessing technique is accomplished upon the depth fields. This preprocessing is done by following several steps (i.e., formation generation layer, erosion, Canny edge detection, contour detection, and binning operations gradually.

Formation Generation Layer: The formation generating layer uses the positions of suspected impediments to decide where the robot should travel in order to produce a specific configuration. The terms "target" and "place" are used throughout the article to refer to an obstacle-free path and a point where the robot should travel based on the position of the obstruction. The generalized format of the formation matrix is depicted in Eq. 1. The robot measures the distance d from the upcoming obstacles in its way in order to move to a certain direction (i.e., either left or right depending on the condition arises from the flag bit). The assessment of distance measurement is shown in Eq. 2. An outline of distance measurement of our robot bot is shown in Fig. 2a. The location and target are calculated using a distance cost table. The creation of a distance cost table based on formation shape is depicted in Fig. 2b. While moving to a certain direction the robot takes it decision based the distance from the cost table (i.e., formation matrix of distance).

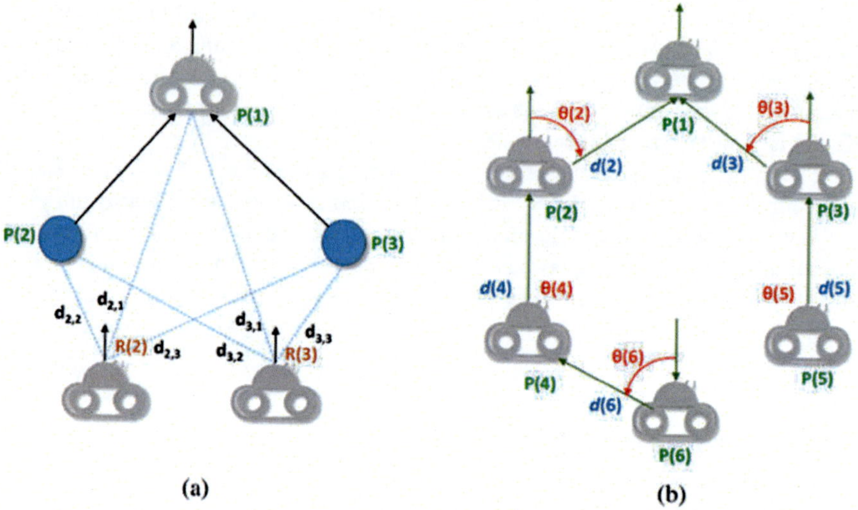

Fig. 2 **a** Measurement of distance from the obstacle, **b** measuring the angle while movement of the robot

$$F(M) = \begin{bmatrix} P(1) \\ P(2) \\ P(3) \\ . \\ . \\ . \end{bmatrix} = \begin{bmatrix} T(1)\ d(1)\ \theta(1) \\ T(2)\ d(2)\ \theta(2) \\ T(2)\ d(2)\ \theta(2) \end{bmatrix} \tag{1}$$

$$d_{i,j} = \sqrt{d_j^2 + d_{i,l}^2 - 2d_j d_{i,l} \cos(\varDelta\theta)} \tag{2}$$

Notation: $P(i)$—ith row of the formation matrix, $T(i)$—target, $d(i)$—distance, $theta (i)—angle.

Erosion: The basic idea is to erode the regions of the foreground pixels which are typically the white pixels. It takes two inputs to process further. The first input is the image that is to be eroded and the second one is a set of coordinate points named structuring elements. The second one is also known as the kernel. The use of the structuring element is to determine the precise effect of the erosion on the input image.

Edge Detection: To detect an object coming toward the robot, edge detection is needed to identify the object as an obstacle. Most of the shape information of an image is enclosed in edges. So, in this regard, we have used Canny edge detector methods and then enhance those areas of an image that contain edges. The sharpness of the image is increased in several steps.

- **Noise Reduction**: Edge detection is very much susceptible to noise. So, we have reduced the noise level from the image using proper filtering techniques.
- **Intensity Gradient of the Image**: Having done with the noise removal part, the noise-free image is then filtered with a Sobel kernel to get the first derivative in the horizontal and vertical directions.
- **Non-Maximum Suppression**: In our previous steps, we have reduced noise levels from the image but some unwanted pixels may be included while finding the edges which may not form the necessary edges.

Contour Detection: Contours are a curve joining all the continuous points (alongside the boundary), having the same intensity values. In the process of object, detection contours are a useful tool. It takes three arguments. The first one is the input image, the second one is the contour retrieval mode, and the last one is the contour approximation method. Then, it returns a modified image.
Binning: This is a way to group several continuous values into a smaller number of bins. Binning combines the information of adjacent pixels into a resulting information bin. This operation leads to a reduced resolution.

3.2 Object Avoidance Phase

Obstacles are avoided based on the intensity levels. For different intensity values, different types of decisions are taken. If the intensity level ranges from 80 to less than that, it means that the obstacle is too close to the user. Then, the user is said to be stopped or move in a certain direction. If the intensity level is more than 120, the robot moves to the right or left immediately. If the intensity level is equal to 80, the obstacle is said to be close to the user. The turning of the device to the right or left is done by taking some calculations taken into account. From this part, the task of avoiding the obstacle is done. A pseudo program is depicted in Algorithm 1.

- If the flag bit value is between 0 and 2, it means that the left side of the obstacle is safer to go. So, the "move left" signal is given by the processor unit.
- If the flag bit value is between 1 and 3, it means that the front side of the camera is obstacle-free. So, the "move forward" signal is given by the processor unit.
- If the flag bit value is between 2 and 4, it means that the right side of the user is obstacle-free. So, the signal "move right" is given.

Algorithm 1: Process of Obstacle Avoidance

Call region check function
Analyze the intensity level of the robot environment
if *intensity.level* ≤ 80 **then**
  Obstacle is close to the robot;
else if *intensity.level* ≥ 120 **then**
  Obstacle is in imminent position;
end
Call *movement generation function*
Action: *Divide the robot environment into 5 regions*
foreach *detection region* **do**
  Prepare *a cost table*
  if *flag bit = [0-2]* **then**
    Action: *Move Left*
  else if *flag bit = [2-4]* **then**
    Action: *Move Right*
  else if *flag bit = [1-4]* **then**
    Action: *Move forword*
  end
end

4 Implementation and Result Analysis

Our system has some minimum requirements to run successfully. The main requirements are a Microsoft Kinect 360 camera, a Raspberry Pi unit, a micro SD storage unit, a 12 V battery, two wheels, a bug module, and a boost module. The robotic feature of the proposed system can be achieved by sending the signal to the motor driver attached to the robot. This robot can move forward, right, left, and stop based on the position of the obstacle. The task of navigation is done by sending signals from the Raspberry Pi to the motor driver. The robot contains two wheels that can move right or left. The connection between the robot and the Raspberry Pi is done using the GPIO (general purpose input-output) pins. Pins are arranged in a (2×20) fashion. This provides an interface between the Raspberry Pi and the motor driver. These pins act as a switch that has a high voltage of (3.3 V) and a low voltage of (0 V) to connect the Raspberry Pi to the navigation robot.

The objects that are approaching toward the robot are defined as obstacles based on the intensity values as described in the previous section. Figure 3a shows an object that exists in the way of our moving robot. The Kinect device captured the image and after analyzing the intensity values shown in Fig. 3b, our system has detected the object is at a safe distance and the system generates a soft signal for the robot to move forward. Different types of intensity levels from 0 to 7 are the NumPy (a python library) data to identify the distance from the obstacle. So, our obstacle avoidance algorithm then sends a signal to the robot to move forward as it is a safe state.

When the obstacle is closer than the safe distance shown in Fig. 4a, the robot rotates in a certain direction based on the intensity levels shown in Fig. 4b. The

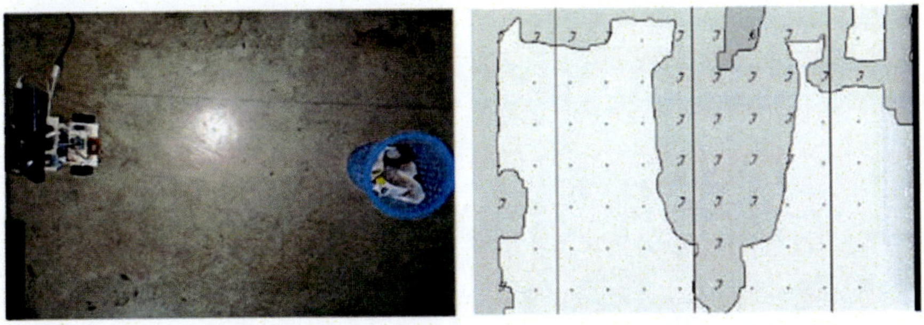

(a) (b)

Fig. 3 **a** An obstacle exists at a safe distance, and **b** NumPy library data for the safe state

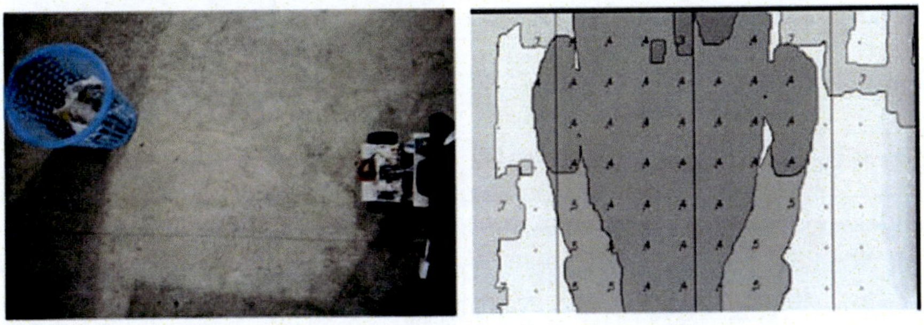

(a) (b)

Fig. 4 **a** An obstacle exists at a nearer distance, and **b** NumPy library data for the nearer state

intensity levels got darker than the previous safe state as the obstacle is nearer to our robot.

When the object is at a collision state shown in Fig. 5a (i.e., the obstacle is imminent), the nearest pixels of the obstacle got even darker shown in Fig. 5b than the previous scenarios. This indicates that a collision might happen if the robot continues to go in the same direction. To avoid this collision, the algorithm sends a collision alert signal. This signal is then sent to the robot through the Raspberry Pi unit. The motor driver takes the signal and rotates at an obstacle freeway by moving its wheels.

We have tested our robot several times with different hurdles to identify any moving or stand-still objects from its surroundings. And, with the help of the Kinect sensor as well as an integrated obstacle avoidance algorithm, our robot has successfully detected obstacles and avoided them by turning its wheels. In our experimental environment, we have found our robot can move at an average speed of 0.43 m/s while avoiding obstacles successfully. On the other hand, the average speed of the proposed LIDAR-based robot [1] was 0.31 m/s. Our robot achieves such greater

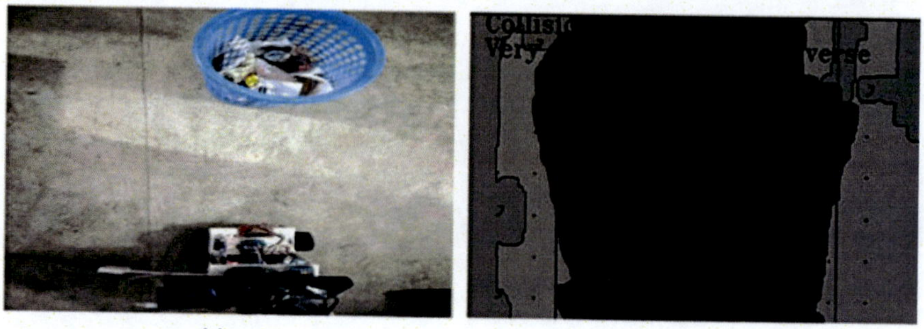

(a) (b)

Fig. 5 **a** An obstacle exists at a collision state, and **b** NumPy library data for the collision state

Table 1 A comparative study among available systems with our proposed framework

Refs.	Hard-wares	Parameters	Efficiency	Convergence	Complexity
[10, 23]	DS (IR, sonar), MC	CDP	Low	Yes	High
[6, 23]	DS (IR, sonar), MC	Target and OD	Low	No	Low
[22]	SSP, high memory	OD	Low	No	Average
[13]	C, SS, P, BB	OP, AD	High	No	High
[19]	ULS, COVS, NIPXI-811108RT, PXi-7954R FPGA	OD and angle	High	No	Low
[20]	LSS, PR	PIE	Medium	Yes	High
[15]	LSS, MP	PIE	Medium	Yes	High
Our model	MKC, R-pi, DM	OP, AD	High	Yes	Low

speed due to the lightweight factor associated with our proposed obstacle avoidance algorithm.

We compare the performance of our robot with other existing obstacle avoidance robots in Table 1 in terms of five parameters. To move faster and avoid the upcoming obstacles toward the robot effectively, we use Raspberry Pi unit as our main processing unit. In addition, our proposed obstacle avoidance algorithm analyze the surroundings of the robot in terms of MKC-360 unit more efficiently than the previous proposed frameworks. Our obstacle avoidance algorithm is capable to identify the distance of the obstacle and thereby process further to take the decision of movement based on the intensity values (i.e., higher the intensity level, higher the probability of collision).

Notation: DS—distance sensor, MC—micro-controller, CDP—current and destination position, SSP—Sonar sensor processor, OD—obstacle distance, AD—angle and distance, C—camera, SS—sonar sensor, P—processor, BB—Beagle board, OP—obstacle position, ULS—Ultrasonic sensor, COVS—camera optical velocity sensor, LSS—laser and Sonar sensor, MP—microprocessor, PIE—prior information of environment, MKC—Microsoft Kinect camera, R-pi—Raspberry Pi, DM—driver motor.

5 Conclusion and Future Works

Our primary target was to develop a lightweight obstacle avoidance robot that would pave the way for blind people. Therefore, we have focused on the lightweight factor of the designing purpose because large and heavy robot faces problems while moving in a narrow space. We have contributed to letting the system function within real environments. This proposed framework largely relies on the Microsoft Kinect camera to sense the environment accurately and to analyze the captured images with its obstacle avoidance algorithm. By using Raspberry Pi as well as Microsoft Kinect together, we have improved the overall system performance. Our proposed system is cost-friendly for everyone and, hopefully, it will help the blind people of our society by reducing the complexity of the navigation problem for visually impaired people. In the future, we want to integrate our robot with a smart cane so that the task of sensing the surroundings becomes more reliable so that it can improve the user-friendly experience level for the blind.

References

1. Baras N, Nantzios G, Ziouzios D, Dasygenis M (2019) Autonomous obstacle avoidance vehicle using lidar and an embedded system. In: 2019 8th International conference on modern circuits and systems technologies (MOCAST). IEEE, pp 1–4
2. Run RS, Xiao ZY (2018) Indoor autonomous vehicle navigation—A feasibility study based on infrared technology. Appl Syst Innov 1(1):4
3. Takizawa H, Yamaguchi S, Aoyagi M, Ezaki N, Mizuno S (2013) Kinect cane: Object recognition aids for the visually impaired. In: 2013 6th International conference on human system interactions (HSI). IEEE, pp 473–478
4. Khan A, Moideen F, Lopez J, Khoo WL, Zhu Z (2012) KinDectect: kinect detecting objects. In: International conference on computers for handicapped persons. Springer, Berlin, Heidelberg, pp 588–595
5. Filipe V, Fernandes F, Fernandes H, Sousa A, Paredes H, Barroso J (2012) Blind navigation support system based on Microsoft Kinect. Procedia Comput Sci 14:94–101
6. Creo LMV, Dacanay GM. Jarque LCP, Umali, CJP, Tolentino ERE (2021) Controlling the bomb disposal robot using Microsoft Kinect sensor. In: 2021 International conference on communication, control and information sciences (ICCISc), vol 1. IEEE, pp 1-6
7. Ganz A, Gandhi SR, Schafer J, Singh T, Puleo E, Mullett G, Wilson C (2011) PERCEPT: indoor navigation for the blind and visually impaired. In: 2011 Annual international conference of the IEEE engineering in medicine and biology society. IEEE, pp 856–859

8. Budiharto W (2015) Intelligent surveillance robot with obstacle avoidance capabilities using neural network. Comput Intell Neurosci
9. Naveen V. Aasish C, Kavya M, Vidhyalakshmi M, Sailaja K (2021) Autonomous obstacle avoidance robot using regression. In: Proceedings of international conference on computational intelligence and data engineering. Springer, Singapore, pp 1–13
10. Prasad A, Sharma B, Vanualailai J, Kumar SA (2020) A geometric approach to target convergence and obstacle avoidance of a nonstandard tractor–trailer robot. Int J Robust Nonlinear Control 30(13):4924–4943
11. Peng Y, Qu D, Zhong Y, Xie S, Luo J, Gu J (2015) The obstacle detection and obstacle avoidance algorithm based on 2-d lidar. In: 2015 IEEE international conference on information and automation. IEEE, pp 1648–1653
12. Deac MA, Al-doori RWY, Negru M, Dănescu R (2018) Miniature autonomous vehicle development on raspberry pi. In: 2018 IEEE 14th international conference on intelligent computer communication and processing (ICCP). IEEE, pp 229–236
13. Sunehra D, Jhansi B, Sneha R (2021) Smart robotic personal assistant vehicle using raspberry pi and zero UI technology. In: 2021 6th International conference for convergence in technology (I2CT). IEEE, pp 1–6
14. Sezer V, Gokasan M (2012) A novel obstacle avoidance algorithm: "Follow the Gap Method". Robot Auton Syst 60(9):1123–1134
15. Xie Y, Zhang X, Meng W, Zheng S, Jiang L, Meng J, Wang S (2021) Coupled fractional-order sliding mode control and obstacle avoidance of a four-wheeled steerable mobile robot. ISA Trans 108:282–294
16. Zhang W, Cheng H, Hao L, Li X, Liu M, Gao X (2021) An obstacle avoidance algorithm for robot manipulators based on decision-making force. Robot Comput-Integr Manuf 71:102114
17. Oroko J, Ikua B (2012) Obstacle avoidance and path planning schemes for autonomous navigation of a mobile robot: a review. In: Sustainable research and innovation proceedings, vol 4
18. Zhu Y, Zhang T, Song J, Li X (2012) A new hybrid navigation algorithm for mobile robots in environments with incomplete knowledge. Knowl-Based Syst 27:302–313
19. Kumari CL (2012) Building algorithm for obstacle detection and avoidance system for wheeled mobile robot. Glob J Res Eng
20. Tian S, Li Y, Kang Y, Xia J (2021) Multi-robot path planning in wireless sensor networks based on jump mechanism PSO and safety gap obstacle avoidance. Future Gener Comput Syst 118:37–47
21. Yufka A, Parlaktuna O (2009) Performance comparison of bug algorithms for mobile robots. In: Proceedings of the 5th international advanced technologies symposium, Karabuk, Turkey, pp 13–15
22. Li G, Yamashita A, Asama H, Tamura Y (2012). An efficient improved artificial potential field based regression search method for robot path planning. In: 2012 IEEE international conference on mechatronics and automation. IEEE, pp 1227–1232
23. Chen KH, Tsai WH (2000) Vision-based obstacle detection and avoidance for autonomous land vehicle navigation in outdoor roads. Autom Constr 10(1):1–25

Surface Electromyogram (S-EMG) Spectrogram Analysis of Human Arm Activity Towards Interpretability and Classification

Pritam Chakraborty, Biswarup Neogi, and Achintya Das

Abstract Spectrogram analysis of Surface Electromyogram (S-EMG) signal towards interpretability and classification of active/inactive muscle during common arm movement activity has been studied in this article. EMG signals from four common muscles (i.e. Biceps, Deltoids, Flexion and Triceps) from the different movements have been recorded, and corresponding raw S-EMG signals have been processed using signal processing techniques. A detailed observation has been sketched with the probable application for the diagnosis of neurodegenerative diseases and rehabilitation research.

Keywords Surface-electromyogram (S-EMG) · Envelop detection · Spectrogram analysis · Interpretation of muscle activity · Muscle classification

1 Introduction

Spectrogram analysis of surface S-EMG signal paves one of the efficient way of understanding muscle association during many human daily life activity [1]. An EMG signal recorded during locomotive action is a rundown of potentials from the muscle fibers due to the generation of an electromagnetic space around the active muscle, thus detection, dissention and study of S-EMG signal gives an overall proficiency of active and inactive muscle fibers results toward early diagnosis of neuro-degenerative diseases and also beneficial for physiotherapists providing assistants for the rehabilitation [2]. Attempts to put on quantitative information from EMG recording extensively investigated representing the signal as a function of frequency. The spectral

P. Chakraborty (✉)
St. Mary Technical Campus Kolkata, Kolkata, West Bengal 700126, India

B. Neogi
JIS College of Engineering, Kalyani, West Bengal 741235, India

A. Das
Kalyani Government Engineering College, Kalyani, West Bengal 741235, India

M. S. Kaiser et al. (eds.), *Proceedings of Trends in Electronics and Health Informatics*, Lecture Notes in Networks and Systems 376,
https://doi.org/10.1007/978-981-16-8826-3_25

mechanism of the S-EMG signal are compacted toward the lower frequency component throughout a sustained muscle contraction and classification of this normalized phenomenon has been studied toward applicability of EMG signal for diagnostic purposes [3]. The EMG signal offers useful information that can help to understand the human locomotion but raw EMG signal provided information in inherent form incorporated with noise. Thus the recorded EMG signal traverse through Envelop detector, takes the high frequency signal as input and provides an output which is the envelop of the original signal, filtering is being performed to smooth the original output. The statistical analysis and pattern classification of Electromyography signal from biceps and triceps of a paralysis person generated using discrete lower arm movement, contributes the controlling of prosthetic arm with minimal mental effort [3]. The biological data mining for deep learning was shown in [4], with a thorough application perspective using machine learning. Knowledge based data base using Surface EMG toward characterization of muscle activity using digital signal processing module is shown in [5].

In this present literature, we are considering arm action during daily activity and corresponding muscle responses have been studied. The movements are operated in presence of load i.e. using wright training fitness dumbbell of 2 kg and 4 kg, to observe the response or more specifically fluctuations of potentials inside muscle neurons. Influence of weight and drive of specific muscle (i.e. Flexor, Biceps, Triceps and Deltoid) during arm action i.e. Elbow Flexion, Extension of Fore arm and Shoulder Abduction, will be analyzed. During recording of the EMG signal under the study potential divisions and amplitude measure over weight training time period was kept constant for achieving accurate response pointer for each muscle response [3].

2 Methodology

2.1 *Participant*

An assemblage of ten students from the department ECE of JIS College of Engineering, Kalyani, West Bengal including five male and five female candidates within age of 20–22 years, average weight of 70 ± 5 kg (male) and 50 ± 5 kg (female) enthusiastically took part in this commotion under the direction of Dr. Biswarup Neogi, Associate Professor, HOD, Department of ECE, JIS College of Engineering. All participated candidates have been chosen on a prior condition that they were free from any muscular-skeletal injury in their medical history.

2.2 EMG Signal Data Acquisition

Non-invasive gelled surface electrodes with recording area of 37.55 mm^2, attached with 24″ colored cable ideally suited for Acoustic Entreated Potential (AEP) and Nerve Conduction Training (NCP) positioned in couples above the skin surface analogous to the muscle fibers i.e. Flexor, Biceps, Triceps and Deltoid, under observation during specific movement analysis using EMG Electrode Conductive gel ® which acts as an interface between skin surface and electrodes with an electrode gap of 200 mm. These electrodes are then connected to RMS EMG EpMK2 recorder. Assuming motor control evenness of the both body sides we are using participants right dominant sites for our analysis [5].

2.3 Noise Elimination

An un-cleaned raw surface EMG signal sensing Motor Unit Action Potential (MUAPs) contains unescapable noise [6]. The noise in EMG can originate from numerous bases i.e. intrinsic noise in the electronics apparatus, ambient noise from electromagnetic emission, active motion, integral uncertainty of the EMG signal and Cross talk due to undesired EMG signal from neighboring un-measured muscle tendons [7].

2.3.1 Motion Artifacts

Motion artifacts originate due to electrode arrangements on skin surface and electrode wires. Noise created due to motion variants in Surface EMG signal ranges within 0–20 Hz do provide significant information on activation rate of specified motor unit, however, information content in signal in this range is not of interest, in case of body vibration analysis artifact noise is unavoidable [8]. In circumstances, where this conditions are neglected are processed out using high pass filter [9].

2.4 Processing of S-EMG Signal

Raw EMG signal provides useful information when it is quantified. S-EMG signals are the amalgamation of several motor unit events, thus it requires decomposition of the signal to reveal important information affecting to muscle stimulation and motor unit shooting. Disintegration of S-EMG signal are done using wavelet spectrum matching and finding out the principle constituents of the wavelet coefficients. During a robust muscle contraction, additional motor unit potential will fire up at equal time overlapping [10].

Once, interference induced in the S-EMG signal by the lower frequency components or because of high frequency noise, spectrum matching technique is at times reflected to be much operative than its wavelet equivalent [11].

3 Experiment

Muscle activation for different arm movements are outlined in this section. The S-EMG signal of particular muscle is recorded on the basis of relation to human arm movement and position of the surface electrode placed above the skin is done in accordance with the result of a European research project SENIAM protocol [12].

For the present study we are considering, three basic movements from our daily life i.e. Extension of Fore arm, Elbow Flexion, Shoulder Abduction. First, extension of forearm movement gives us the idea about straightening movement of arm i.e. forearm is extended from fold position to straight position as shown in Fig. 1a. In this situation there is an increase in angle between ventral surfaces. Second, the flexion of elbow joint is just opposite to the extension of forearm and angle decreases between ventral surface and increases between dorsal surface Fig. 1b. Third, in abduction movement the arm moves away from the mid line or center of the body and are parallel to length of torso furthermore, raised in the tors Fig. 1c a right angle is created between midline of the body and arm, further it rotates and make a right angle with the previous position. Figure 1d, shows anatomical plane of human body along which the movement has been considered and blue and green dot marker point representing the position of the Surface EMG electrode. Figure 1e, presents the lab overview of data acquisition of S-EMG signal at JIS College of Engineering, Department of ECE, Kalyani, West Bengal-741235, using RMS EMG EpMK2 recorder.

3.1 *Envelop Detection and Analysis of S-EMG Signal*

Muscle activity recognition is achieved by looking into amplitude inception of the EMG envelop. Excluding physical examination of raw S-EMG data, most usual practice is the digitization and discretization of the signal. The S-EMG signal envelop (i.e. the refined signal is attained using low pass filtering of the full wave rectified signal) is used as it permits modest understanding and comparatively informal muscle inception and interruption detection is done using threshold or more detailed curve shape analysis [13].

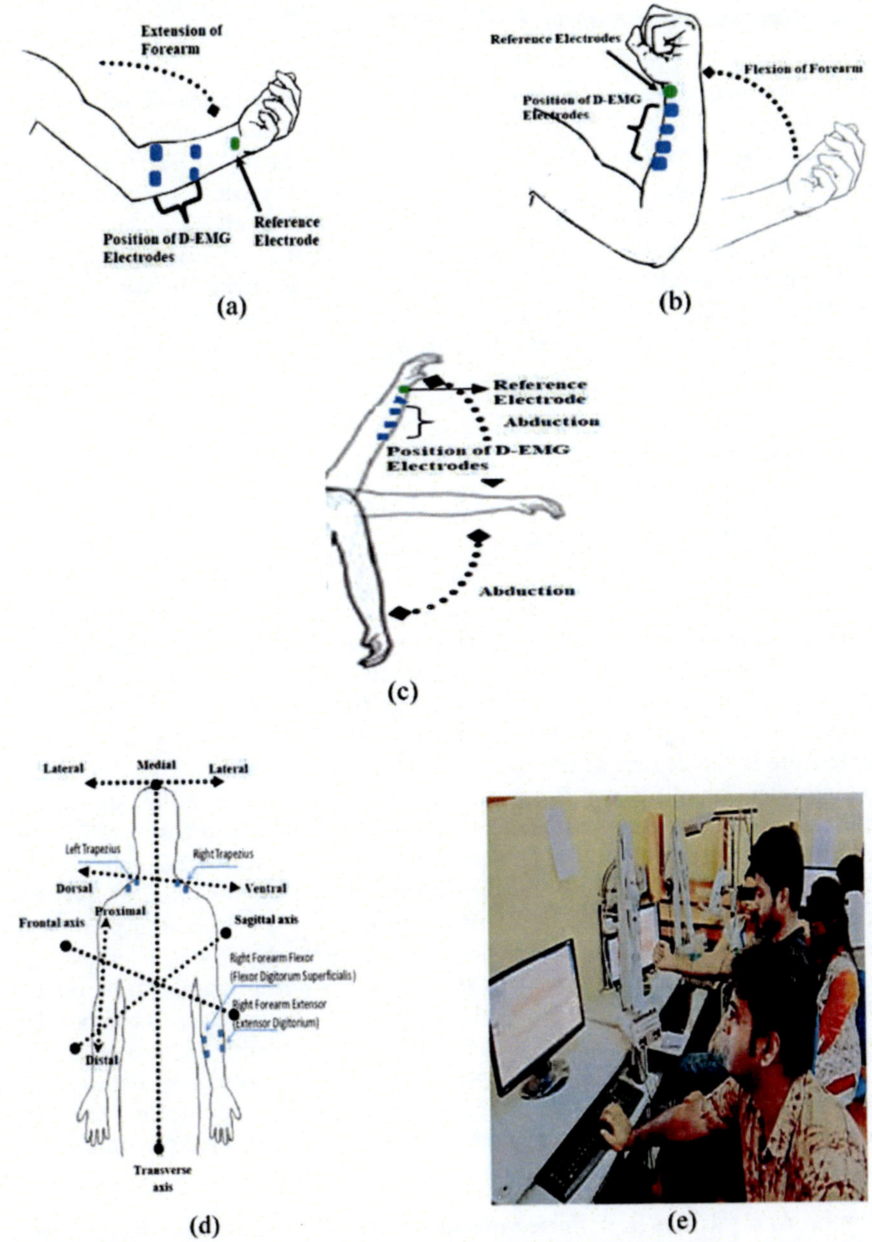

Fig. 1 **a** Extension of forearm, **b** flexion of forearm, **c** abduction movement, **d** anatomical plane of upper human body and **e** the lab overview of data acquisition of S-EMG signal using RMS EMG EpMK2 recorder

3.2 *Spectrogram Analysis of S-EMG Signal*

Spectrogram analysis can be viewed as a visual representation of spectrum of frequencies, and is inspired by the limitation of Fast-Fourier transform to gratify non-stationary signal spectral characteristic in time domain [14]. The frequency of a particular frequency component is represented in color band. The observations for each movement is recorded for 3 s, while the actual reflection for the active movement range is considered 0–1.4 s. The rest part of the signal is considered as noise incurred while synchronization of the two EMG recorders. Comparison of the recorded S-EMG signal within equal time intervals and the incremental response due to incorporation of movement have been taken into consideration [15–18].

4 Result and Discussion

4.1 *Extension of Forearm*

During the extension of forearm, muscle that run along the frontal part of the forearm after the elbow to hand. The impact on the Bicep muscle due to the movement tends to increase, this can be visualized by looking into the spectrogram, Fig. 2a. A specific mucle response can be seen at the initial movement phase with maximum peak amplitude of 140 μV and as the time progress when we are coming back to relax state there is the decline in response, which can be viewed as a justification that during extension of forearm Bicep muscle comes into picture. In Fig. 2b, Deltoid muscle activation or the impact of deltoid muscle is minimal in extension of forearm with peak amplitude 60 μV and spectrogram of the muscle signal validates the observation. Figure 2c, Flexor muscle activates during the extension of fore arm and we can clearly visualize in the spectrogram there is a blue spectrum which denotes that during relaxation phase flexor muscle is coming to rest as fast as it got activated. Figure 2d, Tricep muscle is showing a prominent response to movement with maximum amplitude approximately 250 μV but as the movement is approaching near saturation the muscle action potential is declining bringing the muscle at rest.

From the observations of Fig. 2(a)–(d), we can infer that during Extension of forearm Bicep and tricep muscle is active where as deltoid and flexor muscle are minimally active. Such characterization plays a crucial role toward classification of active and minimally active muscle during specific movement.

Similar Analysis Has Been Performed for Elbow Flexion and shoulder abduction movement leading toward observed muscle activation. We found some attention-grabbing observation, when we increase the load amplitude of activating muscle is increasing, leading and relation time of the muscle also increases.

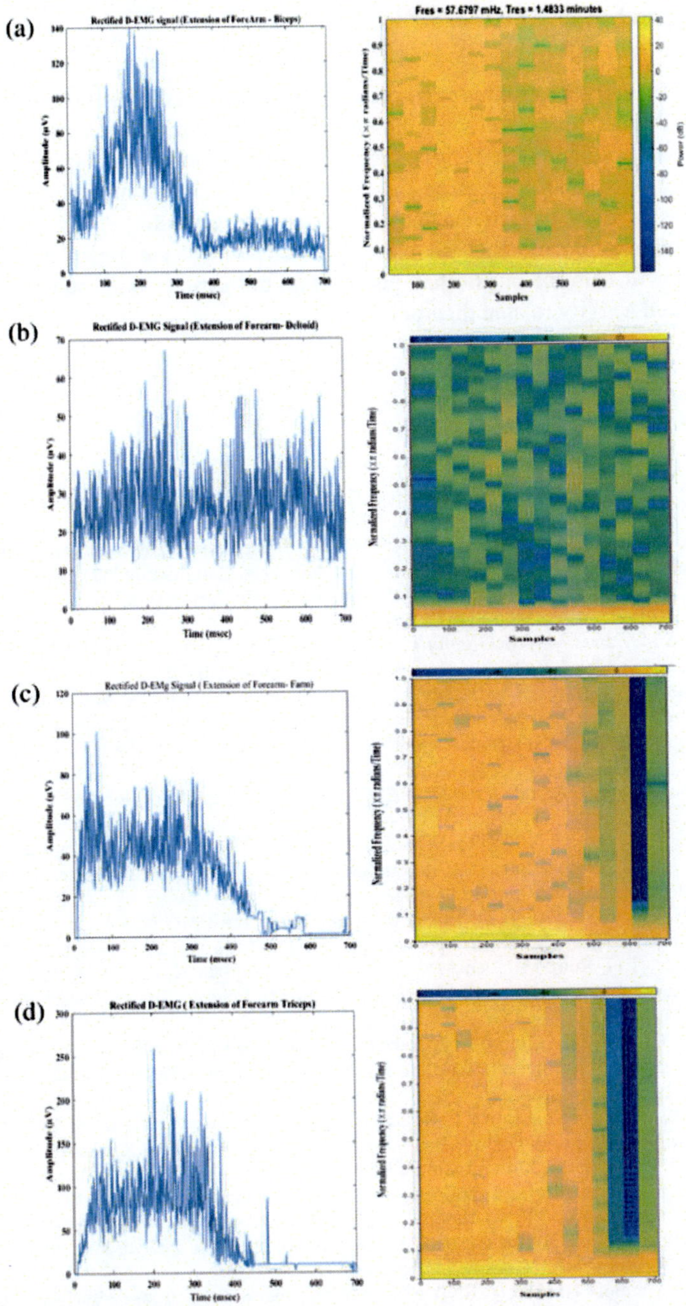

Fig. 2 **a** Rectified S-EMG signal for Biceps and corresponding spectrogram, **b** S-EMG signal and spectrogram for deltoid muscle; **c** S-EMG signal and spectrogram for fore arm, and **d** S-EMG signal and spectrogram for triceps, during extension of forearm movement using 2 kg load

5 Conclusion

In this article, envelop amplitude and spectrogram analysis of Diagnostic-EMG signal has been studied, peak envelop of the signal detected during the signal processing showed muscle activation during activity and muscle relaxation can be concluded from the minimal amplitude value and corresponding spectrogram plot justifies the result. Thus, inactive and active muscle classification can be done using this approach and principle component analysis based classification of the muscle with specific movement will help the physiotherapist to treat the patients with neuro-generative disorders and activity related disorder.

References

1. Basmajian JV, de Luca CJ (1985) Muscles alive: their functions revealed by electromyography. Williams & Wilkins, Baltimore ©1985
2. Kleissen RF, Buurke JH, Harlaar J, Zilvold G (1998) Electromyography in the biomechanical analysis of human movement and its clinical application. Gait Posture 8(2):143–158
3. Hamilton-Wright A, Stashuk DW (2005) Physiologically based simulation of clinical EMG signals. IEEE Trans Biomed Eng 52(2):171–183
4. Mahmud M, Kaiser MS, McGinnity TM et al (2021) Deep learning in mining biological data. Cogn Comput 13:1–33. https://doi.org/10.1007/s12559-020-09773-x
5. Chakraborty P, Neogi B, Das A, Jin Z (Reviewing editor) (2020) Knowledge based database of arm-muscle and activity characterization during load pull exercise using diagnostic electromyography (D-EMG) signal. Cogent Eng 7:1. https://doi.org/10.1080/23311916.2020.1849942
6. Duchene J, Hogrel J (2000) A model of EMG generation. IEEE Trans Biomed Eng 47(2):192–201
7. Karlsson S, Nystrom L (1995) Real-time system for EMG signal analysis of static and dynamic contractions. In: Proceedings of 17th international conference of the engineering in medicine and biology society, vol 2, pp 1347–1348
8. Kale SN, Dudul SV (2009) Intelligent noise removal from EMG signal using focused time-lagged recurrent neural network. Appl Comput Intell Soft Comput 2009(Article ID 129761):12
9. Chowdhury RH, Reaz MB, Ali MA, Bakar AA, Chellappan K, Chang TG (2013) Surface electromyography signal processing and classification techniques. Sensors (Basel, Switzerland) 13(9):12431–12466
10. De Luca CJ, Donald Gilmore L, Kuznetsov M, Roy SH (2010) Filtering the surface EMG signal: movement artifact and baseline noise contamination. J Biomech 43(8): 1573–1579. ISSN 0021-9290
11. Fratini A, Cesarelli M, Bifulco P, Romano M (2009) Relevance of motion artifact in electromyography recordings during vibration treatment. J Electromyogr Kinesiol 19(4):710–718
12. Raez MB, Hussain MS, Mohd-Yasin F (2006) Techniques of EMG signal analysis: detection, processing, classification and applications. Biological Procedures Online 8:11–35
13. Go SA, Coleman-Wood K, Kaufman KR (2014) Frequency analysis of lower extremity electromyography signals for the quantitative diagnosis of dystonia. J Electromyogr Kinesiol: Off J Int Soc Electrophysiol Kinesiol 24(1):31–36
14. Freriks B, Hermens HJ (1999) SENIUM 9: European recommendations for surface electromyography, results of the SENIAM project. Roessingh Research and Development b.v.
15. Márquez-Figueroa S, Shmaliy YS, Ibarra-Manzano O (2020) Optimal extraction of EMG signal envelope and artifacts removal assuming colored measurement noise Biomed Signal Process Control 57:101679, ISSN 1746-8094

16. Zawawi TNST, Abdullah AR, Shair EF, Halim I, Rawaida O (2013) Electromyography signal analysis using spectrogram. In: 2013 IEEE student conference on research and development, pp 319–324
17. Too J, Abdullah AR, Saad NM et al (2019) Exploring the relation between EMG pattern recognition and sampling rate using spectrogram. J. Electr. Eng. Technol. 14:947–953
18. Joshi D, Nakamura BH, Hahn ME (2015) High energy spectrogram with integrated prior knowledge for EMG-based locomotion classification. Med Eng Phys 37(5):518–24

An Atypical Approach Toward PTSD Diagnosis Through Speech-Based Emotion Modeling Using CNN-LSTM

M. Josephine Mary Juliana, Gnanou Florence Sudha, and R. Nakkeeran

Abstract Post-Traumatic Stress Disorder (PTSD) remains a stigma in today' society as it is a portrayal of an individual who refrains from exiting an ended trauma. This research approaches PTSD from an emotion recognition viewpoint with the aid of Deep Learning Algorithms. PTSD diagnosis is usually done by a psychiatrist by means of administering an assessment tool in the form of a questionnaire. However, scores based on questions are not accurate and in addition disturb the patients making them unsettled and perturbed. Speech signals are a form of non-stationary signals, which is a universally preferred biomarker in emotion recognition. For this research, emotional speech is taken from the RAVDESS database and Mel spectrogram features are extracted and classified using the Convolutional Neural Network with Long Short-Term Memory deep learning algorithm. Consecutively emotions falling under both high and low arousal category are chosen and marked as PTSD cases and the other emotions are taken as controls. The performance parameters of the CNN LSTM classifier are computed on a per emotion basis. Results demonstrate that, superior performance with average classification accuracy of 98.68% for PTSD diagnosis is achieved outperforming existing counterparts.

Keywords Post-traumatic stress disorder · Trauma · Speech emotion recognition · MFCC and Mel spectrogram

1 Introduction

Trauma is the representation of the violation of all that a person holds to be either dear or sacred. Traumatic events are usually so terrible that they could not be uttered aloud as well are unspeakable. There may also be cases where the survivor of the trauma

---

M. Josephine Mary Juliana (✉) · G. F. Sudha
Puducherry Technological University, Puducherry, India
e-mail: julianabenno27@pec.edu

R. Nakkeeran
Pondicherry University, Puducherry, India

M. S. Kaiser et al. (eds.), *Proceedings of Trends in Electronics and Health Informatics*, Lecture Notes in Networks and Systems 376,
https://doi.org/10.1007/978-981-16-8826-3_26

sometimes may wish to speak, however the community is unwilling and unable to bear witness to their trauma thus pushing the survivor to silence. A lingering trauma is commonly referred to as Post-Traumatic Stress Disorder (PTSD). PTSD is as severe as any other Psychiatric disorder as the traumatic thoughts and those memories start to impede the brain's natural process of recovery from the traumatic incident. These become stuck points in the brain inhibiting the mental reintegration that may be needed for the healing to occur. PTSD characterizes isolation from the society in the foreground and hence PTSD diagnosis is conventionally done via administration of questionnaires. However, this is an improper approach as it would be causative in pushing the individuals back to the traumatic thoughts.

A biomarker is a biological feature that could be used to diagnose the presence of any disease or disorder. The identification of an effective biomarker is vital for any research as its tailoring would make it a signature for diagnosis. Speech is an excellent non-invasive biomarker for Emotion Recognition and Psychiatric Disorder Diagnosis. Psycho-Emotional state assessment can be performed by analysis of speech signals as it is the most adept and promising form of real-time analysis. Definite psychogenic state patterns can be diagnosed from speech characteristics by processing this non-stationary signal to detect the embedded emotions. Disturbed communication is said to be a hallmark for several mental illnesses as these could be diagnosed through the linguistic and acoustic analytic techniques that objectify communication. Although Speech Processing could greatly aid assessment of mental health issues, they have least been employed on account of their prominent obstacle namely the need for comprehensive and transdiagnostic studies [1].

Speech Emotion Recognition (SER) systems are automated computerized methods having large clinical relevance which is demonstrated via the in-vivo link it establishes with the classic 'language regions' of the brain. While it comes to the linguistic analysis, the relation it establishes with the candidate genes can identify several psychiatric disorders. In general, there are two approaches toward SER, namely the linguistic approach and the non- linguistic one. The former deals with the textual part while the latter addresses the non-verbal content [2]. Thus, the difference between reading one's voice with respect to listening to one's words is of paramount importance when it comes to speech-based Emotion Recognition in general and psychiatric disorder diagnosis in particular as these non-verbal speech sounds provide subtle yet powerful clues to what the speaker means.

The major challenges encountered by SER systems are as follows: The emotional states do not have clear cut boundaries and therefore its expression too varies from person to person. Secondly the speaking styles and rates of speakers vary with individuals and also with places, as native speakers may have different accents than others. Therefore, selecting speech features that do not have the impact of speaking style, region or culture is of utmost importance. For extraction of such features, speech signals are converted from time domain to frequency domain. Following this, selection of relevant features is carried out and importantly a suitable classifier model is applied so as to recognize the emotions.

This paper discusses an entirely different approach of PTSD diagnosis through Speech-based emotion recognition. The speech samples used in the study are those from a database consolidating sets of enacted emotional speech and the proposed model shows superior performance in diagnosing PTSD.

The paper is organized in the following manner: Sect. 2 delineates the existing work related to the work presented in this paper. Section 3 briefs the details of the Proposed work, giving the details about the emotional speech database used, tool description, extraction of speech features for Speech Emotion Recognition, and details of the classifier algorithm that offered superior performance. Section 4 presents in detail the results obtained from the proposed model and other classifiers that were used for comparison. Finally, the paper is concluded explaining the reasons for the better performance of the CNN-LSTM classifier model with Mel spectrogram features.

2 Related Work

Miao et al. [3] enumerate the guidelines facilitating the diagnosis of PTSD, also listing down the treatment procedures ranging from psychological intervention to pharmacological treatments. According to the author, diagnostic procedure involves identification of clusters of symptoms following an event of exposure to extreme stressors. Knowledge on probable symptoms greatly supports diagnosis as discussed in Shalev and Douglas Bremner [4] where the author identifies the prescribed symptoms such as avoidance of any form of reminder to the traumatic event, sleeplessness, frequent feeling of reliving the trauma along with listing the neurological and biological changes caused by PTSD and the treatment to the disorder in the form of pharmacological therapy and psychotherapy are covered in David Kinzie [5].

Bryant [6] reviews the PTSD as described by the Diagnostics & Statistics Manual (DSM) as well as by the International Classification of Diseases (ICD). The paper briefs the risk factors associated with the disorder and the effective treatment for the same. The DSM-5, the latest edition published by The American Psychiatric Association (APA) categorizes PTSD under Trauma & Stressor related disorders. This disorder characterizes a person with the failure to recover from the traumatic event, who relives and re-experiences the terrific event, symptomatically experiencing nightmares, flashbacks and avoids even at the slightest reminder that could virtually bring back the trauma. Thus, an affected individual personifies a heightened reactivity to stimuli and therefore always remains anxious and depressed.

Victoria and Diane [7] investigated the conflicting effects of Angry and Fearful facial expressions in PTSD. According to the author PTSD can be manifested as a hyper vigilance for threat in the form of threatening stimuli. In this work the participants were made to view blocks of face stimuli in a pseudo randomized order and their responses are recorded by administering the Combat Exposure Scale (CES) and the Aggression Questionnaire (AQ). Barbano et al. [8] differentiated PTSD from anxiety and depression through data collected using the clinician administered PTSD scale for DSM IV applying the diagnostic rule of ICD-10 and ICD-11. They also addressed the co-occurring disorders by means the Structural Clinical Interview for DSM IV also measuring the depression severity by administering the Beck Depression Inventory.

In Shalev et al. [9], the responses to the CAPS Questionnaire were analyzed for assessing the existence/risk of onset of PTSD in recent trauma survivors. The Mann–Whitney tests and χ^2 tests were used for continuous risk predictions and categorical risk predictions respectively. The logistic regression model was obtained and the area under the receiver operating characteristic curve (AUC) was computed to assess the model's performance. While in Worthington et al. [10] the prospective prediction of onset of PTSD was performed from data collected through personal interviews, the statistical analyses were performed in R, with the feature selection being conducted using a Gradient Boosting Machine (GBM) algorithm. Three classifier techniques were employed namely, the classification trees, penalized logistic regression and Bayesian Additive Regression Trees (BART) all offered an accuracy around 92.03%.

Ben-Zion et al. [11] conducted an exhaustive study on multi-domain potential biomarkers for PTSD severity detection in recent trauma survivors. The study concludes that the biomarkers taken from the structural MRI and the functional MRI describing the cingulate cortices' volumes, the amygdala's functional connectivity with the insula and thalamus and other neural and cognitive potential biomarkers differentiated the clusters associated with PTSD.

Zhang et al. [12] worked on the structural and resting-state functional MRI (rs-fMRI) scans, which were taken as the input and the gray matter volume (GMV), amplitude of low-frequency fluctuations (ALFF), and regional homogeneity were extracted as classification features, the extracted features were combined by a multi-kernel combination strategy and fed to a support vector machine (SVM) classifier which was trained to distinguish the subjects at individual level. The performance of the classifier was evaluated using the leave-one-out cross-validation (LOOCV) method and it offered accuracies of 89.19%.

In Etkin et al. [13], the fMRI connectivity was analyzed to reveal a form of treatment resistant PTSD. Statistical analyses were performed on the collected data using IBM's SPSS software. Generalized linear mixed models, except for the treatment outcome prediction analyses were deployed. All tests and post hoc analyses were corrected for multiple comparisons using two-sided tests.

Zandvakili et al. [14] computed the Principal Component Analysis and least-angle regression (LARS) which were used to identify relationships between PTSD's symptoms severity and brain networks and found that brain network connectivity predicted PTSD symptom profiles. The goodness of fit for total PTSD Check List PCL-5 and that for intrusion, cognition and reactivity symptoms were computed. The findings demonstrated links between PTSD symptoms and the neural network connectivity patterns.

Cheng et al. [15] detailed on the approach of affective recognition toward Major Depressive Disorder. Affective computing [16] or Affect recognition could be called as a comprehensive process that incorporates various aspects including the mechanism of emotion, acquisition of the emotional information, recognition of the emotional pattern, modeling and understanding the emotions followed by its synthesis and expression.

Grazianno [17] studied and established the link between PTSD and steroidogenesis diagnosis. The endocannabinoid target PPAR-α is one among many neuronal targets discovered recently to enhance steroidogenesis. A bio-signature for stress-induced disorder detection here is the crosstalk between the endocannabinoid system and the biosynthesis of neurosteroids. This acts as a pivotal complement to the current practice of assessing the disorder that may either based on self-reported symptoms or psychiatrist assessments.

A review on the Deep Learning algorithms used in research is explained in Durstewitz et al. [18], facilitating Psychiatric Disorder Diagnosis utilizing clinician provided labels for defining an upper bound on the system's performance.

Chen et al. [19] discusses about the popular 'Ekman's six emotion model comprising of seven emotions namely, Fear, Joy, Sadness, Contempt, Disgust and Surprise from which evolved the six emotion model which is now adapted by Researchers in this domain. In this, 'contempt' emotion was dropped, and among these, four basic emotions, namely, Fear, Anger, Joy and Sadness are categorized as outcomes of three core affects namely Reward, Punishment and Stress. In this, the first two are a result of stress while the next comes with reward and the last with punishment. Here the universal emotions are Anger, Joy, Sadness and Neutral [20].

Low et al. [21] reviewed the techniques that perform automated assessment of psychiatric disorders through speech. This review puts forth evidence of research that have focused on employment of acoustic features of speech to detect depression and schizophrenia. For emotion recognition through speech, the process of formulation of speech is paramount, so also the nuances about different emotions.

Lado-Codesido et al. [22] conducted a multi-center clinical trial on patients with Schizophrenia and Schizoaffective disorder as an attempt to study the efficacy of vocal emotion recognition in aiding the diagnosis of the disorder. Statistical analysis was performed using SPSS and ANOVA computation was made.

In Issa et al. [23] The Ryerson Audio Visual Database for Speech and Song (RAVDESS) and couple of other databases were used to perform Speech Emotion Recognition and a classification accuracy of 71.61% was achieved on Deep Convolutional Neural Network (CNN) classifier. Although accuracies vary from one database to another, this is the highest recorded regarding RAVDESS.

Speech samples, obtained from warzone-exposed veterans were taken so as to perform PTSD diagnosis. This was achieved by recording the audio responses to the CAPS Questionnaire and were fed to the Random Forest classifier post feature extraction. The receiver operating characteristic curve had an area under the curve (AUC) of 0.954 showed an overall correct classification rate as 89.1% in Marmar et al. [24].

Thus, from the exhaustive study of the existing research works, it is inferred that among the several biomarkers for PTSD diagnosis, the most non-intrusive one is from vocal emotions. Secondly, existing PTSD diagnosis from speech samples and Deep Learning algorithms have not established high accuracy in classification and diagnosis. This paves the way for developing a new model for detection of PTSD from speech with better accuracy. Therefore, in this paper, an innovative methodology for PTSD detection through Speech Emotion Recognition is proposed which exploits the efficacy of Artificial Intelligence by incorporating the Convolutional Neural Network with Long Short-Term Memory (CNN-LSTM).

3 Proposed Work

In this section, the stages of PTSD diagnosis adopted in this work, along with the database and tool used are described. Figure 1 is functional and is descriptive of the workflow adopted in this research from the input speech signal taken from the database to the classification of emotions as PTSD disorders or normal controls.

3.1 Database Used

The major barrier in incorporating AI into Psychiatric Disorder Diagnosis is that for a DL Algorithm, to offer excelling performance they need databases with huge number of samples, but when the sample size becomes small, it poses a severe challenge toward finding solutions that could generalize to the population very well. Huge sample sizes are always an oasis when it comes to Psychiatric diagnosis [25]. For this research work, the Ryerson Audio-Visual Database for Emotional Speech and Song (RAVDESS) was utilized. The RAVDESS, as proposed by Livingstone and Russo (2018) is a voluminous database holding close to 7356 files occupying 24.8 GB. Databases are generally categorized based on the type of emotional speech samples they carry namely natural, enacted and elicited [26], here the RAVDESS contains enacted emotional audio datasets vocalized by 24 professional actors comprising of a group of 12 male and 12 female actors, found to utter 2 lexically matched statements in a neutral North American accent. This archive incorporates expressions of seven emotions namely calm, happy, sad, angry, fearful, surprise and disgust, each of which is produced at 2 distinct levels of emotional intensity namely 'normal' and

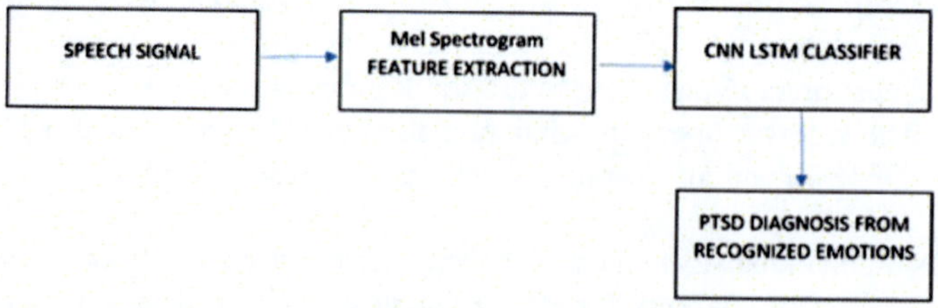

Fig. 1 Block diagram of methodology adopted for PTSD diagnosis

'strong' with an additional neutral expression. This is available in 3 modality formats: video-only, audio-only, audio–video.

For this research the second format is employed as it is a Speech Emotion Recognition analysis. The audio- only files of RAVDESS also have 2 sub classes, the speech file and the song file. For this work the data in speech format is chosen. Each RAVDESS file has a unique file name carrying a 7 parts numerical identifier defining the stimulus characteristics. The statements which vocalize the emotion are 'Dogs are sitting by the door' and 'kids are talking by the door'. Figure 2 shows the wave plots corresponding to different emotional speech samples.

The bar charts representing the ratios of the number of speech samples used in this work with respect to the emotions, gender and intensity from the RAVDESS dataset are shown in Fig. 3a–c.

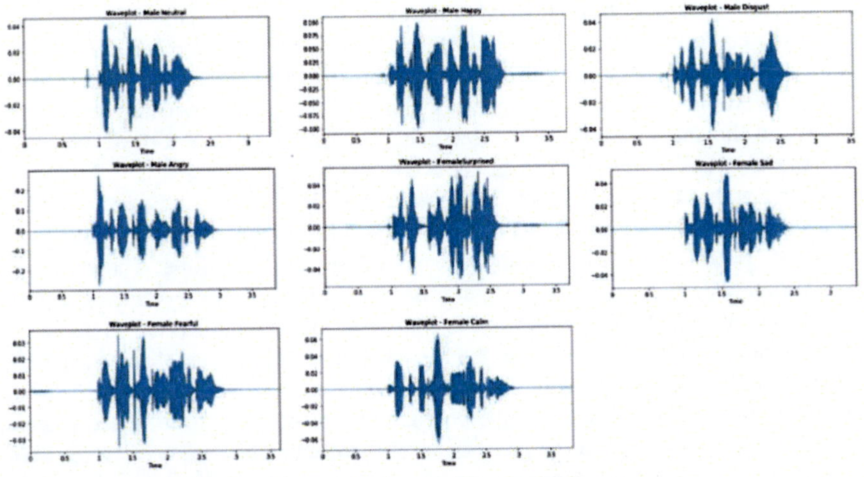

Fig. 2 Wave plots corresponding to different emotional speech samples

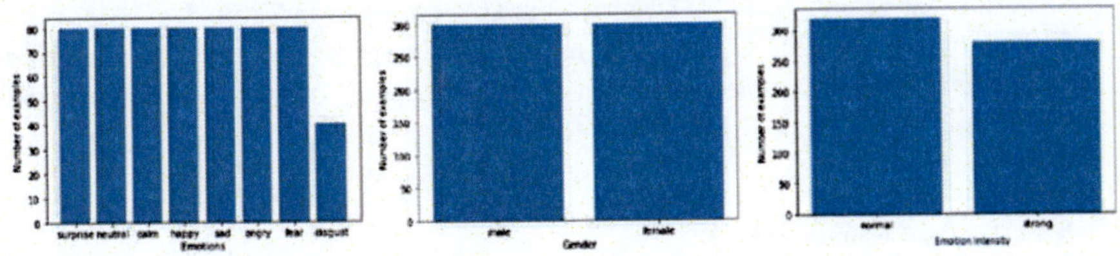

Fig. 3 **a–c** Bar plot of number of emotional speech samples taken per emotion, per gender, per intensity

3.2 Tool Used

The tool used in this research is Python version 3.6.0, an open-source software, with the codes written on the Jupyter notebook. Several prominent Python libraries were installed using the *pip install* and *conda install* commands. The important libraries include Numpy, Pandas, Librosa, Matplotlib, Tensorflow, Sklearn and Seaborn.

3.3 Feature Extraction

For this work, three features are extracted from the speech samples to be given as input to the classifier. As speech signal is a non-periodic signal whose frequency components vary with time, the spectrum of these signals needs to be represented over time using the Short Time Fourier Transform (STFT). Thus, an audio signal is mapped from time domain to frequency domain using FFT and by performing this on overlapping windowed segments and converting the frequency axis to log scale, and the color dimensions to decibels, the spectrogram is formed. Next, the Mel spectrogram is obtained in which the frequencies are converted into Mel scale.

Along with Mel spectrogram, Mel Frequency Cepstrum Coefficients (MFCC) features were also extracted. MFCC provides information about rate changes in different spectral bands, describing the overall spectral envelope. These cepstral parameters offer robust performance compared to other spectral parameters even in a noisy environment. In addition to the Mel spectrogram and MFCC features, the chromagram is also extracted from the speech signal. It is a time-chroma representation which is obtained by aggregating all information related to a given chroma in a local time window into a single coefficient. Shifting this time window across the speech signal results in the production of a sequence of chroma features being spread out across the twelve chroma bands.

Table 1 shows the number of features extracted, with mean and standard deviation for each feature class. This comprises of 12 chromagram pitch classes, 128 Mel spectrogram bands and 40 MFC Coefficients as mentioned in Table 1.

A total of 1440 audio samples are represented with a score of 180 numerical features extracted per sample. Figure 4a–d show the plots of the Spectrogram, Mel Spectrogram, MFCC and Chromagram for two emotions 'happy' and 'angry'.

Table 1 Details of features extracted

Feature class	Number of features extracted in each class	Minima	Maxima	Mean	Standard deviation
Mel spectrogram	128	0.000	136.103	0.201	1.665
MFCC	40	−822.737	96.946	−14.212	94.106
Chromagram	12	0.320	0.864	0.650	0.820

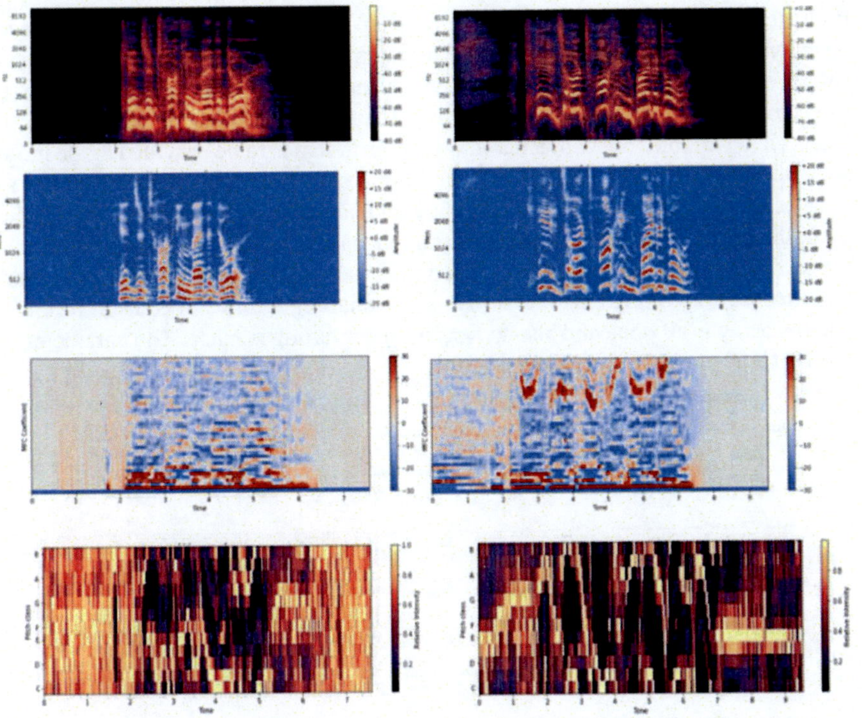

Fig. 4 Emotions 'happy' & 'angry' **a** Spectrogram, **b** Mel spectrograms, **c** MFCC coefficients, **d** Chromagram for emotions

3.4 Convolutional Neural Network

The extracted features are now input to the Convolutional Neural Network (CNN) which is a Deep Learning Algorithm. The architecture is much analogous to the pattern in which the neurons are connected. Thus, the CNN is simply a multi-layered neural network that detects complex features in data. The CNN implies its brilliance by being successful in capturing spatial and temporal dependencies from any given set of input [27]. Although several activation functions such as the sigmoid, tanh are available, ReLU is used because it offers optimal performance over speech signals. The neural network is built with all vital layers including the input layer, convolutional layer, max pooling and average pooling, flatten and dropout etc., wherein the dropout layer is generally placed after the activation function, but for ReLU it is placed above. Pooling is done as a merging process in order to reduce the data size. Flattening is a process done so as to convert the data into a 1D array to pass it over as input to the subsequent fully connected layer. This is done by appending each subsequent row to the one that precedes it. Next the dropout is a process implemented on either all or any of the hidden layers in the neural network thereby preventing overfitting.

Following this, batch normalization is done so as to normalize the inputs to each layer on a feature-by-feature basis. This attempts to solve the internal covariate shift problem, thus performing the tasks of normalization of the input value as well as scaling and shifting them. Consecutively, one hot encoding is done where the categorical variables are converted into such form that is to be provided to the model so as to facilitate better prediction. Then the Exploratory Data Analysis (EDA) is done as to gain preliminary understanding and acquaintance to the dataset and thus eyeballing it. Finally Ridge Regression and Stochastic Gradient Descent optimization are carried out to minimize the loss function. Lastly, redundancy reduction, anomaly elimination, converting data into arrays and reshaping it into a 3D tensor, format of Numpy array is all done and also hyperparameter tuning is made. The parameters of the 1D CNN classifier are shown in Fig. 5.

Layer (type)	Output Shape	Param #
conv1d (Conv1D)	(None, 250, 64)	704
conv1d_1 (Conv1D)	(None, 241, 128)	82048
max_pooling1d (MaxPooling1D)	(None, 30, 128)	0
dropout (Dropout)	(None, 30, 128)	0
conv1d_2 (Conv1D)	(None, 21, 128)	163968
max_pooling1d_1 (MaxPooling1	(None, 2, 128)	0
dropout_1 (Dropout)	(None, 2, 128)	0
flatten (Flatten)	(None, 256)	0
dense (Dense)	(None, 256)	65792
dropout_2 (Dropout)	(None, 256)	0
dense_1 (Dense)	(None, 8)	2056

Total params: 314,568
Trainable params: 314,568
Non-trainable params: 0

Fig. 5 Description of CNN layers and corresponding parameters

3.5 *Convolutional Neural Network and Long Short-Term Memory*

The Long Short-Term Memory (LSTM) is a profound component of the Recurrent Neural Networks (RNN) [28]. Inputs that possess spatial structures such as images, audio and video cannot be modeled using the LSTM. In the CNN-LSTM, the LSTM model is sandwiched between the CNN model and the dense layer, which in turn is a fully connected layer.

Our model's architecture is designed in such a manner that it possesses 4 convolutional blocks thus offering a 4D CNN model, wherein the first convolutional block comprises of one input channel, sixteen output channels with a kernel of size 3, stride and padding one each. Following this, comes the 2D Batch Normalization followed by the ReLU activation function, a 2D max pooling layer and a dropout layer. Here the kernel is a filter in the CNN model that extracts features from the input. It is a matrix that moves over the input data, performing dot product with the sub region of input data and gets the output as a matrix of dot products. The stride is nothing but a parameter of the network's filter which is said to modify the amount of movement over the data and finally padding refers to the conventional zero padding technique. The second convolutional block accommodates sixteen input channels i.e. the output of the previous convolution block and thirty-two output channels, kernel, stride, padding and other layers as the earlier block. Following it come the third and fourth convolutional blocks wherein the former has thirty-two input channel and sixty-four output channels respectively while the latter has sixty-four input and output channels respectively and all other layers as earlier. Next comes the Bidirectional LSTM block in the architecture followed by convolutional embedding where the flattening is done but for batch dimension followed by the LSTM embedding. This architecture is found to offer superior performance when compared to other architectures, offering the highest test accuracy of 98.68%.

4 Results and Discussion

Features extracted from all the eight emotions inclusive of neutral are fed as input to the classifier to be categorized. For the proposed model, only Mel spectrogram feature was used. Emotions could be categorized as, valence and arousal [29]. Valence refers to affectivity or in other words the cause of the emotion. Emotions that come under positive affectivity are surprise and joy while those that fall under negative affectivity category are anger and sadness. Arousal refers to the effect created by any particular emotion, example how calm or soothing as well as on the contrary, how agitating or exciting the emotion is. Feeling of agitation or anxiety is what a survivor of a trauma encounters. It is an experience of fear, sorrow as well an untargeted anger ultimately ending up in disgust giving a disinterest for instance in performing day today activities and living life. Thus, these emotions with a negative affectivity

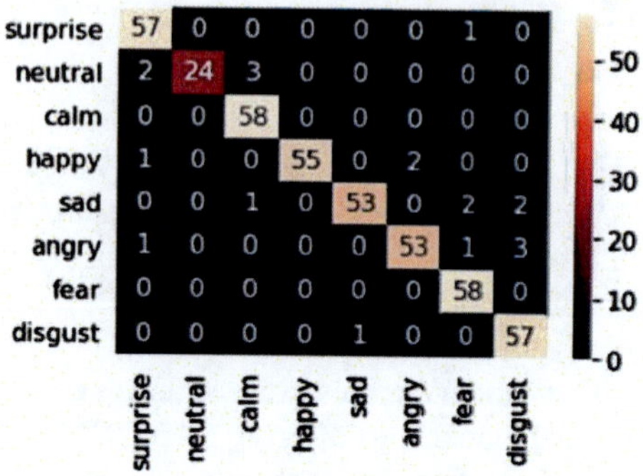

Fig. 6 Confusion matrix of proposed model using Mel spectrogram features and CNN LSTM classifier

or valence as well as falling under both high and low arousal categories are to be categorized as PTSD is classified under Trauma and Stressor related disorder by the DSM V. On the other hand, emotions with positive valence portray non-stressed individuals or controls.

The confusion matrix of the proposed model is shown in Fig. 6 using which the performance of the proposed CNN-LSTM classifier with audio features is shown in Table 2.

From the below table, the efficiency of the proposed PSTD diagnosis system using CNN-LSTM in classifying PTSD subjects and controls is calculated. The emotions pertaining to stress and anxiety viz., sadness, anger, fear and disgust are used for classification resulting in individual classification accuracies of 98.62%, 98.39%, 99.08%, 98.62% respectively. The proposed model produces an average accuracy of 98.68% in correctly classifying PTSD. For computing the classification accuracy of controls, the other emotions excluding neutral namely, happiness, surprise and calm are used, each contributing a classification accuracy of 99.31%, 98.85% and 99.08% respectively, thus collectively offering an average of 99.08% accuracy. Other parameters such as sensitivity, specificity, precision and F1 score also computed, show good performance of the proposed PTSD detection model.

Figure 7 shows the correlation matrices which are square matrices displaying the correlation coefficients between the variables. These matrices give the data related to the ratio of the data samples correctly classified or misclassified with respect to the variable concerned. Figure 8 is the loss plot, which is a curve that is often used to debug the neural network's training process, giving the direction in which, the network learns. It therefore shows the training and validation error over the number of iterations/epochs of the model. The accuracy curve is the contrast of the loss curve when one decays exponentially the other raises. Here the training and validation accuracies would be displayed, the gap between which is the indication of overfitting.

Table 2 Performance parameters of proposed model using CNN LSTM classifier with only Mel spectrogram features

Emotion	True positive	True negative	False positive	False negative	Accuracy	Sensitivity	Specificity	Precision	F1 score
Surprise	57	373	4	1	0.9885	0.9828	0.9894	0.9344	0.9580
Neutral	24	406	0	5	0.9885	0.8276	1	1	0.9057
Calm	58	373	4	0	0.9908	1	0.9894	0.9355	0.9667
Happy	55	377	0	3	0.9931	0.9483	1	1	0.9735
Sad	53	376	1	5	0.9862	0.9138	0.9973	0.9815	0.9464
Angry	53	375	2	5	0.9839	0.9138	0.9947	0.9636	0.9381
Fear	58	373	4	0	0.9908	1	0.9894	0.9355	0.9667
Disgust	57	372	5	1	0.9862	0.9828	0.9867	0.9194	0.9501

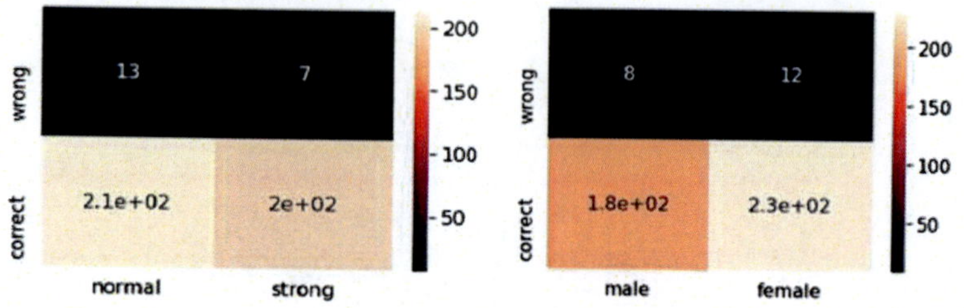

Fig. 7 Correlation between **a** gender and correctness, **b** emotional intensity and correctness

Fig. 8 Loss plot

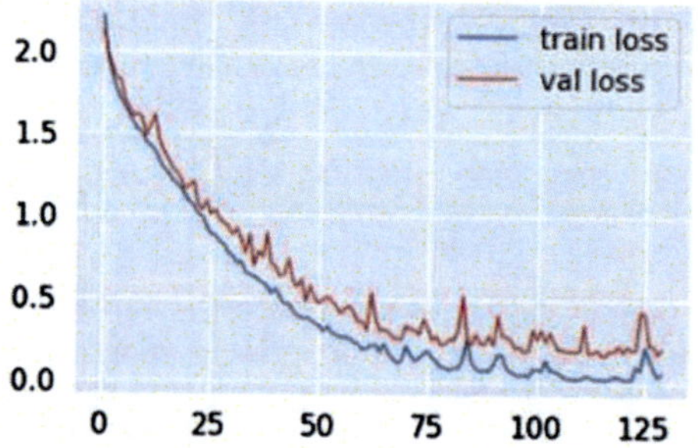

4.1 Comparison with Other Traditional Classifiers

In order to study the efficacy of the proposed model for PTSD diagnosis, comparison with K-Nearest Neighbors (KNN), Random Forest (RF), Gaussian Naïve Bayes, Support Vector Machine (SVM), Multi-Layer Perceptron (MLP) and Convolutional Neural Networks (CNN) was studied.

For all the machine learning classifiers, the three genres of features namely, Mel Frequency Cepstral Coefficients (MFCC), Mel Spectrogram-based features and Chromagram-based features were extracted and then the data was fed independently to the classifier models and executed, and their results are tabulated.

K-Nearest Neighbors: K-Nearest Neighbor (KNN) is a supervised machine learning algorithm that functions based on the assumption that similar entities exist in close proximity. It is based on the fact that similarity could be attributed as proximity/closeness/distance vector. It offered a classification accuracy of 53.33%.

Random forest classifier: Random Forest (RF) is also a machine learning algorithm. It has been inspired from the Decision Tree Algorithm but for the difference is that it contains large number of standalone individual decision trees. Each single tree in the forest splits out a prediction category/class and thereby the class with utmost votes ultimately becomes the mode's prediction. Accuracy of 52.50% was only achieved for PTSD

Gaussian Naïve Bayes: This algorithm is a machine learning (ML) algorithm and is a variant of Naïve Bayes, following the popular Gaussian Normal Distribution supporting continuous data. The algorithm is a direct approach toward modeling the probability of interest, which in this case, is modeled using a linear function applying a sigmoid function on top of it. Poor accuracy of 18.33% only could be achieved.

Support Vector Machine: The Support Vector Machine (SVM) is yet another supervised Machine Learning Algorithm which works by constructing a hyperplane in the multi-dimensional space in order to separate different classes. It works by generating an optimal hyperplane in an interactive manner that could be employed to minimize the error and finds a maximum marginal hyperplane which is used to divide the dataset into classes. Classification accuracy of 45% accuracy was obtained for the speech emotion database used in this work.

Multi-layer Perceptron: A Multi-Layer Perceptron (MLP) is a neural network with the input and output layers being fully connected layers and multiple hidden layers. This classifier, when unscaled offers an accuracy of 80.21% over the training set and 50% over the test set. When minmax scaling is deployed the score changes to 72.50% and 49.17% respectively and for standard scaling the score rises to 99.58% and 66.67% respectively. Thus, the performance of MLP is better when compared to the previous classifiers but is not optimal. This is quite expected because most of the hyperparameters chosen by grid search are default with sklearn's MLP.

Convolutional Neural Network: For the CNN, the Mel spectrogram was computed, from which 13 MFCC features were extracted. Along with this, 2 out of the 12 element chroma vector of the chromagram was extracted. From these prominent spectral features and statistical parameters were computed and given as input to the classifier. Although the CNN being a Deep Learning algorithm is expected to outperform all other Machine Learning algorithms mentioned earlier, the CNN too did not succeed in achieving a high classification accuracy and yielded only 58.33% accuracy. Table 3 gives the comparison between all the seven classifiers, their performances and the features extracted.

Considering the KNN, although its functionality is versatile in implementing it for classification problems rather than regression, it gets slower and less effective as the volume of data increases. In this work the number of prediction classes as high as 8 emotions are to be categorized and also the amount of data is comparatively huge, thus becoming a leading cause for its limited performance offering an accuracy of 53.33%. On the other hand, though Random Forest algorithm, is built on the powerful fundamental concept called the wisdom of crowds, these uncorrelated models produce ensemble predictions with higher accuracy when compared to individual predictions, thus making it more difficult to interpret and also curtailing the algorithm from working with unknown difference between sample and population, making it more suitable for regression than classification, hence offering limited performance of 52.50% in this work.

The Gaussian Naïve Bayes algorithm offers the poorest performance yielding an accuracy of 18.33% as it encounters the zero-frequency problem wherein a zero probability is assigned to any categorical variable whose category isn't available with the training set but not with the test set thus producing wrong estimations. When taking the SVC into consideration, it is again not suitable for large sets of data and also does not offer robust performance in noisy environments and also when

Table 3 Performance comparison of all the classifiers deployed

Si. No.	Classifier algorithm	Feature(S) extracted	Emotion recognition accuracy (%)
1	K-nearest neighbors (KNN)	MFCC features (40), Mel spectrogram features (128) and Chromagram features (12)	53.33
2	Random forest (RF)		52.50
3	Gaussian Naïve Bayes		18.33
4	Support vector machine (SVM)		45
5	Multi-layer perceptron (MLP)		66.67
6	Convolutional neural networks (CNN)	MFCC features (13), Chromagram features (2), spectral features and statistical features of the above	58.33
7	Proposed convolutional neural networks with long short-term memory (CNN-LSTM)	Mel spectrogram	95.40

the target classes are overlapping, however in Speech Emotion Recognition, many emotional expressions are conveyed only with a ray of difference between them and so it is obvious that it has offered only 45% accuracy.

The Multi-Layer Perceptron, also called as the vanilla Neural Network offered a maximum of 66.67% accuracy but still suffers from a drawback that the number of total parameters has a possibility to grow too high and also becomes insufficient as it encounters redundancy at high dimensions. Finally, the CNN, which is a Deep Learning Algorithm offered 58.33% accuracy but in turn requires high computation power and also it suffers from a dependency issue. CNN also depends on the initial parameter tuning for avoiding the local optima. Thus, it needs considerable amount of initialization according to the problem we have at hand and its data requirements may either end up with overfitting or underfitting.

On the contrary, the CNN LSTM combination offers innumerable advantages as it exploits the efficacy of CNN as well that of the LSTM which is a vital component of the RNN. While the CNN is capable of extracting the effective features from a given data, the LSTM is capable of finding the interdependence within the data if it is a time series one. It also possesses the capability of detecting the best model that is suitable for the relevant data on its own. Thus, it offered superior performance giving 95.40% emotion recognition accuracy. Thus, the efficiency of the proposed model with Mel spectrogram features and CNN LSTM classifier for classifying PTSD cases is 98.68% thus offering superior performance.

The proposed model incorporating the CNN-LSTM was evaluated in comparison with the other Machine Learning and Deep learning approaches attempted for PSTD research. Table 4 data tabulates the approach of this research alongside other methods

Table 4 Comparison of Speech Emotion Recognition approaches for diagnosis of Disorders in research

Sl. No.	Work	Biomarker used	Approach	Accuracy
01	Issa et al. [23]	Speech	Speech emotion recognition using deep convolutional neural network (CNN) classifier on the Ryerson audio visual database for speech and song (RAVDESS)	71.61%
03	Marmar et al. [24]	Speech	Speech samples obtained from warzone-exposed veterans captured as responses to CAPS and PTSD Diagnosis using Random forest classifier	89.1%
04	Proposed Model	Speech	An atypical approach to PTSD Diagnosis through speech emotion recognition using convolutional neural network classifier with long short-term memory (CNN-LSTM)	98.68%

adopted earlier by other researches toward Speech Emotion Recognition and PTSD diagnosis.

5 Conclusion

In this work seven classifier algorithms were compared to perform Emotion Recognition from Speech signal and thereby quantify the existence of PTSD in an indirect way. Among these the Deep Learning Algorithms, CNN LSTM offers superior performance offering highest classification accuracy with limited features. The usual sphere of approach taken by researchers is, looking for biological markers such as changes in neural structures and function, genomic markers or immune function markers. Such biomarkers usually come with coupled drawbacks on accuracy, patient burden and cost. Speech has been used by Mental Health Care providers for over years as a diagnostic tool. Such speech-based diagnostic techniques serve as an attractive and potential approach while serving as an alternative for diagnosing different psychiatric disorders and PTSD, in particular. Speech, being a non-intrusive and inexpensive biomarker, also facilitates data collection to be done remotely and non-invasively. Individuals suffering from Psychiatric Disorders display changes in speech and thus the impressions of their voice quality facilitate the diagnosis. This research is an Automated Speech Analysis technique wherein, Speech is used as an attractive candidate, aiding PTSD diagnosis wherein, the CNN-LSTM classifier has demonstrated encouraging specificity and sensitivity on a 'Per Emotion' bases using only Mel Spectrogram features. The LSTM layer in this network is adopted for learning the long-term dependencies from the learned local features. Thus, the combination of CNN and LSTM takes the advantage of the strengths of both the networks while overcoming their shortcomings. On comparing its performance with the other ML and DL classifiers, the CNN-LSTM achieves excellent performance on the Speech Emotion Recognition task outperforming all traditional approaches on the selected RAVDESS Database.

References

1. Low DM, Bentley KH, Ghosh SS (2020) Automated assessment of psychiatric disorders using speech: a systematic review. Laryngoscope Invest Otolaryngol 5:96–116
2. Anagnostopoulos CN, Iliou T, Giannoukos I (2015) Features and classifiers for emotion recognition from speech: a survey from 2000 to 2011. Artif Intell Rev 43:155–177
3. Miao XR, Chen QB, Wei K et al (2018) Post-traumatic stress disorder: from diagnosis to prevention. Mil Med Res 5(32):1–7
4. Shalev AY, Douglas Bremner J (2016) Posttraumatic stress disorder: from neurobiology to clinical presentation. In: Bremner JD (ed) Posttraumatic stress disorder
5. David Kinzie J (2015) Post-traumatic stress disorder, edn 2. International Encyclopedia of the social & behavioral sciences, pp 702–706
6. Bryant RA (2019) Post-traumatic stress disorder: a state-of-the-art review of evidence and challenges. World Psychiatry 18:259–269
7. Victoria A, Diane S (2019) Angry and fearful face conflict effects in post-traumatic stress disorder. Front Psychol 10:136
8. Barbano AC, Grauer E, Lowe SR et al (2019) Differentiating PTSD from anxiety and depression: lessons from the ICD-11 PTSD diagnostic criteria. Depress Anxiety 36(6):490–498
9. Shalev AY, Gevonden M, Ratanatharathorn A et al (2019) International consortium to predict PTSD. estimating the risk of PTSD in recent trauma survivors: results of the international consortium to predict PTSD (ICPP). World Psychiatry 18(1):77–87
10. Worthington MA, Mandavia A, Richardson R (2020) Prospective prediction of PTSD diagnosis in a nationally representative sample using machine learning. BMC Psychiatry 20(532):1–12
11. Ben-Zion Z, Zeevi Y, Keynan NJ et al (2020) Multi-domain potential biomarkers for post-traumatic stress disorder (PTSD) severity in recent trauma survivors. Translation Psychiatry 10(1):208
12. Zhang Q, Wu Q, Zhu H et al (2016) Multimodal MRI-based classification of trauma survivors with and without post-traumatic stress disorder. Front Neurosci 10:1–9
13. Etkin A, Maron A, Marmar CR et al (2019) Using fMRI connectivity to define a treatment-resistant form of post-traumatic stress disorder. Sci Transl Med 11(486):1–12
14. Zandvakili A, Barredo J, Swearingen HR et al (2020) Mapping PTSD symptoms to brain networks: a machine learning study. Transl Psychiatry 10(195):1–8
15. Cheng X, Wang X, Ouyang T, Feng Z (2020) Advances in emotion recognition: link to depressive disorder. Mental Disord
16. Swain M, Routray A, Kabisatpathy P (2018) Databases, features and classifiers for speech emotion recognition: a review. Int J Speech Technol 21:93–120
17. Pinna G (2018) Biomarkers for PTSD at the interface of the endocannabinoid and neurosteroid axis. Front Neurosci 12(482). 6:1–9
18. Durstewitz D, Koppe G, Meyer Lindenberg A (2019) Deep neural networks in psychiatry. Mol Psychiatry 24:1583–1598
19. Chen L, Mao X, Xue Y, Cheng LL (2012) Speech emotion recognition: features and classification models. Digit Signal Process 22(6):1154–1160

20. Koduru A, Valiveti HB, Budati AK (2020) Feature extraction algorithms to improve the speech emotion recognition rate. Int J Speech Technol 23:45–55
21. Low DM, Bentley KH, Ghosh SS (2020) Automated assessment of psychiatric disorders using speech: a systematic review. Laryngoscope Invest Otolaryngol 5(1):96–116
22. Lado-Codesido M, Méndez Pérez C, Mateos R et al (2019) Improving emotion recognition in schizophrenia with "VOICES": an on-line prosodic self-training. PloS One 14(1)
23. Issa D, Demirci MF, Yazici A (2020) Speech emotion recognition with deep convolutional neural networks. Biomed Signal Process Control 59:1–11
24. Marmar CR, Brown AD, Qian M (2020) Speech-based markers for posttraumatic stress disorder in US veterans. Depress Anxiety 36:607–616
25. Durstewitz D, Koppe G, Meyer-Lindenberg A (2019) Deep neural networks in psychiatry. Mol Psychiatry 24:1583–1598
26. Wang J (2018) Detecting postpartum depression in depressed people by speech features. Lect Notes Comput Sci 10745:433–442
27. Akcay MB, Oguz K (2020) Speech emotion recognition: emotional models, databases, features, preprocessing methods, supporting modalities, and classifiers. Speech Commun 116:56–76
28. Fayek HM, Lech M, Cavedon L (2017) Evaluating deep learning architectures for speech emotion recognition. Neural Netw 92:60–68
29. Khalil RA, Jones E, Babar MI, Jan T, Zafar MH, Alhussain T (2019) Speech emotion recognition using deep learning techniques: a review. IEEE Access 7:117327–117345

Effective Independent Component Analysis Algorithm (EICA) for Blind Source Separation of Mixed Images for Biomedical Applications

Nishant Tripathi, Raghvendra Singh, and Utkarsh Pandey

Abstract When dealing with medical applications like X-Rays, EEG, MRI and analyzing individual image component into individual images objects and thereby evaluating the exact image and process it the primary purpose is to convert analysis of images into information. The most basic problem encountered to this procedure is to present the database of mixed images or sample images patch during its analysis i.e. during image segmentation or de-noising for knowing the exact information provided through the mixed or individual sample of images. Independent component analysis (ICA) is new algorithmic approach in Image segmentation of investigate and is being applied for their mutually exclusive statistical PSNR in independent separation images. Independent component analysis is primarily a procedure class from the concept of BSS which is a theoretical concept given for the image and sound representation. In this paper we have developed an analytical approach for an effective distributive algorithmic approach for ICA-based blind source separation for separating out individual component from a mixed picture with maximum PSNR. In blind source separation (BSS) produces after simulation in MATLAB all original images from the observed mixtures. Independent Component Analysis (ICA) is built retrieve individual values called components from a non-regular combination called mixture which are more statistically independent from one another as possible (preferably non-Gaussian higher statistical calculations). The paper will be divided into 4 sections with ICA-BSS introduction, basic theoretical and mathematical model approach for image segmenting or image de-noising from mixed sample picture followed by simulation results followed by conclusion. The simulation of mixed images has been done in MATLAB.

Keywords Independent component analysis (ICA) · Blind source separation (BSS) · Image de-noising · Peak signal to noise ratio (PSNR)

N. Tripathi (✉) · R. Singh · U. Pandey
Department of Electronics and Communication Engineering, Pranveer Singh Institute of Technology, Kanpur, India

M. S. Kaiser et al. (eds.), *Proceedings of Trends in Electronics and Health Informatics*, Lecture Notes in Networks and Systems 376,
https://doi.org/10.1007/978-981-16-8826-3_27

1 Introduction

Basically, the whole problem in image de-noising or segmentation lies in their representation and then simulating them. The idea is to have problems like mixed images picture or a noisy picture from which, we have to estimate or find the original image in close proportion to the original individual image without knowing the proportion of the image content in the mixed sample. Blind source separation (BSS) and Independent Component Analysis (ICA) [1, 2] is a now scope in image analysis especially telemetry and biomedical image/signal data. The main objective solved by ICA [3] is to obtain independent object or source from unknown linear combinations without prior knowledge of un-observed mixed source signals. ICA first decorrelate the signal (2nd and higher order statistics) and lessens higher-order statistical dependencies [4, 5]. This helps the produced components after simulation to be as much independent as possible. ICA was projected to answer the task which is to separate the mixed image/signals and recover the original sources [4, 6].

In the whole process the concept is to mix individual images in an unknown manner in MATLAB taking some sample images/signal (3 in the present paper) in single mixture, and then find out the individual image/signal from the mixture sample. After each simulation Peak Signal to Noise Ratio (PSNR) is computed in MATLAB of each individual image/signal one before the combination and one after ICA-based extraction. In Biomedical signal processing, ICA [3] is a method for unscrambling a multi-variate image/signal into small independent non-Gaussian sub-components signals which are statistically independent. In modern day to day applications ICA is extensively used in biomedical signal processing, electroencephalographic (EEG) and magnetoencephalographic (MEG) data analysis [7–9]. ICA retrieve individual outputs which are called independent components. These results are obtained by exploiting the statistical independency of the retrieved output which are estimated components. There are basic two descriptions of statistical independence for ICA:

- Minimizing Mutual Information [I (X, Y)]
- Maximizing the Non-Gaussian nature in retrieved output after ICA.

1.1 Pre-processing Before ICA Estimation

There are few pre-processing steps before applying the algorithm for retrieving individual output/component

(a) **Kurtosis**—the fourth-order cumulants
(b) **Negentropy**—subtract the mean to create a zero-mean signal
(c) **Centering**—Make vectors Non-zero mean variable
(d) **Whitening**—Eigen value decomposition.

The important part of the algorithm result also depends upon few more constraints as during mixing of the sample images. The first thing is that if noisy or non-desired component is on higher side then PSNR after ICA extraction will lower for individual component while if the noisy component is lower in the mixed proportion, then the PSNR after ICA extraction of individual component will higher.

1.2 Mathematical Modeling

Suppose **M is** the arbitrary course vector whose rudiments are in the combinations $m_1, \ldots, m_n$, and similarly 's' is a random directional vector (component) with matrix elements ($s_1, \ldots, s_n$). Assume '**V**' is a matrix with elements different 'v_{ij}'. Taking the case of vector–matrix notation, 'mixing model' is

$$\mathbf{v} = \mathbf{Ms}. \tag{1.1}$$

$$\mathbf{V} = \sum m_i s_i \tag{1.2}$$

$\mathbf{V} = \sum m_i s_i$ is the part of the outcome termed as Independent component analysis or ICA-based model. The independent components (retrieved output individual PSNR) cannot be directly detected. The whole combination mixing is unknown, both *m*, *s* is unknown. So, it is evident and must underline a basic threshold to provide assumption of both *m*, *s* bits.

First basic assumption is 's_i' are statistically *independent (2nd order).* Then, after approximating the matrix **M**, calculate its inverse, '**I**', and get the independent component

$$\mathbf{s} = \mathbf{Iv} \tag{1.3}$$

After calculating all the parameters and doing preprocessing independency of latent variable needs to be processed, so that PSNR after ICA estimation must uncorrelated and should be on a higher side.

1.3 Independency of Latent Variable Needed to Be Estimated with the Following Steps Mathematically

Technically, independency of two different extracted versions can be estimated by mutually exclusiveness and can be defined by the probability density function and then finding the entropy or 2nd order statistical value [2, 3, 6]. Consider $p\ (y_1, y_2)$ are the joint PDF of a_1 and a_2.

$$P_1(a_1) = \text{Joint integral of } p(a_1, a_2)\mathrm{d}a_2 \text{ and same for } a_2 \tag{2.1}$$

a_1 and a_2 are independent if the joint pdf is factorizable exclusively like

$$p(a_1, a_2) = p_1(a_1)p_2(a_2). \tag{2.2}$$

The same definition can be used to derive as Given two functions, k_1 and k_2, we always have

$$E\{k1(a1)k2(a2)\} = E\{k1(a1)\}E\{k2(a2)\}. \tag{2.3}$$

1.4 *Uncorrelated Variables Are Only Partly Independent*

If their covariance is zero, then the observed data is said to be uncorrelated.

$$E\{a_1a_2\}--E\{a_1\}E\{a_2\} = 0 \tag{2.4}$$

And If the variable quantity is independent, then they are uncorrelated also [10, 11].

$$h_1(a_1) = y_1 \text{ and } h_2(a_2) = a_2. \tag{2.5}$$

2 ICA Basic Approximation/Estimation Principal

The most important feature in approximating the ICA model is its Non-Gaussian nature. In almost all statistical theory, random variables are mostly assumed to have Gaussian as their PDF distributions. Let us now assume that the data vector ‘s’ is distributed according to the ICA data model

$$y = i^T s \tag{3.1}$$

where **i** is a vector to be determined. So, for the sake of Non-Gaussian nature to achieve peak or attain maximum value of ‘$\mathbf{i}^T\mathbf{s}$’ gives us one of the independent components. For several independent components’ estimations, calculated all local maxima.

2.1 Measures of Non-Gaussianity

Kurtosis: It is nothing but a fourth-order cumulants. The kurtosis of s is classically defined by

$$\mathrm{Kurt(s)} = E\{s^4\}^{-3}\left(E\{s^2\}\right)^2 \tag{3.2}$$

Basic assumptions: 's' is of unit variance; kurtosis is non-zero for Non-Gaussian Variable Quantity.

Negentropy

The entropy of a random variable can be understood as degree of information that the observation of the variable stretches.

$$H(Y) = -P(Y = p_i)\log(Y = p_i) \tag{3.3}$$

$$H(\mathbf{y}) = -\int f(\mathbf{y})\log f(\mathbf{y})d\mathbf{y}. \tag{3.4}$$

The definition of differential entropy, called Negentropy. Negentropy J is defined as follow

$$J(\mathbf{y}) = H(\mathbf{y}_{\mathbf{gauss}}) - H(\mathbf{y}) \tag{3.5}$$

where **y** *gauss* is a Gaussian random variable of the same covariance matrix as **y**.

2.2 Algorithm Proposal

$$i^+ = E\{s\,g(i^T s)\} - E\{g'(i^T xs)\}I$$

$$i = i^+/\|w^T\|$$

where I^* is a column.

$$I^+ = C^{-1}E\{S\,g(I^T S)\} - E\{g'(I^T S)\}I$$
$$I* = I^+/I^+C\,I^+$$

where $c = \{SS^T\}$ is the covariance matrix of mixed data.

3 Algorithm Proposal for ICA Extraction (EICA)

(i) Initialize the weight vector w (with random values).
(ii) Let $i^{+} = E\{s\, g\, (i^{T}\, s)\} - E\, \{g\, (i^{T}\, s)\}\, i\ldots$, where g is the derivative of G.
(iii) Let $i = i^{+}/|i|$;
(iv) If not converged, return to step 2 (Fig. 1).

3.1 *Final Algorithm/Iteration that Has Been Obtained is as Follows*

- Center the data;
- make its mean zero;
- Choose an initial orthogonal vector Quantity 'I';
- Place $k = 1$;
- Place and estimate $i_i\,(k) = E\{(s_i\hat{}\,(i_i(k-1)^{T} s_i\hat{})^{3}\} - 3i_i\,(k-1)$;
- Place and estimate $i_i\,(k) = i_i\,(k)/\|i_i\,(k)\|$;
- If not converged then place $k = k + 1$;
- go to step no. v;
- Make the counter and iteration $i = i + 1$;
- When $i<$ no. of sample values of signals, go back to step iv.

4 Simulation Steps

In this particular algorithmic approach, the simulation is being done with three independent sources of different kurtosis values as three different images are mixed in an unknown proportion. In the present MATLAB simulation results a total of three signals are generated randomly. The separated signal is improved and retrieved using Effective ICA Algorithm. A total selection of five different images of 256 * 256 resolute dimension in RGB format and then it is being converted into gray scale format which are named as: Cameraman one (Cam-1), Cameraman two (Cam-2), Bank, Lena and Monkey (Monk) to examine the results, through MATLAB simulation.

The very basic approach has been used to recover from a mixed sample the original distinguished images by using the concept of BSS using the algorithm provided through the use of ICA. A total of 9 different samples have been made through the different combinations of the images being considered for the simulation purpose to estimate the results through application of the proposed algorithm (Table 1).

All the above given image samples have been thoroughly simulated in MATLAB applying the proposed algorithms and the simulation results have been shown through the figures and comparison results related to PSNR of the cases using first the original image PSNR and then finding the PSNR obtained through the proposed algorithm

Table 1 Image mixture combination

S. No.	Sample No	Image Combinations
1	Sample-1	Lena, Cam-1, Bank
2	Sample-2	Cam-2, Bank, Lena
3	Sample-3	Monk, Cam-1, Bank
4	Sample-4	Cam-1, Cam-2, Bank
5	Sample-5	Lena, Cam-1, Cam-2
6	Sample-6	Monk, Cam-1, Cam-2
7	Sample-7	Monk, Cam-1, Lena
8	Sample-8	Lena, Monk, Bank
9	Sample-9	Monk, Cam-2, Bank

of the same image from a mixed sample. To compute the peak signal to noise ratio, between the original image A and the mixed or separated image B.

$$\text{Peak Signal to Noise Ratio(PSNR)} = 10\log(M * N)^2/\text{MSE}$$

$$\text{Mean Square Error} = 1/MN\sum_{i=1}^{M}\sum_{i=1}^{N}(B\,(i,\ j)--A\,(i,\ j))^2$$

4.1 Sample Wise Simulation in MATLAB

See Figs. 2, 3, 4, 5, 6, 7, 8, 9, 10 and 11.

Figures 2, 3, 4, 5, 6, 7, 8, 9, 10 and 11 containing different combination and mixture of 3 sample images and then ICA extracted images in MATLAB.

(Tables 2, 3, 4, 5, 6, 7, 8, 9 and 10 showing Individual PSNR before mixing of individual Sample Image before mixing, and then ICA retrieved PSNR from the mixture of images).

4.2 Result Analysis

After studying the output results from different samples of sample-1 to sample-9 shown, we noticed that the PSNR of the individual images before mixing and the PSNR of the images after recovering from mixed samples through proposed algorithm is approximately 91% close the original PSNR. A brief table has been provided to see the efficiency obtained through different Cases of mixed sample (Table 11).

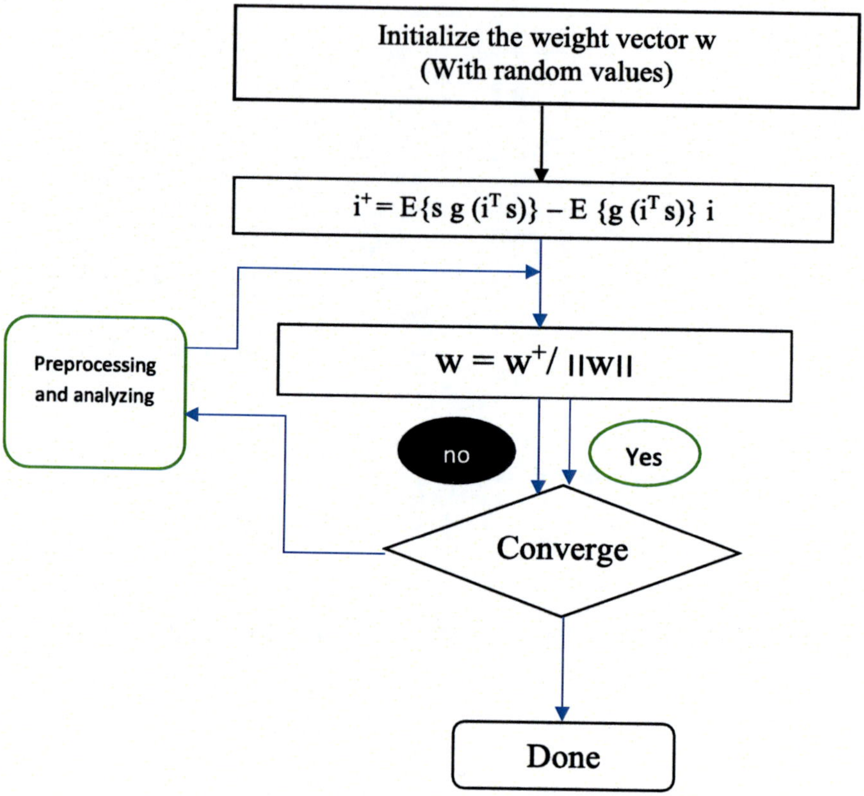

Fig. 1 EICA algorithm flowchart

From all the results obtained from the simulations of previous different Cases numbered from Sample-1 to Sample-9, it has been observed that the proposed algorithm based on Independent Component Analysis in this report is efficient enough to extract the individual images from a mixed sample with greater accuracy and all 9 Cases have shown it. It is evident from the resultant table, which is the summary of all simulation results that all the previous simulations based on ICA have the potential to recover individual images from a noisy image sample or a mixed image sample patch. The overall efficiency in recovering original desired image from noisy image environment is around 91% in taking the average of all the cases. If n1, n2, n3 are the respective efficiencies of different samples, so the resultant efficiency (N) obtained is:

$$N = \frac{n1 + n2 + n3 + \cdots + n9}{9} = 91\%$$

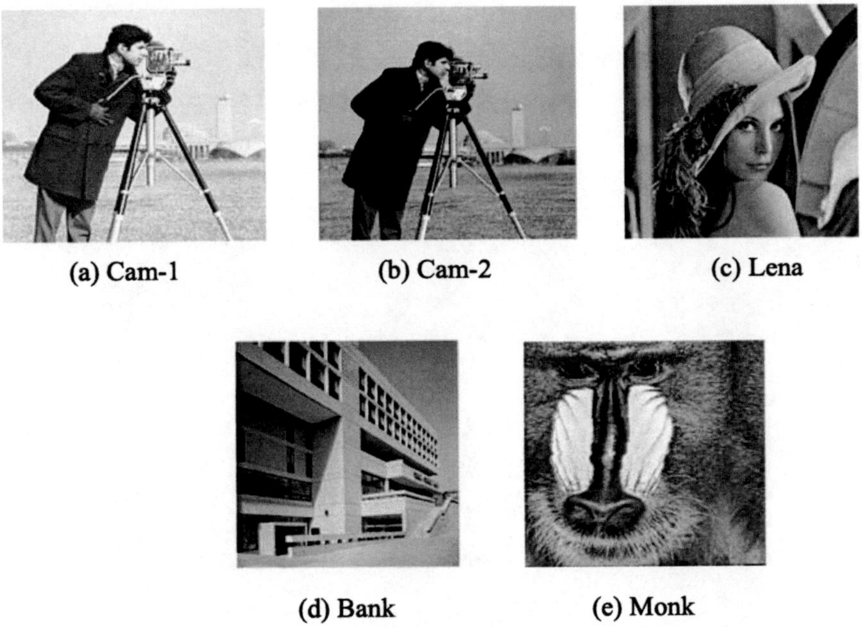

Fig. 2 Various images taken for the simulation

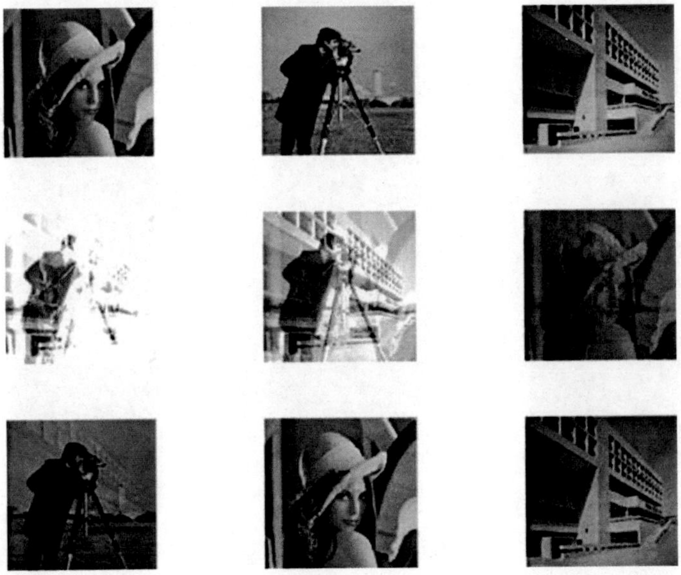

Fig. 3 Sample-1 (images of Lena, Cam-1, Bank)

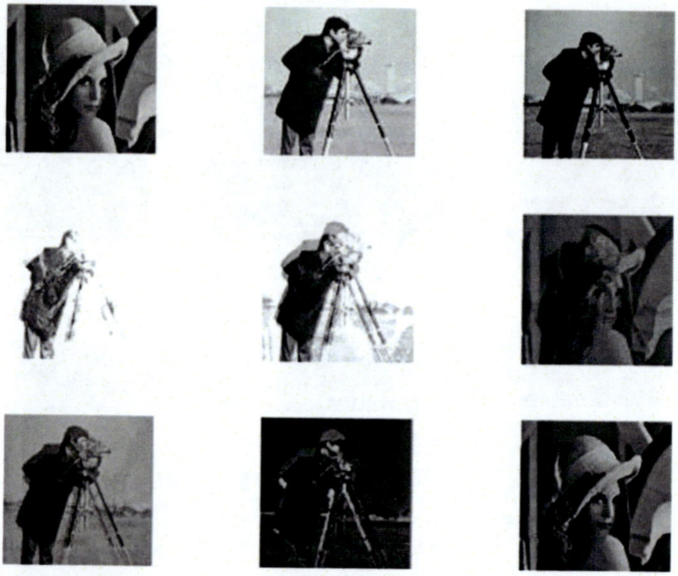

Fig. 4 Sample-2 (images of Lena, Cam-2, Bank)

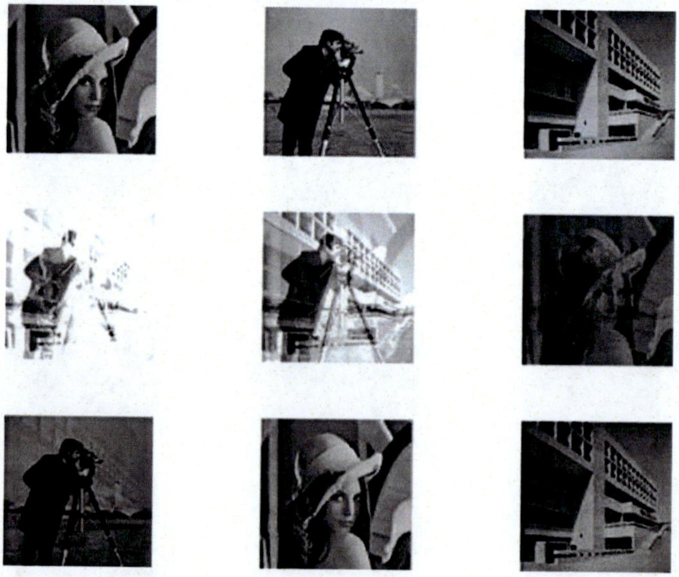

Fig. 5 Sample-3 (image of Cam-1, Monk, Bank)

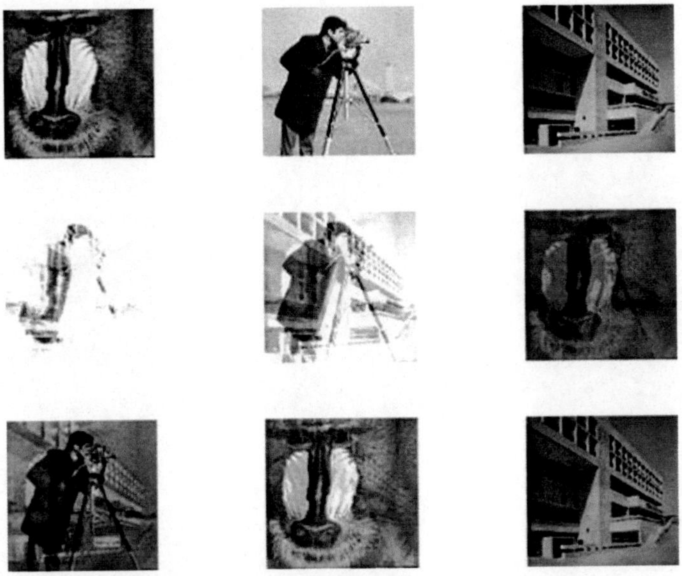

Fig. 6 Sample-4 (images of Bank, Cam-1, Cam-2)

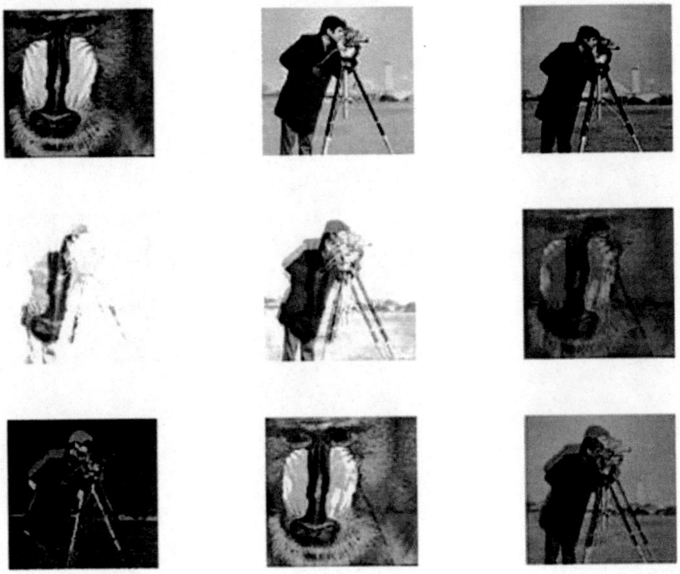

Fig. 7 Sample-5 (images of Lena, Cam-1, Cam-2)

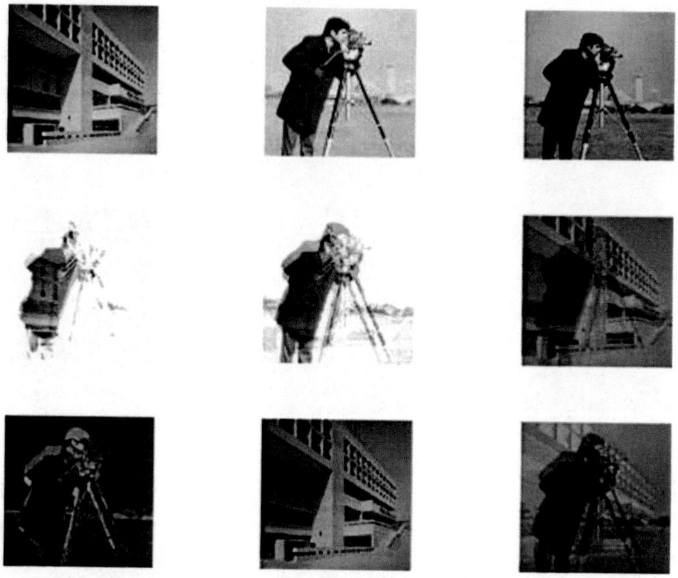

Fig. 8 Sample-6 (images of Monk, Cam-1, Cam-2)

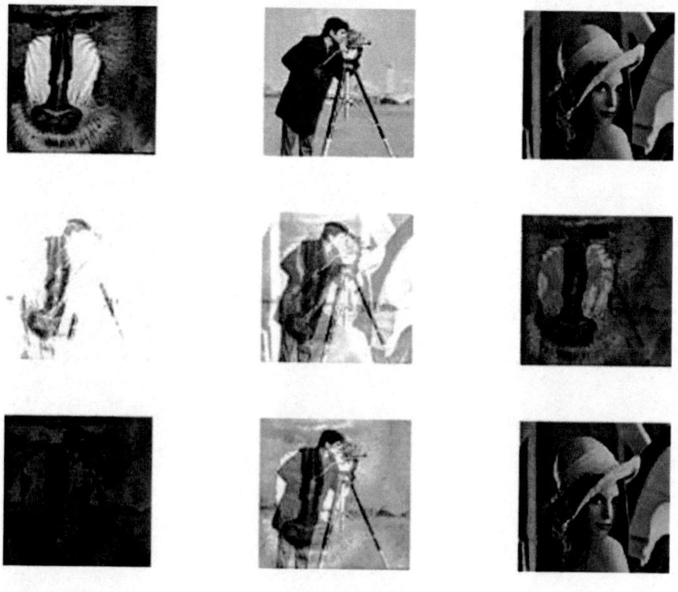

Fig. 9 Sample-7 (images of Monk, Cam-1, Lena)

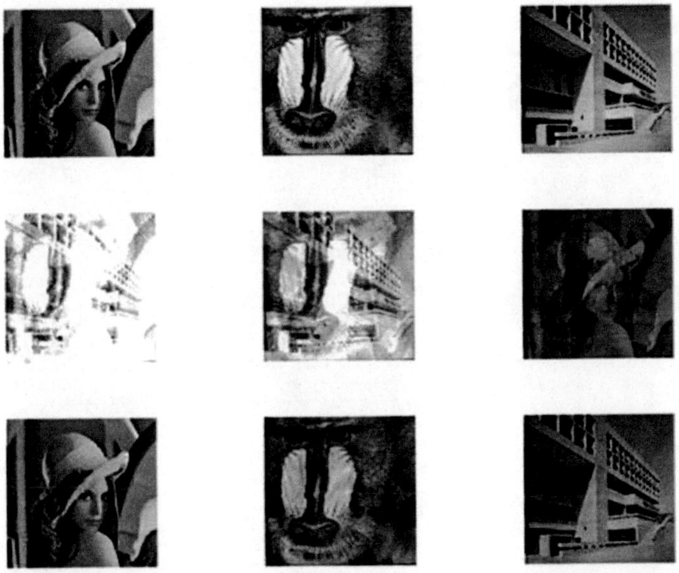

Fig. 10 Sample-8 (image of Lena, Monk, Bank)

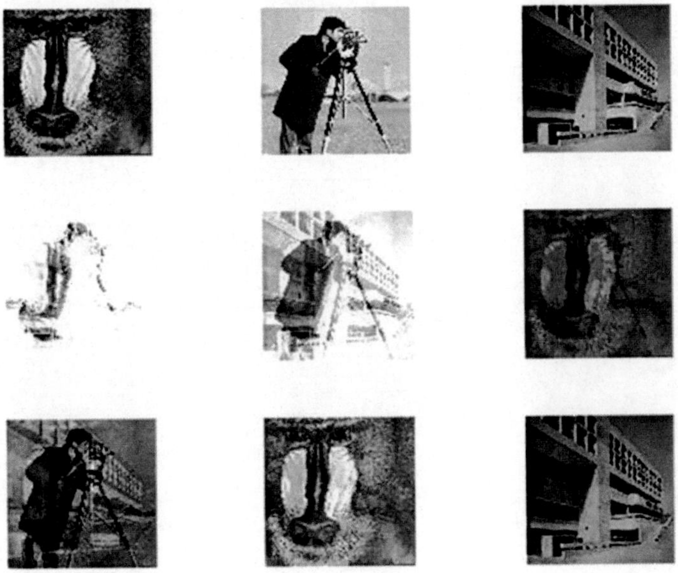

Fig. 11 Sample-9 (images of Monk, Cam-2, Bank)

Table 2 Individual PSNR before mixing of individual sample Image before mixing, and then ICA retrieved PSNR from the mixture of images

S. No.	Image names	Original image PSNR	ICA separated algorithm PSNR
1	Lena	28.490	39.3749
2	Cam-2	27.4194	15.0428
3	Bank	27.6976	27.6696

Table 3 Individual PSNR before mixing of individual sample Image before mixing, and then ICA retrieved PSNR from the mixture of images

S. No.	Image names	Original image PSNR	ICA separated algorithm PSNR
1	Lena image	27.6976	23.9547
2	Cam-1 image	25.9391	26.4505
3	Bank image	28.2490	43.8037

Table 4 Individual PSNR before mixing of individual sample Image before mixing, and then ICA retrieved PSNR from the mixture of images

S. No.	Image name	Original PSNR	ICA separated algorithm PSNR
1	Monk	27.1123	10.11
2	Cam-1	27.2348	21.91
3	Cam-2	25.12	16.15

Table 5 Individual PSNR before mixing of individual sample Image before mixing, and then ICA retrieved PSNR from the mixture of images

S. No.	Image names	Original image PSNR	ICA separated algorithm PSNR
1	Cam-1	27.6976	22.6695
2	Monk	27.6252	26.9914
3	Bank	25.9391	24.9435

Table 6 Individual PSNR before mixing of individual sample Image before mixing, and then ICA retrieved PSNR from the mixture of images

S. No.	Image names	Original image PSNR	ICA separated algorithm PSNR
1	Lena	28.2490	16.7656
2	Cam-1	27.4194	22.0011
3	Cam-2	25.9391	18.23

Table 7 Individual PSNR before mixing of individual sample Image before mixing, and then ICA retrieved PSNR from the mixture of images

S. No.	Image names	Original image PSNR	ICA separated algorithm PSNR
1	Bank	27.4434	15.1213
2	Cam-1	27.1223	19.1218
3	Cam-2	25.9391	17.2326

Table 8 Individual PSNR before mixing of individual sample Image before mixing, and then ICA retrieved PSNR from the mixture of images

S. No.	Image name	Original PSNR	ICA separated algorithm PSNR
1	Cam-1	28.2490	12.5671
2	Lena	25.9391	23.3421
3	Monk	27.6252	19.1211

Table 9 Individual PSNR before mixing of individual sample Image before mixing, and then ICA retrieved PSNR from the mixture of images

S. No.	Image name	Original PSNR	ICA separated algorithm PSNR
1	Lena	29.3417	28.1211
2	Monk	26.3423	24.0098
3	Bank	27.9391	26.9870

Table 10 Individual PSNR before mixing of individual sample Image before mixing, and then ICA retrieved PSNR from the mixture of images

S. No.	Image name	Original PSNR	ICA separated algorithm PSNR
1	Bank	27.2424	24.1244
2	Cam-2	28.1245	18.9211
3	Monk	27.1212	25.2345

Table 11 Final conclusion table

S. No.	Sample No.	Original PSNR (average)	ICA recovered PSNR (average)	Efficiency (approx.) (%)
1	Sample 1	26.9234	26.2322	97
2	Sample 2	27.5443	25.2312	95
3	Sample 3	26.2423	24.1231	93
4	Sample 4	26.3445	23.2233	90
5	Sample 5	27.2322	23.1987	88
6	Sample 6	26.2213	22.9887	87
7	Sample 7	26.7885	21.45411	85
8	Sample 8	28.2422	26.0992	92
9	Sample 9	28.0011	22.9299	87

5 Conclusion

After studying the results obtained the final conclusion is that Independent Component Analysis-based image segmentation, de-noising approach, filtering process and extracting the individual features is quite simpler than other approach of image processing. The results obtained from the algorithm have provided simpler and a faster approach to find out the individual images from a mixed sample with greater accuracy. The algorithm being proposed here has been shown to have 91% efficiency, but it is good enough to extract information from noisy environment in many application cases as: Biomedical signal processing especially for EEG data analysis, MEG Data analysis, Tissue Cancer treatments, E-Ray data interpretation along with Face Recognition, Image de-noising, Satellite Image Resolution, speech processing.

References

1. Olshausen et al (1998) Emergence of simple cell receptive field properties by learning a sparse code for natural images Nature-A Tech Rev Mag 381:607–609
2. Hyvarinen (1999) The fixed point algorithm and maximum likelihood estimation for Independent Component analysis. IEEE Trans Neural Netw 10(3):626–634
3. Hyvarinen (1999) Guassian moments for noisy independent component analysis. IEEE Signal Process Lett 6(6):145–147
4. Comon P (1994) Independent component analysis: a new concept. ELSEVIER, Signal Process 36:287–314
5. Lee et al Independent component analysis using an extended infomax algorithm for mixed sub-Gaussian and super-Guassian sources. Neural Comput 11(2):417–441
6. Amari S et al (1996) A new learning algorithm for blind source separation. Adv Neural Inf Process Syst 8:757–763
7. Usman K, Juzoji H, Nakajima I, Sadiq MA (2004) A study of increasing the speed of the independent component analysis (ICA) using wavelet technique. In: Proceedings international workshop on enterprise networking and computing in healthcare industry (HEALTHCOM 2004), 28–29 June, pp 73–75
8. Moussaoui R, Rouat J, Lefebvre R (2006) Wavelet based independent component analysis for multi-channel source separation. In: Proceedings IEEE international conference on acoustics, speech and signal processing, (ICASSP 2006), vol 5, 14–19 May, pp V645–V648
9. Sadeghi MH, Aghabozorgi MR, Sadeghi MT (2008) Removing reflection from image using ICA. Int Symp Telecommun, IST 2008:815–820
10. El-khaimy SE et al (2003) blind separation of mixed images using higher order statistics. In: Twentieth national radio science conference, Cairo, Egypt
11. Choi S et al (2005) Blind source separation and Independent component analysis: a review. Neural Inf Process-Lett Rev 6(1)
12. Hyvarinen A et al (1997) A fast fixed point algorithm for independent component analysis. Neural Comput 9:1483–1492
13. Hyvarinen (1998) Independent component analysis in the presence of Guassian noise by maximizing joint likelihood. Neuro Comput 22:49–67
14. Ristaniemi et al (1999) On the performance of BSS in CDMA downlink. In: Proceedings international workshop on independent component analysis and signal separation (ICA'99), Aussois, France, pp 437–449
15. Hyvarinen A, A survey on independent component analysis. Neural Comput Surv 2:94–128
16. Hyvarinen Sparse code shrinkage: denoising of non-Guassian data by maximum likelihood estimation. Neural Comput 11(7):1739–1768
17. Li Y et al (2000) Comparison of blind source separation algorithms. Adv Neural Netw Appl, WSES, p 18–21
18. Saruwatari H, Kawamura T, Shikano K (2001) Fast-convergence algorithm for ICA-based blind source separation using array signals processing. In: Proceedings of the 11th IEEE signal processing workshop on statistical signal processing, pp 464–467
19. Rajkishore P, Hiroshi S, Kiyohiro S (2005) Blind separation of speech by fixed-point ICA with source adaptive negentropy approximation. IEICE Trans Fundam, pp 1683–1692

20. Moussaoui R, Rouat J, Lefebvre R (2006) Wavelet based independent component analysis for multi-channel source separation. In: Proceedings IEEE international conference on acoustics, speech and signal processing (ICASSP 2006) vol 5, 14–19 May, pp V645–V648
21. Saruwatari H, Kawamura T Shikano K (2001) Fast-convergence algorithm for ICA-based blind source separation using array signals processing. In: Proceedings of the 11th IEEE signal processing workshop on statistical signal processing, p 464
22. Huang Q, Wang S, Liu Z (2007) Improved image feature extraction based on independent component analysis, vol 34. Opto Electronic Press, pp 123–125
23. Li H, Zhao Q, Zhao J, Xiao B (2009) Blind separation of noisy mixed images based on wiener filtering and independent component analysis. In: 2nd International congress on image and signal processing, CISP'09. IEEE, pp 1–5
24. Huang Q, Wang S, Liu Z (2007) Improved image feature extraction based on independent component analysis. Opto Electronic 34(1):123–125
25. Acharaya DP et al (2008) A review of independent component analysis technique and their application. IETE Tech Rev 25(6)
26. Liu Y et al (2009) Blind Source separation based on Fast-ICA. In: 9th International conference on hybrid intelligent system. IEEE Computer Society
27. Ma C, Wang L (2010) Review of ICA based fixed-point algorithm for blind separation of mixed images. In: 4th International conference on bioinformatics and biomedical engineering (iCBBE), pp 1–3
28. Taizi S et al (2011) Least square independent component analysis. Neural Comput 23(1):284–301
29. Duan L et al (2012) A neural image compression approach based on independent component analysis and visual saliency detection. Research Article, Adv Sci Lett 5(1–4), American Scientific Publisher
30. Tripathi N, Sharma AK (2013) Efficient algorithm based on blind source separation independent component analysis using MATLAB. Int J Electron Commun Technol 4(6), pp 14–20
31. Gupta MS et al (2019) Progression on spectrum sensing for cognitive radio networks: a survey, classification, challenges and future research issues. J Netw Comput Appl 143:47–76
32. Gupta MS et al (2020) Energy efficient transmission trends towards future green cognitive radio networks (5G): progress, taxonomy and open challenges. J Netw Comput Appl 168, Art. no. 102760
33. Gupta MS et al (2020) Application aware networks' resource selection decision making technique using group mobility in vehicular cognitive radio networks. Vehicular Commun 26

GSR Signals Features Extraction for Emotion Recognition

Kuryati Kipli, Aisya Amelia Abdul Latip, Kasumawati Lias, Norazlina Bateni, Salmah Mohamad Yusoff, Nurul Mirza Afiqah Tajudin, M. A. Jalil, Kanad Ray, M. Shamim Kaiser, and Mufti Mahmud

Abstract Over the years, the recognition of emotion has become more efficient, diverse, and easily accessible. In general, emotion recognition is conducted in four main steps which are signal acquisition, preprocessing, feature extraction, and classification. Galvanic skin response (GSR) is the autonomic activation of sweat glands in the skin when an individual gets triggered through emotional stimulation. The paper provides an overview of emotion recognition, GSR signals, and how GSR signals are analyzed for emotion recognition. The focus of this research is on the performance of feature extraction of GSR signals. Therefore, related sources were identified using combinations of keywords and terms such as feature extraction, emotion recognition, and galvanic skin response. Existing emotion recognition methods were investigated which focused more on the different feature extraction methods. Research conducted has shown that feature extraction method in time–frequency domain has the best accuracy rate overall compared to time domain and frequency domain. Current GSR-based technology also has the potential to be improved more toward the implementation of a more efficient and reliable emotion recognition system.

K. Kipli (✉) · A. A. A. Latip · K. Lias · N. Bateni · N. M. A. Tajudin
Faculty of Engineering, Universiti Malaysia Sarawak, 94300 Kota Samarahan, Malaysia
e-mail: kkuryati@unimas.my

S. M. Yusoff
Faculty of Cognitive Sciences and Human Development, Universiti Malaysia Sarawak, 94300 Kota Samarahan, Malaysia

M. A. Jalil
Department of Physics, Faculty of Science, Universiti Teknologi Malaysia, 81310 Skudai, Johor, Malaysia

K. Ray
Amity School of Applied Sciences, Amity University, Jaipur, Rajasthan 303001, India

M. Shamim Kaiser
Institute of Information Technology, Jahangirnagar University, Savar, Dhaka 1342, Bangladesh

M. Mahmud
Nottingham Trent University, Clifton Lane, Nottingham NG11 8NS, UK

M. S. Kaiser et al. (eds.), *Proceedings of Trends in Electronics and Health Informatics*, Lecture Notes in Networks and Systems 376,
https://doi.org/10.1007/978-981-16-8826-3_28

Keywords Emotion recognition · Galvanic skin response · Feature extraction

1 Introduction

Emotion recognition is a method applied in understanding human behavior and is generally performed by signal processing [1]. Emotion recognition is applied in various fields such as engineering, medical, physics, psychiatric, and many more. Understanding emotions is important because emotions affect the way we proceed with our daily activities such as decision making, communication, recognition, and perception [2].

Latest developments in biomedical devices enable researchers to accomplish emotion recognition by measuring physiological signals, for example, galvanic skin response (GSR), electrocardiogram (ECG), heart rate variability (HRV), and electroencephalogram (EEG) [2]. This method utilizes the interaction between biological and psychosocial factors [3] by measuring generated signals from autonomic arousal such as the changes in level of blood pressure, heart rate, and variation in skin conductance [4].

GSR, also defined as electrodermal activity (EDA), is defined as electrodermal activity. GSR has shown that it is an efficient biomarker that uses the autonomic activation of sweat glands in the skin when triggered through emotional stimulation. Stimulus can be in the form of audio-visual, videos, music, and even arithmetic stimulation [5]. Sweat secretion is an activity of the body that cannot be controlled consciously since it is mainly driven by the autonomic nervous system to satisfy behavioral demands [5]. In a study by [6], the sweat glands function as variable resistors. The variation in the conductance level when sweat is secreted is useful biomarkers for the identification of different classes of emotions.

The aim of this paper is to review the literature on emotion recognition methods based on GSR signals and GSR signal processing pipeline. The focus will be on the feature extraction methods and evaluation of the performance of existing work using different feature extraction methods.

1.1 Background of GSR Signals

The measured skin conductance is categorized into two components which are the skin conductance response (SCR) and skin conductance level (SCL). SCL is referred as the tonic level which represents the baseline of skin conductance (SBL). The level varies in a gradual manner, where the rising and declining depend on the individual skin moisture, hydration, or autonomic regulation [5]. SCR is known as the phasic level, and it represents the phasic change in the skin conductance [6]. This response shows significant faster alterations as it is sensitive toward certain emotionally arousing stimulus [5]. As stated in [4], the electrical variation observed

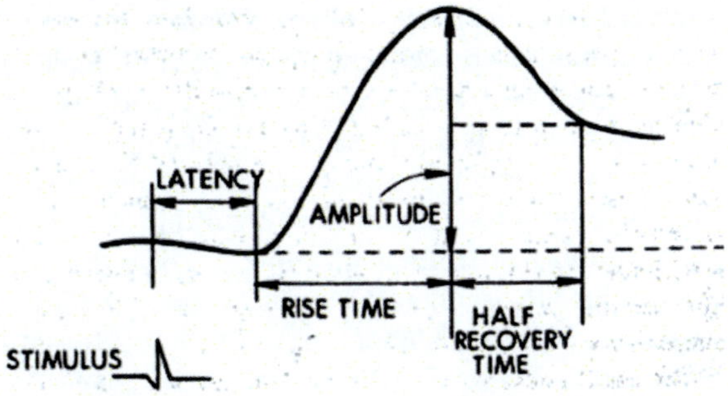

Fig. 1 Typical GSR signal waveform adapted from [10]

or measured at the surface of the human skin varies with each individual depending on several factors.

There are two different approaches when it comes to emotion recognition, and it depends on the scale and scope decided by the researchers. The first approach would be mapping of individual emotions, and the second approach is representation of emotion on multidimensional spaces. In most research studies, basic emotion comprises of happy, fear, surprise, sad, anger, and disgust [7]. These emotions are based on a two-dimensional plan (bipolar model) known as the valence bipolar model [8].

The measurement of skin conductance over time is represented by the two components, SCL, and SCR. SCL refers to the tonic component, while SCRs represent the short-term phasic responses or in another term, reactive phasic component. A "non-specific" SCR (NS-SCR) is known as the response that appears in the absence of a stimuli. GSR signals in general show approximately fast level increments and accompanied by comparatively slower level decrements, gradually return to the baseline level [9]. In other words, these measurements vary in its amplitude, latency, and duration. A typical GSR waveform is shown in Fig. 1.

2 GSR Signal Processing

According to [11–13], the process of emotion recognition using GSR is divided into four main steps which are signal acquisition, preprocessing, feature extraction, and classification.

Preprocessing is a step that mainly involves noise reduction and sampling processes. It is an important step for the elimination of noise from the acquired raw data signals. This helps in reducing any interference exist within the signals and thus increases the accuracy of the desired results [7]. A preprocessed GSR signal ensures that the signal is ready and accessible for further analysis and feature extraction.

After the preprocessing of the GSR signals, useful information is then extracted from the signals to be used in pattern classification for the detection of different states of emotions. This process is referred as feature extraction. Feature extraction is described as the process of transforming raw data signal into a list of measurable features, and this process can be categorized into three groups which are frequency based, time based, and time–frequency based [14].

Classification is the process of predicting the class of given data points and is last step in emotion recognition. One of the most significant factors that affects the suitability of a classification algorithm with regards to an unidentified dataset is the training time. Examples of classifiers that are commonly used for emotion recognition are quadratic discriminant analysis (QDA), decision tree, support vector machines (SVM), random forest (RF), Naïve Bayes, and k-nearest neighbor (kNN).

2.1 *GSR Feature Extraction*

Several feature extraction methods for the emotion recognition based on GSR signals have been proposed in recent studies. The methods can be categorized into time domain feature extraction, frequency domain feature extraction, and time–frequency domain feature extraction.

Time Domain Feature Extraction

The method extracting features of GSR signals in the time domain is a common preceding step applied before combining with other feature extraction methods. In most research, the time domain extracted features consist of statistical parameters of the signals during approximately long recordings, and this includes basic features such as standard deviation, mean value, root mean square (RMS), and higher order statistics (HOC) features such as kurtosis and skewness [9]. There are other studies that focus on attributes of event-related short-term responses, and this refers to features such as SCR amplitude, mean SCR rise time, or sum of SCR areas [15, 16]. Similarly, in a study [17], the identification of GSR measures includes SCL; the change in SCL; frequency of NS-SCRs; SCR rise and half recovery time; the latency and amplitude of SCR; SCR habitation which refers to the number of stimuli occurring before no response, and lastly, the slope of SCR habitation [10]. Several studies such as [17, 18], and [19] have found that SC increases when arousal level increases. However, it is not definite when it comes to the relationship between SC and valence level [17] had reported that in most studies, SC is unable to distinguish positive valence from negative valence stimuli. However, in another research, it was found that any increment in the magnitude of SC is related with negative valence [20].

Frequency Domain Feature Extraction

Although the transitory properties of GSR signals are more efficiently evaluated by analyzing the signal's frequency domain representation, there has only been a few research on the predictive capability of the GSR features linked to the frequency domain compared to time domain features [9]. The frequency domain in signal processing is a coordinate system which describes the frequency characteristics of the signals. A frequency spectrogram describes between the relationship between the amplitude and frequency of the signal [21]. A study by [22] had found that frequency domain analysis demonstrated superior efficiency in detecting transient components of SCR compared to the conventional amplitude analysis. According to [23], GSR signals differ greatly with frequency due to distinctive rates of physiological processes. Examples of frequency domain features are signal magnitude area, peak frequency, peak amplitude, variance, kurtosis, skewness, and harmonics summations [9]. Other known frequency domain techniques include empirical mode decomposition (EMD) and intrinsic mode functions (IMFs).

Time–Frequency Domain Feature Extraction
For extracting features in time–frequency domain, wavelets transform has been found suitable since GSR signals shows non-stationary behavior. An example of one of the most common time–frequency domain feature extraction technique is the discrete wavelet transform (DWT). DWT is an effective technique based on time–frequency domain for feature extraction because of its inherent multiresolution approach to signal analysis [24]. This technique involves the projection of signals onto a basis of wavelet functions which separates the fine-scale and large-scale information of the desired signals [25]. This technique is suitable to analyze GSR signals as the amplitude, frequency, and phases of GSR signals changes over time compared to Fourier transformation technique. A study by [11] also stated that for non-stationary signals, DWT helps in overcoming the shortcomings of Fourier transformations. Furthermore, this technique is less prone to getting affected noises or any other interference [11]. Another well-known time–frequency domain technique is matching pursuit (MP). This algorithm was first proposed by [26].

2.2 *Performance of Emotion Recognition Using Different GSR Signals Feature Extraction Methods*

For achieving a maximum recognition rate of emotion from GSR signals, researchers have proposed different combinations of preprocessing, feature extraction and classification methods. This section mainly discusses the comparison of different GSR feature extraction methods and respective recognition accuracy. Table 1 shows a summary of the emotion recognition methods from recent studies on GSR signals and the achieved recognition accuracy.

Based on the table, most of the studies used either videos or audio-visual as the stimuli for their experiment. In general, those type of stimuli yield higher accuracy when compared to stimuli in the form of images.

The recognition rates vary across different studies depending on the type of features extracted and what methods were used for the extraction. For time domain features, generally statistical features, high order statistics, and SCR features are extracted. As for frequency domain features, there were several methods introduced in studies such as Fourier transform, Welch's power spectral density (PSD), and

Table 1 Performances of existing emotion recognition methods using GSR signals

<table>
<tr><th>Paper info (authors)</th><th>Stimulus</th><th>Subjects</th><th>Signals</th><th>Feature extraction method</th><th>Classifiers</th><th colspan="2">Recognition rate (%)</th></tr>
<tr><td rowspan="4">[27]</td><td rowspan="4">Images</td><td rowspan="4">5</td><td rowspan="4">GSR</td><td rowspan="4">Time domain features</td><td rowspan="4">Quadratic discriminant (QDA)</td><td colspan="2">Half:train, half:test</td></tr>
<tr><td colspan="2">55</td></tr>
<tr><td colspan="2">Leave one out (LOO)</td></tr>
<tr><td colspan="2">51.66</td></tr>
<tr><td>[28]</td><td>Videos</td><td>35</td><td>SCR</td><td>Fourier transform</td><td>SVM</td><td colspan="2">85.75</td></tr>
<tr><td rowspan="9">[29]</td><td rowspan="9">Videos</td><td rowspan="9">Not stated</td><td rowspan="9">GSR</td><td rowspan="9">Welch's power spectral (PSD) and statistical features</td><td rowspan="9">SVM, Naïve Bayes, and kNN</td><td colspan="2">Happy and sad</td></tr>
<tr><td>PSD</td><td>Statistical</td></tr>
<tr><td>100</td><td>100</td></tr>
<tr><td colspan="2">Happy and neutral</td></tr>
<tr><td>PSD</td><td>Statistical</td></tr>
<tr><td>80.30</td><td>83.13</td></tr>
<tr><td colspan="2">Sad and neutral</td></tr>
<tr><td>PSD</td><td>Statistical</td></tr>
<tr><td>100</td><td>81.61</td></tr>
<tr><td rowspan="4">[11]</td><td rowspan="4">Videos</td><td rowspan="4">32</td><td rowspan="4">GSR</td><td rowspan="4">Time domain features, DWT, and EMD</td><td rowspan="4">DT(148), RF, and kNN</td><td colspan="2">Arousal</td></tr>
<tr><td colspan="2">81.81</td></tr>
<tr><td colspan="2">Valence</td></tr>
<tr><td colspan="2">89.29</td></tr>
<tr><td rowspan="4">[9]</td><td rowspan="4">Videos</td><td rowspan="4">37</td><td rowspan="4">SCR</td><td rowspan="4">Time domain features, DWT, and SWT</td><td rowspan="4">SVM, and RBF kernel</td><td colspan="2">Arousal</td></tr>
<tr><td colspan="2">85.75</td></tr>
<tr><td colspan="2">Valence</td></tr>
<tr><td colspan="2">83.9</td></tr>
<tr><td>[4]</td><td>Audio-visual</td><td>39</td><td>GSR</td><td>Data lagging and data labeling</td><td>SVM, and RBF kernel</td><td colspan="2">75.65</td></tr>
<tr><td>[30]</td><td>Audio-visual</td><td>27</td><td>GSR</td><td>Time–frequency domain analysis</td><td>SVM</td><td colspan="2">57.69</td></tr>
<tr><td rowspan="4">[31]</td><td rowspan="4">Music</td><td rowspan="4">457</td><td rowspan="4">SC</td><td rowspan="4">Deep hybrid neural network and residual bidirectional GRU networks</td><td rowspan="4">SVM</td><td colspan="2">Arousal</td></tr>
<tr><td colspan="2">60.22</td></tr>
<tr><td colspan="2">Valence</td></tr>
<tr><td colspan="2">60.66</td></tr>
</table>

empirical mode decomposition (EMD). As for time–frequency domain features, examples of existing methods are discrete wavelet transform (DWT) and statistical wavelet transform (SWT).

In most cases, time domain features extraction method is used as a preceding step before combining with other techniques to achieve a high recognition rate. In some cases such as [27], only time domain features extraction method was used, and the features extracted were mean, standard deviation, mean of derivative, and the features extracted due to consider the importance of average variation and deviation. This was only able to yield low recognition rates (below 50%).

Das et al. [29] proposed a time domain extraction technique with statistical features and was able to yield high recognition rates with the highest being 100% for happy and sad emotions. Features extracted were mean, median, mode, variance, kurtosis, and skewness. Das et al. [29] also applied a frequency domain technique named Welch's power spectral density (PSD). Both techniques were able to produce high recognition rates with the highest being 100%. The limitation of the method used in [29] is that it analyzed emotions by taking all three mutually exclusive emotional states only which were neutral, happy, and sad. Besides this, it is also known that the Welch's PSD method has a reduced spectral precision.

In [11] and [9], both studies applied combined time domain feature extraction with DWT which is time–frequency based. The main difference between the method used by the two studies is that [9] further extract the signals using the stationary wavelet transform (SWT) technique, while [11] applied EMD. The combination of techniques used in [9] for feature extraction was able to contribute an accuracy up to 85.75% and 83.9% for arousal and valence, respectively. SWT is a technique that is shift invariant, redundant, and linear. More efficient sampling rates can be provided for low-frequency bands if compared to the standard DWT technique [32]. A previous study had successfully applied the SWT technique to denoise EDA signals efficiently, and less computational complexity was required [33]. In [11], the combination of time domain feature extraction, DWT, and EMD was able to contribute an accuracy up to 81.81% for arousal and 89.29% for valence. Without EMD, the accuracy achieved was only 71.53% for arousal and 71.04% for valence [11]. The limitation of the EMD technique is that it takes around 50–60 iterations, which means that in real-time implementations, it would produce high system latency.

There are certain studies that only used one method for feature extraction. In [28], only Fourier transform was performed for feature extraction but it was able to reach a recognition rate of 85.75%. Although this study only used Fourier transform for the feature extraction method, it was still able to reach a high accuracy. A study by [8] stated that the Fourier transform method leads to inefficient exemplification functions that are well localized in time. Meanwhile, [30] used only time–frequency domain method for feature extraction, and the recognition rate achieved was 57.69%. [15] used the MP technique for feature extraction and was able to achieve an average recognition rate of 100%.

The study by [4] proposed a method called the lagging and labeling technique for feature extraction. This method prepares and frames the input data into time series. In the study, the researchers concluded that the required number of lags to form relevant data for classification is 40, and this was able to contribute an accuracy of 75.65%. [31] proposed a feature extraction method based on deep hybrid neural networks. To remove the characteristics, it consists of time distributed one-dimensional convolutional neural network (1D CNN) layers. This extraction technique was able to contribute an accuracy up to 60.22% for arousal and 66.66% for valence.

For classification, support vector machine (SVM) is the most widely used classifier for emotion recognition on GSR signals. In [28, 31], and [30] classifier SVM was used meanwhile in studies such as [9] and [29], and other classifiers such as Naïve Bayes and k-nearest neighborhood (kNN) were also tested together with SVM for comparison purposes. In general, most studies that used SVM were able to achieve notable recognition rates. The efficiency of the classifiers used depends on how it is applied and combined with prior preprocessing and feature extraction techniques.

3 Conclusion and Recommendation

This paper presented an overview of existing emotion recognition methods on GSR signals which focused on the feature extraction step. Based on the research, it was found that feature extraction methods can be further grouped into three types which are time domain, frequency domain, and time–frequency domain features.

This paper also compared the performance of the different feature extraction methods in terms of accuracy rate. From the comparison, the time–frequency domain feature extraction method has shown the most favorable, and it is also the most complex since it involves wavelets transform. Since time–frequency domain feature extraction method has shown the best performance, future work could focus on developing a simpler process for this complex technique that would yield the same or better performance. In addition, more types of features such as the entropy domain features and time–frequency domain features that involve complex processes should be investigated using the research method applied in this project.

References

1. Sebe N, Cohen I, and Huang TS (2004) Chapter 1 multimodal emotion recognition. Rev Lit Arts Am, pp 981–256
2. Kumar J, Kumar JA (2015) Machine learning approach to classify emotions using GSR. Adv Res Electr Electron Eng 2(12):72–76
3. Sarchiapone M, Gramaglia C, Iosue M, Carli V, Mandelli L, Serretti A, Marangon D, Zeppegno P (2018) The association between electrodermal activity (EDA), depression and suicidal behaviour: a systematic review and narrative synthesis. BMC Psychiatry 18(1):22. https://doi.org/10.1186/s12888-017-1551-4.PMID:29370787;PMCID:PMC5785904
4. Setyohadi DB, Kusrohmaniah S, Gunawan SB, Pranowo P, Prabuwono AS (2018) Galvanic skin response data classification for emotion detection. Int J Electric Comput Eng. 8:4004–4014
5. Govoni NA (2012) Galvanic skin response. Dict Mark Commun. https://doi.org/10.4135/9781452229669.n1404

6. Eesee AK (2019) The suitability of the Galvanic skin response (GSR) as a measure of emotions and the possibility of using the scapula as an alternative recording site of GSR. In: 2nd International conference on electrical, communication, computer, power, and control engineering ICECCPCE19, pp 13–14
7. Bulagang AF, Weng NG, Mountstephens J, Teo J (2020) A review of recent approaches for emotion classification using electrocardiography and electrodermography signals. Inf Med Unlocked 20:100363. https://doi.org/10.1016/j.imu.2020.100363
8. Goshvarpour A, Abbasi A, Goshvarpour A (2017) An accurate emotion recognition system using ECG and GSR signals and matching pursuit method. Biomed J 40(6):355–368. https://doi.org/10.1016/j.bj.2017.11.001
9. Shukla J, Barreda-Angeles M, Oliver J, Nandi GC, Puig D (2019) Feature extraction and selection for emotion recognition from electrodermal activity. IEEE Trans Affect Comput 3045. https://doi.org/10.1109/TAFFC.2019.2901673
10. Swangnetr M, Kaber DB (2013) Emotional state classification in patient-robot interaction using wavelet analysis and statistics-based feature selection. IEEE Trans Hum-Mach Syst 43(1):63–75. https://doi.org/10.1109/TSMCA.2012.2210408
11. Ayata D, Yaslan Y, Kamasak M (2017) Emotion recognition via galvanic skin response: comparison of machine learning algorithms and feature extraction methods. Istanbul Univ—J Electr Electron Eng 17(1):3129–3136
12. Greco A, Valenza G, Citi L, Scilingo EP (2017) Arousal and valence recognition of affective sounds based on electrodermal activity. IEEE Sens J 17(3):716–725. https://doi.org/10.1109/JSEN.2016.2623677
13. Perez-Rosero MS, Rezaei B, Akcakaya M, Ostadabbas S (2017) Decoding emotional experiences through physiological signal processing. ICASSP. In: IEEE Int Conf Acoust Speech Signal Process—Proc, pp 881–885. https://doi.org/10.1109/ICASSP.2017.7952282
14. Domínguez-Jiménez JA, Campo-Landines KC, Martínez-Santos JC, Delahoz EJ, Contreras-Ortiz SH (2020) A machine learning model for emotion recognition from physiological signals. Biomed Signal Process Control 55:101646. https://doi.org/10.1016/j.bspc.2019.101646
15. O'Connell RG, Bellgrove MA, Dockree PM, Lau A, Fitzgerald M, Robertson IH (2008) Self-alert training: volitional modulation of autonomic arousal improves sustained attention. Neuropsychologia 46(5):1379–1390. https://doi.org/10.1016/j.neuropsychologia.2007.12.018
16. Coley AA (1999) Qualitative properties of scalar-tensor theories of gravity. Gen Relativ Gravit 31(9):1295–1313. https://doi.org/10.1023/A:1026776808535
17. Dawson ME, Schell AM, Filion DL (2016) The electrodermal system. In: Handbook of psychophysiology, 4th edn. pp 217–243. https://doi.org/10.1017/9781107415782.010
18. Mandryk RL, Atkins MS (2007) A fuzzy physiological approach for continuously modeling emotion during interaction with play technologies. Int J Hum Comput Stud 65(4):329–347. https://doi.org/10.1016/j.ijhcs.2006.11.011
19. Nakasone A, Prendinger H, Ishizuka M (2005) ProComp infiniti bio-signal encoder. In: Proceedings 5th international workshop on bio-signal interpretation, pp 219–222
20. Amershi S, Conati C, Maclaren H (2006) Using feature selection and unsupervised clustering to identify affective expressions in educational games. In: Proceedings of the workshop on motivation and affect. Issues 8th international conference on intelligent tutoring systems, pp 21–28
21. Wen T, Zhang Z (2017) Effective and extensible feature extraction method using genetic algorithm-based frequency-domain feature search for epileptic EEG multiclassification. Med (United States) 96(19):1–11. https://doi.org/10.1097/MD.0000000000006879
22. Shimomura Y, Yoda T, Sugiura K, Horiguchi A, Iwanaga K, Katsuura T (2008) Use of frequency domain analysis of skin conductance for evaluation of mental workload. J Physiol Anthropol 27(4):173–177. https://doi.org/10.2114/jpa2.27.173
23. Ghaderyan P, Abbasi A (2016) An efficient automatic workload estimation method based on electrodermal activity using pattern classifier combinations. Int J Psychophysiol 110:91–101. https://doi.org/10.1016/j.ijpsycho.2016.10.013

24. Mallat SG (2009) A theory for multiresolution signal decomposition: the wavelet representation. Fundam Papers Wavelet Theory I(7):494–513
25. Bruce LM, Koger CH, Li J (2002) Dimensionality reduction of hyperspectral data using discrete wavelet transform feature extraction. IEEE Trans Geosci Remote Sens 40(10):2331–2338. https://doi.org/10.1109/TGRS.2002.804721
26. Mallat SG (1993) Zhang Z (1993) Matching pursuits with time-frequency dictionaries. IEEE Trans Signal Process 41(12):3397–3415. https://doi.org/10.1109/78.258082
27. Khalili Z, Moradi MH (2009) Emotion recognition system using brain and peripheral signals: using correlation dimension to improve the results of EEG. In: Proceedings of the international joint conference on neural networks, pp 1571–1575. https://doi.org/10.1109/IJCNN.2009.5178854
28. Ménard M, Richard P, Hamdi H, Daucé B, Yamaguchi T (2015) Emotion recognition based on heart rate and skin conductance. PhyCS 2015—2nd international conference on physiological computing proceedings, pp 26–32. https://doi.org/10.5220/0005241100260032
29. Das P, Khasnobish A, Tibarewala DN (2016) Emotion recognition employing ECG and GSR signals as markers of ANS. Conf Adv Signal Process CASP 2016:37–42. https://doi.org/10.1109/CASP.2016.7746134
30. Wei W, Jia Q, Feng Y, Chen G (2018) Emotion recognition based on weighted fusion strategy of multichannel physiological signals. Comput Intell Neurosci 2018(1). https://doi.org/10.1155/2018/5296523
31. Susanto IY, Pan TY, Chen CW, Hu MC, Cheng WH (2020) Emotion recognition from galvanic skin response signal based on deep hybrid neural networks. In: ICMR 2020—proceedings 2020 international conference on multimedia Retrieval, pp 341–345. https://doi.org/10.1145/3372278.3390738
32. Nason GP, Silverman BW (1995) The stationary wavelet transform and some statistical applications, pp 281–299
33. Shukla J, Barreda-Ángeles M, Oliver J, Puig D (2018) Efficient wavelet-based artifact removal for electrodermal activity in real-world applications. Biomed Signal Process Control, 42(April):45–52. https://doi.org/10.1016/j.bspc.2018.01.009

Development of Mobile Application for Detection and Grading of Diabetic Retinopathy

Kuryati Kipli, Lee Yee Hui, Nurul Mirza Afiqah Tajudin, Rohana Sapawi, Siti Kudnie Sahari, Dayang Azra Awang Mat, M. A. Jalil, Kanad Ray, M. Shamim Kaiser, and Mufti Mahmud

Abstract The key to preventing blindness caused by diabetic retinopathy (DR) is regular screening and early recognition during its early stages. Currently, DR grading is done manually by ophthalmologists and trained graders where the process is time-consuming. Therefore, this paper aims to develop a mobile app that can provide DR detection and grading without a professional or doctor. The patients will be referred to ophthalmologists if further evaluations are required. This research builds an image classification within a mobile application by using deep learning techniques which utilized the Google AI technologies: Google TensorFlow and Google Cloud Platform (Cloud AutoML and Cloud storage). Image classification is performed in two layers which involve DR detection and grading. A total of 12,062 fundus images are chosen from the dataset collected and undergo image preprocessing. The preprocessed images are used to train the model in TensorFlow and Cloud AutoML, respectively. The model will be implemented into the mobile application after being trained with high accuracy. The final test accuracy for the MobileNet pretrained model is 82.9%, while averaging precision for the model of Cloud AutoML is 75%. Further research is required to improve the stability of this algorithm and mobile app for real clinical environment settings.

K. Kipli (✉) · L. Y. Hui · N. M. A. Tajudin · R. Sapawi · S. K. Sahari · D. A. A. Mat
Department of Electrical and Electronics, Faculty of Engineering, Universiti Malaysia Sarawak, 94300 Kota Samarahan, Malaysia
e-mail: kkuryati@unimas.my

M. A. Jalil
Department of Physics, Faculty of Science, Universiti Teknologi Malaysia, 81310 Skudai, Johor, Malaysia

K. Ray
Amity School of Applied Sciences, Amity University, Jaipur, Rajasthan 303001, India

M. Shamim Kaiser
Institute of Information Technology, Jahangirnagar University, Savar, Dhaka 1342, Bangladesh

M. Mahmud
Nottingham Trent University, Clifton Lane, Nottingham NG11 8NS, UK

M. S. Kaiser et al. (eds.), *Proceedings of Trends in Electronics and Health Informatics*, Lecture Notes in Networks and Systems 376,
https://doi.org/10.1007/978-981-16-8826-3_29

Keywords Diabetic retinopathy · Image classification · Mobile application · Google TensorFlow · Google cloud platform · Cloud AutoML

1 Introduction

Software development of DR in mobile devices is in demand because mobile devices having the portability and lightweight advantages. Instead of a computer, mobile devices have been implemented with high-resolution cameras in the current trend. A smartphone provided more advanced computing capabilities and connectivity which allows the user to use a specific platform to install and run more advanced applications. The accessibility of programs for a smartphone such as build-in camera and gallery enables users to obtain the desired image more easily than desktop as desktop require setup and additional hardware before capturing process.

According to National Diabetes Registry Report 2020, 1,698,683 diabetic patients are enrolled in the National Diabetes Registry 2020. In 2020, out of 88,457 patients audited for retinopathy, 11.52% have been diagnosed with DR [1]. DR is the most common cause of blindness among the working-age population globally including in Malaysia. DR has been recognized as a microvascular disease where retinal abnormalities such as vascular bleeds or leaks of fluid eventually lead to one's vision distortion [2]. The retina damage occurred due to the microvascular complication of diabetes mellitus.

Usually, it does not have any symptoms for the early stages of DR. So, most of the patients will not notice the presence of DR. The frequency for the screening of DR decreases due to the lack of awareness among the patients. A clinical specialized visit is required for the diagnosis of DR since the grading of DR is mostly done manually by expertise such as ophthalmologists and trained graders. Thus, the process of diagnosis of DR required a lot of time, and this will lead to some patients suffer vision loss before they are being diagnosed. Lack of effective and regular screening is one of the problems in the management of DR. Effective screening is important for the early detection and treatment of DR as it can help to prevent blindness or slow down the progress of DR.

To solve the problems stated above, a mobile solution for DR is proposed. This mobile solution enables to prevent the growth of blindness in Malaysia and even the world as the diagnosis of DR can be done easily without the need of professionals. The mobile application is designed to classify the retinal images by utilizing the Google AI technologies which are Google TensorFlow and Google Cloud Platform. The retinal images are captured by using a smartphone's camera with external tools such as an ophthalmoscope. The main objective of this research work is to develop a mobile application that can provide detection and grading of DR. The patients must refer to ophthalmologists if further evaluations are required.

The main expected outcome for this research work is the mobile application that can automatically detect and grade DR. The mobile application provides a real-time evaluation that uses a smartphone's camera to capture the images of the DR with a specific external tool such as an ophthalmoscope for the detection and grading of DR.

2 Methodology

The process involved consists of the collection of a bunch of fundus images, image preprocessing, image classification, and mobile application development. Figure 1 illustrated the flowchart of the overall process for the proposed system.

Firstly, the desired retinal image dataset must be collected. Dataset plays an important role in deep learning techniques as this technique requires a large amount of data. In this research, the dataset is obtained from an open-source retinopathy screening

Fig. 1 Flowchart of the overall process of the proposed research

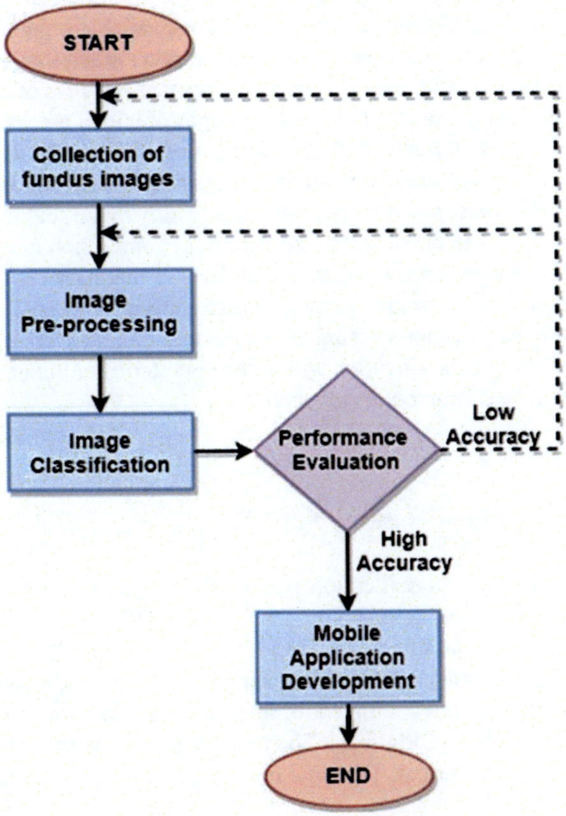

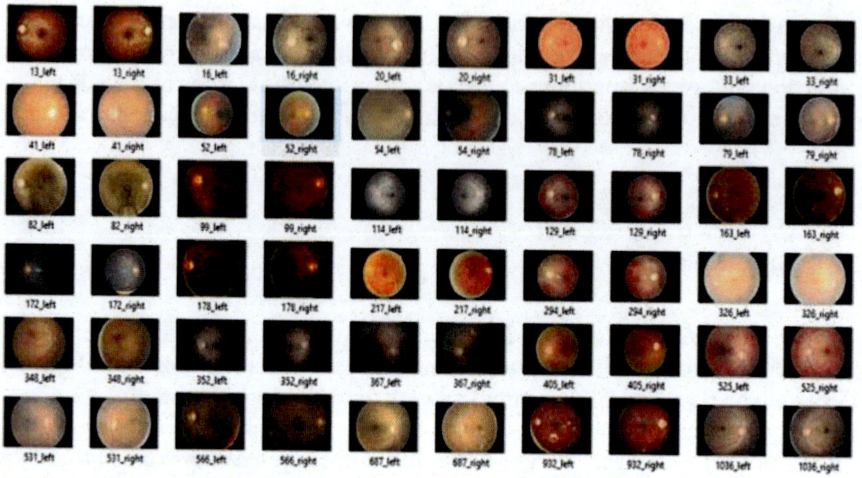

Fig. 2 Samples of fundus images for DR

platform, EyePACS in Kaggle that is available on an official Web site [3]. Figure 2 shows some samples of the retinal fundus images collected. The dataset obtained is present in multiple zip files which contain five files of training images and seven files of testing images. The fundus images obtained are sorted according to the patient's ID and provided a CSV file with five classes graded by the clinician.

The next step is image preprocessing. The image preprocessing techniques used in this research are image smoothing and image scaling. Image smoothing is needed to filter the noise and make the images smoother. For image scaling, the images in the dataset are resized to 224 × 224, so that they can be feed into the classification model. open source computer vision library (OpenCV) module is used to perform the image preprocessing with Python.

Image classification will be the next step after image preprocessing, and the details will be discussed in sub-section A.

2.1 Image Classification

The image classification part is divided into two layers which are detection and grading. The detection of DR is either DR (1) or no DR (0), whereas the grading of DR is classified into five levels which are no DR (0), mild non-proliferative DR (1), moderate NPDR (2), severe NPDR (3), and proliferative DR (4). Google AI technologies are utilized for image classification which are Google TensorFlow and Google Cloud Platform. The total number of fundus images used for grading of DR is 12,062 images. The total fundus images used in each level for the grading of DR are no DR (0) 2818 images, mild NPDR (1) 2443 images, moderate NPDR (2) 5220 images, severe NPDR (3) 873 images, and PDR (4) 708 images.

For Google TensorFlow, a pretrained model of MobileNet is being selected and configuration is required before trained the model. Input image resolution and relative size of the model are configurable in the model. For input image resolution, four options are 128,160,192, or 224px. Higher classification accuracy results in a longer processing time with higher image resolution. The size of the model is configured according to the fraction toward the largest size of the model. A virtual environment that implements TensorFlow API is created for the model training. MobileNet pretrained model is trained and evaluated in TensorFlow. The programming language used in TensorFlow is Python. TensorFlow is an open-source software library that will be used to train and evaluate the models. Model is a visual database that contains specialized convolutional neural networks (CNN) framework in the computer vision field.

Cloud storage and a cloud-hosted classification model will be implemented into the application. Google cloud platform (GCP) is the solution that has been selected for this research. The services that are used in this work are Cloud AutoML and Cloud storage. Before being implemented into the app, the project has to be created on the GCP Console with billing and enable the Cloud AutoML and Storage APIs for grant access. From the GCP Console, the AutoML Vision platform is accessed for the creation of the model. A new dataset for the model is created on the AutoML Vision page. Then, the retinal fundus images are uploaded to the AutoML Vision page, and the fundus images is being labeled after the image is uploaded. Next, the model is trained and created once training is completed. After the model is created, the model can be used in the application by using coding to make a prediction. By using the representational state transfer application programming interface (REST API), the application can generate the prediction from the trained model by uploading the image. In this research, Google Cloud AutoML API allowed us to train a model on the cloud in a simpler way. This method overcome the limitation of mobile phones to run huge prediction models that required large computation power. Performance of the MobileNet pretrained model is evaluated by several factors which are training accuracy, validation, cross-entropy, and test accuracy.

2.2 *Mobile Application*

Figure 3 illustrated the development of the mobile application. First, the mobile application is designed then comes the implementation of the mobile application. After the model has been trained and created, the model will be implemented into the mobile application. Xcode is selected to implement the mobile application. It is a native integrated development environment (IDE) for developing Apple's product Operating System. Xcode is built on Objective C and Swift. As the research is developing a machine learning model in the application, native IDE is more suitable compared to hybrid framework software development kit because native IDE has

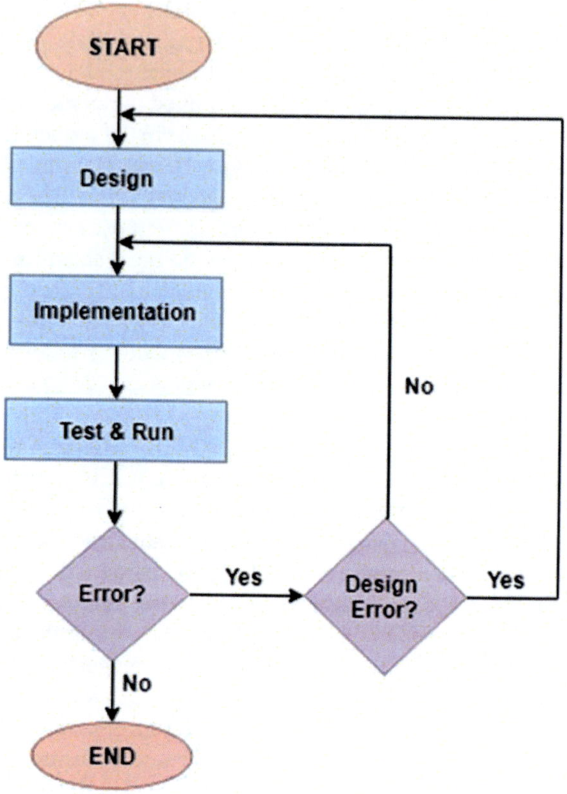

Fig. 3 Flowchart of the mobile application development

more features and supports more external libraries. In the case of this project, the TensorFlow-experimental library is required for our model's operation. Swift is the native programming language for iOS which is used in Xcode. After implementation, the mobile application will be tested and run to ensure if it functions well without error. If there is an error occurred, then, it detects the error and debugs the errors.

3 Results

Figure 4 indicates the progress of the training and validation accuracy of the trained model. The *x*-axis shows the training step which is set to 50,000 steps. Training accuracy is the accuracy of model prediction with the correct label in the current training batch in which each batch chooses ten random training images for training. Validation accuracy is the accuracy of the model predicting the randomly selected images from a different set. From Fig. 4, the training and validation accuracy is proving that the trained model is not overfitted.

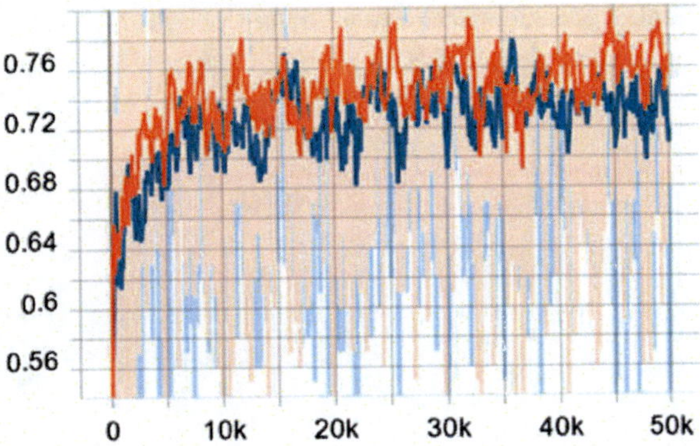

Fig. 4 Accuracy graph of the trained model

Upon completing the training for detection of DR, the final validation accuracy evaluation is proceeded based on a bundle of images from the validation dataset. The final validation accuracy of the MobileNet model is 82.9% while the final training and validation accuracy are both 74% as shown in Fig. 4.

During the grading of DR, the initial results indicate that confusion occurs as most images are validated as level 2. Thus, due to the imbalance number of fundus images used for the training process, the images used for level 2 are decreased to 2721. A total of 9563 images are used for training, and 951 images are used for testing. For the model trained in Google Cloud AutoML for the grading of DR, the averaging precision is 75% as shown in Fig. 5. From the confusion matrix created from the AutoML evaluation tab, the model is proven that it can classify each class of labels correctly with little confusion as given in Table 1.

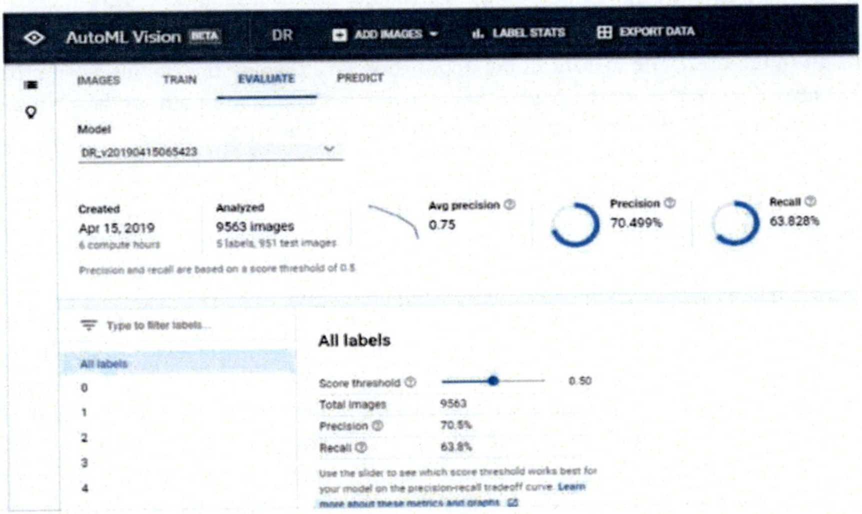

Fig. 5 Training results presented by Cloud AutoML

Table 1 Confusion matrix of the trained model in Google Cloud AutoML

True label \ Predicted label	2	1	0	3	4
2	61.2%	22.0%	10.4%	4.9%	1.5%
1	17.8%	61.0%	20.7%	-	0.4%
0	3.7%	6.6%	89.7%	-	-
3	43.2%	3.4%	1.1%	44.3%	8.0%
4	23.5%	3.7%	-	17.3%	55.6%

For the development of the application on iOS, the Xcode 10 and iPhone were utilized. The application is designed to capture the retina by using the smartphone's camera with auto-detection of fundus image. Figure 6 illustrated the design and the process flow of the mobile application. In the main interface of the application, the user is allowed to access the history of the fundus image with grade and the screening model. In screening mode, the fundus image is taken by the camera with the AV foundation framework on iOS. The MobileNet model is implemented to detect and auto-capture the fundus image in this phase. After the application capture the retina image, diagnosis on the image is run by the detection model initially. If the image was taken and it shows that it is detected with DR, then the image will proceed to the grading phase by uploading the image into Google Cloud AutoML. The result of the captured fundus images is displayed on the screen after classification is done. The grading phase would proceed once the device is connected to the network. The screening tool is designed to capture the fundus image through a mobile phone's camera with the aid of an external tool and classifies the image and then displays the result to the user. The history in the application will display the fundus image that has been analyzed from the past. Fundus image is then stored with the label of the result with the ability to share the results via email or another method.

4 Discussion

A powerful neural network is required, so that high accuracy classification can be achieved although the patterns between different levels/classes/labels are alike. Thus, the deep neural network is chosen in this research. MobileNet is implemented in the mobile application for the detection of DR, while the AutoML model is used for classification through the Cloud AutoML API for Internet-connected devices. AutoML is used in this work to solve the limited power of the mobile phone. Although classification models can be implemented into the mobile device with conversion nowadays, the performance of the model on cloud and computer is still better than

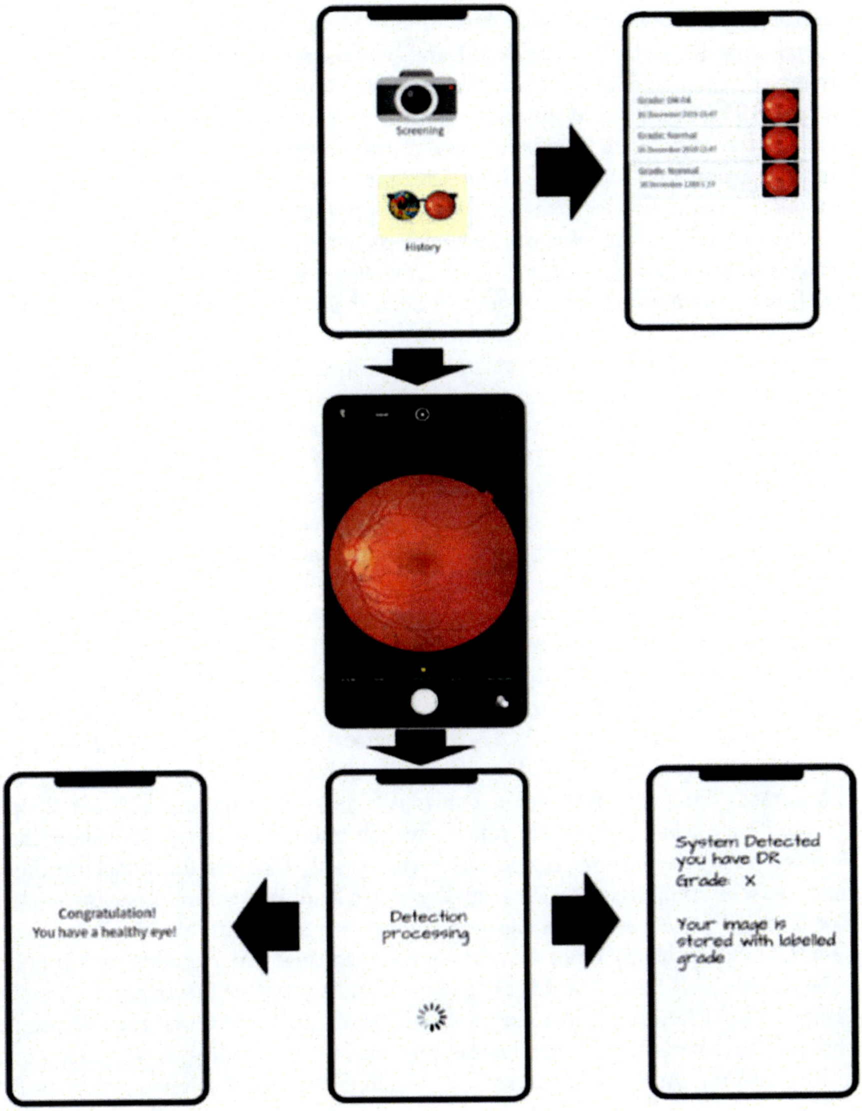

Fig. 6 Process flow of the mobile application

on mobile due to the computational power. Thus, the grading of the DR phase that is predicted by AutoML requires a high-performance model with a high demand for computational power.

MobileNet_v1_1.0_224 is the pretrained model that used in this work. The input image size is 224px * 224px. The pretrained model can cut off the time for training the model. MobileNet is suitable because it is a lightweight deep neural network for efficient on-device vision. The architecture of MobileNet is light due to the usage of depth-wise separable convolution. Depth-wise separable convolution reduces the number of parameters and reduces the multiplication of floating points during the operation. This results in MobileNet requiring less computational power to operate. In model training, much time is required to train a large DNN from scratch. Thus, transfer learning is a technique that reuses the lower layers of the existing neural network to accomplish the same task which is applied for this research.

To ensure the performance of the model, overfitting checking is required. Overfitting occurs due to the model memorized the data instead of learned the data. From Fig. 4, if the validation accuracy graph's trend is not similar to the training graph's trend, it is said that the model is overfitting.

Hyperparameters such as learning rate, batch size, number of epochs, and network architecture might affect the accuracy of the model. Unluckily, there is no direct method of tuning the hyperparameter for a neural network to its best performance, thus, trial and error is applied. The hyperparameter of the model tuned is the learning rate and the network architecture. It is tricky to find a good learning rate as a learning rate that is set too high may lead to diverging but setting too low may cause the training to take a long time or be stuck onto a local minimum. Thus, in the final training, the learning rate is set at 0.01.

Quality of training data affected the performance of the model as model detection is based on the pattern from input data. The selected dataset consists of noise as the data is collected from multiple sources and examined by only one grader. There might be an occurrence of human error when labeling. For the grading phase, the model accuracy is very low at 23.2% than planned initially. We concluded that the accuracy of the model is affected by the quality of the retina image and the network architecture. The pretrained model that is selected only supports 224px * 224px of input image while each of the images for the training dataset having more than 3000px * 4000px which are good resolution images. To feed into the model, the input image must be compressed to a low-quality image leading to difficulty in grading the fundus image as the features for each grade show only slight differences. Therefore, a powerful model with big input data supported is required to perform the task leading to the selection of Cloud AutoML. Cloud AutoML is a service that is provided in the Google Cloud Platform. It is a machine learning model builder that enables people who are not experts in machine learning to train a high-quality model through an online platform. As Google research on machine learning has been going on for several years, Google research technology has made the models achieve faster and accurate predictions.

5 Conclusion

The smartphone is an easy way for everyone to use as a diagnostic tool of DR. We have developed an iOS mobile app integrated with a cloud-based and mobile-based classification model into the app engine. Google AutoML model in the Google Cloud platform has been applied successfully. Google Cloud Platform's tool and services have been making the research to be accomplished. The first result produce may not exceed the expected result. The mobile application for the detection and grading of DR has been successfully built. MobileNet model achieved test accuracy of 82.9% for detection of DR while the AutoML model has a 75% of averaging precision for grading of DR. For further improvement, the model will be retrained with an extra training set or other procedure which will improve the accuracy of the detection and grading system.

Acknowledgements The authors would like to thank University Malaysia Sarawak (UNIMAS) and Ministry of Science Technology and Innovation (MOSTI), Malaysia, for supporting this research through Technology Development Fund 1 (TDF05211383).

References

1. Ministry of Health Malaysia (2021) National diabetes registry report 2020
2. Zago GT, Andreão RV, Dorizzi B, Ottoni E, Salles T (2019) Diabetic retinopathy detection using red lesion localization and convolutional neural networks. Comput Biol Med. https://doi.org/10.1016/j.compbiomed.2019.103537
3. Kaggle (2015) Diabetic retinopathy detection. https://www.kaggle.com/c/diabetic-retinopathy-detection/data. Accessed 16 Feb 2019

Toward Deep Learning-Based Automated Speed and Line Change Detection System in Perspective of Bangladesh

Abdullah-Al-Mahmod, Sabbir Ahmed Usmani, Mohammad Abdus Salam, Md. Foyjul Haque Somrat, and M. Shamim Kaiser

Abstract In the smart city, major crossing and most part of the road will be under the CCTV surveillance system. This influenced the community to investigate a vision-based speed and line change detection system for traffic management in the city, ensuring both road safety and efficient road design. In this paper, we proposed a deep learning model for detecting vehicle type, speed and abrupt line change using the CCTV footage in real-time. The faster region-based convolutional neural network (fr-CNN) model is chosen in this scenario, which demonstrates amazing performance in object detection. The model is trained and validated using data acquired from a self-created traffic dataset from Dhaka. According to the results of the performance evaluation, the suggested fr-CNN model for moving vehicle status detection system outperforms the mobile-net single-shot multibox detection technique in terms of overall performance.

Keywords Object detection · CNN · Single-shot multibox detection · Road-traffic · Open CV · Tensor flow

1 Introduction

Countries' growth and development rely on futuristic concepts they adopt and technologies they implement to improve people's quality of life. Converting megacities of a developing country to smart cities can be one of the initial steps toward that. One of the crucial facts to be noticed here is the value lies in how technologies are used in this conversion of cities rather than how much technology is available.

A combination of machine learning, IoT, and automation is needed to be allowed for various applications in process of converting an ordinary city to a smart city.

Abdullah-Al-Mahmod · S. A. Usmani · M. A. Salam · Md. Foyjul Haque Somrat
Department of ICE, Bangladesh University of Professionals, Dhaka 1212, Bangladesh

M. A. Salam · M. Shamim Kaiser (✉)
Institute of Information Technology, Jahangirnagar University, Savar, Dhaka 1342, Bangladesh
e-mail: mskaiser@juniv.edu

M. S. Kaiser et al. (eds.), *Proceedings of Trends in Electronics and Health Informatics*, Lecture Notes in Networks and Systems 376,
https://doi.org/10.1007/978-981-16-8826-3_30

An example would be inclusion of smart traffic management toward deep learning-based automated speed and line change detection systems. A developing country like Bangladesh will be highly benefited if it can adopt this smart city concept and introduce smart traffic management to its highly crowded main cities.

In the past few decades, traffic jam has become one of the main challenges for the government and the people who lives in the urban areas of Bangladesh where most of the motorist's visits. Particularly at the peak time of business hours traffic scenario become very congested in places like office area, industrial area, downtown, etc. Because of unplanned rise of population and private transportation in metropolitan cities in Bangladesh, people face traveling delays, work hour losses, even road accidents.

Remedy against this issue can be implementation of smart traffic management which can begin with collecting traffic congestion information, identifying the reason for the cognition such as detecting specific vehicles that are overspeeding, illegally changing lanes and effectively apply traffic law against them. This paper discussed a concept where a simple hardware setup can detect speed and lane change of specific types of vehicles toward the deep learning-based system in perspective of Bangladesh.

2 Literature Review

Many research works have been proposed in detecting object and classify vehicles using machine learning approach.

Al-Abaid [1] mostly used MATLAB codes to process their work of controlling traffic on road by counting the number of vehicles and managing the traffic signal lights. Though the authors have not shed any light on measuring vehicle's speed or illegal lane changes.

AI Banna et al. [2] use deep CNN learning and transfer learning both approaches to identify camera model. The authors of this paper propose a deep convolutional neural network and transfer learning approach for extracting features from an images dataset.

Arinldi et al. [3] used RCNN, SVM, GMM methodological techniques in their research of classifying and estimating speed of different types of vehicles. But they did not explore the area of traffic rule violating lane change detection of vehicles.

Biswas et al. [4] used UAV and optical camera to detect speed of vehicles on the ground from the moving platform in the air by utilizing faster R-CNN, CSRT, FBIA, SSIM, etc. Authors of this research have not mentioned any detail on identifying specific vehicles or detecting illegal lane changes.

Javadi et al. [5] have developed a comprehensive mathematical model to obtain the probability density function of the vehicle's speed. Researchers of this paper concentrate on measuring speed of different vehicles, but they have not focused on other aspects like identifying vehicle type or detecting violating traffic rules like lane change.

Kaiser et al. [6] evaluate the performance of an artificial neural network-based maximum power point tracker (MPPT) which can be used for solar electric vehicles. Digital signal processor (DSP), proportional-integral derivative (PID) or proportional-integral (PI) controllers were also used to complete the overall process by the researchers.

Luvizon et al. [7] utilized SIFT, KLT and MHI algorithms to measure the speed of vehicles that circulates in urban areas via number plate identification. Other than using lots of assumptions in their approached system, authors of this paper have not unveiled any technique to identify vehicles nor detecting unlawful lane change of vehicles.

Makwana et al. [8] described a basic method of measuring vehicle speed by calculating data from starting reference point to end reference point. Researchers of this paper mainly focus on the overall concept of vehicle identification and speed measurement. They did not properly describe any specific methodology or share any hardware implementation detail either.

Miah et al. [9] focused on machine learning (ML) techniques to diagnose and detect neurodegenerative diseases. Researchers of this paper completed a comparative study of the performance of several ML techniques, including support vector machine, logistic regression, artificial neural network and many more.

Rad et al. [10] utilized CVS, a novel algorithm, and MATLAB to complete their work process. The main focus of their work was measuring the speed of various types of vehicles with coordination and calibration of a camera module that is mounted on a freeway. Other than focusing on the velocity of the vehicle, authors of this paper have not unveiled any technique to identify the vehicles or attempt to detect lane change.

Ranjit et al. [11] implemented vector-valued function and motion vector techniques to estimate the velocity of moving vehicles. Other than identifying vehicle's velocity, researchers of this paper have not described any process of identifying specific vehicles or how they change lanes illegally.

Sajib et al. [12] proposed a cost-effective, faster vehicle detection model that can be implemented for real-time applications. They have used VDL, BOF, BOVW and SVM to complete their research. Unfortunately, the authors of this paper have not described any speed measuring or illegal lane change detection process other than identifying vehicles fast.

Shahrear et al. [13] implemented YOLOv3 and OpenCV both types of algorithms in their license plate recognition-based traffic signal violation detector. Researchers of this paper have not shared any idea about more important traffic rule violations like overspeeding or illegal lane changing.

Shaikat et al. [14] use OpenCV library to identify and detect speed of different types of vehicles in online and offline mode. But the authors have not clearly mentioned how to implement their model in the real world.

Shamrat et al. [15] have developed an automatic Web-based traffic rules violation detection system where vehicles can be identified with help of Raspberry Pi. The main flaw of the research is its dependency on the Internet. Researchers of this paper concentrate on designing the system to identify the vehicles but did not concentrate on major issues like usage of low-resolution camera Raspberry camera or interruption of connectivity.

Suhao et al. [16] used DNN technique to classify and detect different types of vehicles from videos or images. Authors of this paper have not clearly mentioned any reality-based implementation procedure neither did they focus on measuring speed of the vehicles or lane change detection.

Tabassum et al. [17] utilized YOLO model to classify 15 vehicles on Bangladeshi roads. In spite of this, the authors have not estimated vehicle speeds nor have they discovered vehicle traffic law violations through sudden line changes.

Tania et al. [18] utilize the state-of-the-art pre-trained models of convolutional neural network (CNN) to perform the assay-type detection of an enzyme-linked immunosorbent assay (ELISA) and lateral flow assay (LFA). The authors of this paper take initiative to define colorimetric assay types from the eyes of a machine and perform any colorimetric test using deep learning.

A conventional deep learning-based traffic rule violating vehicle identification model must identify vehicle type (such as car, bus, truck and bike), line change and their speed in real time. However, to the best of our knowledge, we have found that none of the published articles have not considered all of these mentioned features in the traffic rule, violating vehicle identification model.

3 Proposed System Model

Before moving to the software part, from the image below, a hypothetical hardware implementation can be seen. For this paper, a single camera has been used to capture the raw videos, but in proper installation, one camera will be required for each lane at a specific angle. Electric post poles, over bridges, etc., can be used as the primary base for these cameras. To get conti1nuous video feed, these cameras have to be connected with the Internet and hardware requirement-wise power supply (Fig. 1).

3.1 rf-CNN Model

It is a deep convolutional network that is used for object detection. The network quickly and accurately predict location of different objects. rf-CNN's process begins with generating region proposal, then by using ROI pooling layer, a fixed-length feature vector is extracted. Next, the feature vectors get classified using rf-CNN. Finally, the class scorers of detected objects returned to their bounding-boxes (Fig. 2).

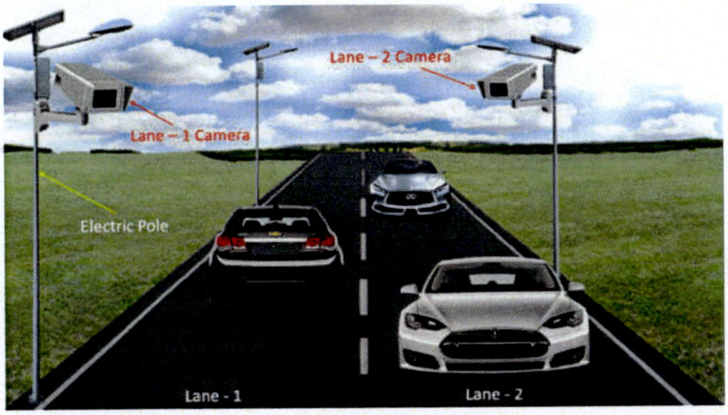

Fig. 1 Conceptual representation of system implementation

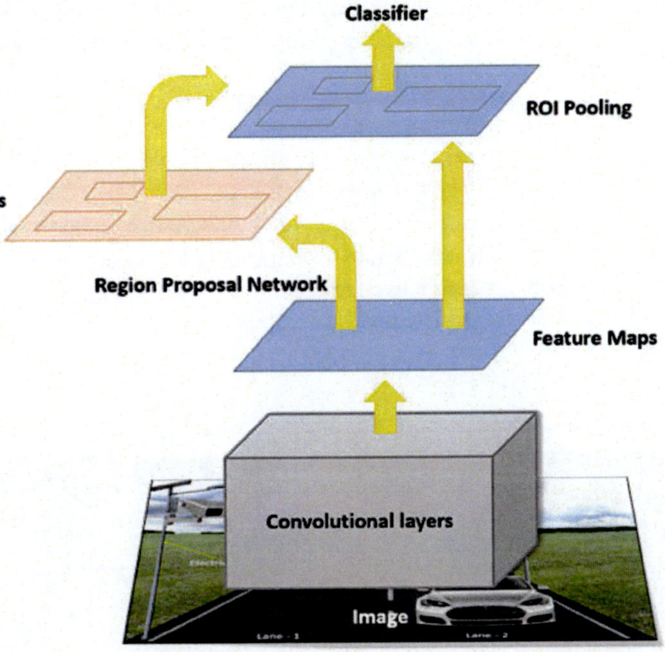

Fig. 2 The architecture of rf-CNN

3.2 *Identify Image from CCTV Footage*

First, the AVI format captured videos are extracted into single frames, and then they get converted into RGB images. Then the RGB's get converted into grayscale images. Reason behind converting to grayscale is minimizing information required for each pixel. To identify the vehicles even faster and measuring speed within a limited time, converting images into binary is helpful. So for this project, all the grayscale images are converted into binary images.

3.3 *Image Preprocessing*

Removing unnecessary areas of the video by OpenCV masked operation is the next step. Here, OpenCV help by reducing the portion that the camera has to look at. Another advantage of background masking is that it helps to specify dedicated lane for each camera (Fig. 3).

3.4 *Identifying Vehicle Type*

This process starts with subtracting backgrounds by separating reference frames where GMM model is used on each frame of the collected videos to identify moving objects. These objects get detected by clusters of moving pixels which get formed (Fig. 4).

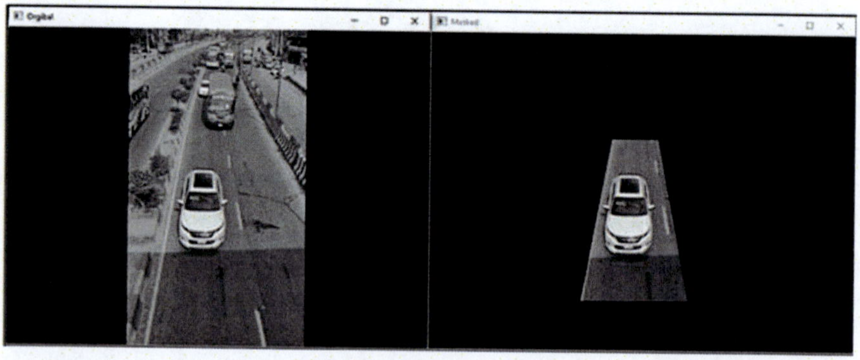

Fig. 3 Background masking

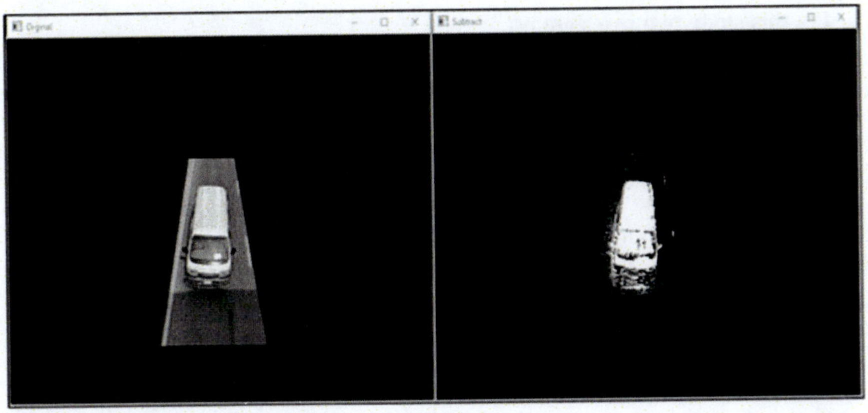

Fig. 4 Substracting backgrounds

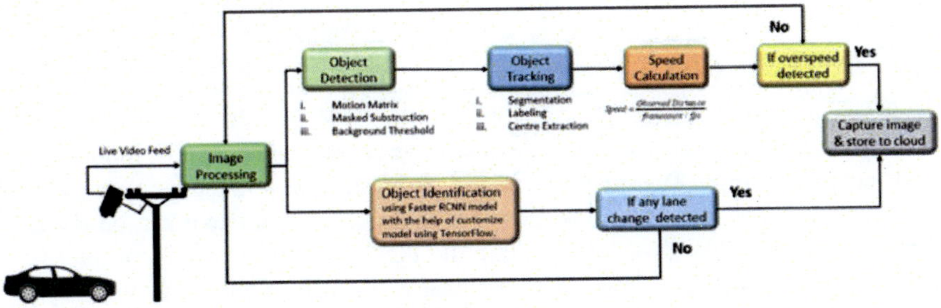

Fig. 5 Flow diagram of vehicle detection, speed measuring and storing

3.5 *Measuring Speed of Vehicles*

The flow diagram of Fig. 5 shows the overview of the proposed methodology where tracking specific types of vehicles, measuring their speed, sending and storing these records to the database are described. The cycle begins from "Image processing" where cameras capture the live video feeds. Then in "Object detection" and "Object Tracking," moving vehicles get separated from the background and unwanted objects around them via subtraction and other techniques. After that in "Speed Calculation" phase, speed of every identified vehicle gets detected and if any violation like over speed gets detected, it "Capture image and store to the cloud" for future usage.

In speed measuring step, all the vehicles get tracked from live video feed simultaneously. Here, all the centroid values are stored into a track structure that is created for this model. Speed of each identified vehicle is calculated as,

$$Speed = (ObservedDistance)/((FrameCount)/fps)$$

For this study two cases are used:

1. If (Current.centroid = Initial Position) by which the frame count started for any specific vehicle and initialize the corresponding structure variable to hold the frame count. 2. If (Current.centroid = Final Position) by which the final frame count get stored in the respective variable and calculate the total frame traversed by that vehicle in order to reach from initial position to final position.

$$Speed(i) = (Distance)/((totalframes)/fps)$$

From the above equation, speed(i) denotes the speed of the vehicle. frame per second is mentioned as fps. Total frames are the number of frames traversed over the distance. Speed here is calculated in the number of pixels traveled per second unit; it is converted into kilometer per hour (km/h) unit. This conversion is implemented by taking the actual distance measure of the area covered by the camera view.

3.6 Detecting Line Change

As mentioned previously for this project, a single camera and a specific model is used to detect lane change. The model is trained with four types of vehicle data so that it can detect car, bus, van and truck these four vehicles, this number can be changed. The model works like this, let's assume the lane that the camera is monitoring is specified for a car only. Now if any car passes through this lane, then the system detects it as normal. But if any bus, van or truck gets identified on this lane, the system will identify them as illegal lane changers and will capture an image of that vehicle instantly to send it at specific cloud storage.

4 Results and Discussion

The purpose of the project is to design a system that can reduce traffic jam and road accidents through its systematic approach. This paper describes a system which is specially designed for developing and underdeveloped countries by integrating efficient models, workable algorithms, commonly available hardware and smart technologies.

After compilation of all methodological steps above, some desired findings were generated. The first finding is about identifying the vehicles. The research team tagged and trained the system to identify four main types of vehicles which are car, bus, van, and truck. Subcategories like minibus, mini truck and micro-bus were included in the main categories to avoid conflicts. Developing a system to identify specific types of vehicles was one of the main targets of this research. The system identified 85% of the vehicles it was trained to identify. The system will be able to identify more types of vehicles if needed as per demand and the identification percentage will remain the same.

Table 1 Dataset used in this project after filtarization

Sl	Vehicle type	No. of vehicle
1	Car	83
2	Bus	68
3	Truck	39
4	Van	35
	Total	225

Table 2 Performance evaluation of the speed detection by the fr-CNN

Vehicle count	Speed (actual)	Speed (Estimated)	Error (in %)
1	26.8	27	0.7
2	26	27	3
3	21	20	5
4	25.3	27	6
5	27	28.9	6
6	23	23.8	3
7	22	21.3	3
8	28	57	50
9	22	22.5	2
10	26	25.3	2

4.1 Dataset

Every research project is unique from its own point of view and need personalized modifications. There are lots of vehicle datasets available on internet, but as per our requirements and perspective, most of them did not match properly. Our raw video footage collection get hampered several times because of lockdown situation in Bangladesh. We collect video footage from several points that we selected earlier. Finally, the dataset we used in this project in given in Table 1.

4.2 Speed Detection

In Table 2 the comparison between real-time speed and the proposed model detected speed is provided. From this table, the percentage of speed difference can be identified.

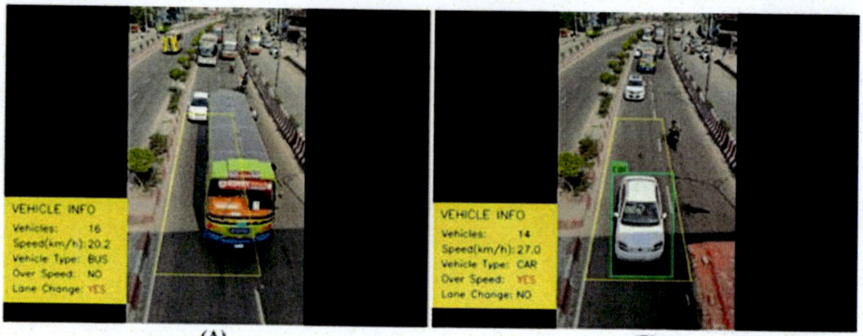

(A) (B)

Fig. 6 Lane change detection

4.3 Line Change Detection

Finding of the vehicle's line change comes next. This proposed system is trained to separate lanes for a specific vehicle. Whenever any other type of vehicle appears in that lane, the system successfully identifies the vehicle as an intruder for that exact lane. So far, this line change detecting success percentage is 85%. Lane change in this proposed system is dependent on object detection. The accuracy of detecting lane change gets higher when the accuracy of detecting an object is precise (Fig. 6).

The proposed system identified the left lane for private cars only. Now from the above "Image A," it is clearly shown that the system detects a lane change while a bus is passing through the lane. But when a car is passing the lane as per image B, the lane change is showing NO sign. So these images show the model is working perfectly to identify lane change.

5 Conclusion

Converting crowded and over populated cities of Bangladesh to smart cities where deep learning-based traffic management system will minimize traffic jam, road accident and air pollution is not just a dream anymore. The conversion may take some time, but it is possible by taking small step toward it by implementing projectes like this one which is described above.

This research tried to design a system that detects vehicles that are violating traffic rules and causing issues like traffic jam and road accidents. A few issues were raised while working on the project, but alternative ways are also get founded and the final result shows an accuracy rate of 85% in vehicle identification and lane change detection. Speed measurement of the vehicles also shows sufficient accuracy. Conceptually, it is an expendable field as well where improvement and integration both are possible in related future projects.

References

1. Al-Abaid SAF (2020) A smart traffic control system using image processing: a review. J Southwest Jiaotong Univ 55(1)
2. Al Banna MH, Haider MA, Al Nahian MJ, Islam MM, Taher KA, Kaiser MS (2019) Camera model identification using deep CNN and transfer learning approach. In: 2019 international conference on robotics, electrical and signal processing techniques (ICREST). IEEE, pp 626–630
3. Arinaldi A, Pradana JA, Gurusinga AA (2018) Detection and classification of vehicles for traffic video analytics. Procedia Comput Sci 144:259–268
4. Biswas D, Su H, Wang C, Stevanovic A (2019) Speed estimation of multiple moving objects from a moving uav platform. ISPRS Int J Geo Inf 8(6):259
5. Javadi S, Dahl M, Pettersson MI (2019) Vehicle speed measurement model for video-based systems. Comput Electr Eng 76:238–248
6. Kaiser MS, Aditya SK, Mazumder RK (2006) Performance evaluation of a maximum power point tracker (mppt) for solar electric vehicle using artificial neural network
7. Luvizon DC, Nassu BT, Minetto R (2016) A video-based system for vehicle speed measurement in urban roadways. IEEE Trans Intell Transp Syst 18(6):1393–1404
8. Makawana B, Goel P (2013) Moving vehicle detection and speed measurement in video sequence. Int J Eng Res Tehnol (IJERT), str pp 3534–3537
9. Miah Y, Prima CNE, Seema SJ, Mahmud M, Kaiser MS (2021) Performance comparison of machine learning techniques in identifying dementia from open access clinical datasets. In: Advances on smart and soft computing. Springer, pp 79–89
10. Rad AG, Dehghani A, Karim MR (2010) Vehicle speed detection in video image sequences using cvs method. Int J Phys Sci 5(17):2555–2563
11. Ranjit S, Anas S, Subramaniam S, Lim K, Fayeez A, Amirah A (2012) Real-time vehicle speed detection algorithm using motion vector technique
12. Sajib MSR, Tareeq SM (2018) Real time feature based vehicle detection and classification from on-road videos. Dhaka Univ J Appl Sci Eng 4(2):91–101
13. Shahrear R, Rahman MA, Islam A, Dey C, Zishan MSR (2020) An automatic traffic rules violation detection and number plate recognition system for Bangladesh. AIUB J Sci Eng (AJSE) 19(2):87–98
14. Shaikat AS, Saleheen RU, Tasnim R, Mahmud R, Mahbub F, Islam T (2019) An image processing and artificial intelligence based traffic signal control system of dhaka. In: 2019 Asia Pacific conference on research in industrial and systems engineering (APCoRISE). IEEE, pp 1–6
15. Shamrat FJM, Mahmud I, Rahman AS, Majumder A, Tasnim Z, Nobel NI (2020) A smart automated system model for vehicles detection to maintain traffic by image processing. Int J Sci Technol Res 9(02):2921–2928
16. Suhao L, Jinzhao L, Guoquan L, Tong B, Huiqian W, Yu P (2018) Vehicle type detection based on deep learning in traffic scene. Procedia Comput Sci 131:564–572
17. Tabassum S, Ullah MS, Al-Nur NH, Shatabda S (2020) Native vehicles classification on Bangladesh roads using CNN with transfer learning. In: 2020 IEEE region 10 symposium (TENSYMP). IEEE, pp 40–43
18. Tania MH, Lwin KT, Shabut AM, Abu-Hassan KJ, Kaiser MS, Hossain MA (2019) Assay type detection using advanced machine learning algorithms. In: 2019 13th international conference on software, knowledge, information management and applications (SKIMA). IEEE, pp 1–8

Automated Acute Lymphocytic Leukemia (ALL) Detection Using Microscopic Images: An Efficient CAD Approach

Tahmina Akter Sumi, Mohammad Shahadat Hossain, and Karl Andersson

Abstract Leukemia, which is caused by the excessive and aberrant reproduction of white blood cells, completely destroys the immune system of our body and leads to death. Among four different types of leukemia, the progress of acute lymphocytic leukemia is rapid and becomes fatal even in weeks if it is kept untreated. So, early diagnosis of ALL is quite necessary. In manual methods, pathologists diagnose ALL by the microscopic test of blood specimen or bone marrow test. Though this is the most efficient process to diagnose ALL, it is a time-consuming matter. In this case, computer-aided diagnosis (CAD) may be considered as a great associative diagnostic tool for ALL identification. Numerous supervised and unsupervised machine learning algorithms have been proposed for ALL detection for years. This paper concerns with establishing a CNN- based CAD system for automated ALL detection from the microscopic blood images which is collected from ALL-IDB dataset. In this regard, at first the images have been preprocessed applying median filter and histogram equalization for the purpose of reducing the noise and enhancing the image. Being smaller in size, data augmentation has been applied on the dataset which increases the images by including slightly modified copies of images that already exist in the dataset. Finally, the modified images are passed through a CNN model for training purpose where feature extraction and classification are performed by convolution, ReLU, pooling layer, and a fully connected layer. Here, the dataset is also trained using some pretrained model to show a comparison of our model with other models. It is observed that our proposed model results as a well fitting model with 100% training accuracy and 97.89% testing accuracy which is promising.

Keywords Acute lymphocytic leukemia · Computer-aided diagnosis · Median filter · Histogram equalization · CNN

T. A. Sumi (✉) · M. S. Hossain
Department of Computer Science and Engineering, University of Chittagong, Chittagong, Bangladesh

K. Andersson
Pervasive and Mobile Computing Laboratory, Luleå University of Technology, Skellefteå, Sweden

M. S. Kaiser et al. (eds.), *Proceedings of Trends in Electronics and Health Informatics*, Lecture Notes in Networks and Systems 376,
https://doi.org/10.1007/978-981-16-8826-3_31

1 Introduction

Leukemia, also written as leukaemia, is a Greek word which means white blood cell [5]. It originates in the bone marrow and after that causes excessive numbers of abnormal blood cells. So, leukemia can be considered as a type of cancer which mainly makes bad effect on the blood, lymphocyte system, and bone marrow [23]. Blood generally comprises four types of elements, namely white blood cells (WBCs), red blood cells (RBCs), platelets, and plasma [8]. Leukemia is related to the white blood cells (WBCs) which yields a large number of aberrant WBCs and damages the immune system of our body. Leukemia is subdivided into two categories based on the growth rate which are acute (rapidly increases the immature blood cells) and chronic (spreads slowly). Additionally based on which blood cell is affected, the disease is classified into two categories, namely lymphoblastic (produces lymphocytes) and myeloid (produces other WBCs, RBCs, and platelets). Therefore, combining these sub-categories, leukemia is categorized into four different types such as acute lymphoblastic leukemia (ALL), acute myelogenous leukemia (AML), chronic lymphoblastic leukemia (CLL), and chronic myelogenous leukemia (CML). In our study, we have focused on the acute lymphoblastic leukemia (ALL) detection from the microscopic blood images. ALL caused by the over regeneration of immature white blood cells in the bone marrow is generally noticed in children [10].

ALL is diagnosed by hematologists manually from blood test by checking the presence of blast cells or calculating the number of WBC to check whether there is too many or too few white blood cells. But this process has some drawbacks. Only blood test is not enough to fruitfully detect ALL. A bone marrow aspiration and biopsy are also performed in this case. But these are really time-consuming matter moreover not highly accurate. On the contrary, this problem of manual diagnosis can be overthrown by automated diagnostic systems. Furthermore, the hassle of medical professional can be assuaged and accurate, and fruitful result can be provided comparing with manual diagnosing. Therefore, a computer-aided detection approach can be a effective diagnostic tool in case of ALL detection. So in this paper, an efficient CAD approach has been proposed for ALL detection considering the drawbacks mentioned above and for reducing the hassle of medical diagnosis.

Several CAD approaches have been introduced for ALL detection from the microscopic blood images since years. For classification, most of the research works used traditional machine learning algorithm [9, 32, 33]. However, comparing with other traditional machine learning algorithm, CNN which is a deep learning approach proved to perform better in case of image classification [7, 12, 27, 34]. In this study, we have applied CNN on the microscopic blood images collected from a public dataset (ALL-IDB). Our main goal behind this research work is to gain a better accuracy in detecting ALL which tends to lessen the error rate of treating the ALL patient. In this regard, at first the images are prepossessed by applying median filter for reducing the noise and histogram equalization for increasing the sharpness of images. Since the dataset (ALL-IDB) is relatively smaller in size, the number of images has been increased using the augmentation technique. Finally, the dataset is passed through convolutional neural network(CNN) for training purpose. Finally, a classification part is conducted to identify the blood images as healthy or ALL blast cell.

The following sections of this paper are organized as follows: Sect. 2 describes the previous works based on ALL detection. Section 3 depicts the entire methodology where whole CNN model used in this paper has been illustrated broadly. Section 4 is about the result of our research, and finally Sect. 5 is about conclusion and future work.

2 Literature Review

In case of ALL detection, several research works have been conducted since ages. In these studies, different machine and deep learning algorithm have been presented for ALL detection.

Kumar et al. [19] in 2018 have presented a model for ALL identification where they have utilized KNN and Naive Bayes classifier. In this research, they have used 60 sample images for ALL detection which is quite low. They have achieved an accuracy of 92.8% which can be further improved. Jothi et al. [16] at first have segmented the images by BSA-based clustering. After that, ALL has been identified using decision tree, KNN, NB, LDA, SVM and ensemble random undersampling boost. In this case, SVM and decision tree have showed a better accuracy. In [21], S. A. Kareem et al. have proposed a proficient selection and feature extraction process to detect ALL where the classification has been performed by KNN using Euclidean distance. The best accuracy they have found by this research is 92.5%. Ahmed et al. [2] have worked on leukemia classification where they have categorized ALL vs healthy samples, and thereafter, they have classified the subtypes of leukemia. In this research, they have used CNN for classification and achieved 88.25% accuracy for ALL vs healthy classification and 81.74% accuracy in case of subtypes of leukemia classification. Thanh et al. [35] in 2018 showed a decent accuracy of 96.60% using CNN where they have used ALL-IDB1 dataset for the diagnosis of leukemia. In [25], the authors have utilized the ALL-IDB1 and ALL-IDB2 datasets to detect ALL. However, in this research, SVM was applied for the classification of ALL vs healthy samples where the accuracy of this classification was 89.81%. In [1], ALL-IDB1 dataset has been employed for ALL detection based on cell energy features where SVM was applied for the classification. The authors attained 94.00% accuracy in this case. In [38], the authors have utilized ALL-IDB2 dataset for ALL detection where KNN method has been employed for classification with 96.25% accuracy.

Among some very recent studies, Janaki [15] in 2020 established computer-aided diagnosis to detect leukemia using the microscopic image of blood. Here the authors entailed a preprocessing technique which is adaptive filtering, a segmentation step to segment WBCs from blood image and feature extraction where features, i.e., entropy, energy, and correlation had been extracted from the segmented WBCs. Finally, Gaussian feature convolutional visual recognition had been utilized for classifying WBCs as normal or abnormal. The authors obtained 95.59% accuracy after implementation. Nikitaev et al. [26] in the same year proposed another computer-aided diagnosis system for identifying the abnormal cells from bone marrow image. Here two segmentation techniques (histogram analysis and watershed) were applied to separate the nucleus. After the feature extraction, KNN, SVM, and random forest have been applied individually for classification. The result the authors gained after implementation was 89, 85, and 80% which is not much satisfactory and can be improved. Continuously, Bodzas et al. [11] in 2020 have proposed a three-phase filtration algorithm for segmentation. Furthermore, 16 features have been extracted from the segmented images, and thereafter, SVM classifier has been used for the recognition of leukemic cells. The authors claimed an accuracy of 96.72% in their study of leukemia detection.

After analyzing all the previous works that have been established in case of ALL detection, it can be said that an improvement in ALL detection is necessary. So, in this research, we have tried to recover the lacking and to improve the result of ALL identification using CNN which is a multilayer neural network model as CNN can optimize filters utilizing automated learning which helps to achieve a superior performance [22].

3 Methodology

3.1 Dataset

The dataset for ALL detection has been collected from a public source named ALL-IDB [20]. It contains peripheral blood images from the ALL affected patient and healthy individuals. These samples have been collected from M. Tettamanti Research Center, Monza, Italy. This dataset is more reliable as it is labeled by expert oncologists. The ALL-IDB dataset consists of two groups: ALL-IDB1 and ALL-IDB2.

- ALL-IDB1: ALL-IDB1, which is the first group of ALL-IDB dataset, contains 108 microscopic blood images (49 images of patients and 59 images of healthy person). The resolution of the first 33 images of ALL-IDB1 dataset is 1712 × 1368. However, the rest images of this group have a resolution of 2592 × 1944. The images have been taken with different magnifications where the microscopic ranging is from 300 to 500.
- ALL-IDB2: ALL-IDB2 is the aggregation of cropped images of the normal and abnormal cells which are collected from ALL-IDB1 dataset. This dataset consists of 260 images where the 50% images represents blast cells.

We have considered the first group which is ALL-IDB1 in this research for ALL detection.

3.2 Preprocessing

Image preprocessing is required to clean the image data before the model training and inference. The microscopic blood images are generally corrupted by various noises and also may have some blurred regions. So in this research, a preprocessing technique has been applied to diminish the noise and make a better view of the image data for efficient result.

Different filtering techniques are used in image preprocessing for reducing the noise. Here, we have employed median filter on the dataset for removing the noise and making the images smooth. Further we have utilized histogram equalization on the dataset for enhancing the contrast of the images. The histogram equalization is accomplished on a small area of an image. It increases the contrast of each small area of that image. This enables CNN to analyze the dataset in a better way. Figure 1 illustrates resulted images after applying median filter and histogram equalization.

3.3 Augmentation

Data augmentation is a process of increasing dataset by combining slightly modified copies of data that already exist. This process helps to reduce overfitting by maximizing the size of dataset which increase the efficiency of the architecture. The features of a large dataset can be easily extracted while it is quite challenging in case of a dataset containing insufficient data. However, data augmentation can boost the model accuracy when the dataset is insufficient.

Since the ALL-IDB1 dataset is limited (108 images in a whole) for deep learning approach, it may lead to overfitting. That is why we have applied some data augmentation techniques to maximize dataset. For this augmentation, ImageDataGenerator has been utilized here. The settings for image augmentation that we utilized have been illustrated in Table 1.

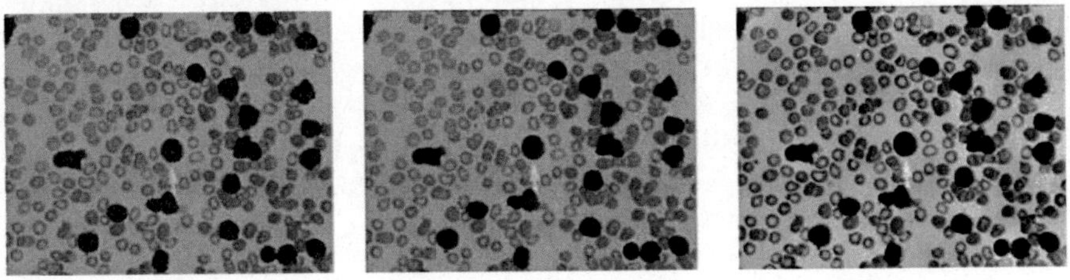

a b c

Fig. 1 Preprocessing steps: **a** Initial microscopic blood image. **b** Median filter effect on image. **c** Histogram equalization effect on image

Table 1 Data augmentation settings

Augmentation techniques	Range
Rotation	25
Width shift	0.10
Height shift	0.10
Zoom	0.40
Horizontal flip	True
Fill mode	Nearest

3.4 CNN Model

After performing the data augmentation on the training dataset, images are passed on to the CNN which is a deep learning model. CNNs are proficient in learning the raw data automatically [3, 6, 29, 40]. A typical convolutional neural network starts with several layers, i.e., convolutional, activation, and max pooling layer, and thereafter finally at the end, a fully connected layer is used. Our proposed model includes two components, namely feature extraction and classification. The convolutional, activation, and pooling layers serve the feature extraction part, and the classification part is executed by fully connected layer.

Feature extraction In the feature extraction part, at first the convolutional layer containing 32 filters of 3×3 kernel size is applied. The features are then passed through the ReLU activation function followed by batch normalization which generate low-level features of convolution. A pooling layer with 3×3 pool size is employed to minimize the spatial dimension. To alleviate the overfitting problem, a dropout layer is utilized which works by disconnecting nodes randomly from layer to layer.

Therefore, the convolutional layer is applied twice along with ReLU and batch normalization. In this case, after applying the first convolutional layer, the filter size increases from 32 to 64. However, the second convolutional layer does not make any change in the filter size, but it helps to learn richer set of features. Therefore, the filter size remains 64. A pooling layer is again applied, but this time the pool size is reduced to 2×2 so that the spatial dimension does not get reduced promptly.

The convolutional layer, ReLU activation function, and pooling layer are applied for the final time. Here, again the convolutional layer and ReLU activation function are applied twice. This helps to increase the filter size from 64 to 128. The pool size of the pooling layer remains same as before which is 2×2. A dropout layer of 25% is applied for the final time.

Classification A fully connected layer and ReLU function is employed here, and since there are two categories of output, a sigmoid function has been applied for classifying the images. The dense (1024) is employed as fully connected layer which is further followed by ReLU and batch normalization. The sigmoid activation function is applied just after the fully connected layer to classify the images as "healthy" or "patient" categories.

$$\text{Sigmoid}(x) = \frac{1}{1 + \mathrm{e}^{-\theta^T x}}$$

4 Result

The outcomes after implementing our model on ALL-IDB1 dataset have been explained in detail in this section. The result after applying fivefold cross-validation has been illustrated. In addition, we have also shown the comparison of our proposed model with other traditional models and previous works.

4.1 K-fold Cross-Validation

The K-fold cross-validation is a resampling method which is used for utilization of different train and test data. It also reduces the overfitting problem and helps to improve generalization capacity. In this research, we have attempted fivefold cross-validation for assessing our model. In Table 2, the training and testing accuracies after applying fivefold cross-validation have been demonstrated where individual accuracy for each fold is added. The average (98.53% training and 93.53% testing) and best (100% training and 97.89% testing) accuracies are also added in the table which are calculated from the fivefold cross-validation. Figure 2 graphically represents the curve of accuracy vs epoch for fivefold cross-validation on ALL-IDB1 dataset. Here each fold is highlighted using different colored line.

Table 2 Data augmentation settings

Fold	Training accuracy (%)	Testing accuracy (%)
1	100	96.30
2	98.20	97.58
3	97.15	89.34
4	97.34	86.55
5	100	97.89
Average accuracy	98.53	93.53
Best accuracy	100	97.89

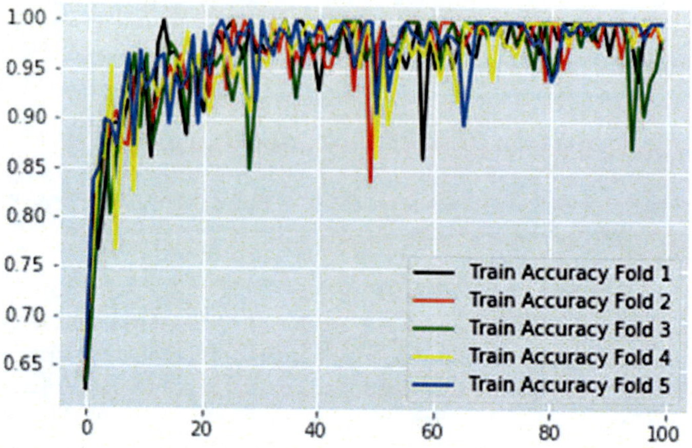

Fig. 2 Accuracy versus epoch for fivefold cross-validation

4.2 Performance Metrics

To test the efficacy and to assess the overall performance of our proposed model, we have attempted several performance measures, i.e., recall, precision, and $F1$-score. The mathematical expression for these performance metrics is illustrated in Table 3. Here, TP refers to the true positive rate, FP refers to the false positive rate, TN refers to the true negative rate, and FN refers to the false negative rate.

It is exhibited from Table 4 that for healthy sample, the precision is 93%, recall is 100%, and $F1$-score is 96%, while in case of ALL, the precision is 100%, recall is 95%, and $F1$-score is 97%.

Figure 3 shows the confusion matrices after implementing our model on ALL-IDB1 dataset.

Table 3 Data augmentation settings

Measures	Derivations
Precision	$\frac{TP}{TP+FN}$
Recall	$\frac{TP}{TP+FN}$
$F1$-score	$2.\frac{Precision\ .\ Recall}{Precision+Recall}$

Table 4 Different parameters

Performance Measures	Healthy	ALL	Macro average
Precision	0.93	1.00	0.96
Recall	1.00	0.95	0.97
$F1$-score	0.96	0.97	0.97

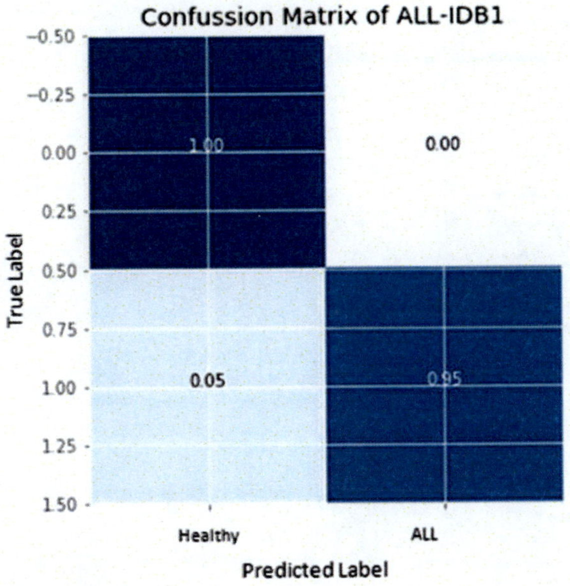

Fig. 3 Model accuracy and model loss

4.3 Comparison of Proposed Model

This section is about the comparison of our proposed model with other pre-trained models like Inception-v3, ResNet50, Xception, VGG-16, VGG-19, and MobileNetV2. Here, a comparison and discussion of our study with various previous works have also been highlighted.

From Table 5, it is clear that the VGG-19 and VGG-16 are under fitting model as the training accuracy is less than the testing accuracy, where the Xception, InceptionV3, ResNet50, and MobileNetV2 are overfitting models since the difference between training and testing accuracy is much greater. However, comparing with all these models CNN can be acknowledged as wellfitting model with training accuracy 100% and testing accuracy 97.89%.

Table 5 Comparison of results

Models	Training accuracy	Training loss	Testing accuracy	Testing loss
Proposed model	1.00	0.0189	0.9789	0.0754
VGG-19	0.7031	0.5842	0.8030	0.5757
VGG-16	0.7188	0.5961	0.7424	0.5878
InceptionV3	0.7273	0.5349	0.6212	0.6596
Xception	0.9922	0.2245	0.4697	0.6519
ResNet50	0.9766	0.1234	0.3485	0.7260
MobileNetV2	1.00	0.1450	0.4545	0.9026

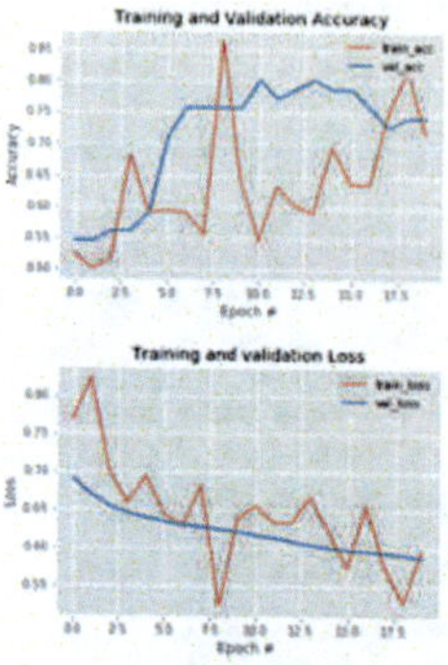

VGG-16 acc and loss

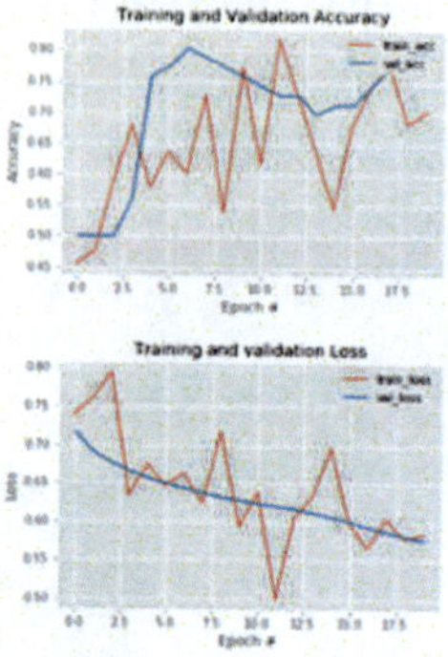

VGG-19 acc and loss

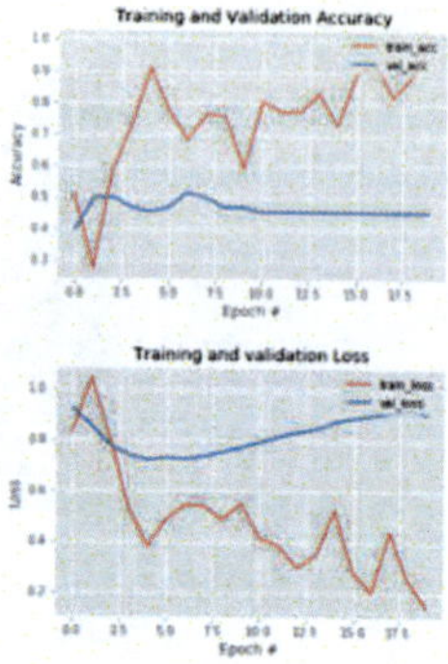

MobileNetV2 acc and loss

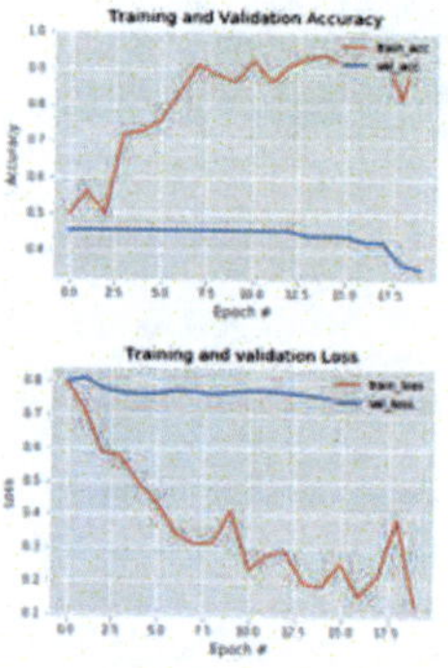

ResNet50 acc and loss

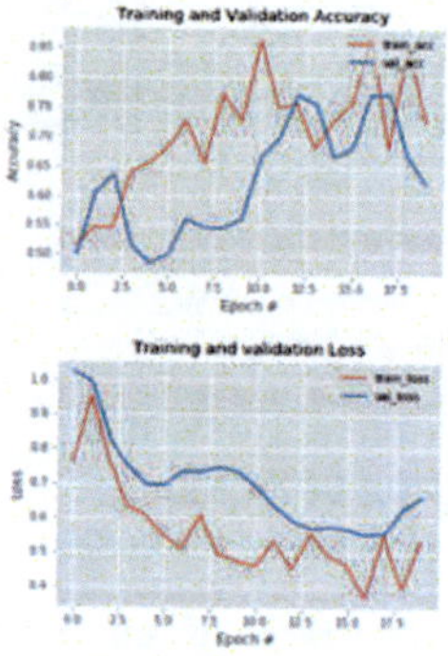

InceptionV3 acc and loss

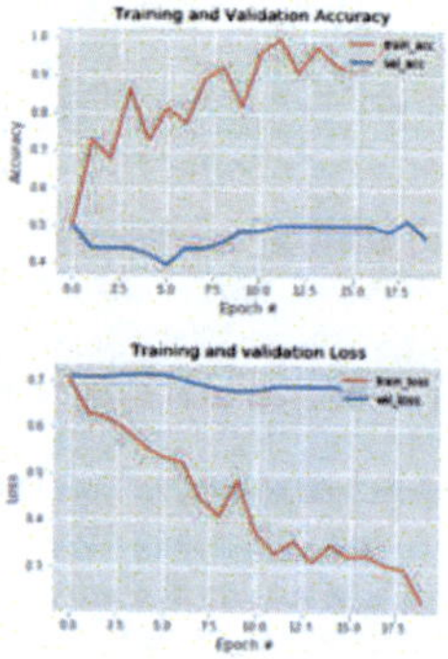

Xception acc and loss

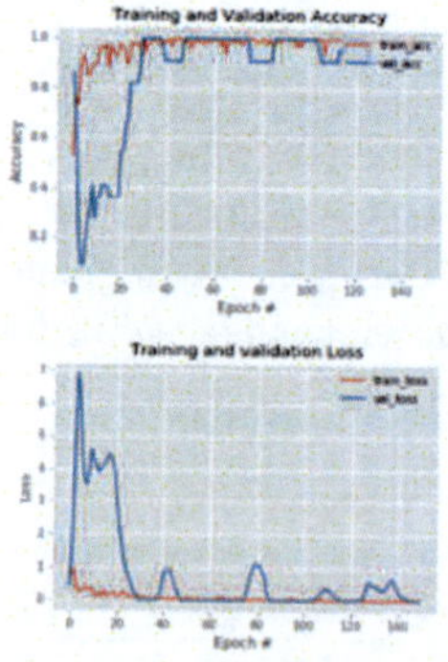

Prop osed model acc and loss

Fig. 4 Accuracy and loss curve of proposed model and other traditional models

Table 6 Comparison with previous works

Reference	Dataset	Classifier	Accuracy (%)
Singhal and Singh [32]	ALL-IDB	SVM	89.72
Bhattacharjee et al. [9]	ALL-IDB	KNN	95.23
Singhal and Singh [33]	ALL-IDB	KNN	93.84
Sahlol et al. [30]	ALL-IDB	KNN	95.67
Sahlol et al. [31]	ALL-IDB	SVM	96.11
Mohapatra et al. [24]	ALL-IDB	SVM	95
Ahmed et al. [2]	ALL-IDB	CNN	88.25
Tuba and Tuba [36]	ALL-IDB2	GAO-based methods	93.84
Al-jaboriy et al. [4]	ALL-IDB1	GA and ANN	97.07
Thanh et al. [35]	ALL-IDB1	CNN	96.60
Agaian et al. [1]	ALL-IDB1	Cell energy feature with SVM	94.00
Moshavash et al. [25]	ALL-IDB1, ALL-IDB2, Dr. Juan Bruno Zayas Alfonso Hospital, Santiago de Cuba	Two ensemble classifiers with SVM	89.81
Proposed method	ALL-IDB1	CNN	97.89

In Fig. 4, the curve of accuracy and loss function of our models as well as other models is illustrated.

In Table 6, a comparison of our proposed approach to other previous works has been illustrated in brief. Here, the classification techniques with the dataset that have been used in the previous papers with their performance are mentioned. As we can see, our proposed methods outperform all the previous works with 97.89% accuracy.

5 Conclusion and Future Work

The possibility of a successful cancer treatment primarily increases when it is detected early. ALL which is the most ordinary kind of blood cancer can be detected by examining the bone marrow and blood samples. But this process of detecting ALL takes time a lot moreover it may be error prone. So, a CAD approach for automatic ALL detection may be considered as a great associative diagnostic tool. In this research, a CAD approach is proposed for the ALL detection where microscopic blood images have been used. As the blood image samples are full of noise, a median filter and histogram equalization have been applied for enhancing the image quality. Being smaller in size, augmentation technique has been applied on the dataset which increases the size of it. A deep learning method has been adapted for classifying the image. It is observed that the proposed model outperforms the other models.

In future, we will use the established model to find other abnormalities in the blood. Moreover, this research aims at collecting more sample of blood images as the dataset is smaller in size. This will make the diagnosis of ALL more accurate and effective. However, a belief rule-based expert system will also be applied to make the system more efficient [13, 14, 17, 18, 28, 37, 39].

References

1. Agaian S, Madhukar M, Chronopoulos AT (2018) A new acute leukaemia-automated classification system. Comput Methods Biomech Biomed Eng Imaging Vis 6(3):303–314
2. Ahmed N, Yigit A, Isik Z, Alpkocak A (2019) Identification of leukemia subtypes from microscopic images using convolutional neural network. Diagnostics 9(3):104
3. Ahmed TU, Hossain S, Hossain MS. ul Islam R, Andersson, K (2019) Facial expression recognition using convolutional neural network with data augmentation. In: 2019 Joint 8th international conference on informatics, electronics & vision (ICIEV) and 2019 3rd international conference on imaging, vision & pattern recognition (icIVPR). IEEE, pp 336–341
4. Al-jaboriy SS, Sjarif NNA, Chuprat S, Abduallah WM (2019) Acute lymphoblastic leukemia segmentation using local pixel information. Pattern Recogn Lett 125:85–90
5. B Kekre H, B Patankar A, Ramesh Galiyal H (2013) Segmentation of blast using vector quantization technique. Int J Comput Appl 72(15):20–23
6. Basnin N, Nahar L, Hossain MS (2020) An integrated CNN-LSTM model for micro hand gesture recognition. In: International conference on intelligent computing & optimization. Springer, pp 379–392
7. Basnin N, Sumi TA, Hossain MS, Andersson K (2021) Early detection of Parkinson's disease from micrographic static hand drawings. In: International conference on brain informatics. Springer, pp 433–447
8. Bennet MA, Diana G, Pooja U, Ramya N (2019) Texture metric driven acute lymphoid leukemia classification using artificial neural networks. Int J Recent Technol Eng 7(6S3):152–156
9. Bhattacharjee R, Saini LM (2015) Robust technique for the detection of acute lymphoblastic leukemia. In: 2015 IEEE power, communication and information technology conference (PCITC). IEEE, pp. 657–662
10. Bibi N, Sikandar M, Ud Din I, Almogren A, Ali S (2020) IOMT-based automated detection and classification of leukemia using deep learning. J Healthcare Eng 2020
11. Bodzas A, Kodytek P, Zidek J (2020) Automated detection of acute lymphoblastic leukemia from microscopic images based on human visual perception. Front Bioeng Biotechnol 8:1005
12. Islam MZ, Hossain MS, ul Islam R, Andersson K (2019) Static hand gesture recognition using convolutional neural network with data augmentation. In: 2019 Joint 8th international conference on informatics, electronics vision (ICIEV) and 2019 3rd international conference on imaging, vision & pattern recognition (icIVPR). IEEE, pp 324–329
13. Islam RU, Hossain MS, Andersson K (2020) A deep learning inspired belief rule-based expert system. IEEE Access 8:190637–190651
14. Jamil MN, Hossain MS, ul Islam R, Andersson K (2019) A belief rule based expert system for evaluating technological innovation capability of high-tech firms under uncertainty. In: 2019 Joint 8th international conference on informatics, electronics & vision (ICIEV) and 2019 3rd international conference on imaging, vision & pattern recognition (icIVPR). IEEE, pp 330–335
15. Janaki R (2020) Detection of leukemia in microscopic white blood cell images using gaussian feature convolutional visual recognition algorithm. J Critic Rev 7(3):173–180
16. Jothi G, Inbarani HH, Azar AT, Devi KR (2019) Rough set theory with Jaya optimization for acute lymphoblastic leukemia classification. Neural Comput Appl 31(9):5175–5194

17. Kabir S, Islam RU, Hossain MS, Andersson K (2020) An integrated approach of belief rule base and deep learning to predict air pollution. Sensors 20(7):1956
18. Karim R, Andersson K, Hossain MS, Uddin MJ, Meah MP (2016) A belief rule based expert system to assess clinical bronchopneumonia suspicion. In: 2016 Future technologies conference (FTC). IEEE, pp 655–660
19. Kumar S, Mishra S, Asthana P et al (2018) Automated detection of acute leukemia using k-mean clustering algorithm. In: Advances in computer and computational sciences. Springer, pp 655–670
20. Labati RD, Piuri V, Scotti F (2011) ALL-IDB: The acute lymphoblastic leukemia image database for image processing. In: 2011 18th IEEE international conference on image processing. IEEE, pp 2045–2048
21. Madhloom HT, Kareem SA, Ariffin H (2012) A robust feature extraction and selection method for the recognition of lymphocytes versus acute lymphoblastic leukemia. In: 2012 International conference on advanced computer science applications and technologies (ACSAT). IEEE, pp 330–335
22. Mahmud M, Kaiser MS, McGinnity TM, Hussain A (2021) Deep learning in mining biological data. Cogn Comput 13(1):1–33
23. Mohammed ZF, Abdulla AA (2021) An efficient cad system for all cell identification from microscopic blood images. Multimedia Tools Appl 80(4):6355–6368
24. Mohapatra S, Patra D, Satpathy S (2014) An ensemble classifier system for early diagnosis of acute lymphoblastic leukemia in blood microscopic images. Neural Comput Appl 24:7–8:1887–1904
25. Moshavash Z, Danyali H, Helfroush MS (2018) An automatic and robust decision support system for accurate acute leukemia diagnosis from blood microscopic images. J Digital Imaging 31(5):702–717
26. Nikitaev V, Pronichev A, Polyakov E, Chernysheva O, Serebryakova I, Tupitsyn N (2020) Bone marrow cells recognition methods in the diagnosis of minimal residual disease. Procedia Comput Sci 169:353–358
27. Progga NI, Hossain MS, Andersson K (2020) A deep transfer learning approach to diagnose covid-19 using X-ray images. In: 2020 IEEE international women in engineering (WIE) conference on electrical and computer engineering (WIECON-ECE). IEEE, pp 177–182
28. Rahaman S, Hossain MS (2013) A belief rule based clinical decision support system to assess suspicion of heart failure from signs, symptoms and risk factors. In: 2013 International conference on informatics, electronics and vision (ICIEV). IEEE, pp 1–6
29. Rezaoana N, Hossain MS, Andersson K (2020) Detection and classification of skin cancer by using a parallel CNN model. In: 2020 IEEE international women in engineering (WIE) conference on electrical and computer engineering (WIECON-ECE). IEEE, pp 380–386
30. Sahlol AT, Abdeldaim AM, Hassanien AE (2019) Automatic acute lymphoblastic leukemia classification model using social spider optimization algorithm. Soft Comput 23(15):6345–6360
31. Sahlol AT, Kollmannsberger P, Ewees AA (2020) Efficient classification of white blood cell leukemia with improved swarm optimization of deep features. Sci Rep 10(1):1–11
32. Singhal V, Singh P (2014) Local binary pattern for automatic detection of acute lymphoblastic leukemia. In: 2014 Twentieth national conference on communications (NCC). IEEE, pp 1–5
33. Singhal V, Singh P (2016) Texture features for the detection of acute lymphoblastic leukemia. In: Proceedings of international conference on ICT for sustainable development. Springer, pp 535–543
34. Sumi TA, Hossain MS, Islam RU, Andersson K (2021) Human gender detection from facial images using convolution neural network. In: International conference on applied intelligence and informatics. Springer, pp 188–203
35. Thanh T, Vununu C, Atoev S, Lee SH, Kwon KR (2018) Leukemia blood cell image classification using convolutional neural network. Int J Comput Theory Eng 10(2):54–58
36. Tuba M, Tuba E (2019) Generative adversarial optimization (GOA) for acute lymphocytic leukemia detection. Stud Inf Control 28(3):245–254

37. Uddin Ahmed T, Jamil MN, Hossain MS, Andersson K, Hossain MS (2020) An integrated real-time deep learning and belief rule base intelligent system to assess facial expression under uncertainty. In: 9th International conference on informatics, electronics & vision (ICIEV). IEEE Computer Society
38. Umamaheswari D, Geetha S (2018) A framework for efficient recognition and classification of acute lymphoblastic leukemia with a novel customized-kNN classifier. J Comput Inf Technol 26(2):131–140
39. Zisad SN, Chowdhury E, Hossain MS, Islam RU, Andersson K (2021) An integrated deep learning and belief rule-based expert system for visual sentiment analysis under uncertainty. Algorithms 14(7):213
40. Zisad SN, Hossain MS, Andersson K (2020) Speech emotion recognition in neurological disorders using convolutional neural network. In: International conference on brain informatics. Springer, pp 287–296

Zero-Contact Novel Corona Virus (Sars-Cov-2) Patient Monitoring and Management System Using IoT

Ankit Jain, Raghvendra Singh, and S. K. Bhalla

Abstract Entire world is passing through the corona virus disease (COVID-19) outbreak badly. According to the WHO, corona virus affects respiratory system. This corona virus majorly spreads when someone comes in contact with an infected person and respiratory droplets that generates by coughing or sneezing play major role in spreading the infection. These respiratory droplets can spread infection when inhaled by someone or contaminate hands and surfaces in contact. During the treatment of such infectious disease, the safety of healthcare workers becomes the matter of primary concern as they are directly involved during the process of diagnosis as well as treatment and care of COVID-19 patients; hence, they are always open to infection, and their chances of getting infected with SARS-CoV-2 virus become very high. A lot of challenges hospitals and staff are facing, and few of them need to be addressed technologically. In present work, in this paper, we have proposed a Bluetooth and IOT-based wireless healthcare monitoring system. The proposed system can be utilized to get real-time online physiological conditions of a patient. Doctors can monitor their COVID-19 patients remotely. A robotic trolley could be pressed into service (serve or fulfill the patient need) in hospital in order to remove direct connection and minimize the risk of spreading infection between healthcare workers who are directly involved in treating COVID-19 patients. This system continuously monitors the real-time temperature and pulse rate of the patient and send data remotely to the doctors. A medicine reminder system also reminds the patient about the medicine with date and time through voice system.

Keywords COVID-19 · Node MCU · DS18B20 temperature sensor · RTC · Robotics trolley · Pulse sensor

---

A. Jain (✉) · R. Singh
Department of Electronics and Communication Engineering, PSIT, Kanpur, U.P., India

S. K. Bhalla
Department of Electrical Engineering, PSIT, Kanpur, U.P., India

M. S. Kaiser et al. (eds.), *Proceedings of Trends in Electronics and Health Informatics*, Lecture Notes in Networks and Systems 376,
https://doi.org/10.1007/978-981-16-8826-3_32

1 Introduction

Corona virus disease (COVID-19) is rapidly spreading all over the world. Corona viruses are found in large groups and have potential to make humans and animals ill. Seldom, animal corona viruses can develop and cause people to infect, and then, further, spreading between people happen such as has been observed with MERS and SARS. Initially, the outbreak of novel corona virus disease (COVID-19) was reported in Hubei Province of China, in Wuhan city in a seafood market in December, 2019, has now spread more than 214 countries/territories/areas worldwide. On 30th January, 2020, WHO declared this outbreak as a "Public Health Emergency of International Concern" (PHEIC), and subsequently, WHO declared COVID-19 a pandemic on 11th March, 2020 [1].

Initially, in a hospital in Wuhan, the covid patients were reported to have symptoms like high fever, excessive fatigue, dry cough, and cold [2], but later, patients were admitted having serious or even fatal pneumonia [3]. Clinical presentations were found to resemble SARS-CoV-2 to a great extent. Patients with severe illness developed ARDS and required ICU admission and oxygen therapy.

The main source of infection was the people himself only who got infected by the novel corona virus infection. On other hand, if a healthy person touches or comes in contact with an infected surface and after that he or she touches his or her eyes, nose, or mouth, is likely to be infected [4]. The median incubation period by study was calculated approximately to be 5.1 days (95% CI, 4.5–5.8 days), and 97.5% of those who develop symptoms will do the same within 11.5 days (CI, 8.2–15.6 days) of infection. These approximate calculations suggest that under conservative assumptions, 101 out of every 10,000 cases (99th percentile, 482) will develop symptoms after 14 days of active monitoring or quarantine [5].

According to a review study [6], the prime source of the disease is not known yet, and it is suspected that the virus was transmitted through bat to an intermediate host and then to humans. The primary symptoms of COVID-19 infection are tiredness, fever, and dry cough. The incubation period of the disease is about 2–14 days, which is considered to be an important parameter for planning to prevent disease outbreak.

HCWs are at the vanguard of the epidemic response, and they need to be supported. Healthcare workers are likely to be in contact with patients and colleagues who have a typical, few, or no symptoms while still being highly contagious [7, 8]. Healthcare workers have to face various challenges while treating covid patients. They experience significant burdens from corona virus infections, including SARS-CoV-2. The infection risk can be reduced by using PPE kit and infection control training, while certain exposures may lead to increase the infection risk [9].

It becomes important to ensure the safety of fellow clinicians, nursing staff, paramedical, and support staff. Transmission of disease happens from person to person, and moreover, there is no information that how much contagious the virus is, and how fast it could spreads. Hence, a lot of challenges are there in treatment and management of such infectious disease. Apart from keeping staff safe, the other challenges are scarcity of personal protective equipment (PPE), lesser availability of test kits, and supplies, inadequate staff to take care of COVID-19 patients. Scarcities of essential supplies, like no-touch infrared thermometers, disinfectants and cleaning supplies, inflated prices for supplies. Office of the Inspector General (OIG) at the Department of Health and Human Services (U.S) reported that the hospitals where covid patients are being treated which includes testing and management of patients as well are facing the most significant challenge to keep their staff safe from infection [10, 11].

Infection prevention control (IPC) is considered to be a significant and essential part of clinical management of patients and should be activated at time when the patient gets entry to the emergency department of the hospital. It is required to apply routinely the standard precautions in all domains of healthcare facilities. Regular hand wash at small time intervals, use of PPE kit in order to avoid direct contact with patients' blood, body fluids, secretions are the basic requirements of standard precautions. Prevention of needle-stick or sharps injury, protected waste management, cleaning and disinfection of used equipment, and environment cleaning are also included in same. In a study done on 222 medical staff who were sent to Wuhan city for support, it was found that zero occupational infection is major goal to attain among all healthcare workers who are deployed at front line. This could be accredited by several reasons. Complete site training and electronic infection prevention reminder and control programs were conducted mainly, while prevention of infection and control programs were strictly followed, and constant monitoring was done [12].

According to a survey done through an app called Symptom Study app during March 24 and April 23, 2020 with 2,135,190 people from USA and UK [13], it was observed during survey that healthcare workers who were on front had a threefold increased risk of getting infected with COVID-19 infection, as compared to common people belonging to general community. As an example, in a study done just within two weeks after the first Dutch case was detected [14], a considerable number of healthcare workers were found to be infected with SARS-CoV-2. The common symptoms were high fever, cold, and problem related to respiratory systems. This infection was suspected to be caused by acquirement of the virus from the community. This study verifies the dangerous behavior of SARS-CoV-2 virus.

Maharashtra Chief Minister Uddhav Thackeray's office on Twitter shared a video on July 08, 2020, In this video, it is shown that at Podar Hospital in Worli, Mumbai during the treatment of COVID-19 patients a robotic trolley has been taken in to service in order to minimize direct contact between healthcare workers and COVID-19 patients so that the risk of spreading infection among medical staff while treating COVID-19 patients gets reduced. This robotic trolley was called "Gollar," and the major use of this trolley was to distribute medicine to the COVID-19 patients [15]. A study [16] on design restraint for designing implantable microstrip antenna (MSA) for body-centric communication suggested an approach to design implantable MSA used for body-centric communication. It also reported a multilayer MSA for medical implant communication services (MICS) band.

2 Features of the Proposed System

The system consists of many features. These incorporated features are useful in reducing the chances of getting infected of health workers and doctors as well with this highly infectious corona virus. The system makes use of node MCU Wi-Fi module to attach with Internet. This combination is helpful as real-time data can be displayed, and the same can be observed and accessed over Internet using IOT technology from anywhere in the world. The incorporated features are being summarized below.

Patient can send predefined requirement to the ward boy/doctor/relatives by a Bluetooth. We can get the picture and voice message on the cell phone using android app, regarding requirement of the patient. We have one panic button also for any emergency. To serve or fulfill the patient need, a robotic trolley can be employed in order to help in maintaining zero contact and reducing the risk of spread of infection among health workers who are involved in treating COVID-19 patients.

This system will continually monitor the patient's temperature and pulse rate over IOT remotely, and the information is displayed on LCD also. This system is equipped with RTC which can be used to display the real time with date on LCD. This system also has medicine reminder system with voice alert.

Block diagram of the robotic trolley is shown in Fig. 1a, and block diagram of the control panel is shown in Fig. 1b.

3 Material and Methods

In order to overcome the defined problem, we propose a model which is designed by making use of control engineering. We also intend to incorporate many other useful features to the proposed model so that its utility is enhanced. The development of hardware of the overall proposed system is done by adopting step-by-step methodology. The major aim behind the development of the model is to acquire data from external devices like sensors and to manipulate it to attain a specific output.

In Table 1, the sensors/modules and components are being listed below which are used in the development of the hardware for the present model.

Circuit diagram of the robotic trolley has been shown in Fig. 2a, and circuit diagram for control panel is shown in Fig. 2b.

The methodology is as follows.

There are 14 buttons available on control panel, out of which 10 buttons are used to send the information regarding requirement of the patient. Whenever the patient will press the button, the device shares the picture and voice message via Bluetooth using android application to the ward boy/doctor/relatives, etc. These dedicated messages will also be displayed on LCD, and messages will be announced on speaker also through predefined saved voice in SD card.

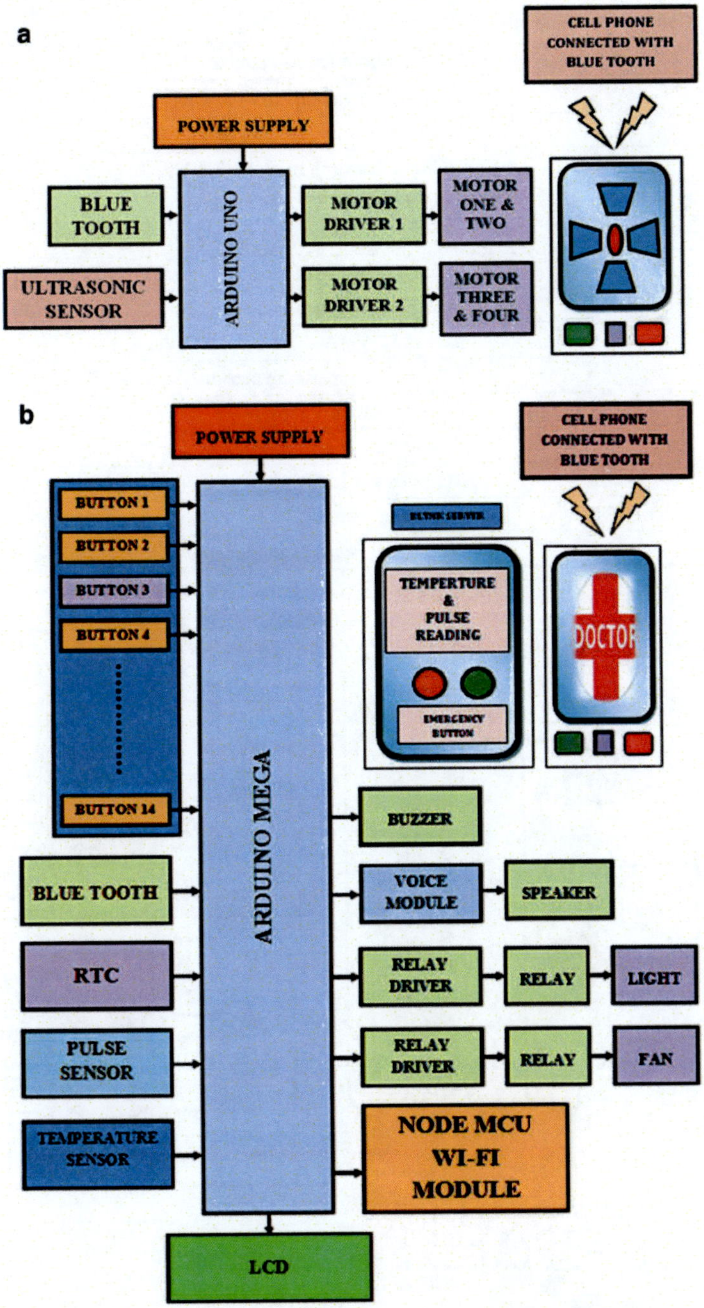

Fig.1 **a** Block diagram of the robotic trolley, **b** block diagram of the control panel

Table 1 Major components required for the proposed system

S. No.	Sensors/modules/components
1	Arduino Mega and Arduino UNO
2	LCD (16 × 2)
3	HC-05 Bluetooth module (3.3 V)
4	Node MCU-12E Wi-Fi module
5	RTC (Real-time clock) DS3231
6	Voice module with speaker
7	Push buttons (push to on)
8	Relays 12 V/1A
9	DS18B20 temperature sensor
10	Pulse sensor (5 V)
11	Buzzer 12 V/1A
12	Motor driver L298
13	Ultrasonic sensor
14	Active and passive components

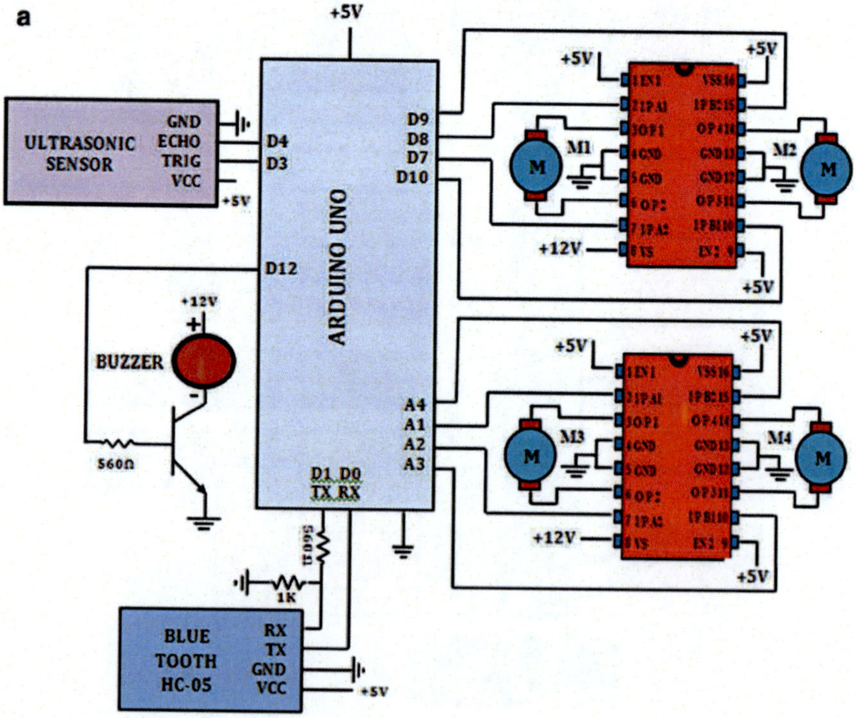

Fig. 2 **a** Circuit diagram of the robotic trolley, **b** circuit diagram of the control panel

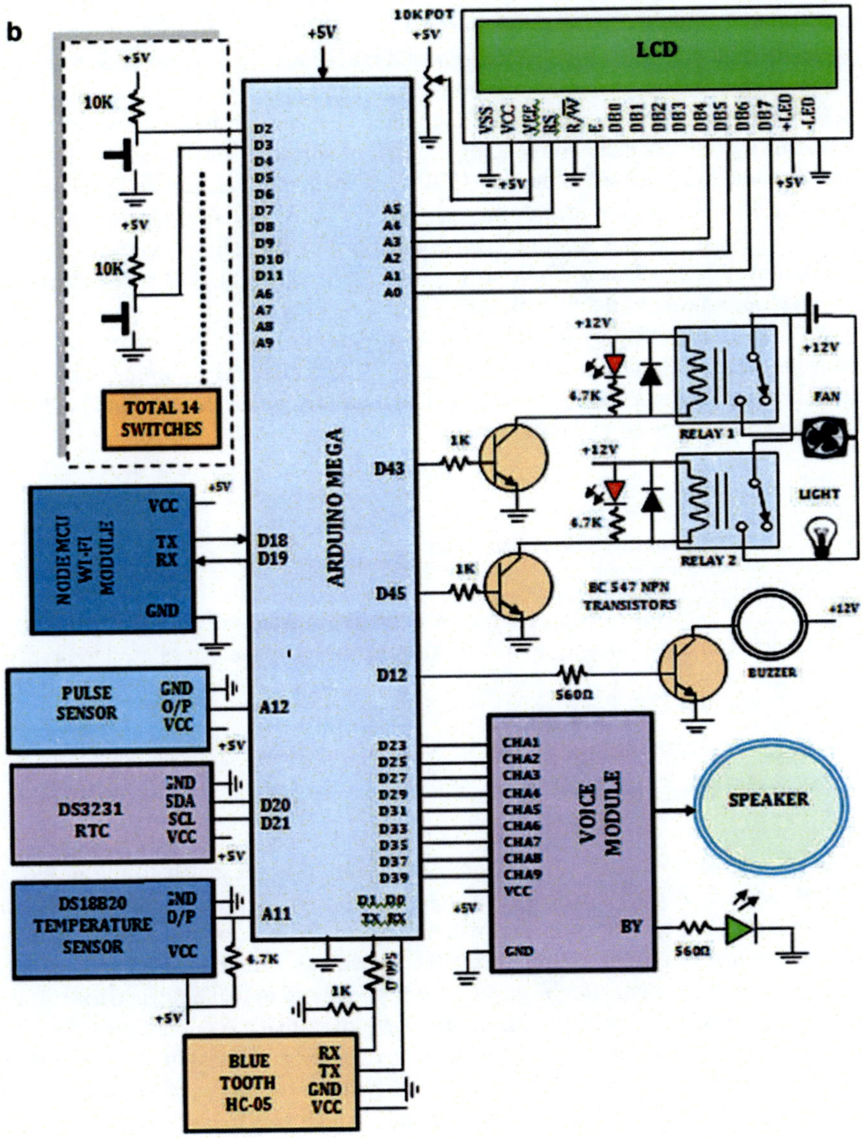

Fig. 2 (continued)

We are using DS18B20 temperature sensor and pulse sensor for checking the temperature and pulse rate of the patient. One button is dedicated for checking pulse rate of the covid patient. Temperature value is continually monitored on the Blynk server. These two parameters will be displayed on the LCD, and we can also send this data wirelessly through Blynk server to anywhere in the world.

One panic button is especially dedicated to any emergency situation on the control panel. Two buttons are dedicated for light and fan, so patient can also operate his/her fan and light. We use two relay to operate light and fan.

To fulfill the patient requirements, a robotic trolley will be used in order to help in maintaining zero contact and reducing the risk of spread of infection among health workers who are involved in treating COVID-19 patients. This trolley has obstacle-avoiding feature. We are using ultrasonic sensor to avoid any obstacle within the range of 25 cm. We will operate this robotics trolley by cell phone using android application through Bluetooth. Two motor driver module (L298) will be used to operate four wheels of the four motor.

RTC is used to display the real time with date on LCD. This system also has medicine reminder system with voice alert. We can customize the medicine time and medicine name in coding. Patient will be reminded about the time and medicine through voice followed by buzzer sound.

4 PCB Implementation and Circuit

Figure 3a, b show lower and upper view of PCB for robotics trolley. Figure 3c, d show lower and upper view of PCB for control panel. DipTrace was used to prepare this PCB.

5 Results and Discussion

In this work, an electronic and eco-friendly solution is presented to the problem related to the COVID-19 patient management. This will help in eliminating direct contact between health worker and patient so that the risk of spreading infection among medical staff while treating COVID-19 patients will be reduced.

The proposed system after its development was tested in real time, and the results found were satisfactory and up to the mark. As we know that it is important to measure temperature and pulse rate of covid patients frequently, and the system is capable of measuring these parameters accurately over Blynk server through IoT. The system has also an added feature of medicine reminder which was found to work well and reminds the patient through voice message. Patient was able to send the predefined requirement to the ward boy/doctor/relatives by a Bluetooth, and the picture and voice message on the cell phone using android app, regarding requirement of the patient, were also successfully sent. Panic button for emergency was also working.

The devised robotic trolley in order to fulfill the patient need was tested with different payloads and was found that it is capable to bear payload up to 5 kg. To serve or fulfill, the a robotic trolley can be employed in order to help in maintaining zero contact and reducing the risk of spread of infection among health workers who are involved in treating COVID-19 patients.

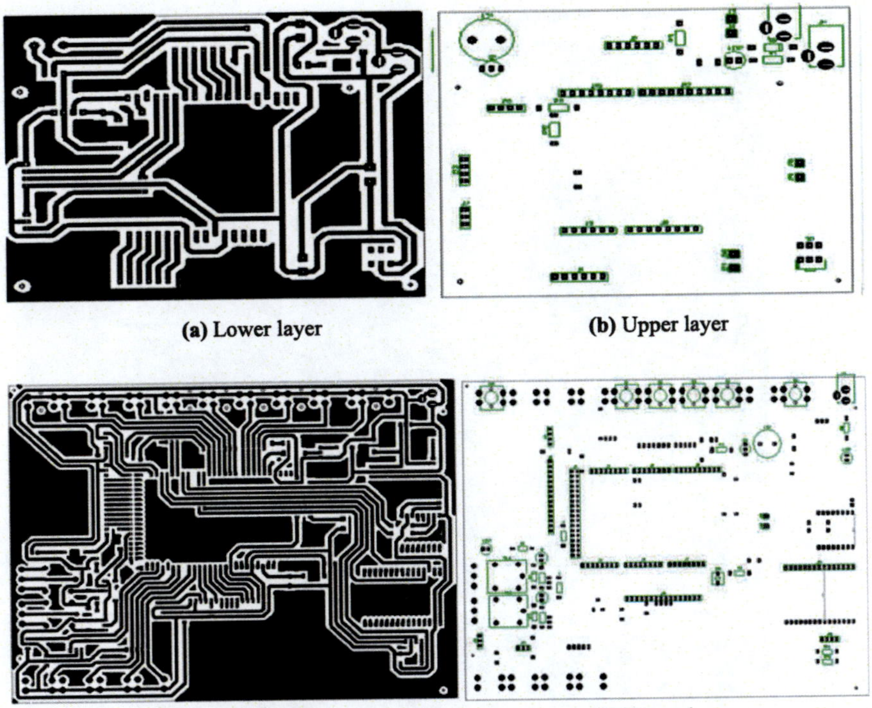

(a) Lower layer **(b)** Upper layer

(c) Lower layer **(d)** Upper layer

Fig. 3 PCB prepared using DipTrace

The original PCB for robotics trolley is shown in Fig. 4, and an original picture of prepared system is shown in Fig. 5. In order to check the compatibility of the system, the real-time temperature and pulse rate of a patient were tested. The real-time values thus obtained are shown in Fig. 5 and were found to be in good agreement with the

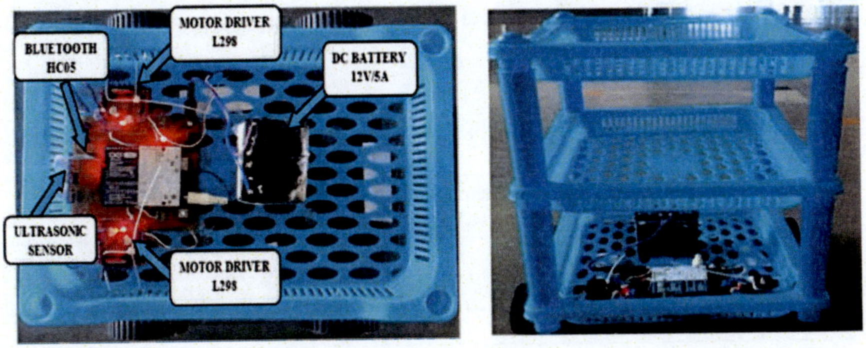

Fig. 4 Robotics trolley for covid patient

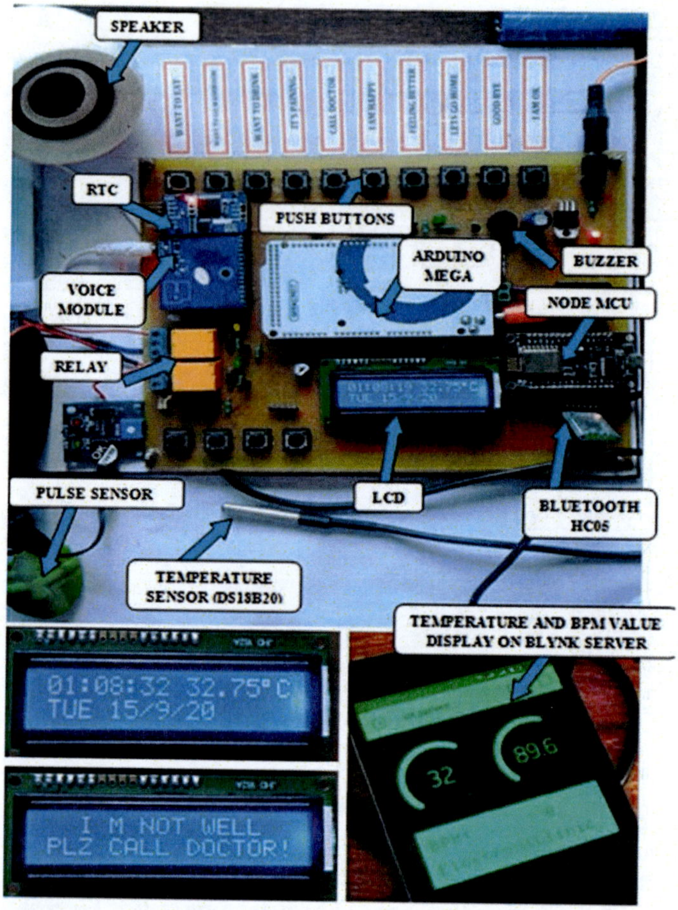

Fig. 5 Original pictures of the prepared system

values obtained by using thermometer and pulse Oximeter. The comparison can be seen in Table 2 given.

Table 2 Comparison of real time values of temperature and pulse rate with thermometer and pulse oximeter

S. No.	Real-time temp. value in °F	Real-time pulse value in BPM	Thermometer reading in °F	Oximeter reading in BPM
1	96.53	82	96.5	82
2	95.50	81	95.5	82
3	96.60	85	96.5	84

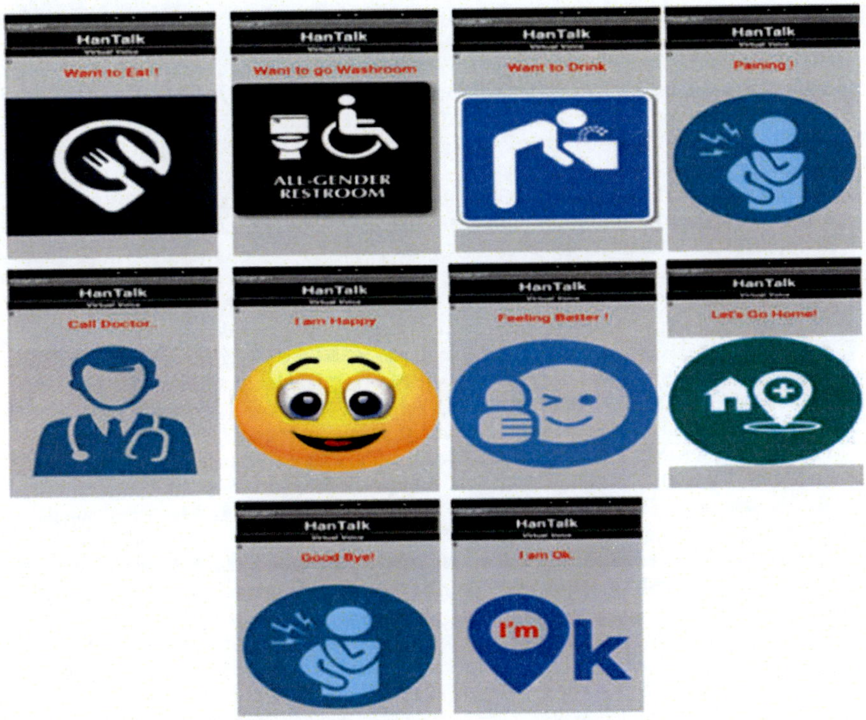

Fig. 6 Picture messages on android application

When we press the button on control panel, the following picture message with voice has been displayed on our android application (Fig. 6).

6 Conclusions

Infected patients and contaminated surroundings work as a source of infection. In present work, we have tried to find out the solution so that the contact between healthcare workers and infected patients can be minimized. Here, we have devised an automated robotic trolley which can be considered as one of the possible solution or measure in direction to stop the spread of infection through contact. This robotic trolley is low cost and can be used during the treatment of COVID-19 patients. During the care-taking process of infected patient which involves food and medicine delivery, the chances of healthcare workers to get infected become higher; at this point, this robotic trolley could be helpful to a great extent in order to minimize the interaction between health worker and infected patient.

References

1. https://www.mohfw.gov.in/pdf/ClinicalManagementProtocolforCOVID19.pdf
2. Paules CI, Marston HD, Fauci AS (2020) Coronavirus infections-more than just the common cold. JAMA 323(8):707–708. https://doi.org/10.1001/jama.2020.0757PubMedGoogle Scholar Crossref
3. Huang C, Wang Y, Li X et al (2020) Clinical features of patients infected with 2019 novel coronavirus in Wuhan, China. Lancet. 2020;395(10223):497–506. https://doi.org/10.1016/S0140-6736(20)30183-5PubMedGoogle Scholar Crossref
4. Hospitals Report Challenges in responding to the COVID-19 Pandemic, a report released by the U.S. Department of Health and Human Services (HHS). https://ascopost.com/news/april-2020/ hospitals report challenges in responding to the covid-19 pandemic/
5. Tong X, Ning M, Huang R et al (2020) Surveillance of SARS-CoV-2 infection among frontline health care workers in Wuhan during COVID-19 outbreak. Immunity, inflammation and disease. 8(4):840–843
6. Garosi VH, Tanhaie S, Chaboksavar F et al (2021) An overview of 2019 novel coronavirus COVID-19 pandemic: A review study. J Educ Health Promot 10:280. https://doi.org/10.4103/jehp.jehp_1403_20. eCollection 2021
7. Xu H, Rebaza A, Sharma L et al (2020) Protecting health-care workers from subclinical coronavirus infection. Lancet Respir Med. 8:e13
8. Hudson B, Toop L, Mangin D, Brunton C, Jennings L, Fletcher L (2013) Pandemic influenza A(H1N1)pdm09: risk of infection in primary healthcare workers. Br J Gen Pract 2013; pmid:23735413
9. Chou R, Dana T, Buckley DI, Selph S, Fu R, Totten AM (2020) Epidemiology of and risk factors for corona virus infection in health care workers. Ann Intern Med. pmid:3236954
10. Lauer SA, Grantz KH, Bi Q et al (2020) The incubation period of corona virus disease 2019 (COVID-19) from publicly reported confirmed cases: estimation and application. Ann Intern Med 2020 https://doi.org/10.7326/M20-0504
11. CDC COVID-19 Response Team (2020) Characteristics of Health Care Personnel with COVID-19-United States, February 12–April 9, 2020. CDC Morbidity and Mortality Weekly Report. April 2020. https://cdc.gov/mmwr/volumes/69/wr/mm6915e6.htm. Accessed Aug 5 2020
12. Yu P, Zhu J, Zhang Z, Han Y (2020) A familial cluster of infection associated with the 2019 novel corona virus indicating possible person-to-person transmission during the incubation period. J Infect 2020. https://doi.org/10.1093/jiaa077
13. Nguyen LH, Drew DA, Graham MS (2020) Risk of COVID-19 among front-line health-care workers and the general community: a prospective cohort study. www.thelancet.com/public-health 5
14. Kluytmans MBA, Pas S, Bentvelsen RG, Bijllaardt W, Oudheusden AJG, van ijen MML, et al SARS-CoV-2 infection in 86 healthcare workers in two Dutch hospitals in March 2020. Med RXiv. https://doi.org/10.1101/2020.03.23.20041913
15. https://www.ndtv.com/mumbai-news/coronavirus-robotic-trolley-gollar-serves-food-water-to-covid-19-patients-at-mumbai-hospital-22588453321
16. Love J, Raghvendra S, Sanyog R, Kanad R (2018) Stacked arrangement of meandered patches for biomedical applications. Int J Syst Assur Eng Manag 9(1)

Distributed and Hierarchical Clustering Techniques Comparison in Wireless Camera Sensor Networks

Nishant Tripathi and Kamal Kumar Sharma

Abstract Most of the applications of modern-day communication, viz., military navigation, home automations, agricultural land security, and many more are totally dependent upon wireless sensor industry. Therefore, a very important task is to establish and operate the wireless sensor networks in such a way that the lifeline of the network is long and it should not be very power consuming or non-reliable. Most of the researchers have shifted their goal post if they are working in sensor-based field to optimize the energy, power, and life span with reliability consideration of sensor-based networks (camera-based or non-camera-based). So, in this paper, the primary focus will be to review all those techniques which can optimize the power consumptions, energy, and overall improvement in lifeline of the network. Since, clustering is cast-off for making the networks more scalable, stable, efficient, reliable, and energy efficient. This helps in minimizing the effective cost of implementation and maintenance of the networks also. The paper will overview wireless sensor networks at first, then the issues that impact the design of any type of wireless sensor networks (camera/ad hoc/nonvisual). After the introduction of the mentioned terms, the next part provides formidable comparison between different clustering techniques used for the implementation of different kinds of wireless networks. The conclusion covers the comparison of different clustering techniques leading to the need of cooperative communication.

Keywords Wireless camera sensor networks (WCSNs) · Cluster heads (CHs) · Energy · Power · Sensor nodes (SNs)

N. Tripathi (✉)
School of Electronics and Electrical Engineering, Lovely Professional University, Phagwara, India

N. Tripathi · K. K. Sharma
Pranveer Singh Institute of Technology, Kanpur, India
e-mail: kamal.23342@lpu.co.in

M. S. Kaiser et al. (eds.), *Proceedings of Trends in Electronics and Health Informatics*, Lecture Notes in Networks and Systems 376,
https://doi.org/10.1007/978-981-16-8826-3_33

1 Introduction

Sensor networks based on wireless transmissions whether camera-based or non-camera-based (WSN/WCSN) [1] are the combination of electronic devices of miniature size (in micrometer) [1–3], i.e., member sensors nodes (SNs). SNs within a WSN/WCSN transmit and receive the information packets using channel as wireless link (BSs) [1]. A base station (BS) is utilized for the purpose of relay the information to the desired end user/system. Information packets which can be SNR or E/N can traverse down the network in single hope or can be multihop [4–6]. Wireless sensor networks or wireless camera sensor networks (WSNs/WCSNs) are of two types: proactive and reactive networks [2]. A proactive network is of a passive architecture and well suitable for data aggregation. This type is based on regular interval basis for information packet transmission. But in reactive networks, member sensor nodes reply instantly and only to variations in the relevant parameters of attention. Reactive networks are more useful continuous signaling from the member sensor nodes without any gap. The important fact to reminisce is that any wireless network (camera/non-camera-based) has drastically affected the domain area applications and stability factor of the networks. Therefore, it is desirable to attain numerous design goals and objectives before implementing and getting the network operational. It is because of the fact that in any wireless camera or non-camera sensor networks, the primary goals or objectives to be achieved could be small size of member sensor node, optimum clustering profiling, easier cluster head election criteria with optimum low cost, easier configurability, significantly scalable, high throughput with better reliability, better fault diagnosis and tolerance ability, excellent security and QoS with optimum power consumption, etc. [1, 6–10].

1.1 *Traffic Patterns in WSNs/WCSNs*

In difference to traditional networks, the wireless sensor networks (WSNs)/wireless camera sensor networks (WCSNs) display single unequal traffic topology of the data packet routing. The primary cause of this is that wireless sensor networks WSNs/wireless camera sensor networks (WCSNs) [1, 2] normally collect data and then member sensor nodes of a given cluster obstinately send their data to the base station. Furthermore, different usage area/domain can provide several shapes and types of traffic topology for data packet flow (Fig. 1; Table 1).

1.2 *Some of the Key Points to Address in Designing a Wireless Sensor Network (Camera/Non-camera-Based)*

See Fig. 2 and Table 2.

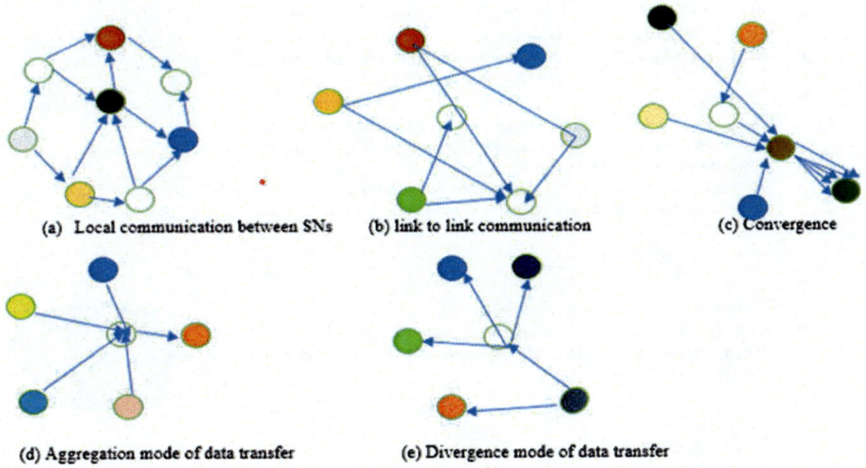

Fig. 1 Traffic patterns in wireless sensor networks/wireless camera sensor networks

Table 1 Application areas with respect to wireless sensor categories

Application areas	Types of sensors used	Examples
Environmental	Symbiotic	1. Agriculture 2. In the detecting tropical or dense forest climatic issues 3. Disaster management pollution detection
Military	Obtrusive	1. In monitoring and updating ammunition records of nearby friendly force posts or bases 2. Targeting and analyzing the movements of enemy posts and movements 3. Border protection and security surveillance 4. Making records and assessments on war Battlefield observation
Health-based	Bio-hybrid symbiotic	1. Tissue movement observation, like cancer tissue status 2. Maintain and monitor the records of patients such as heartbeat or blood pressure
Home-based	Symbiotic parasitic	1. Automation for home security and management 2. Smart appliances entertainment
Industrial	Parasitic obtrusive	1. Environmental control in office buildings 2. early detection of possible threats 3. Managing inventory control

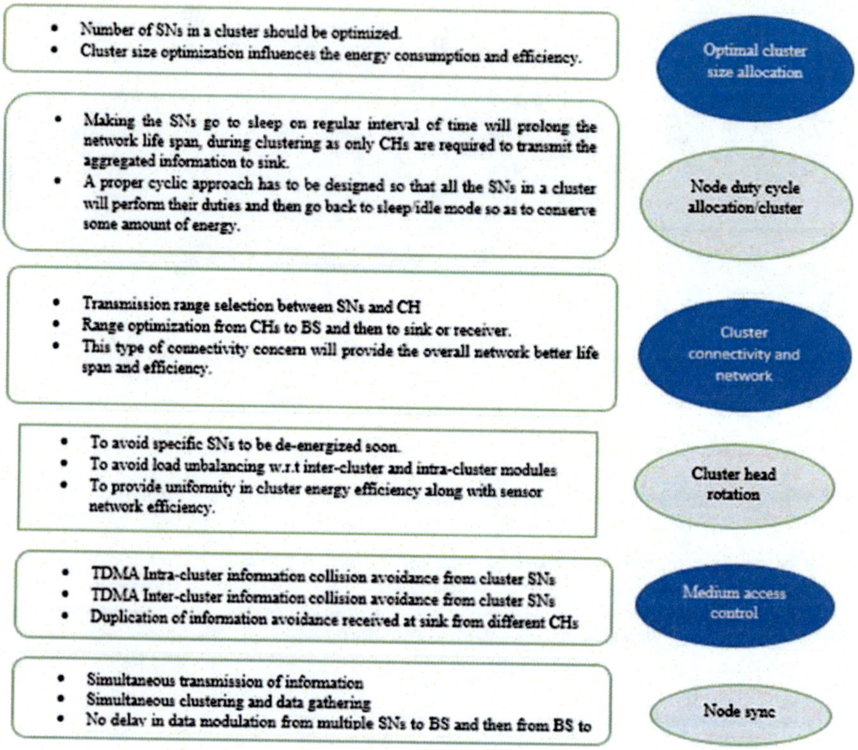

Fig. 2 Shows key issues in designing a sensor network camera-based or non-camera-based

1.3 Clustering

Clustering [1] techniques can determine numerous goalmouths slanting with power budget. The centralized clustering [11] techniques have drawbacks of powered base stations on higher side [2, 3], [39]. It is also recognized that distributive techniques/protocols work on residual energy factor [9, 10]. Clustering in wireless sensor networks or wireless camera sensor networks is scheme to diminution the energy expense per member sensor node [1, 12–14]. Energy per member sensor nodes reduction also impacts the overall power requirement [4, 9, 15] and load balancing of the cluster in WCSN [2, 11]. Power requirement decrement with appropriate matching can lead to stable and prolonged network life [16], [38, 37]. The special condition in the group assembly of the sensors is that in place of all the member sensor nodes transmitting their respective Eb/No, only the assembly group head (which is a member sensor node elected for transmitting called cluster head (CH)) will transfer the aggregated information [1, 2, 7, 11]. A hierarchical network [1, 9, 17] is more efficient than the flat network [1, 2]. Nonflat approach is called hierarchical method [1, 2] utilized in grouping of member sensor nodes called clustering [12, 18]. In

Table 2 Parameters for improving the life of sensor nodes and overall life span of sensor networks

Parameter of research	Working explanation
Deployment model of nodes	Checks the overall performances of the enables routing techniques/protocols in either deterministic or un-deterministic approach
Information/data gathering module	Any routing protocols/techniques or even clustering techniques get influenced through the information/data collection and aggregation modules and the formats, time, nature of the data report model which are highly related to the energy consumptions with SNs route stability from SNs to CHs to BS and then to the sink from each cluster
Fault tolerance/diagnosis	One of the important aspects is to avoid duplicity of the information and yet provide several levels of redundancy which may be required fault tolerance redundant network
Data aggregation and collection	Data aggregation from different SNs should be correlated and data fusion makes the transmitted data size smaller
Reliability and QoS	Reliability is the assurance of data transmission from source to destination but there has to optimization between life time of each sensor and assurance of data transfer as longer the life span, the reliability of data transfer decreases
Network clustering module	Clustering techniques have to be wisely chosen so as to make sure that overall network performance does not degrade

the hierarchical methodology, cluster heads (CHs) are typically at higher level. CHs collect and concise the received information packets from different member sensor nodes (Eb/No) from member sensor nodes which are lower level in terms of energy. The received information packet at cluster head will be further transmitted to the base/sink for further post processing of the information received form the member sensor nodes [12, 18].

1.4 *Performance of Clustering Protocols Is Captured on Following Parameters*

Time to network partition is the effective time for first sensor node (SN) to become energy-less or with insufficient energy for transmission, the network confined by a cluster is said to be partitioned. Dead node will replicate that roughly different routes from the given network have invalid state to show [8, 14].

Average lifetime of sensors most effective parameter to check for the network partition and check for the overall efficiency of the network with its stability [14].

Average delay/packet is average time taken by the data packet to migrate to the sink from source.

Throughput for the network is termed as totality of data packets acknowledged at base station divided by the time taken during overall aggregation, processing, regenerating (if any), and doing the simulation.

Average energy of a data packet a system of measurement to check performance of clustering protocols applied on the network.

Average power is amount of power consumed on an average during the data packet aggregation at CH and transmitting the same to the sink along with the pre-processing and post-processing on the overall information getting transmitted [17, 19].

Standard deviation load/cluster is tested for several sensor nodes deployments. Changing the number of transmitting gateways and clustering are the two methodologies to calculate standard deviation of load/cluster [14, 17, 19].

1.5 Types of Clustering Methodologies

Distributed algorithms elect cluster head (CHs) from member sensor nodes (SNs) within a cluster based on certain dynamic criteria. Cluster heads are updated after next iteration of protocol.

Power base clustering algorithms contemplate remaining battery life of sensor nodes or residual network life time. Approximately, some of the power-based protocols are HEED and TEEN [17, 20] use multi-hop basis and cluster to cluster communication at times. Typically used for path navigated for transferring sensed packet information.

Multilevel clustering is advanced approach in which head of cluster heads (CHs) is to be selected. This methodology shows a dynamic hierarchy within cluster heads (CHs).

Clustering methodology/techniques with their key feature and parameters comparison table with their advantages and disadvantages (Tables 3 and 4).

There are few more clustering techniques which are PSO-based and neural-based in nature. These clustering are advance methodology based on meta-heuristic approach. Almost all the meta-heuristic clustering technique does give a simple mathematical model to generate cluster head in a cluster within a wireless sensor network. But, the overall logic to do is somewhat complicated in nature. Also, the LEACH, PEGASIS, HEED, EECH, and Housdorff clustering [1, 2, 11, 12, 14] have been on an advanced stage of research nowadays with more stability in their implementation. These modern advancements in the basic standard clustering technique are based on mainly the cluster head selection methodology, by incorporating some of the probabilistic model or nature-based model with the prior ones. The simulation results have shown a great improvement in the optimum power consumption and energy degradation, as after merging two or more key feature of different clustering modules, the overall life span of the wireless sensor network have shown improvement and stable communications.

Table 3 Shows analytical comparison between various clustering techniques

S. No	Clustering methodology	Parameter consideration/key features	Pros	Cons
1	Direct transfer protocols (DTP)	Non-clustering approach Individual SNs transfer Member sensor nodes transmit directly to sink/receiver Data aggregation not needed Low life of network Good for small network Good for less dense network	Easy implementation Lesser cost per network design	Energy wastage Lesser life span of network
2	Static clustering protocols	Grouping of SNs is permanent/static Only one cluster head is permanently selected for data aggregation and data transfer Due to permanent selection of a single cluster head, if CH energy dissipates and sensor node dies out, then transmission stops	Network implementation is easy Lesser energy wastage than DTP Typically, longer life span of network	Still life span is not good Power mismanaged
3	Minimum energy transfer protocol [3, 15]	Grouping of sensor nodes is static in nature Cluster head is selected only once, but has the check of a minimum energy threshold criteria Energy available (SN) $\geq$ referenced threshold energy, SN will be CH Data fusion is done for making data optimal	Network implementation is easy Optimum energy is used Better life span of sensor networks	Throughput is average lacks stability

(continued)

Table 3 (continued)

S. No	Clustering methodology	Parameter consideration/key features	Pros	Cons
4	Distributed cluster protocol: LEACH: low energy adaptive clustering hierarchy [1–3]	Grouping of sensor nodes in dynamic nature Sensor heads are dynamically selected or elected based upon certain parametric value Every SN can become CH within a cluster In this first, CHs are elected which is setup phase and secondly data aggregation, data fusion, data transfer, idle and non-idle state allocations of sensor nodes are indicated which is steady state	Better network coverage Optimum energy use Flexible network Easier modification Better throughput	Stability problem modifications needed for better throughput
5	EECH-energy efficient hierarchical clustering [2, 3, 17]	Dynamic clustering algorithm Hierarchy of CHs showing if number of levels in hierarchy increases, energy saving increases Multilevel hierarchy clustering algorithm uses stochastic geometry to obtain lower parameter for minimum energy consumption	Better network coverage Flexible Better throughput	Complex design Lacks stability in long Run Load balancing is problem
6	HEED: hierarchical energy efficient distribution [1, 2, 5, 16]	Dynamic randomized clustering algorithm Two parametric choices for minimum energy consumption First parameter is available energy of SNs while the second is cost of intra-cluster communication leads to cluster head selection	Better load balancing Energy consumption is low Better throughput	Stability is an issue Life span is moderate

(continued)

Table 3 (continued)

S. No	Clustering methodology	Parameter consideration/key features	Pros	Cons
7	PEGASIS: power-efficient gathering in sensor information systems [2, 3]	Extended and modified version of LEACH Greedy algorithm-based two step clustering technique Cluster head is accountable for transmission of the aggregated data to the BS	Better network coverage Optimum energy use Flexible network Easier modification Better throughput Better throughput than LEACH at times	Stability problem Life span is moderate
8	GABEEC:genetic algorithm-based energy efficient clustering [3, 21]	Cluster-based approach like LEACH. Static cluster creation [16, 22–24] New cluster or remaking of clusters is not executed after each round of communication [16] CH election is outstanding energy of present CH and along with other SNs in the cluster	CH selection is optimal Energy wastage is minimum Better life span Implementation is simple	Load balancing is improper Not good for very large network
9	PSO:particle swarm optimization [1–3]	Meta-heuristic optimization [1–3], Neighboring topology of the different particle swarms is based on the imitation of the different societies [3, 15, 21] Long range of iterations Mathematical module-based	Better network coverage Better fault tolerance Reliability is high Energy consumption is moderate	Improper load balancing Complex architecture

(continued)

Table 3 (continued)

S. No	Clustering methodology	Parameter consideration/key features	Pros	Cons
11	Firefly algorithm [21, 25]	Bio-inspired technique Non-linear optimization-based technique Algorithm is centralized LEACH protocol is utilized alongside	Better network coverage Better fault tolerance Reliability is high Efficient lower data/energy rate	Stability is not so good Power optimization is difficult
12	HBMO: honey bee Mating optimization [3, 16, 21]	Expected clustering approach Two steps-based First cluster making 2nd step CH election 2nd step again in 2 steps: 1st is premiere phase 2nd is steady state	Better network coverage Better fault tolerance Lower data/energy rate	Stability is not so good Power optimization is difficult
13	Deterministic energy efficient algorithm	Effective energy consumption Better transmission rate of data packets CH election is on the outstanding energy (OE) of each node Cluster heads (CHs) represent their roles and responsibilities using carrier sense multiple access-media access control	Minimum confusion in electing CH Better network coverage	Stability issue
14	CREEP [14]: cluster head restricted energy efficient protocol [14, 19]	Assumption is some are energy advanced nodes and the remaining are standard nodes with some energy level difference between the 2 types Multiple-hopping is applied	Optimum life span Cost effective implementation	Complex structure CH formation is tricky

(continued)

Table 3 (continued)

S. No	Clustering methodology	Parameter consideration/key features	Pros	Cons
15	Stable election protocol (SEP) [9, 15, 19]	Heterogeneous-aware protocol Spread the time interval first node passing out Weighted election probabilities concepts Each node can be cluster head based on outstanding energy in each node Extends the stable region Better throughput	SEP is more resilient than LEACH Produces better stability	Improper load balancing Complex implementation
16	M-SEP: modified stable election protocols [3, 21]	Network is heterogeneous Different energy levels of member SNs Two aggregators on either side of sink CHs guide the packet data to the sink Cluster heads compute the remoteness from sink to aggregator Increased lifetime and stability of the network due to heterogeneous nature	M-SEP is better than SEP Longer stability Better network coverage	Improper load balancing Complex implementation
17	HEC: heterogeneous-aware energy efficient clustering [5, 7, 11, 14]	Multi-hop network Heterogeneous clustering method Energy is optimized as primary objective Energy is optimized with three ways of definite clustering scheme Advanced nodes are made cluster heads first, then all nodes may participate to become CH in second, and in third phase, direct transmission without making CH is done	Longer Coverage Better throughput Better energy dissipation	CH election is difficult Improper load balancing of SNs

(continued)

Table 3 (continued)

S. No	Clustering methodology	Parameter consideration/key features	Pros	Cons
18	DEEC: distributed energy efficient clustering	Heterogeneous clustering method Multi-hop network Increase stability and life time of network CH election basis is P (RE)/ P (overall energy of network) SNs with energy (initial) or RE will be more likable for CH election	Efficient Reliable Lower energy consumption	Complex architecture Stability issues
19	EDEEC: enhanced distributed energy efficient clustering	Increased heterogeneous prospects Concepts of super node is introduced with very high initial energy Multi hop network Increase stability and life time of network	Efficient Reliable Lower energy consumption Better network coverage Stable for a good time period	Complex architecture
20	MED-DEEC: modified enhanced developed DEEC	Distributed heterogeneous methodology Distribution decision gives two criteria, a number of SNs to become cluster heads and some group of SNs to remain non-CH during entire transmission Performance is better with respect to effective life time Data to energy ratio is increased by quarter value at least as that of LEACH	CH election is easy Energy consumption is lower Network implementation is easy	Complex architecture Cluster formation is difficult due to distributed nature

Table 4 Showing energy and reliability level comparison of different clustering techniques

	Technique/algorithms	Simulation tool	Energy efficient level	Reliability in data transmission	Power optimization level	Complexity in implementation	Throughput level of network
1	O-LEACH	MATLAB	Medium	Better	Better	LOW	Moderately efficient
2	LEACH-C	MATLAB	Medium	Medium	Medium	LOW	Moderately efficient
3	HEED	MATLAB	Better	Better	Better	LOW	Better than LEACH
4	EEHC	MATLAB	Metter	Medium	Better	LOW	Better than LEACH and HEED
5	PEGASIS	MATLAB	Medium	Good	Better	Medium	Very efficient
6	PANEL	MATLAB	Medium	Good	Better	Medium	Very efficient
7	TEEN/APTEEN	MATLAB	Good	Good	Medium	Medium	Better than EEHC but lower than PANEL
8	PSO-based	MATLAB	Good	Good	Good	Medium	Very efficient
9	Firefly algo	MATLAB	Better	Medium	Good	Medium	Very efficient
10	HBMO	MATLAB	Better	Good	Good	HIGH	Efficient than PGASIS
11	Housdorff algo	MATLAB	High	High	Medium	HIGH	Efficient than HBMO
12	DEEC	MATLAB	Moderate	Good	Good	Medium	Better than EEHC but lower than PANEL
13	HEC	MATLAB	Moderate	Good	Medium	Medium	Very efficient
14	SEP	MATLAB	Medium	Good	Medium	Medium	Very efficient
15	MED-DEEC	MATLAB	Good	Good	Good	HIGH	Better than SEP

(continued)

Table 4 (continued)

	Technique/algorithms	Simulation tool	Energy efficient level	Reliability in data transmission	Power optimization level	Complexity in implementation	Throughput level of network
16	M-SEP	MATLAB	Better	Medium	Medium	Medium	Better than MED-DEEC
17	CREEP	MATLAB	Better	Medium	Medium	HIGH	Moderately efficient
18	DEC	MATLAB	Medium	Low	Medium	LOW	Moderately efficient

Note: Simulation tool has not been thoroughly explained in respective articles but all the algorithms can be simulated in MATLAB

2 Conclusion

We need to understand that wireless sensor networks have now become more of a picture/video-oriented information network. These networks are termed as wireless camera sensor networks. Since normal information processing within a network does leads to so many complications as stated above and key parameter to address all the relevant issues such as energy consumption. Overall life of network, power consumption, load balancing, and stability have a common answer clustering. Almost 2 decades have passed just to given more optimum results for the sensor networks with the help of clustering, and we have almost 30 plus clustering techniques/algorithms/methodologies. Based on the fundamental clustering techniques, which are still very good to provide optimum energy consumption and lower average power LEACH, PEGASIS, and HEED have got to be the benchmarks while introducing modern-day meta-heuristic and probability-based mathematical solutions can be incorporated together with the formers to provide more stable network. Since the evolvement of cooperative communication because of the limited bandwidth available for all the different areas of communications, viz., military, biomedical, telemetry, telecom, navigation, and many more, the optimum selection of clustering technique has got to be the main concern before designing any wireless sensor network or wireless camera sensor networks. It is because wireless camera sensor networks will consume larger bandwidth as compared to normal ad hoc or WSN, so the cooperation is needed among multiple domains of communication to properly utilize the available frequency spectrum. This requirement leads to more power sensitive issues, sensor nodes energy consumption issues, overall network life span issues with load balancing. The effective solutions to these problems have two key answers, first better routing methods and second better clustering techniques. So, the study of all these clustering methodologies is more relevant in the context of modern-day wireless communication, and the outline of the study gives a clear picture that fundamental distributed hierarchical clustering techniques like LEACH, PEGASIS, EECH, and HEED have to be merged with PSO-based or neural-based model to provide better results.

References

1. Wang J, Zhang X (2020) Cooperative MIMO-OFDM-based exposure-path prevention over 3D clustered wireless camera sensor networks. IEEE Trans Wirel Commun 19(1)
2. Xie L, Zhang X (2013) "D clustering-based camera wireless sensor networks for maximizing lifespan with Minimum coverage rate constraint. In: Proceedings of IEEE GLOBECOM, Atlanta, GA, USA, 2013, pp 298–303
3. Sirisha G, Babu RB, Rao KR (2016) Establishing path quality management in wireless sensor networks through cluster head determination. Indian J Sci Technol 9(5)
4. Attarzadeh N, Mehrani M (2011) A new three-dimensional clustering method for wireless sensor networks. Glob J Comput Sci Technol 11(6). version 1.0

5. Chong C-Y, Kumar S (2003) Sensor networks: evolution, opportunities, and challenges. Proc IEEE 91(8):1247–1256
6. Xu L, Delaney D, O'Hare G, Collier R (2013) The impact of transmission power control in wireless sensor networks. In: International symposium on network computing and applications (NCA). IEEE, pp 255–258
7. Del Coso A, Spagnolini U, Ibars C (2007) Cooperative distributed MIMO channels in wireless sensor networks. IEEE J Sel Areas Commun 25(2):402–414
8. Rathi N et al (2012) A review on routing protocols for application in wireless sensor networks. Int J Distrib Parallel Syst (IJDPS) 3(5)
9. Kirichek R, Paramonov A, Koucheryavy A (2015) Flying ubiquitous sensor networks as a queening system. In: Proceedings, international conference on advanced communication technology, ICACT 2015, Phoenix Park, Korea, July 01–03, 2015
10. Akyildiz I, Su W, Sankarasubramaniam Y, Cayirci E (2002) Wireless sensor networks: a survey. Comput Netw 38(4):393–422
11. Wang J, Zhang X (2014) AQ-DBPSK/DS-CDMA based energy-efficient and interference-mitigation scheme for 3D clustered WCSNs with minimum coverage rate constraint. In: Proceedings IEEE MILCOM, Baltimore, MD, USA, pp 305–310
12. Nosratinia A et al (2004) Cooperative communication in wireless networks. IEEE Commun Mag
13. Parmar J et al Study of wireless sensor networks using LEACH-TEEN and APTEEN routing protocols. Int J Sci Res (IJSR) ISSN (Online): 2319-7064
14. Kiwan H et al (2013) Hierarchical networks: routing and clustering (a concise survey). In: 2013 26th IEEE Canadian conference of electrical and computer engineering (CCECE)
15. Hooggar M, Mehrani M, Attarzadeh N, Azimifar M (2013) An energy efficient three-dimensional coverage method for wireless sensor networks. J Acad Appl Stud 3(3)
16. Younis O, Krunz M, Ramasubramanian S (2006) Node clustering in wireless sensor networks: recent developments and deployment challenges. IEEE Netw 20(3):20–25
17. Brust MR, Frey H, Roth Kugel S, Adaptive multi-hop clustering in mobile networks. In: Proceedings of the 4th international conference on mobile technology, applications, and systems and the 1st international symposium on computer human interaction in mobile technology. ACM, 2007, pp 132–138
18. Wang J, Zhang X (2015) Cooperative MIMO-OFDM based multi-hop 3D clustered wireless camera sensor networks. Proc IEEE Wirel Commun Netw Conf (WCNC) 2015:1350–1355
19. Baker D, Ephremides A (1981) The architectural organization of a mobile radio network via a distributed algorithm. IEEE Trans Commun 29(11):1694–1701
20. Murugesan S (2008) Harnessing green it: principles and practices. IT Prof 10(1):24–33
21. Lin CR, Gerla M (1997) Adaptive clustering for mobile wireless networks. IEEE J Sel Areas Commun 15:1265–1275
22. Deosarkar BP, Yadav NS, Yadav RP (2008) Cluster head selection in clustering algorithms for wireless sensor networks: a survey. In: 2008 International conference on computing, communication and networking, pp 1–8
23. Zhao M, Yang Y, Wang C (2015) Mobile data gathering with load balanced clustering and dual data uploading in wireless sensor networks. IEEE Trans Mob Comput 14(4):770–785
24. Xu L, O'Hare G, Collier R (2014) A balanced energy-efficient multi-hop clustering scheme for wireless sensor network. In: 7th IFIP wireless and mobile networking conference (WMNC)
25. Nayak P, Devulapalli A (2016) A fuzzy logic-based clustering algorithm for WSN to extend the network lifetime. IEEE Sens J 16(1):137–144
26. Jain P et al (2017) The comparison between Leach protocol and Pegasis protocol based on lifetime of wireless sensor networks. Int J Comput Sci Mob Comput 6(12):15–19
27. Abakumov P, Koucheryavy A (2014) The cluster head selection algorithm in the 3D USN. In: Proceedings, international conference on advanced communication technology, ICACT 2014, Phoenix Park, Korea
28. Hai DT, Son LH, Le VT (2017) Novel fuzzy clustering scheme for 3D wireless sensor networks. Appl Soft Comput J. https://doi.org/10.1016/j.asoc.2017.01.021

29. Amis AD, Prakash R, Vuong TH, Huynh DT (2000) Maxmin d-cluster formation in wireless ad hoc networks. In: INFOCOM 2000. Nineteenth annual joint conference of the IEEE computer and communications societies. Proceedings. IEEE, vol 1. IEEE, pp 32–41
30. Arboleda LMC, Nasser N (2006) Comparison of clustering algorithms and protocols for wireless sensor networks. In: 2006 Canadian conference on electrical and computer engineering, May 2006, pp 1787–1792
31. Abbasi AA, Younis M (2007) A survey on clustering algorithms for wireless sensor networks. Comput Commun 30
32. Kumarawadu P, Dechene DJ, Luccini M, Sauer A (2008) Algorithms for node clustering in wireless sensor networks: a survey. In: 2008 4th International conference on information and automation for sustainability, pp 295–300

Electronics

Comparative Study of Different Material Tri-Gate MOSFET with Dielectric Material

Rani Kiran, Imran Ullah Khan, and Yusra Siddiqui

Abstract In this paper, a near investigation of the design of the TG MOSFET tri-gate metal oxide semiconductor field effect transistor device utilizes the SILVACO TCAD. SILVACO TCAD will be widely utilized for circuital plan and authorization. Device simulator system ATLAS is utilized. ATLAS tool, utilizes a single-material-gate (SMG), a double-material- gate (DMG), and three-material-gate (TMG) tri-gate MOSFET (TGMOSFET), respectively, with hafnium dioxide HfO_2 as dielectric materials are utilized. It shows a traditional model and better DC, AC execution of the tri-material-gate design, creates a high drive flow of the three-material-gate TGMOSFET with dielectric, and shows better electrical qualities contrasted with other device structures. In this paper, all the device boundaries of single-, dual-, and tri-material-gate TGMOSFETs are determined exhaustively, and HfO_2 and SiO_2 are dielectrics. HfO_2 is utilized to expand the gate capacitance in the device, subsequently expanding the drive current. Therefore, the presentation of the device can be improved. Analyze electrical boundaries like electric field, surface potential, electronic mobility, and flow thickness with HfO_2 as a dielectric. A correlation of channel flow, transconductance, and output conductivity between these models with dielectric is contemplated.

Keywords MOSFET · Tri-gate MOSFET · SMG · DMG and TMG

R. Kiran · I. U. Khan (✉) · Y. Siddiqui
Department of Electronics & Communication Engineering, Integral University, Lucknow, India
e-mail: iukhan@iul.ac.in

R. Kiran
e-mail: kiranphd@student.iul.ac.in

Y. Siddiqui
e-mail: yusra@student.iul.ac.in

M. S. Kaiser et al. (eds.), *Proceedings of Trends in Electronics and Health Informatics*, Lecture Notes in Networks and Systems 376,
https://doi.org/10.1007/978-981-16-8826-3_34

1 Introduction

Si CMOS has been a standard IC plan innovation for a very long time. Throughout the long term, the industry has progress ground in growing planar CMOS, and the VLSI industry is searching for MOSFETs with a length of less than 20 nm. Because of the diminished device size, another 3D MOS structure should be created with great protection from short channel effects (SCEs). Double-gate (DG) silicon MOSFET is a promising device with higher drive current and preferred SCEs authority over bulk hardware [1–4]. The change from double-gate to tri-gate (TG) structures gives higher drive flows and preferable insusceptibility to SCEs over DG MOSFETs. Intel created TG device with a high on-off current proportion and consequently high force proficiency, making them more force effective than any planar semiconductor. These gadgets smother SCEs and work on the control of channel flows in the device. Diminishing the thickness of the oxide to a most extreme level can bring about an increment in leakage current. In this way, replacing SiO_2 with a dielectric material will essentially lessen these restrictions. In this paper, hafnium dioxide (HfO_2) is utilized as a dielectric and has great transmitted character [5, 6].

2 MOSFET Basics

MOSFET or metal oxide semiconductor field effect transistor was developed to conquer the disadvantage of field effect semiconductor, like slow activity, high drain resistance, and moderate input impedance. Metal oxide field effect semiconductors, normally alluded to as MOSFETs, are electronic device used to switch or enhance circuit voltages. It is a voltage control device, worked from three terminals. MOSFET terminals are named sources, gate, drain, and body (Fig. 1).

The p-type semiconductors are the establishment of MOSFET. The two kinds of base are blended in with the profoundly doped of the n-type impurity, which is set apart as n+. From the highly doped regions of the base, terminal source and channel originated. The substrate layer is covered with a layer of silicon dioxide for protection. Thin, insulated protected metal plates are put away on top of silicon dioxide and go about as capacitor. The gate terminal is taken out from the thin metal

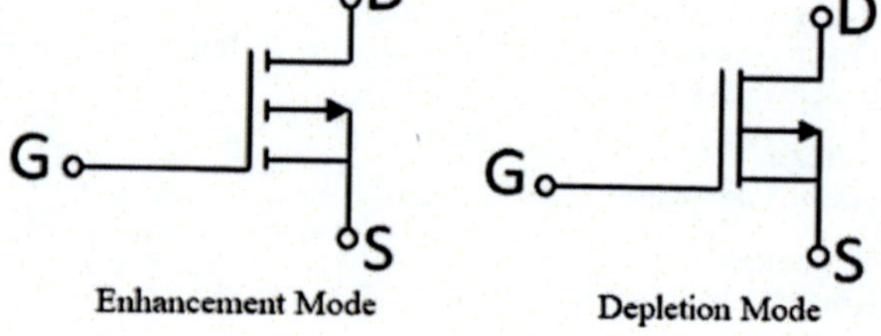

Fig. 1 Symbols of P-channel MOSFET

Table 1 Different MOSFET types

S. No.	MOSFET type	$V_{GS} < 0$	$V_{GS} = 0$	$V_{GS} > 0$
1	P-channel depletion	ON	ON	OFF
2	P-channel enhancement	ON	OFF	OFF
3	N-channel depletion	OFF	ON	ON
4	N-channel enhancement	OFF	OFF	ON

plate. A DC circuit is then framed by associating a voltage source between the two n-type regions. At the point when voltage is applied to the gate, an electric field is produced, changing the width of the channel region, where the electron flows. The more extensive the channel region, the more conductive the device is. There are two kinds of MOSFETs: Enhancement mode and depletion mode. Each type is accessible in n channels or p channels; therefore, in general, four types of MOSFET are there [7]. Table 1 shows the switching feature of the N- channel and P-channel types MOSFET.

MOSFET amplifiers are generally utilized in RF applications. The power supply MOSFET can be utilized to control the DC motor. MOSFET works at a lower voltage with more prominent proficiency. The shortfall of the gate stream brings about a high input impedance bringing about a high exchanging speed.

3 Basics of Tri Gate Structures

Distinctive gate designs and body device are examined, just as how the electric field lines reproduce through the collapse locale related with the intersection. Different gate structures are displayed in Figs. 2 and 3 A, and the electric field line propagates through the consumption area related with the intersection. Their impact on the channel can be diminished by expanding the doping concentration in the channel regions. Unfortunately, in thin device, the doping concentration turns out to be too high (10^{19} cm^{-3}) to work appropriately. In fully doped silicon on insulator (FDSOI) device, the vast majority of the field lines propagate through covered oxides (BOX) prior to arriving at the channel region [8]. By utilizing thin buried oxides and the fundamental ground plane, the short channel effect in FDSOI MOSFETs can be decreased. Notwithstanding, this strategy has the burden of expanding junction capacitance and volume impact [9–11]. A more proficient device arrangement can be gotten by utilizing a double-gate semiconductor structure [12–17].

Figure 2 shows the diverse gate constructions, and Fig. 3 shows a two-dimensional perspective on a single-, double-, and a three-material-gate TGMOSFET, with hafnium dioxide (HfO_2) as the dielectric and silicon dioxide (SiO_2) [18, 19].

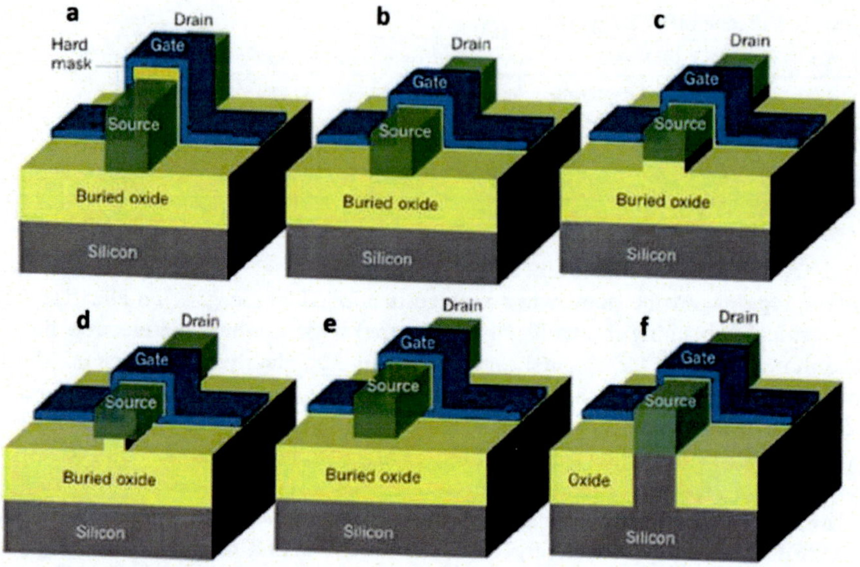

Fig. 2 Different gate structures [8]

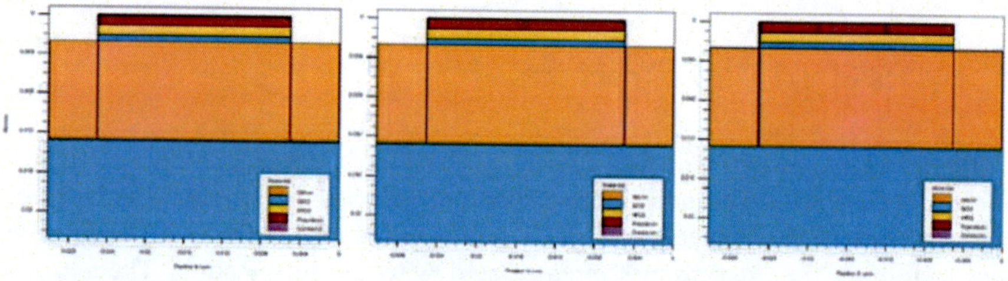

Fig. 3 Two-dimensional view of single-material-gate, double-material-gate, and triple-material-gate TGOSFET

4 Results

Device parameters for single-, double-, and a three-material-gate TGMOSFET, with hafnium dioxide (HfO_2) as the dielectric are as follows:

1. W/L ratio of 1:2, W/L is Channel width/ Channel length
2. Silicon channel thickness: 10 nm for each
3. Oxide thickness 1 nm (without dielectric) and 0.6 nm (with dielectric)
4. Channel doping concentration: 10^{19} cm^2 for each
5. Source and drain doping concentration: 10^{20} cm^2 for each.

Table 2 shows surface potential for single-, dual-, and tri-material-gate TGMOSFET, Table 3 shows total electric field for single-, dual-, and tri-material-gate TGMOSFET, and Table 4 shows surface potential for single-, dual-, and tri-material-gate TGMOSFET with HfO_2 as dielectric, respectively (Table 5).

Figure 4 shows proposed structure, and Fig. 5 indicates the examination of surface potential achievable alongside the perfect factor of the channel for single-, dual-material-gate furthermore, Tri-material-gate TGMOSFETs with HfO_2 as a dielectric with dielectric constant equal to 25 is utilized alongside SiO_2.

In the surface potential, it represents the description of the two stages and three stages of dual- and three-material-gate TGMOSFET. High-quality screening can be achievable in direct devices with dielectrics. In addition. It is also recommended in

Table 2 Surface potential for single-material-gate, dual-material-gate, and tri-material-gate TGMOSFET

S. No.	Distance along the channel (nm)	Surface potential (mV) for SMG	Surface potential (mV) for DMG	Surface potential (mV) for TMG
1	0	625	630	630
2	1	625	635	635
3	2	620	650	650
4	4	600	634	630
5	6	560	630	620
6	8	558	600	590
7	10	558	597	597
8	12	560	560	588
9	16	590	590	590
10	20	610	610	610

Table 3 Total electric field for single-, dual-, and tri-material-gate TGMOSFET

S. No.	Distance along the channel (nm)	Total electric field (V/m) for SMG	Total electric field (V/m) for DMG	Total electric field (V/m) for TMG
1	0	1×10^5	1×10^5	1×10^5
2	1	30×10^5	10×10^5	10×10^5
3	2	60×10^5	50×10^5	50×10^5
4	4	66×10^5	129×10^5	115×10^5
5	6	62×10^5	120×10^5	117×10^5
6	8	62×10^5	110×10^5	110×10^5
7	10	62×10^5	100×10^5	115×10^5
8	12	62×10^5	90×10^5	120×10^5
9	16	7×10^5	7×10^5	7×10^5
10	20	1×10^5	1×10^5	1×10^5

Table 4 Surface potential for single-, dual-, and tri-material-gate TGMOSFET

S. No.	Distance along the channel (nm)	Electron mobility $cm^2/(V.s)$ for SMG	Electron mobility $cm^2/(V.s)$ for DMG	Electron mobility $cm^2/(V.s)$ for TMG
1	0	60	60	60
2	1	40	40	40
3	2	25	25	25
4	4	15	8	8
5	6	12	8	8
6	8	12	8	8
7	10	12	8	8
8	12	12	8	8
9	16	40	40	40
10	20	60	60	60

Table 5 Transfer characteristics for single-, dual-, and tri-material-gate TGMOSFET

S. No.	Gate voltage (V)	Drain current (μA) for SMG	Drain current (μA) for DMG	Drain current (μA) for TMG
1	0	0	0	0
2	0.1	0	0	0
3	0.2	0	0	0
4	0.3	0	0	0
5	0.4	0	0	0
6	0.5	0	2	2.5
7	0.6	0.8	4	5
8	0.7	2	6	7
9	0.8	4	8	9.5
10	0.9	6.5	10.5	12
11	1	9.5	13.5	15
12	1.1	12	16	17.5
13	1.2	14.5	18	20

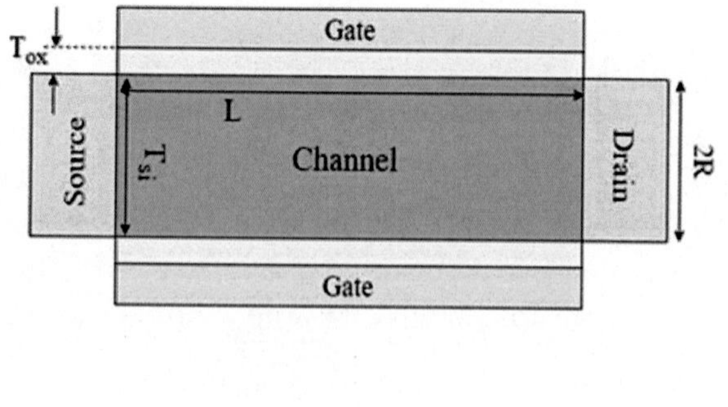

Fig. 4 Proposed structure

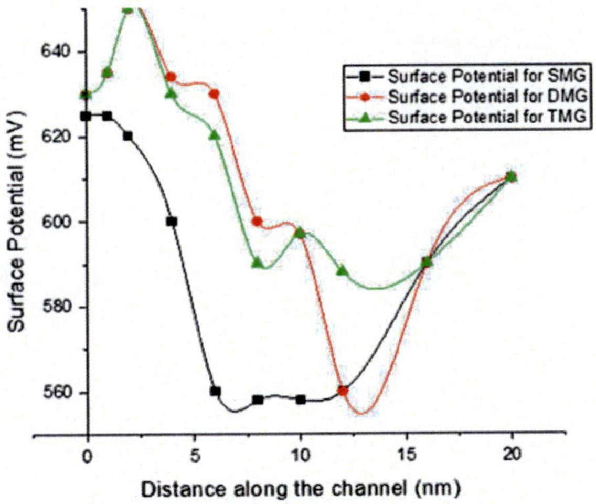

Fig. 5 Surface potential for single-, dual-, and tri-material-gate TGMOSFET

Fig. 5 that the tilt of the surface potential of the channel terminal dielectric device of the three-material-gate TGMOSFET is much smaller than the surface potential of the two- and single-material-gate TGMOSFET. This infers that the three-material-gate development can effectively reduce the degree of electric field near the channel end and by using excessive channel voltage shows a strong impermeability to the short channel effect. Figure 6 depicts the total electric field. It shows the larger electric field area of the gate material with greater working capacity and shows that the three-stage range of the electric field area of the TMG system depends on the unique gate material of the entire gate length. It shows that greater electric field constraints in the entire supply channel region stimulate the development of electrons in the channel.

Figure 7 shows the electron mobility of a single-, dual-, and three-material-gate MOS device having a dielectric. Electron mobility describes how electrons quickly

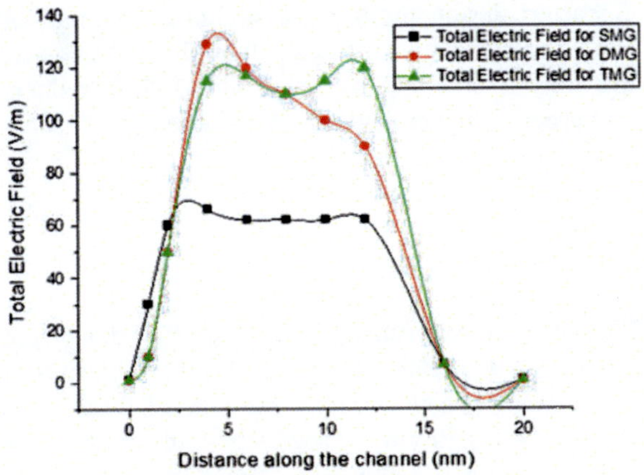

Fig.6 Total electric field for single-, dual-, and tri-material-gate TGMOSFET

Fig.7 Electron mobility for single-, dual-, and tri-material-gate TGMOSFET

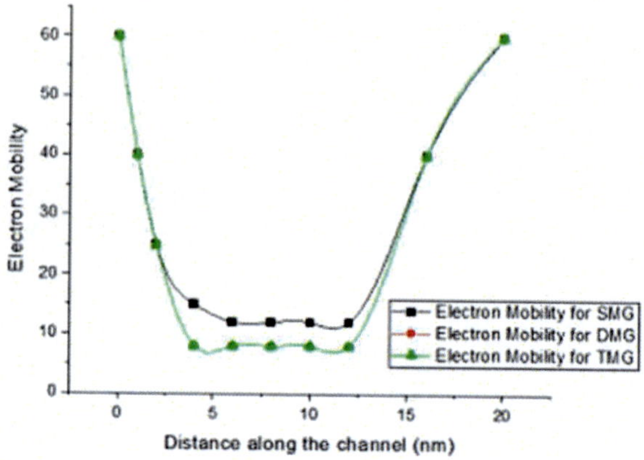

Fig. 8 Transfer characteristic of single-, dual-, and tri-material-gate TGMOSFET

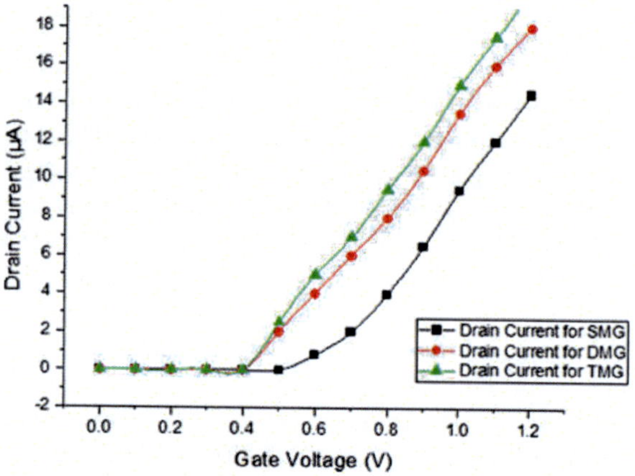

pass through the channel. Figure 8 shows the correlation between the alternating characteristics of single-, dual-, and three-material-gate TGMOSFET devices using HfO_2 as a conventional V_{DS} medium. It can be constant or a value of 1 mV. It seems that for the three-material-gate TGMOSFET, reduction of the short channel effect will produce higher device performance.

5 Conclusion

This comparative result of the TGMOSFET device profile regarding single-, double-, and triple-material-gate TGMOSFET with HfO_2 as dielectric material indicates a decreased model with channel size of 20–25 nm, thickness and width of the channel being 10 nm, respectively, with an thickness of 1.8 nm for the oxide of TGMOSFET and suggests the higher DC and AC implementation of the system for

TMG TGMOSFET with excessive drive current of 1.9 μA for TMGTGMOSFET and suggests a most valuable transconductance of 3.6 μA/V in correlation with different device constructions displaying a finest AC execution of the TMGTG device.

References

1. Dash DK, Saha P, Sarkar SK (2020) 3-D analytical modeling of triple metal tri-gate graded channel high-k SON TFET for improved performance. Silicon J, Springer Silicon 12:2041–2052
2. Saha P, Sarkhel S, Sarkar SK (2018) Compact 3D modeling and performance analysis of dual material tri-gate tunnel field effect transistor. https://doi.org/10.1080/02564602.2018. 1428503, IETE Technical Review, Taylor & Francis 36(2)
3. Banerjee P, Sarkar SK (2017) 3-D analytical modeling of highk gate stack dual-material tri-gate strained silicon-on-nothing MOSFET with dual-material bottom gate for suppressing short channel effects. J Computat Electron, Springer 16(3):631–639
4. Park SJ, Jeon DY, Montès L, Barraud S, Gyu-TaeKim GY, Ghibaudo G (2014) Impact of channel width on back biasing effect in tri-gate MOSFET. Microelectron Eng 114:91–97
5. Gola D, Singh B, Tiwari PK (2018) Subthreshold modeling of tri-gate junctionless transistors with variable channel edges and substrate bias effects. IEEE Trans Electron Devices 65(5)
6. Web Link: Metal-Oxide Semiconductor FET (MOSFET) (uncc.edu)
7. Gola D, Singh B, Tiwari PK (2017) A threshold voltage model of tri-gate junctionless field-effect transistors including substrate bias effects. IEEE Trans Electron Devices 64(9)
8. Chiang T-K (2013) A novel quasi-3-D threshold voltage model for fully depleted quadruple-gate (FDQG) MOSFETs: With equivalent number of gates (ENG) included. IEEE Trans Nanotechnol 12(6):1022–1025
9. Carballo JA, Chan WT, Gargini PA, Kahng AB, Nath S (2014) Itrs 2.0: toward a re-framing of the semiconductor technology roadmap. In: Proceedings of the 2014 IEEE 32nd international conference on computer design (ICCD), Seoul, Korea, 19–22 Oct 2014, pp 139–146
10. Ghani T, Mistry K, Packan P, Thompson S, Stettler M, Tyagi S, Bohr M (2000) Scaling challenges and device design requirements for high performance sub-50 nm gate length planar CMOS transistors. In: VLSI symposium technology digest, pp 174–175
11. Tang X, De VK, Meindl JD (1997) Intrinsic MOSFET parameter fluctuations due torandom dopant placement. IEEE Trans Very Large Scale Integr (VLSI) Syst 5(4):369–376
12. Oh S-H, Monroe D, Hergenrother JM (2000) Analytic description of short- channel effects in fully-depleted double-gate and cylindrical, surrounding-gate MOSFETs. IEEE Electron Device Lett 21(9):445–447
13. Chen Q, Harrell EM, Meindl JD (2003) A physical short-channel threshold voltage model for undoped symmetric double-gate MOSFETs. IEEE Trans Electron Devices 50(7):1631–1637
14. El Hamid HA, Guitart JR, Iniguez B (2007) Two-dimensional analytical threshold voltage and subthreshold swing models of undoped symmetric double-gate MOSFETs. IEEE Trans Electron Devices 54(6):1402–1408
15. Frank DJ, Taur Y, Wong H-SP (1998) Generalized scale length for two-dimensional effects in MOSFETs. IEEE Electron Device Lett 19(10):385–387
16. Young KK (1989) Short-channel effect in fully depleted SOI MOSFETs. IEEE Trans Electron Devices 36(2):399–402
17. Yeh PC, Fossum JG (1995) Physical subthreshold MOSFET modeling applied to viable design of deep-submicrometer fully depleted SOI low voltage CMOS technology. IEEE Trans Electron Devices 42(9):1605–1613

18. Chiang TK (2004) A novel scaling-parameter-dependent subthreshold swing model for double-gate (DG) SOI MOSFETs: including effective conducting path effect (ECPE). Semicond Sci Technol 19(12):1386–1390
19. Fossum JG, Ge L, Chiang M-H, Trivedi VP, Chowdhury NM, Mathew L, Workman GO, Nguyen B-Y (2004) A process/physics-based compact model for nonclasical CMOS device and circuit design. Solid State Electron 48(6):919–926

Performance Characterization of Double Material Gate-All-Around Nanowire MOSFET

Avishisht Kumar and Imran Ullah Khan

Abstract In this work, for the gate dielectric, aluminum oxide is used rather than silicon dioxide and the indium arsenide nanowire is employed in place of silicon nanowire as channel for a cylindrical gate-all-around field-effect transistor (CGAA FET). Silvaco TCAD software-ATLAS simulator was used to illustrate the functioning and performance of the arrangement. On account of high electron velocity, saturation velocity, and low contact resistance, indium arsenide is chosen, while aluminum oxide is preferred due to its higher permittivity. The suggested combination is found to show superior characteristics as per simulation results in comparison with the indium arsenide-silicon dioxide and silicon–silicon dioxide arrangements in CGAA structures. The effect of changes in the radius of nanowire, oxide thickness, and channel length on the transfer characteristics and the final output as well as on performance parameters like maximum transconductance and maximum drain current is analyzed to depict the advantage of the proposed combination.

Keywords Nanowire · MOSFET · GAA · FinFET · Silvaco TCAD

1 Introduction

One of the crucial challenges, in the reduction of MOSFET dimensions for enhanced performance are the short channel effects (SCEs). Primarily, to reduce the short channel effects in order to increase the scalability, unconventional FETs are being considered. Among which multiple gates, Ω-gate, π-gate, FinFET, and gate-all-around field-effect transistors are being preferred in literatures.

The most promising out of these non-classical alternatives for their SCE immunity are the gate-all-around MOSFET structures and hence continually drawing more

A. Kumar (✉) · I. U. Khan
Integral University, Lucknow, India
e-mail: avishish@student.iul.ac.in

I. U. Khan
e-mail: iukhan@iul.ac.in

M. S. Kaiser et al. (eds.), *Proceedings of Trends in Electronics and Health Informatics*, Lecture Notes in Networks and Systems 376,
https://doi.org/10.1007/978-981-16-8826-3_35

focus and attention of the research scholars and professionals [1, 2], and also by virtue of lowered electron scattering, aforesaid structures have remarkable electrostatic gate control. The nanowires used can either be cylindrical or rectangular. Out of the two, the cylindrical ones would be the finer option owing to the fact that rectangular GAA field-effect transistor has lower corner or fringing effects compared to the rectangular nanowires [3, 4].

With the purpose of achieving superior device performance, the literatures propose the use of gate oxide materials with high k and high mobility for channels. On that account, to attain low effective mass and exceptionally high electron mobility InGaAs, SnAs, InAs, etc., III–V semiconductors are preferred as channel materials [5]. Having electron mobility up to 30,000 $cm^{2/}Vs$, saturation velocity of 2×10^7 cm/s, effective mass of 0.023 mo InAs tends to be the most favorable choice. However, properties such as lower leakage current and higher gate capacitance make high k dielectric materials most advocated materials for gate oxides.

Lately, HfO_2, Al_2 $O_{3,}$ etc., materials with high dielectric-k are getting attention as gate oxides.

Do et al. [6] demonstrated that III–V-based semiconductor channel when incorporated with Al_2O_3 as gate oxide while annealing [7] showed no surface defects. Thus, resulting in high quality film of dielectric.

Various research works in literatures are suggested for gate-all-around transistors.

Vertical InAs nanowire GAA structure on Si substrate was proposed by Sofia et al. [1]. Si-nanowires were studied by Xu et al. [3] on GAA structures on bulk Si substrate. HfO_2 has higher permittivity than Al_2O_3, due to aforesaid reasons, Al_2O_3 is preferred. Hence in this work, in as nanowire with Al_2O_3 as gate oxide is envisioned. The suggested device structure realized with the help of Silvaco TCAD software-ATLAS simulator.

Different performance parameters such as transfer characteristics and several figures of merit were also studied. Channel doping, effect of channel length, radius, and oxide thickness were also examined to determine the advantages of the proposed structure results of the simulation were compared to other channel-oxide arrangements.

2 MOSFET and Its Applications

Metal oxide semiconductor FET transistor is an extensively used three terminal (source, gate, and drain) semiconductor device for amplifying signals and switching applications [4, 8]. By far, the most frequently used transistors for electronic devices (both digital and analog) are the MOSFETs.

Varying the width of a channel controls the charge carrier flow from source to drain in MOSFET. The gate is located between drain and source, and the voltage applied over it, governs the width of channel. Considerably, thin layer of metal insulates it from channel.

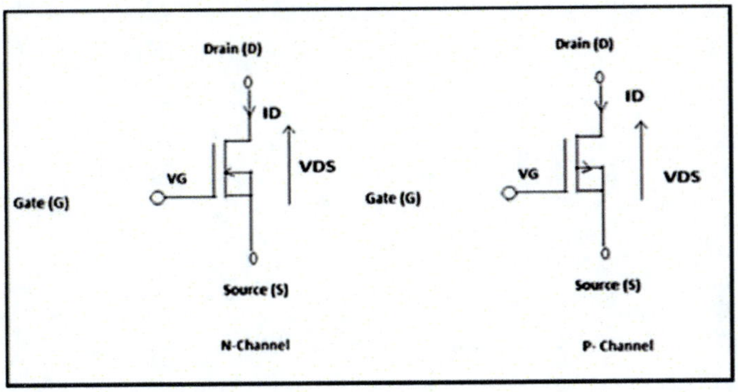

Fig. 1 Depletion mode MOSFET [5]

2.1 Classification of MOSFET Devices

The MOS devices can be of two types:

- Depletion MOSFET
- Enhancement MOSFET.

2.2 Depletion Mode

Maximum flow current is there when the gate voltage is zero. Channel conductivity decreases as the terminal voltage of the gate is rendered positive or negative. Figure 1 shows the depletion MOSFET.

2.3 Enhancement Mode

In this mode, with no voltage at the gate, there is no conduction. As the voltage is increased from zero to some value (threshold voltage), the current starts to increase. Figure 2 shows enhancement mode.

3 SOI Technology

In present scenario, reduction in power consumption and short channel effects has become one of the critical issues in VLSI circuit technology. Fundamental and physical bounds are being encountered with bulk Si devices. The thinning of gate insulators tends to increase the tunneling current, shallow junctions increase the

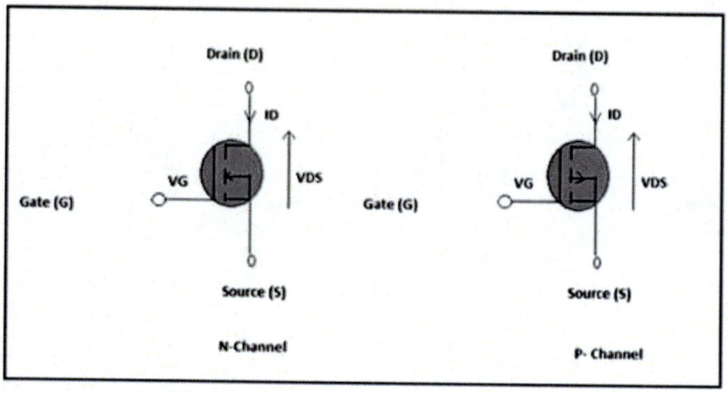

Fig. 2 Enhancement mode MOSFET [5]

leakage current, and the impurity scattering decreases the carrier mobility. These issues become the cause of conventional scaling less viable.

Low capacitance of silicon-on-insulator technology (SOI) permits high speed operations. Ability to endure high voltages and temperatures, decent radiation hardness, are also the virtues of SOI. In addition to the mentioned features, it facilitates flexible design [5, 6, 9, 10].

Compared to bulk Si, SiO_2 layer is just below the surface hence named buried oxide (BOX). It is fabricated by oxidation of silicon or O_2 implantation in silicon. Polycrystalline Si film devices are called as thin film transistors while single crystal Si film on the buried oxide is called SOI device.

For partially depleted and fully depleted, the SOI layer thickness is different. The layer in fully depleted is much less than partially depleted. It is nearly 1/3rd of effective channel length to prevent punch through current. The BOX layer gives SOI MOSFETs many advantages over their bulk Si counterparts. Stated advantages stand typical for both FD- SOI and PD-SOI.

a. ***Drain to substrate capacitance***

Due to the lower dielectric constant of silicon dioxide and negligible thickness of buried oxide, the capacitance is insignificant, rendering improved speed in switching applications.

1/2 to 1/3rd of power consumed by bulk Si devices is consumed by SOI devices at a given access speed.

Hence, they are faster.

b. ***Positive body bias***

In a stacked gate structure, independent body bias makes SOI faster. The negative body bias of transistor on bulk Si decreases the operating speed, and threshold voltage rises in stacked gate structure. However, the positive body bias of stacked SOI MOSFET decreases threshold voltage, and hence, operating speed is raised. Stacked gates reduce the circuit area.

c. ***Latch-up***

Compared to its counterpart (bulk Si), SOI device has no parasitic thyristor that restricts maximum operating voltage, hence SOI device has no latch up issues. Therefore, special circuit design is not required.

d. ***Device isolation and layout area***

BOX separates SOI devices vertically from each other, and an insulator film separates devices. Hence have higher packing density owing to ideal isolation. As a result, devices can be packed closer together than bulk ones. The groove filling process, i.e., shallow trench isolation is simple as the groove is very shallow.

e. ***Good soft-error immunity***

To neutrons, alpha particles, and other particles, SOI devices show superior radiation hardness. Alpha particles generate positive and negative charges in every micron along the trajectory which are adequate to eliminate the DRAM cell memory. Cosmic rays generated neutrons also incorporate soft errors.

f. ***p–n junction leakage***

In SOI devices, p-n junction leakage current is considerably small. The low p-n junction leakage is desirable in applications demanding low stand by power, mobiles phones for example.

Various insulator materials and substrates have been exhibited to form different SOI structures. Silicon-on-oxide, silicon-on-zirconia (SOZ), silicon-on-sapphire (SOS), and silicon-on-nothing are some of the combinations. By far, the most preferred are the oxides for insulators and Si wafer as substrate [7].

4 Short Channel Effects (SCEs)

When electric field lines from drain and source affect the gate control short-channel effects arise [2]. The electric field lines in a bulk device (Fig. 3a) propagate via the depletion regions linked with the junctions. Increase in the doping concentrations of the channel can reduce their effects. However, in small devices, proper functioning is hampered due to larger doping concentration.

In a FDSOI device, (Fig. 3b) before reaching the channel, most of the field lines go through the BOX. Short-channel effects (SCEs) in FDSOI MOSFETs can be reduced by employing a thin buried oxide and a ground plane beneath (Fig. 3c). Unfortunately, the approach has a drawback of increased body effect and junction capacitance [11–15].

A higher competent device configuration is achieved with the help of double-gate structure. The electric field lines cannot reach the channel as they cease on the bottom gate electrode (Fig. 3d).

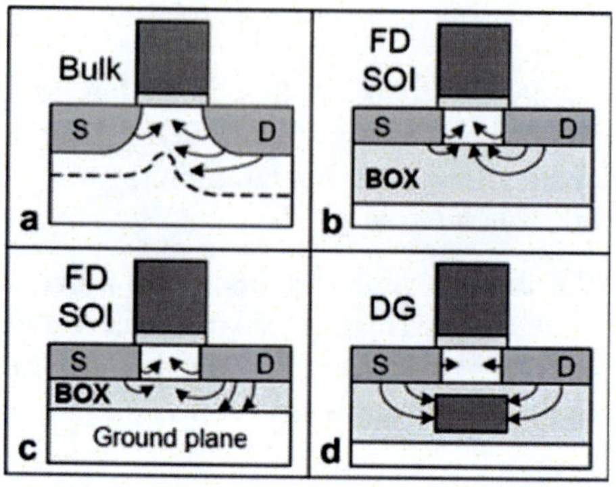

Fig. 3 Electric field lines from drain and source on the channel in different types of MOSFET [4]

5 Results and Discussion

The 3D structure (Fig. 4) projects the DMSG n-channel MOSFET studied in the work. To form the gate terminal, two different materials are chosen (M_1 and M_2) having distinct work functions (ϕ_{m1} and ϕ_{m2}) and lengths L_1 and L_2 are fused together. Hence, total gate length, $L = L_1 + L_2$. The lower work function gate material is kept near the drain to work as screen gate and higher work function material works as control gate and is kept near source end.

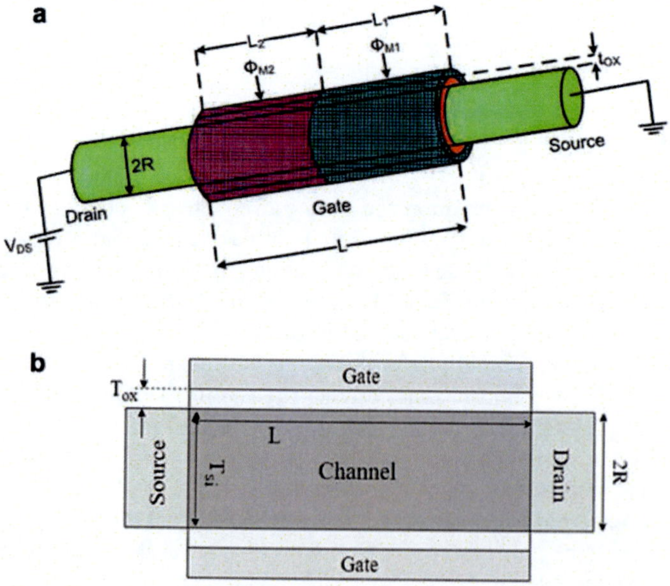

Fig. 4 **a** Three dimensional view DMSG MOSFET, **b** proposed structure on Silvaco

The parameters used in analysis are

Work function of first material gold is $\phi_{m1} = 4.8$ eV, and second material cadmium is ϕ_{m2}=4.0 eV.

Length of first and second material=20nm Gate to source voltage $V_{GS} = 0.5$ Volt Drain to source voltage $V_{DS} = 0.2$ V

Using silicon/silicon-germanium ordered arrangement of atoms in a solid solution superimposed on the solvent crystal lattice epitaxy and an original doping process for tacked wires, four-wire gate-all-around FET. The gate length is about 10 nm for the device. Channel height and width are 10 nm, it is generally based on an electrostatic scale length of 3.3 nm (Figs. 5, 6 and 7; Tables 1, 2 and 3).

ΔV_{Th}= Threshold voltage

ΔV_{DS} = Drain to source voltage

In real fabrication, it is important to decide the core insulator diameter according to application requirements. SiO_2 is the best material to achieve good performance.

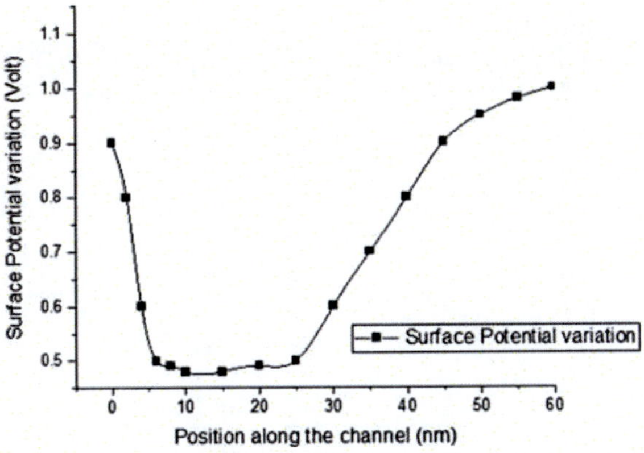

Fig. 5 Position along the channel versus surface potential variation

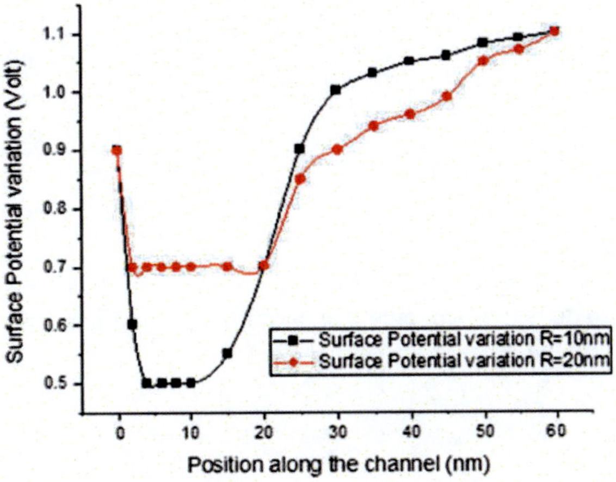

Fig. 6 Position along the channel for radius 10 and 20 nm versus surface potential variation

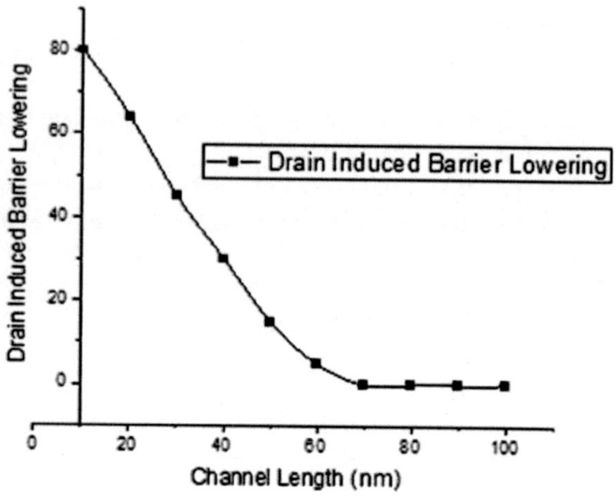

Fig. 7 Position along the channel versus variation of DIBL

Table 1 Position along the channel from the source to the drain versus variation of surface potential

S. No.	Position along the channel (nm)	Surface potential variation (V)
1	0	0.9
2	2	0.8
3	4	0.6
4	6	0.5
5	8	0.49
6	10	0.48
7	15	0.48
8	20	0.49
9	25	0.5
10	30	0.6
11	35	0.7
12	40	0.8
13	45	0.9
14	50	0.95
15	55	0.98
16	60	1.0

Since larger core insulator diameter can reduce on-state current, so the first thing to do is to select core insulator diameter, which enables on-state current to be large enough.

Table 2 Variation of surface potential w.r.t position along the channel from the source side to the drain side for radius 10 and 20 nm, respectively

S. No.	Position along the channel (nm)	Surface potential variation (V) for $R = 10$ nm	Surface potential variation (V) for $R = 20$ nm
1	0	0.9	0.9
2	2	0.6	0.7
3	4	0.5	0.7
4	6	0.5	0.7
5	8	0.5	0.7
6	10	0.5	0.7
7	15	0.55	0.7
8	20	0.7	0.702
9	25	0.9	0.85
10	30	1	0.9
11	35	1.03	0.92
12	40	1.05	0.94
13	45	1.06	0.99
14	50	1.08	1.05
15	55	1.09	1.07
16	60	1.1	1.1

Table 3 Channel length versus drain induced barrier lowering

S. No.	Channel length (nm)	Drain induced barrier lowering
1	10	80
2	20	64
3	30	45
4	40	30
5	50	15
6	60	5
7	70	0
8	80	0
9	90	0
10	100	0

6 Conclusion

Silvaco TCAD is used for analysis. It can be extensively used for circuital design and validation and device simulator ATLAS is used. In Table 1, position along the channel from the source to the drain versus variation of surface potential is analyze. As potential along channel increases, surface potential first decreases and then increases indicates step change near the junction of the two metals in the potential profile responsible for carrier velocity increase tends to carrier transport efficiency increase and hence result in I_{DS} increase. Plot of position versus surface potential at radius 10 and 20 nm, respectively, indicates as radius decreases, minimum value of potential reduces moves it to source side. Table 3 shows channel length and DIBL, drain induced barrier lowering, as channel length increases DIBL reduces and tends to zero referred to lowering of short channel effects.

References

1. Zhang Y, Han K, Jiawei L (2020) A Simulation study of a gate-all-around nanowire transistor with a core-insulator micromachines. MDPI 11(223):1–12
2. Johansson S, Memisevic E, Wernersson L-E, Lind E (2014) High-frequency gate-all-around vertical InAs nanowire MOSFETs on Si substrates. IEEE Electron Dev Lett 35(5):518–520
3. Xu Q, Luo J, Zhou H, Niu J, Liang Q, Zhao C (2012) Performance breakthrough in gate-all-around nanowire n- and p-type MOSFETs fabricated on bulk silicon substrate. IEEE Trans Electron Dev 59(7):1885–1890
4. Cho KH, Yeo KH, Yeoh YY, Suk SD, Li M, Lee JM, Kim M-S, Kim D-W, Park D, Hong BH, Jung YC, Hwang SW (2008) Experimental evidence of ballistic transport in cylindrical gate-all-around twin silicon nanowire metal-oxide-semiconductor field effect transistors. Appl Phys Lett 92(5):052102
5. Cheng Y, Chen CH, Enz C, Matloubian M, Deen MJ (2000) MOSFET modeling for RF circuit design. In: Proceedings of the 2000 third IEEE international caracas conference on devices, circuits and systems (Cat. No.00TH8474). https://doi.org/10.1109/iccdcs.2000.869831
6. Jena B, Ramkrishna BS, Dash S, Mishra GP (2016) Conical surrounding gate MOSFET: a possibility in gate-all-around family. Adv Nat Sci Nanosci Nanotechnol 7(1)
7. Do Q-T, Blekker K, Regolin I, Prost W, Tegude FJ (2007) High transconductance MISFET with a single InAs nanowire channel. Electron Dev Lett 28(8):682–684
8. Jena K, Bhowmick B, Baishya S (2013) Simulation and optimization of a partial gate all around cylindrical tunnel FET. Int J Recent Technol Eng (IJRTE) 2(5):43–45
9. Islam MJ, Hasan MM, Farwah SU, Chowdhury MIB (2014) A novel cylindrical gate all around MOSFET using InAs as channel and HfO_2 as gate oxide. ISTP J Res Electric Electron Eng (ISTP-JREEE), vol special issue on ISTP (IOCRSEM-2014), pp 59–62
10. Kosmani NF, Fatimah AH, Razali MA (2019) A comparison of performance between double-gate and gate-all-around nanowire MOSFET. Indonesian J Electric Eng Comput Sci 13(2):801–807
11. Pal A, Sarkar A (2014) Analytical study of dual material surrounding gate MOSFET to suppress short-channel effects (SCEs). Eng Sci Technol, an Int J 17:205–212
12. Islam MJ, Farwah SU (2016) Silvaco TCAD based analysis of cylindrical gate—all-around FET having indium arsenide as channel and aluminium oxide as gate dielectrics. J Nanotechnol Its Appl Eng 1(1):1–12
13. Singh J, Kumar MJ (2017) A planar junctionless FET using sic with reduced impact of interface traps: proposal and analysis. IEEE Trans Electron Devices 64:4430–4434
14. Tsormpatzoglou A, Dimitriadis CA, Clerc R, Rafhay Q, Pananakakis G, Ghibaudo G (2007) Semi-analytical modeling of short- channel effects in Si and Ge symmetrical double-gate MOSFETs. IEEE Trans Electron Devices 54(8):1943–1952
15. Liang X, Taur Y (2004) A 2-D analytical solution for SCEs in DG MOSFETs. IEEE Trans Electron Devices 51(9):1385–1391

A Comparative Analysis of Different Types of Mixer Architecture for Modern RF Applications

Zohaib Hasan Khan, Shailendra Kumar, and Deepak Balodi

Abstract A correlative analysis of dissimilar mixer architecture is shown in this work which is effectively investigating efficient methods to design the mixer for wide-band with lower power consumption, small size, high noise performance, minimal cost, and high conversion gain (dB). The different mixer's architecture has been mostly using Gilbert cell as it gives better gain, high port to port isolation, and low distortion. Today's communication industry has an increasing demand for low-cost and low-power circuits. Designers are attracted by the development of CMOS technology because it provides compact system and also meets the requirement of low-cost and low-power characteristics.

Keywords Port to port isolation · Cross-coupled · Self-oscillating dual band · Current bleeding down conversion · Transformer coupling cascode topology · Switch circuits · Folded architecture

1 Introduction

Over the last few years, the advancement of electronics and communication technology has led to wireless applications requiring low-power consumption, low-cost, and high integrated circuit design, such as multimedia devices, PAN, and WSN. The wireless components in the RF CMOS field for direct conversion architecture not only provide compact mobile terminals, but also pave the way for low-cost RF solutions (in terms of software and hardware), using the optimum power. In addition, for bandwidth and modern spectrum versatility, RF CMOS components are expected to remain compatible with high data rate multi-standard applications. For such wide range of applications, the noise of RF components needs to be designed as low as

Z. H. Khan (✉) · S. Kumar
Integral University, Lucknow, India

D. Balodi
BBD Engineering College, Lucknow, India

M. S. Kaiser et al. (eds.), *Proceedings of Trends in Electronics and Health Informatics*, Lecture Notes in Networks and Systems 376,
https://doi.org/10.1007/978-981-16-8826-3_36

possible, because end-to-end mobile units seek extremely high signal-to-noise ratio (SNR) performance.

2 RF Mixer Basics and Different Architecture

One of the key components in the radio transmitter and receiver is mixer. All electronic communicating devices have two mixers, one for the transmitter end and the one for the receiver end. Action of any mixer is to accomplish frequency conversion from low to high said as up conversion and from high to low named as down conversion by multiplication of the two signals. In mixture, there are 3 ports, in which 2 input ports are radio frequency (RF) and local oscillator (LO) and 1 port is output intermediate frequency (IF) as shown in Fig. 1.The first port called the RF port carries the input signal from the low noise amplifier, and the 2nd port is the local oscillator input carrier.

The input and output relationship of the mixer may be written as

$$V_{IF} = M V_{RF} V_{LO} \tag{1}$$

Here, V_{IF} is the mixer output known as intermediate frequency output, radio frequency signal is the V_{RF} of low noise amplifier, V_{LO} is voltage signal of local oscillator, and M is the multiplier coefficient.

For instance, let us suppose $V_{RF}(t) = A_{RF}$ Sin$2\pi f_1$ (t) and $V_{LO} = A_{LO}$ Sin$2\pi f_2$ (t), where A_{RF} and A_{LO} are radio frequency and local oscillator amplitudes and f_1 and f_2 are the respective frequency of RF and local oscillator.

The output signal will be multiplication of two signal, i.e.,

$$V_{IF}(t) = A_{RF}\text{Sin}2\pi f_1(t) \times A_{LO}\text{Sin}2\pi f_2(t) \tag{2}$$

Fig. 1 RF mixer model

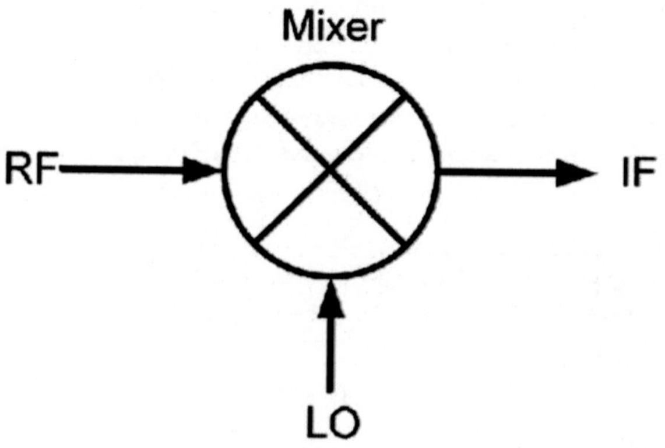

$$V_{IF}(t) = M[\cos 2\pi(f_1 - f_2)t - \cos 2\pi(f_1 + f_2)t] \tag{3}$$

where $M = (A_{RF}\, A_{LO})/2$.

Mixer requires nonlinear devices or time varying devices to get the mixing terms. There are additionally various forms of RF mixer that are needed to be understood. One of the basic fundamental forms relates to the electronic component type active or passive mixer.

Passive mixers: The passive mixer does not require a DC power supply to work. Hence, passive mixer could not give high gain and LO power required is high. A variety of traditional passive mixer architectures can be used to provide better isolation and implementation but they have no gain. Passive mixer is commonly used in high frequency microwave applications because of good noise figure, high linearity, and lower consumption power and good intermodulation. In general, architectures of passive mixer, Schottky diodes are used as switching elements, which have the additional advantage of low on-voltage. For this reason, they need to use balance transformers for most high-performance designs, which will limit the frequency bands, they can operate in [1–3]. In passive mixers, it is important to note that they introduce so-called conversion losses which can have an impact on RF circuit design So there must be a gain stage behind them, so more amplifiers are needed. For example, let us take single diode mixer as passive mixer shown in Fig. 2. The nonlinearity of the diode leads to frequency combining as mixing. Diode current voltage characteristic curve is displayed in the Fig. 3.

Active mixers: Transistors are used as electronic switching element, providing the essential mixing operation. The significant advantage of active architecture is a high gain with reasonable isolation. Unlike passive mixers, active mixers can have a conversion gain, and this will affect the RF design for the item [3] (Table 1).

RF mixers or frequency mixers can also be categorized according to whether they are balanced or unbalanced. This is an important decision to make.

Unbalanced: An unbalanced RF mixer is a basic form of RF mixer which performs the fundamental task of mixing and provides addition or subtraction of input signals to it (RF and LO). Output also comprises significant amplitude of original RF signal in addition with oscillator's component, which in turn results in poor isolation [4, 5]. As there is little isolation between the ports, this can lead to increased levels of

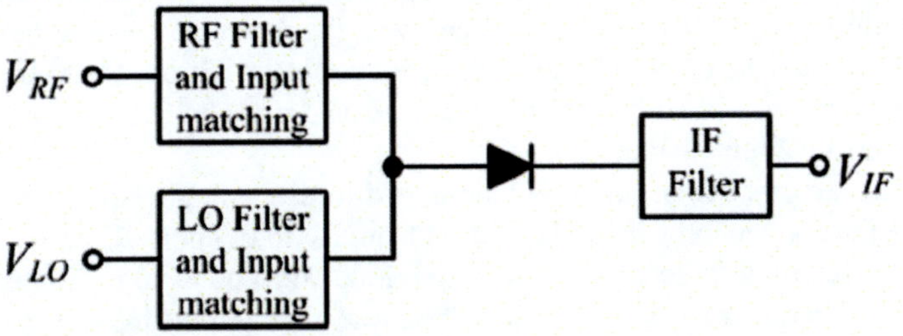

Fig. 2 Mixer with single semiconductor diode

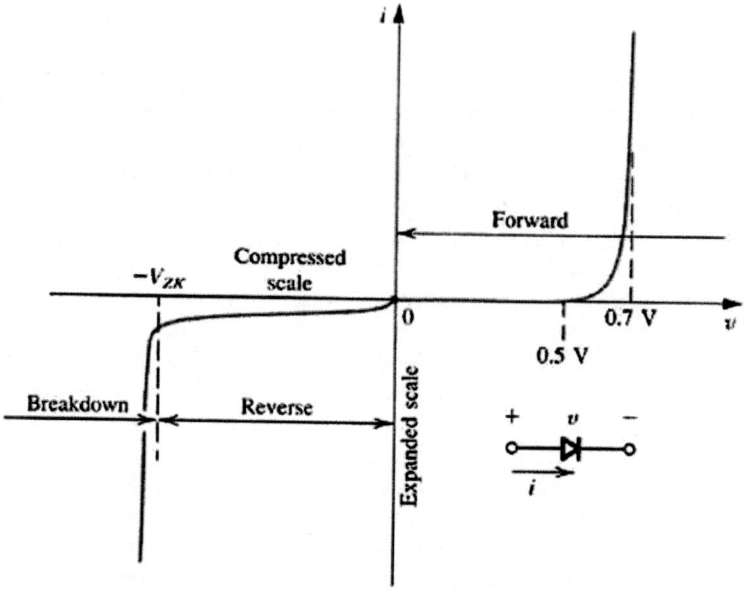

Fig. 3 Diode current voltage characteristic curve

Table 1 A comparison of performance parameter between passive mixer and active mixers

Passive mixer	Active mixer
DC power is not required	DC power is required
Power consumption is low	Power consumption is high
Local oscillator power is high	Local oscillator power is low
Noise performance and noise figure is poor	Noise performance and noise figure is good
Linearity is better	Linearity is average

intermodulation distortion as well as the local oscillator and RF signals being present on the output.

Balanced: A balanced mixer is one in which the ports have a balanced or differential structure. Dependent upon the actual type, there can be isolation between the different ports, and the LO and RF can be suppressed at the IF port. There are different types of balanced mixer: single, double balanced, and triple balanced (more correctly termed a doubly double balanced).

Single Balanced Mixer: It is recommended to use a single balanced mixer for increasing the conversion gain and isolation from RF to LO port, RF to IF port. This architecture requires to accommodate differential form of local oscillator signals, one-ended radio frequency signals, and differential intermediate frequency output, as shown in the Fig. 4. This architecture is superior to other mixers, as it provides high RF to local oscillator and radio frequency to intermediate frequency isolation, conversion

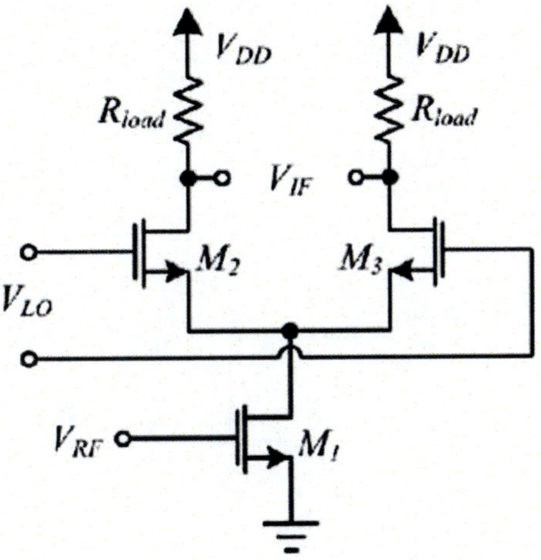

Fig. 4 Single balanced mixer

gain is adjustable, and also it is compact and easy to implement. However, it also has disadvantages. For example, the LO signal may leak to intermediate frequency port, there is no local oscillator noise suppression, so the uneven harmonics appear at the intermediate frequency port which need to be filtered. As this mixer has low IIP3, the RF signal is unbalanced so double balanced mixing came in to picture and is recommended over this mixer.

Double Balanced Mixer: Double balanced mixer operates with differential local oscillator signal as well as differential radio frequency signal. The Gilbert cell is a example of mixer with double balanced architecture as displayed in Fig. 5.

The basic Gilbert cell mixer includes three stages. Transconductance stages M1-M2 convert the differential RF voltage into RF current. In LO switch stage, the cross-coupled switch pairs M3-M4 and M5-M6 achieve a mixing operation similar to a single balanced topology. The connections between the LO terms are anti-parallel to eliminate the second-order terms at the output, but the connections in the RF signal are parallel. The double balanced CMOS Gilbert cell mixer provides large conversion gain, high isolation between all ports low noise figure but also consumes large power, caused by the number of transistors is twice that of a single balanced mixer.

Current bleeding double balanced mixer: If there is no current bleeding technique, then the gain A_v of CMOS is calculated by

$$A_v = (2\,G_m R_L) \div \pi \tag{4}$$

where G_m is RF stage transconductance and R_L is output load stage resistor. So, we can increase the conversion gain when pass high current from the RF, however, this will result in more power consumption. In addition, the voltage margin problem also occurs. The current bleeder transistor as shown in Fig. 6 is encapsulated to solve this issue.

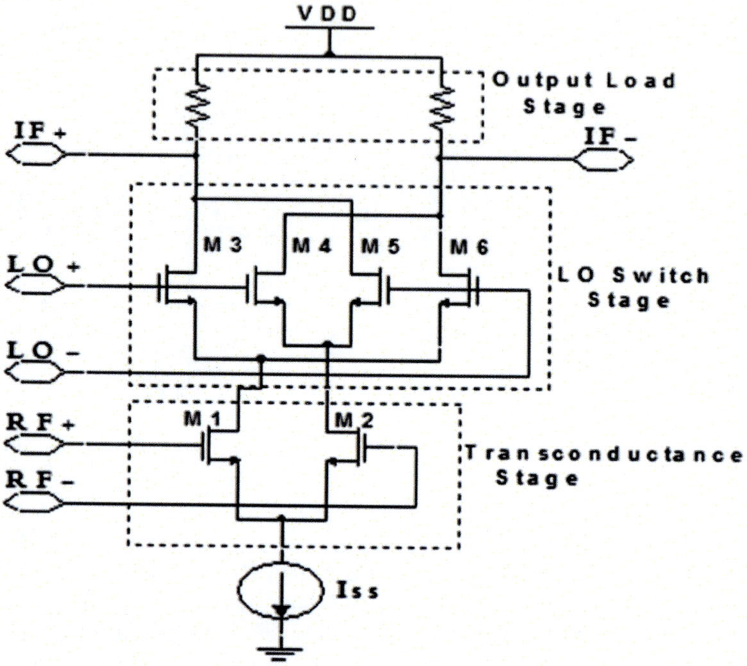

Fig. 5 Mixer with double balanced architecture

Mixer with double balanced and switched biasing technique: One major issue with current bleeding technique is the tail source current which is as a key noise source in the transistor. Noise generated by tail current source causes nonlinearity within the mixer and give rise to additional signals. This can cause issues in circuit design or system in which they are used. To reduce the noise generated by tail current source, we can use switched biasing technique as shown in Fig. 7, where the tail current source is replaced by two identical half sized transistor operated using IF output signal alternatively. It operates periodically in two states such as one is active state and other is inactive state. In active state, it provides a bias current, and in inactive state, the noise and power consumption are reduced [6]. In the wireless communication, devices such as Bluetooth, ZigBee, and Wi-Fi are used for short-distance communication. These battery-powered devices should consume a small amount of power. The double balanced passive mixer with switch bias technology mixer is suitable for low-power applications such as Bluetooth, Wi-Fi, and ZigBee, because the mixer significantly reduces power consumption, and it also has moderate IIP3 and P1dB [7].

Double Balanced Mixer with Cross-Coupled Technique: In the switching nonlinear in the RF front-end module, LO noise gradually spreads and reaches the IF output. A common approach to significantly solve this problem is to choose a differential balanced architecture to suppress noise propagation. A balanced mixer

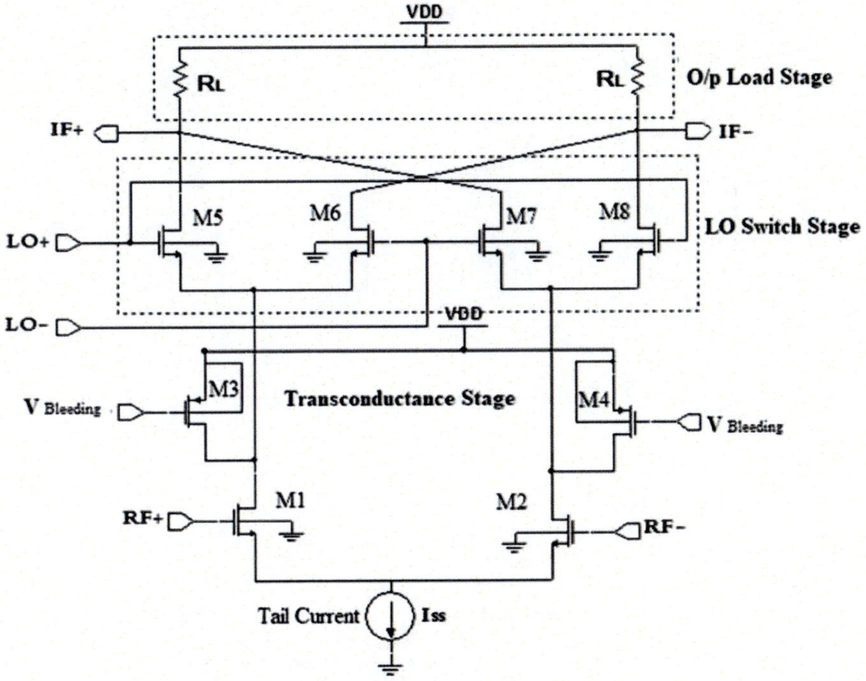

Fig. 6 Double balanced utilizing current bleeding technique

uses a four-port hybrid junction as shown in Fig. 8. The input of this cross-coupled architecture is fed by LO and RF signals. A balanced connection allows the sum of LO and RF to be received at the input of one diode, while the other diode handles the difference between the two. A strict requirement for successful mixing under balanced standards is that the two diodes must have exactly the same characteristics and be closely matched. Since the LO noise remains in phase on the two diodes, it is canceled out.

Switching nonlinear element has limited conduction loss, but reduces the conversion gain, and the value is very different from the ideal mark. If we provide a higher amplitude LO signal, it will result in a high conversion gain, but at will also cause more power consumption.

Folded Double Balanced Down Conversion Mixer: By using current-reuse cross-coupled techniques, the noise figure and current gain performance parameter are improved [8] as shown in Fig. 9. In the folding double balance structure, gain gm and switch-level paths are separated to provide independent bias conditions for the two stages, so gm stage can be biased to achieve high transconductance and reduce noise without affecting bias conditions switching phase. The original unbalanced external input must first be converted to a balanced mode, for which RF and LO baluns (a contraction of balanced-unbalanced) are implemented using on-chip transformers. M1–M2 and M3–M4 are used in the inverter topology, which ultimately

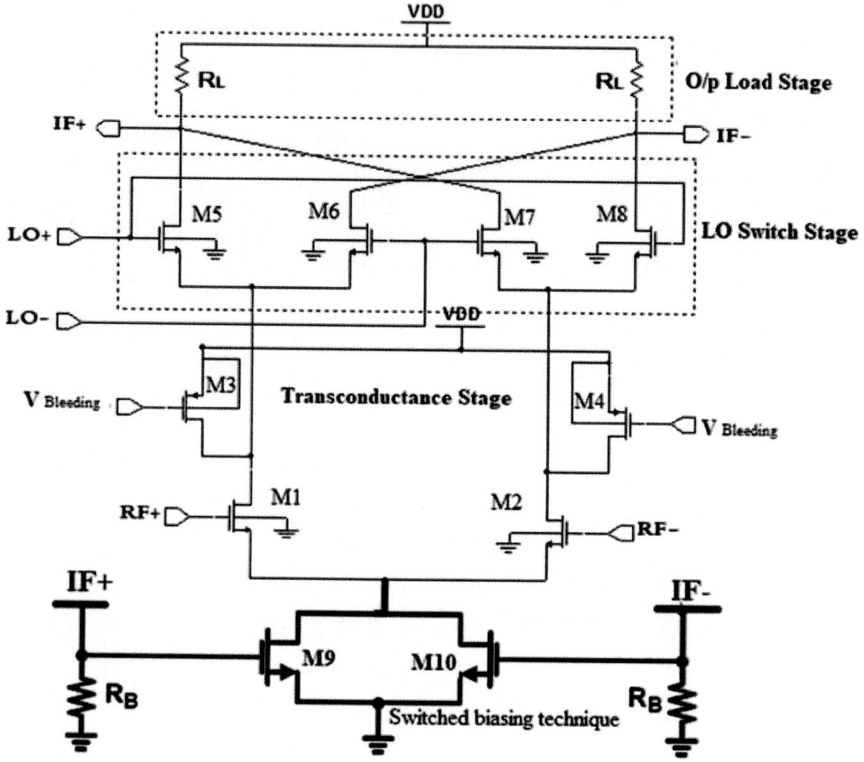

Fig. 7 Double balanced mixer with switched biasing technique

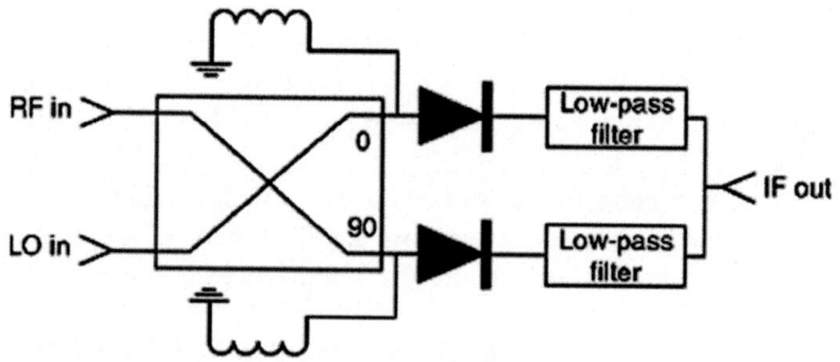

Fig. 8 A double balanced mixer using cross-coupled architecture

provides the phenomenon of current-reuse, thereby providing high transconductance gain gm. Due to the opposite of the differential transistors of the RF stage, the additional advantage of noise in terms of input reference noise is obtained. Due to this, the leakage from LO to RF is significantly reduced and better isolation is achieved.

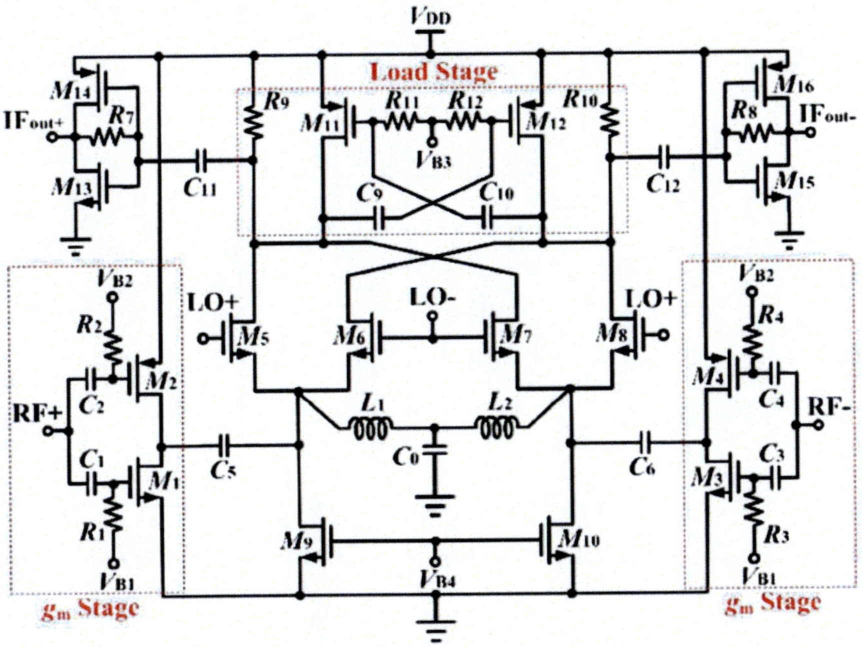

Fig. 9 Folded double balanced down conversion mixer [8]

A 2.4 GHz Bluetooth low energy receiver employing a quadrature RF-to-baseband-current-reuse RF front-end with double balanced current-mode passive mixers architecture, where the DC bias current from a single supply voltage was shared among all the sub-blocks in the RF front-end is developed for low-power low-voltage internet of things applications [9].

3 Comparative Evaluation of Different Architecture

A comprehensive comparison table (Table 2) has been prepared to show the evaluation performance of different mixer architecture technologies. The most important performance parameters are compared for different architecture.

There exists a tradeoff for different performance parameter a from the comparative performance evaluation of different mixer design as seen in Table 2. Among various architecture, the double balanced architecture greatly improves the leakage (LO-RF and LO-IF), thereby providing excellent isolation. In addition, excellent linearity (lower IP1) can be seen. Since this architecture gives a higher conversion gain, so making it the great choice of noisy RF systems, where higher SNR is a strict requirement.

Table 2 Comparative evaluation of the different mixer architecture against some essential parameters

Topology	Unbalanced mixer	Single balanced mixer	Double balanced mixer	Double balanced mixer with current-bleeding technique	Double balanced mixer with switched biased technique	Double balanced mixer with Cross-coupled technique	Folded double balanced down conversion
Conversion gain	High	Low	Large	Large	Low	Moderate	Good
Linearity	Poor	Average	Good	Below average	Moderate	Good	Good
Isolation	High	Average	High	High	High	High	High
Noise figure	High	Average	Low	Below average	Good	Good	Good
Power consumption	Low	Moderate	High	Moderate	Moderate	Moderate	Moderate

4 Conclusion

This paper consists of the comparative analysis of the different down conversion mixers. There are various parameters performance to judge the performance of the mixer. These parameters are gain, noise, linearity, power consumption, etc. There exist trade-offs between these parameters of mixer and it is hard to say if the particular mixer architecture is good or bad. It all depends on the application where we are using the mixer. However, based on our comparative study among the various down conversion mixer, the double balanced current-reuse cross-coupling architecture provides optimized values for all the basic parameters of the RF CMOS mixer.

Acknowledgements This work is an intellectual property of Integral University videos the Manuscript Communication no. IU/R&D/2021-MCN0001256. We would like to acknowledge the Integral University, Lucknow, India for providing an opportunity to carry out this research work.

References

1. Klumperink AM, Louwsma SM, Wienk GJM, Nauta B (2004) A CMOS switched transconductor mixer. IEEE J Solid-State Circuits 39(8):1231–1240
2. Terrovitis MT, Meyer RG (1999) Noise in current-commutating CMOS mixers. IEEE J Solid-State Circuits 34(6):772–783
3. Darabi H, Abidi AA (2000) Noise in RF-CMOS mixers: a simple physical model. IEEE J Solid-State Circuits 35(1):15–25
4. Chang YH, Huang CY, Chiang YC (2012) A 24 GHz down-conversion mixer with low noise and high gain. In: Proceedings of the European microwave integrated circuits conference, pp 285–288
5. Lee SG, Choi JK (2000) Current-reuse bleeding mixer. Electron Lett 36(8):696–697
6. Kim HWMG, An YM, Kang JY, Lee TY (2012) Yun: A Low-Voltage, low-power, and low-noise UWB mixer using bulk-injection and switched biasing techniques. IEEE Trans Microw Theory Tech 60(8):2486–2493
7. Naik SB, Siddharth RK, Chatterjee A, Nithin KY, Vasantha MH, Kini R (2021) A 1 V double-balanced mixer for 2.4–2.5 GHz ISM band applications. IEEE Xplore, Conf. https://doi.org/10.1109/VLSID51830.2021.00048
8. Peng Y, He J, Hou H, Wang H, Chang S, Huang Q, Zhu Y (2019) A K-band high-gain and low-noise folded CMOS mixer using current-reuse and cross-coupled techniques. IEEE Access 7
9. Park B, Kwon K (2021) A 2.4 GHz BLE receiver with power-efficient quadrature RF-to-baseband-current-reuse architecture for low-power IoT applications. IEEE Access 9:62734–62744. https://doi.org/10.1109/ACCESS.2021.3074650
10. Liu Z, Dong J, Chen Z, Jiang Z, Liu P, Wu Y, Zhao C, Kang K (2018) A 62–90 GHz high linearity and low noise CMOS mixer using transformer-coupling cascode topology. IEEE Access 6:19338–19344
11. Huang BJ, Lin KY, Wang H (2009) Millimeter-wave low power and miniature CMOS multicascode low-noise amplifiers with noise reduction topology. IEEE Trans Microw Theory Techn 57(12):3049–3059
12. Lin YS, Lan KS, Wang CC, Chi CC, Lu SS (2016) 6.3 mW 94 GHz CMOS down-conversion mixer with 11.6 dB gain and 54 dB LO-RF isolation. IEEE Microw Wireless Compon Lett **26**(8), 604–606

13. Abdelrheem TA, Elhak HY, Sharaf KM (2003) A concurrent dual-band mixer for 900-MHz/1.8 GHz RF front-ends. Proc 46th Midwest Symp **3**
14. Paco PD, Villarino R, Junkin G, Menendez O, Corrale E (2007) Dual band mixer using composite right/left-handed transmission lines. IEEE Microw Wireless Compon Lett 17(8):607–609
15. Jackson BR, Saavedra CE (2010) A dual-band self-oscillating mixer for C-band and X-band applications. IEEE Trans Microw Theory Techn 58(2):318–323
16. El-Nozahi M, Amer A, Sánchez-Sinencio E, Entesari K (2010) A millimeter-wave (24/31-GHz) dual-band switchable harmonic receiver in 0.18-μm SiGe process. IEEE Trans Microw Theory Techn **58**(11), 2717–2730
17. Mazzanti A, Vahidfar MB, Sosio M, Svelto F (2010) A low phase-noise multi-phase LO generator for wideband demodulators based on reconfigurable sub-harmonic mixers. IEEE J Solid-State Circuits 45(10):2104–2115
18. A D-band gain-boosted current bleeding down-conversion mixer in 65 nm CMOS for chip-to-chip communication. IEEE Microw Wirel Compon Lett 2:143–145
19. Ahn D, Kim DW, Hong S (2009) A K-band high-gain down-conversion mixer in 0.18 μm CMOS technology. IEEE Microw Wireless Compon Lett 19(4)
20. Chang YT, Wu HY, Lu HC (2016) A K-band high-gain downconverter mixer using cross couple pair active load. In: Proceedings of the European microwave integrated circuits conference, pp 377–380
21. Lin DR, Kao KY, Lin KY (2018) A K-band high-gain linear CMOS mixer with current-bleeding neutralization technique. In: Proceedings of the IEEE Asia Pacific microwave conference, pp 267–269
22. Sudhakar KIU, Mittal N (2021) Design and simulation of low power, high gain and high bandwidth CMOS folded cascode OTA using recycling and gm/ID technique. Int Res J Comput Sci (IRJCS) 8:3–3
23. Charan P, Usmani T, Paulus R, Saeed SH (2016) Performance evaluation of AODV protocol for energy consumption and QoS in IEEE 802.15.4 based wireless sensor network using QualNet simulator. Wirel Sensor Netw 8:166–175
24. Yoon DY, Yun SJ, Cartwright J, Han SK, Lee SG (2011) A high gain low noise mixer with cross-coupled bleeding. IEEE Microw Wireless Compon Lett 21(10)
25. Balodi D, Arunima PPA, Govindacharyulu (2019) Low power LC-voltage controlled oscillator with −140 dBc/Hz @ 1 MHz offset using on-chip inductor design in 0.13 mm RF-CMOS process for S-Band application. Circuit World
26. Balodi D, Arunima PPA, Govindacharyulu (2020) Ultra-wideband quadrature LC-VCO using capacitor-bank and backgate topology with on-chip spirally stacked inductor in 13 μm RF-CMOS process covering S-C bands. Microelectron J 104727
27. Darabi H, Chiu J (2005) Anoise cancellation technique in active RF-CMOS mixers. IEEE J Solid-State Circuits 40(12):2628–2632
28. Park J, Lee CH, Kim BS, Laskar J (2006) Design and analysis of low flicker-noise CMOS mixers for direct-conversion receivers. IEEE Trans Microw Theory Techn 54(12):4372–4380
29. Yoon J, Kim H, Park C, Yang J, Song H, Lee S, Kim B (2008) A new RF CMOS Gilbert mixer with improved noise figure and linearity. IEEE Trans Microw Theory Techn 56(3):626–631

Recursive IDMA Receiver with Unequal Power Allocation Scheme for Beyond 5G Networks

Shivani Dixit, Varun Shukla, Priyanka Agarwal, and M. Shukla

Abstract Non-orthogonal multiple access (NOMA) is the solution to accommodate tremendous increase in Internet of things (IoT) applications. In interleave division multiple access (IDMA) systems, NOMA is realized using distinguished interleavers for every user. Here, we suggest a recursive successive interference cancellation (SIC)-based IDMA receiver structure for NOMA systems. With unequal optimum power distribution among multiple users, SIC has been implemented in a recursive manner. Chip-by-chip (CBC) multi-user detection (MUD)-IDMA receiver along with recursive SIC structure has been simulated under different simulation environments. The simulation results suggest the effectiveness of the receiver for dense 5G networks in future.

Keywords Interleave division multiple access · Non-orthogonal multiple access · Unequal power allocation · Recursive successive interference cancellation

1 Introduction

The major boom in IoT devices and their applications has started an active discussion [1, 2] on 5G and beyond 5G wireless network standards. 5G features include [3] ultra-reliable low latency to support autonomous vehicles and enable drone communications. 5G networks also target at enhanced data rates to fulfill massive data rate requirements by new IoT applications. Moreover, enhanced machine type communication is also supported to connect large number of devices in 5G networks.

Conventionally, multiple access to large number of devices is accomplished by frequency division multiple access (FDMA), time division multiple access (TDMA), code division multiple access (CDMA), and orthogonal frequency division multiple

S. Dixit (✉) · V. Shukla
Department of Electronics and Communication Engineering, Pranveer Singh Institute of Technology, Kanpur, Uttar Pradesh, India

P. Agarwal · M. Shukla
Department of Electronics Engineering, Harcourt Butler Technical University, Kanpur, Uttar Pradesh, India

M. S. Kaiser et al. (eds.), *Proceedings of Trends in Electronics and Health Informatics*, Lecture Notes in Networks and Systems 376,
https://doi.org/10.1007/978-981-16-8826-3_37

access (OFDMA), respectively, in 1G, 2G, 3G, and 4G standards [4]. In the above-mentioned classical approaches, orthogonal multiple access (OMA) is gained by orthogonally splitting the wireless resources in frequency, time, code, or in sub-carrier domain. The obvious advantage of OMA design approach is a relatively less complex and low cost receiver design.

However, the third feature of 5G networks, i.e., the massive connection demand by large number of IoT devices cannot be supported by orthogonal splitting of the wireless resources. Along with this, unpredictable channel variations also result in impaired orthogonality among multiple users accessing the same channel resulting in high complexity receivers.

NOMA is the solution to provide optimal capacity to wireless resources as suggested in [5]. In 5G standards, NOMA has been suggested as an optimal way to operate a wireless system with limited orthogonal resources. NOMA overcomes the limited spectrum problem with efficient use of non-orthogonal multiple access, along with the advantage of effective solution for highly time varying channel conditions. The cost paid for this non-orthogonal resource sharing is the highly involved receiver structure with sophisticated decoding algorithms.

As per third-generation partnership project (3GPP) study, co-scheduling of multiple users in NOMA can be implemented with power domain NOMA [6], code domain NOMA [7] and many other NOMA methods [8] along with interleaver-based [4] NOMA method. In power domain NOMA, multiple users are allotted with unequal powers at the transmitter, and an SIC-MUD strategy-based receiver detects the signals of multiple users at the receiver. In code domain NOMA spreading sequences used have very low cross-correlation among them. IDMA is also a potential candidate proposed for interleaver-based NOMA technology. In IDMA, interleaved chips have less correlation resulting in diversity gain as compared to bit interleaved CDMA while performing iterative MUD at the receiver. Further, multiple MUD structures have been suggested in literature to decode the signals of IDMA-based NOMA for spectrum sharing.

Conventional IDMA receiver with equal power allocation to multiple users has been suggested in [9]. Unequal power allocation to multiple users as in power domain NOMA along with CBC-MUD strategy in [10] has demonstrated the performance of IDMA scheme to reach the theoretical limits of capacity. Another method for the optimization of IDMA performance with unequal power allocation among users has been suggested and verified in [11].

SIC-based MUD is the characteristic [8] of any power domain NOMA system. As per SIC strategy, the user with the largest power is detected first and then rest of the users are detected sequentially with the remaining signal which is obtained after removing the large power user signals from the combined signal. In this work, we suggest to improve the performance of existing IDMA system with unequal power allocation among multiple users with a recursive SIC [12] receiver structure. The outcome of the results of recursive SIC-based IDMA receiver has suggested further improvement in the multiple access interference (MAI) cancellation among multiple users in IDMA systems. Of course, the price paid for this is the highly involved receiver strategy to decode the signals in NOMA environment.

The following sections are structured as follows. The next section discusses the basic recursive SIC transceiver structure for users with unequal power allocation for an IDMA system. After this, IDMA-MUD algorithm with unequal power allocation strategy has been explained in detail. Simulation results have been derived for the recursive SIC-based IDMA with unequal power receiver along with plain IDMA with unequal power receiver under multiple simulation conditions. Finally, the main conclusions are summarized to suggest the presented technique as potential candidate for future 5G networks with dense population.

2 Recursive SIC-IDMA Principles

2.1 Recursive SIC Structure

In the suggested recursive SIC-IDMA transmitter, powers to N number of multiple users are allocated using the optimum power allocation strategy in [10]. Then, all users' combined signal is transmitted using the IDMA transmitter principles as suggested in the following paragraph. At the receiver side, to implement recursive SIC-based MUD, all the users are ranked in descending order of their power levels. Further, the strongest user signal is decoded iteratively using CBC-MUD detection strategy of IDMA system. This decoded signal of first user is subtracted from the combined received signal. Subtraction of the strongest user signal from the combined received signal actually removes most of the multiple access interference from the signal for the remaining users. Next from the subtracted received signal, next strongest user signal is decoded iteratively. This process continues till the weakest user signal is decoded. The weakest user signal actually faces minimum multiple access interference with SIC strategy. To make this process recursive, decoded signals of user 2 to user N are combined again and subtracted from the received signal to detect user 1 signal again. This recursive process is repeated for every user to detect each user signal iteratively using IDMA-MUD strategy as follows.

2.2 IDMA Structure

IDMA with equal power allocation scheme [9] and unequal power allocation scheme [10] for multiple users has been tested and verified successfully. In this work, unequal power allocation scheme suggested in [10] has been implemented with random interleavers to distinguish the users. Unequal power allocation along with unique interleavers provides NOMA access to multiple users.

At the transmitter end as shown in Fig. 1, N simultaneous user IDMA signal system, with d_n information bits, which after encoded by a forward error correction encoder results in length M bit stream is considered. Further, as per IDMA algorithm,

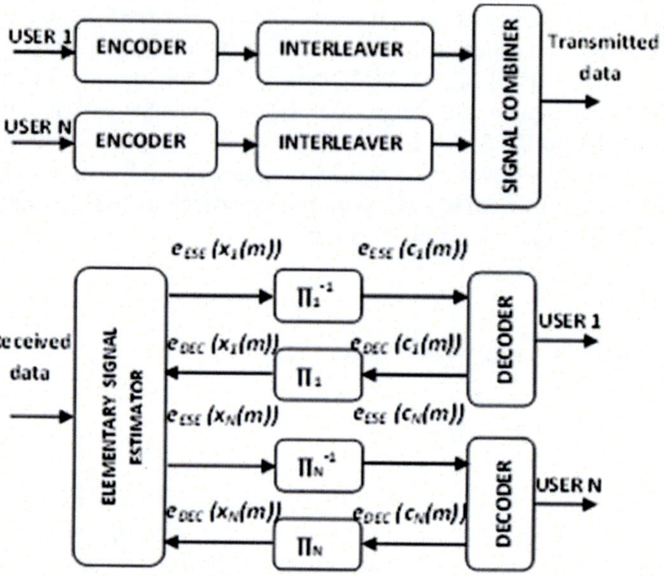

Fig. 1 IDMA transceiver algorithm [9]

user-specific interleaved and spreaded chips with proper power allocation scheme [10] are transmitted through multiple access channel.

For each user *n*, individual chips m of length M sequence can be denoted as $x_n(m) \in \{+1, -1\}$, assuming binary phase shift keying (BPSK) modulation scheme.

As per unequal power allocation suggested in [10], the received signal from all the N users with individual power factor P_n can be expressed as

$$r(n) = \sum_{n=1}^{N} P_n h_n x_n(m) + w(m), \quad m = 1, 2, \ldots M \tag{1}$$

Here, h_n are the channel coefficients for individual user n, with $w(m)$ as additive white Gaussian noise (AWGN) samples of zero mean and variance $\sigma^2 = \frac{N_0}{2}$ [9].

Perfect channel estimation and randomly interleaved chips facilitate chip-by-chip elementary signal estimator (ESE) operation [9] at the receiver for each user.

Considering the individual user's chip, (1) can be written again as,

$$r(n) = P_n h_n x_n(m) + \xi_n(m) \tag{2}$$

Here, $\xi_n(m)$ is the multiple access interference by other users including noise and can be represented as

$$\xi_n(m) \equiv r(n) - P_n h_n x_n(m) = \sum_{i \neq n} P_i h_i x_i(m) + w(m) \tag{3}$$

Gaussian random variable approximation for $\xi_n(m)$ with mean $E(\xi_n(m))$ and variance $\mathrm{Var}(\xi_n(m))$ results in output of ESE for user-n in terms of log-likelihood ratios (LLRs) [9], expressed as

$$e_{\mathrm{ESE}}(x_n(m)) = \frac{2P_n h_n (r(m) - E(\xi_n(m)))}{\mathrm{Var}(\xi_n(m))} \tag{4}$$

After this, LLRs are generated by a posterior probability (APP) decoders [9] for every chip of a particular user n and can be denoted as $\{e_{\mathrm{DEC}}(x_n(m))\forall n, m\}$. An iterative turbo algorithm [9] is applied to the LLRs output of ESE and decoders to get the transmitted information data bits of each user.

3 Simulation Results

As stated above, in this work, an optimum unequal power allocation has been done according to [10] so as to implement recursive SIC receiver. To analyze the receiver, in these MATLAB simulations, bit error rate (BER) of 10^{-4} or less is the target for minimum required bit energy to spectral noise density (E_b/N_0) ratio.

In the following simulations, random interleavers are used to achieve IDMA system. Application of random interleavers provides maximum orthogonality among users as suggested in [9]. Information of each user is convolutionally encoded with rate ½ code and spreading code of length 16 for the transmission over AWGN channel with BPSK signaling. While performing these simulations, iteration count has been taken as 20 for data length of 1024 bits.

Figure 2 shows the BER performance of smallest power user with recursive SIC-IDMA receiver for 32 simultaneous users. Simulations have also been done for non-recursive IDMA receiver with unequal power allocation among same number of 32 users to justify the significant performance improvement of the recursive SIC receiver. Apparently, results of recursive IDMA with unequal power are better than non-recursive unequal power IDMA system. Simulations are also done to show the BER result of IDMA system with equal power among 32 users. Unequal power allocation with recursive receiver improves the results by 2.0 dB with respect to conventional equal power IDMA system with the price of increased complexity.

BER trends for multiple iteration counts have also been simulated in Fig. 3 for the worst power profile users. Results suggest that larger iteration count (20) improves the performance; however, performance is not much inferior even for lesser iteration count (5) for the suggested recursive SIC receiver resulting as compensation for the high complexity of recursive receiver.

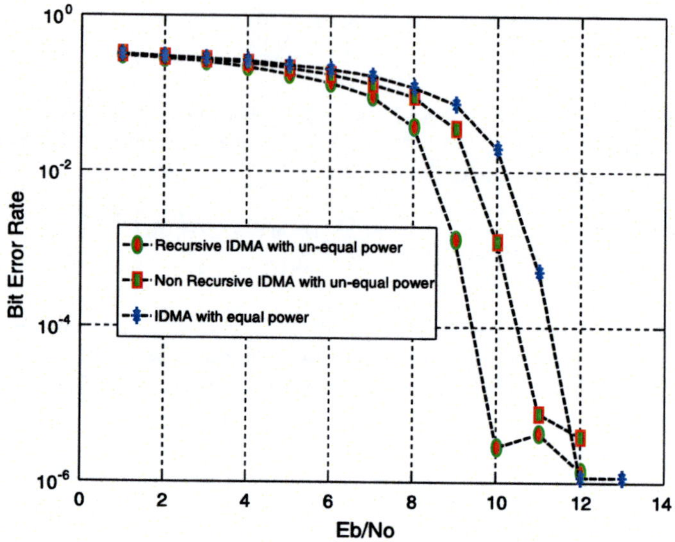

Fig. 2 BER performance of smallest power user with recursive SIC-IDMA receiver for 32 simultaneous users

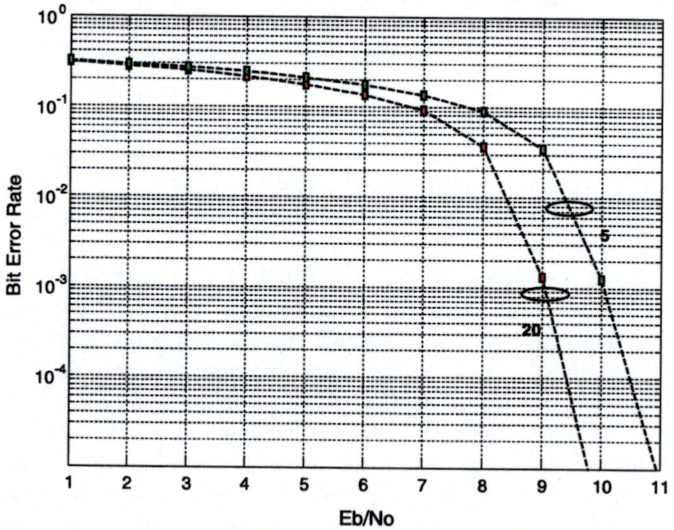

Fig. 3 BER performance of smallest power user with recursive SIC-IDMA receiver for iteration count 5 and 20 for 32 users

4 Conclusions

In this work, we have suggested a recursive SIC receiver structure for an IDMA system with unequal power allocation among multiple users to provide more efficient NOMA to the available spectrum. We concentrated on a recursive receiver structure to improve the performance of unequal power allocation-based IDMA system. With the results of modified receiver algorithm, it has been pointed out that the suggested recursive receiver with unequal power IDMA performs better than simple IDMA with unequal power system. It has also been verified that lesser number of iteration count can result in same performance trends as in plain IDMA system with unequal power allocation assisting complexity of receiver versus performance tradeoffs. The results recommend the method as an appropriate multiple access method for future NOMA systems in beyond 5G networks.

References

1. Dai L, Wang B, Ding Ding Z, Wang Z, Chen S, Hanzo L (2018) A survey of non-orthogonal multiple access for 5G. IEEE Commun Surv Tutor 20(3):2294–2323
2. Osseiran A, Boccardi F, Braun V (2014) Scenarios for 5G mobile and wireless communications: the vision of the METIS project. IEEE Commun Mag 52(5):26–35
3. Boccardi F, Heath RW, Lozano A, Marzetta TL, Popovski P (2014) Five disruptive technology directions for 5G. IEEE Commun Mag 52(2):74–80
4. Makki B, Chitti K, Behravan A, Alouini M-S (2020) A Survey of NOMA: current status and open research challenges. IEEE Open J Commun Soc 1:179–189
5. Wang P, Xiao J, Ping L (2006) Comparison of orthogonal and non-orthogonal approaches to future wireless cellular systems. IEEE Vehicular Tech Mag 1(3):4–11
6. Islam SMR, Avazov N, Dobre OA, Kwak K (2016) Power-domain non-orthogonal multiple access (NOMA) in 5G systems: potentials and challenges. IEEE Commun Surv Tutor 19(2):721–742
7. Duchemin D, Gorce JM, Goursaud C (2018) Code domain non orthogonal multiple access versus ALOHA: a simulation based study. In: 2018 25th international conference on telecommunications (ICT). IEEE, Saint-Malo, France, pp 445–450
8. Aldababsa M, Toka M, Gokceli S, Kurt GK, Kucur O (2018) A tutorial on nonorthogonal multiple access for 5G and beyond. Wirel Commun Mobile Comput 2018(5)
9. Ping L, Liu L, Wu K, Leung WK (2006) Interleave-division multiple-access. IEEE Trans Wireless Commun 5(4):938–947
10. Ping L, Liu L (2004) Analysis and design of IDMA systems based on SNR evolution and power allocation. In: IEEE 60th vehicular technology conference. IEEE, Los Angeles, CA, USA, pp 1068–1072
11. Li K, Wang X, Ping L (2007) Analysis and optimization of interleave-division multiple-access communication systems. IEEE Trans Wirel Commun 6(5), 1973–1983 (2007)
12. Yeo HK, Sharif BS, Adams AE, Hinton OR (2002) Implementation of multiuser detection strategies for coherent underwater acoustic communication. IEEE J Oceanic Eng 27(1):17–27

Low-Power Front End for Continuous-Wave Doppler Harmonic Ultrasonography System

Tanmai Kulshreshtha, Sudhir Kumar Singh, Ruchi Chaurasia, Manish Kumar, and Naimur Rahman Kidwai

Abstract In this paper, we propose system-level improvement in the front end of the continuous-wave (CW) Doppler harmonic ultrasonography (USG) system with less power consumption. The harmonic Doppler signal is used to make a precise visualization of the heart wall tissues under high blood flow. The proposed method alleviates the need for high-order analog filter and the requirement of the high dynamic range of the ADC utilized in the front end. The simulation results also show improvements compared to the existing methods.

Keywords CW Doppler ultrasound · Harmonic imaging · Analog front end

1 Introduction

Ultrasound techniques are widely used in medical imaging. Out of the other imaging modalities, e.g., magnetic resonance imaging (MRI), computerized axial tomography (CAT), positron emission tomography (PET), etc., ultrasonography (USG) is considered least hazardous. The USG system transmits the ultrasound beam (it may be a pulsed wave, PW or a continuous wave, CW) and receives back the echo of this signal [1]. The received signal may be attenuated; therefore, it is required to amplify the received signal in the front-end stage. This signal is then fed to the analog-to-digital converter (ADC), and the digital output is analyzed using digital signal processing (DSP) to display the image or the spectrum. Figure 1 shows the block diagram of the PW and CW ultrasound systems.

There are various modes of ultrasound by which the received signal is displayed in the form of images (in case of B-mode USG in Fig. 1a), or in the form of spectrum (in case of CW Doppler mode USG in Fig. 1b). The PW USG system has single element transducer, whereas the CW USG system has two elements in the transducer. In CW

T. Kulshreshtha (✉) · S. K. Singh · R. Chaurasia · M. Kumar
Pranveer Singh Institute of Technology, Kanpur, India

S. K. Singh · R. Chaurasia · N. R. Kidwai
Integral University, Lucknow, India

M. S. Kaiser et al. (eds.), *Proceedings of Trends in Electronics and Health Informatics*, Lecture Notes in Networks and Systems 376,
https://doi.org/10.1007/978-981-16-8826-3_38

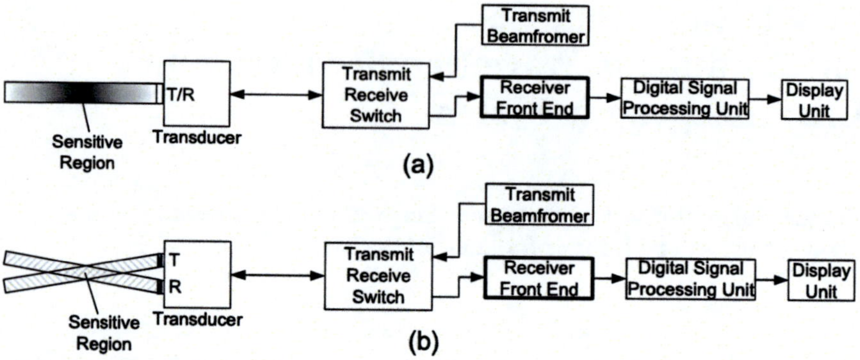

Fig. 1 Block diagram of the PW and CW ultrasound systems

USG, the transmitted signal is a continuous wave with fixed frequency, and velocity of blood is measured depending on the frequency shift of the received signal.

The Doppler mode of ultrasound (both PW and CW) is based on the Doppler effect, which is based on the received signal frequency shift compared to the transmitted signal frequency [2]. This is used to determine the flow of blood and the motion of tissues in the body. The Doppler signal may have a very small amplitude (with a high velocity of 600 m/s) or a high amplitude (with a low velocity up to 10 m/s in systolic phase of the heart).

In harmonic USG system, the frequency of the received echo signal is in the multiple (usually double) of the transmitted signal frequency. This is used to get the improved lateral resolution and therefore the better ultrasound image. This is due to fact that the harmonic signal has the higher frequency and hence the smaller wavelength [3]. In case of B-mode ultrasound imaging, the harmonics are originated from the non-moving tissues and the static micro-bubbles. In Doppler mode, the harmonic signals are generated from the moving tissues or blood particles [4]. The harmonic Doppler signal is used to make the precise visualization of the heart wall tissues under high blood flow. This is possible due to the smaller wavelength of the harmonic signals.

Now, the complexity of the harmonic USG system is to uncover the harmonic signal which is having a very less amplitude in comparison with the fundamental signal. In the existing literature, there are three methods to retrieve the harmonic signal, namely pulse-to-pulse amplitude modulation (PPAM), pulse inversion (PI), and using analog filters. The first two methods need a very high dynamic range of the ADC in the front end, as the fundamental and harmonic signal amplitude difference is considerably large by at least 20 dB. This may result in the saturation of the ADC and thus may lead to the generation of odd harmonic components [5]. Therefore, analog filtering methods have been adopted to reduce the fundamental component only, thereby reducing the required dynamic range of the ADC. As the fundamental component is very high, the high filter order is required to suppress the fundamental.

In this paper, we have proposed another analog filtering approach to mitigate the need of high filter order. We have achieved higher fundamental rejection using lower filter order as compared to the existing methods of analog filtering. This also have benefit of lower power consumption in the front end of the USG system.

This paper is organized as follows: Description of the existing front ends of harmonic USG systems is given in Sect. 2. In Sect. 3, the proposed front end for harmonic USG is reported. Simulation results are presented in Sect. 4, and finally, a conclusion is rendered.

2 Existing Front Ends of Harmonic USG System

To study about harmonic signals received through ultrasound signal, there are three USG systems available in the front end:

(a) PPAM method (pulse-to-pulse amplitude modulation method),
(b) PI method (pulse inversion method), and
(c) using analog filters.

2.1 *PPAM (Pulse-to-Pulse Amplitude Modulation) Method [6]*

In Fig. 2, time gain compensation (TGC) is used with gain amplifiers within variable limits. The purpose of TGC and amplifiers is for applying uniformity in process of image processing. If the signal with lesser amplitude is entered in the body, the nonlinearity components may get missed due to attenuation and amplitude degradation. One signal is received with the harmonic component, whereas the other is

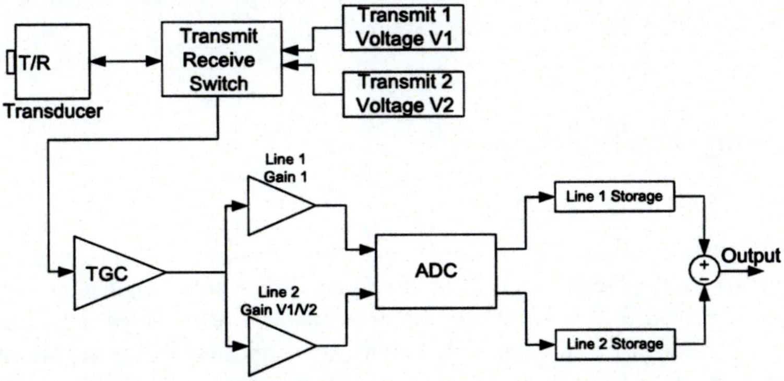

Fig. 2 Block diagram: PPAM method [6]

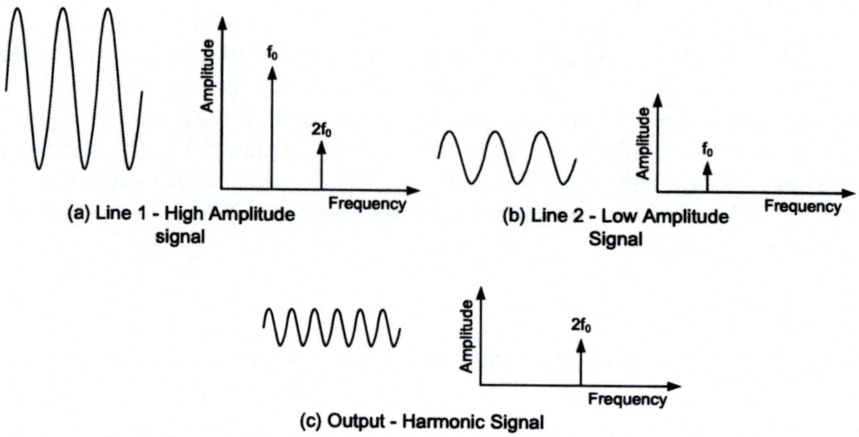

Fig. 3 Working principle of PPAM method for PW USG

without harmonic component. Thus, as a result of subtractions of above two signals shown in line-1 and line-2, it provides only the harmonic component (Fig. 3).

2.2 *Pulse Inversion (PI) Method [7, 8]*

Nonlinearity issues are usually complex in the control systems. Pulse inversion method in Fig. 4a is adopted when the second harmonic has to be added with the signal during the return path, and it is same in the phase. In this case, it is observed that, with respect to the first pulse signal, the second pulse signal is at 180° out of phase. In Fig. 4b, pulse 1 and pulse 2 are in opposite phase. The nonlinearity nature is same for the both pulses. When these two signals are added as a single harmonic signal, the fundamental is canceled, but the nonlinearity (or harmonic component) becomes double as the previous single signal.

2.3 *Using Analog Filtering*

The major drawback with these two methods is that both methods use ADCs with a wider dynamic range. It is measured that the harmonic is 20 decibels less on comparing with the fundamental. Both the signals are as usual digitized by the use of ADC as shown in Fig. 4a. Thus, the converter can reach in saturation due to higher magnitude of the fundamental, and the harmonic can be detected because of its lesser amplitude. Now, this is the major problem that the ADC is saturated in this process, and it generates odd harmonics. This is now the second major problem in identifying the second-order harmonics [5]. If some nonlinearity is removed in this

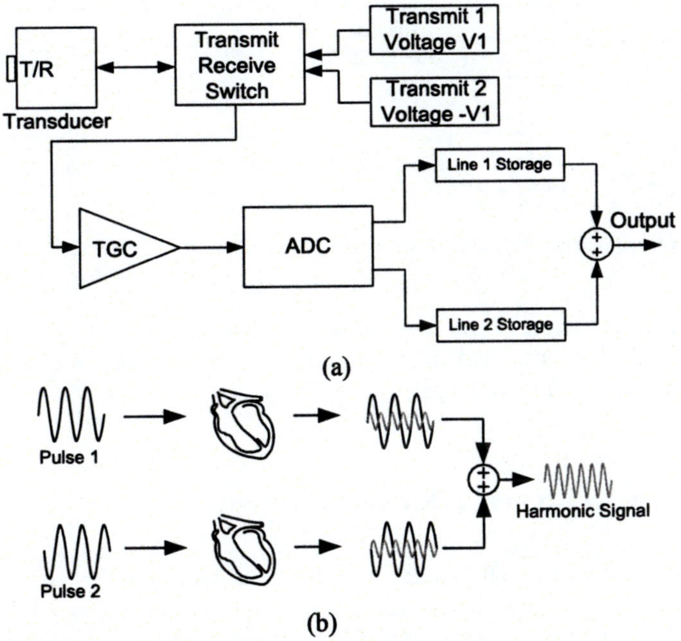

Fig. 4 **a** Block diagram: PI method [8] and **b** its working principle

method, larger power consumption is needed to accomplish it. Now the problem is to find the second harmonic component, and it is only possible if the fundamental component of the signal is canceled out. As after achieving the same, the dynamic range in which harmonic signal resides is required. If we apply a fundamental analog filter and a harmonic analog filter just before the ADC, the process becomes more convenient. According to the frequency essentials, the filter should be selected as to consider the harmonic components and filter the fundamentals one. A band-pass filter is selected which considers only harmonic components and filters all the fundamental components (Figs. 5 and 6).

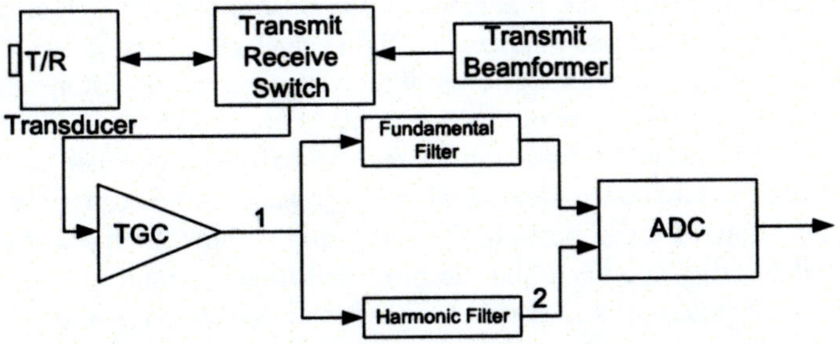

Fig. 5 Block diagram with different fundamental and harmonic analog filters [9]

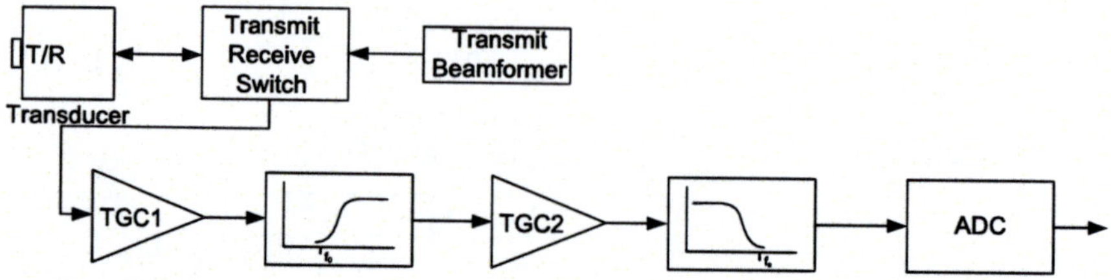

Fig. 6 Block diagram to filter fundamental components and select harmonic [5]

The frequency range of the B-mode and the Doppler mode USG is from 1 to 20 MHz. In the B-mode, bandwidth is around 1–15 MHz, whereas a bandwidth of 200 kHz is sufficient for the Doppler mode [10, 11].

3 Proposed System and Simulation Results

These front ends mentioned in Sect. 2 are basically developed for harmonic USG. The method using analog filtering method is also applicable to the CW harmonic Doppler. CW harmonic Doppler is used to measure the blood flow within the vessel and to characterize the contrast agents. The main issue in the harmonic ultrasound systems using analog filtering is the requirement of the high-order filter to reject the fundamental component before ADC.

Now it is required to build the front end of harmonic USG system, with these main features, with tunable frequency arrangements from 1 to 40 MHz in order to cover both fundamental and harmonic components of ultrasound signal. For the front end of CW Doppler, the required ADC should have a narrowband of 200 kHz. Analog-to-digital conversion should be performed using band-pass sigma-delta modulators instead of pipelined ADC in order to have power efficient front end. The proposed system is developed for the CW harmonic Doppler.

The proposed approach is to apply a band-pass filter at the fundamental frequency and then subtract this in phase from the original signal. This overall filtering is band reject filtering. The problem in the direct filtering approach is the requirement of high-order filter to reduce the fundamental component. As the proposed method deals with the subtraction, the fundamental signal can be easily canceled. Therefore, the proposed method requires lower-order filter compared to the existing approaches. The proposed method also relaxes the high dynamic range requirement of the ADC. Figure 7 shows the proposed front end for the CW harmonic Doppler USG system.

Now, simulations for conventional analog filtering approach and proposed filtering approach are shown for comparison. Figures 8 and 9 show the block diagrams of conventional filtering approach and the proposed filtering approach, respectively. The second-order band-pass filter transfer function is given in Eq. 1 as

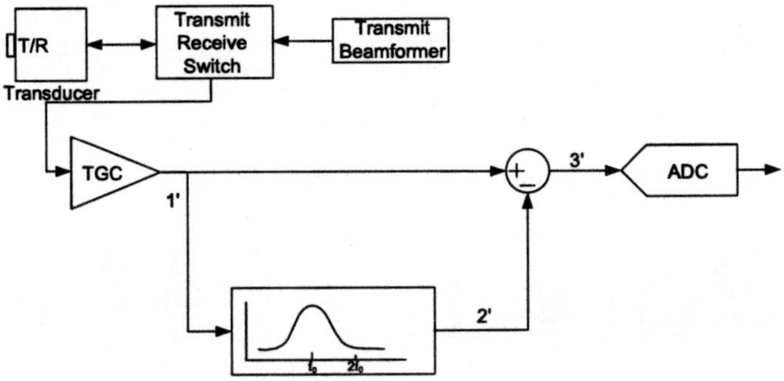

Fig. 7 Proposed front end for CW harmonic Doppler

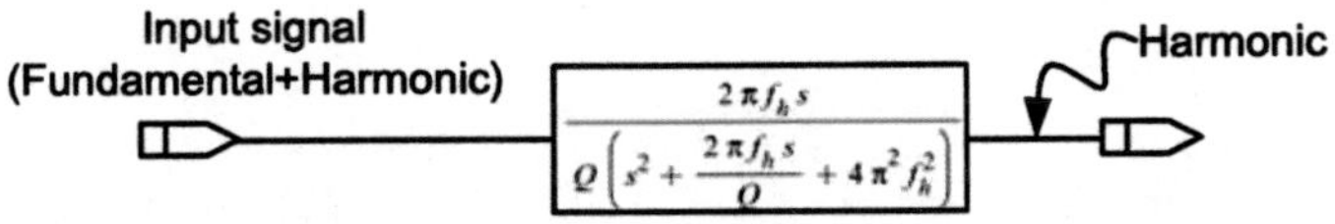

Fig. 8 Conventional filtering method used in [8] for CW harmonic Doppler system in Simulink

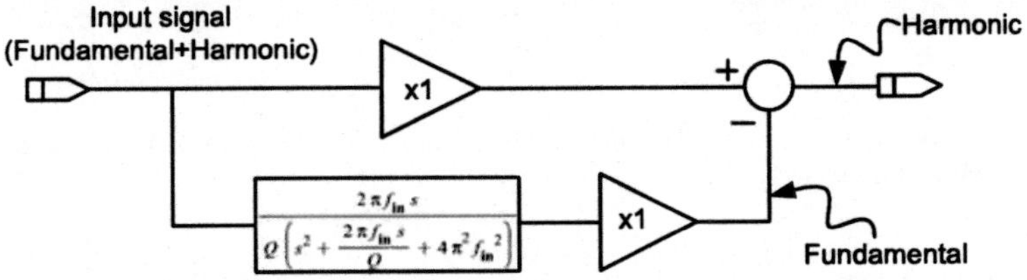

Fig. 9 Proposed filtering method for CW harmonic Doppler system in Simulink

$$H(s) = \frac{\frac{\omega}{Q}s}{s^2 + \frac{\omega}{Q}s+^2} \tag{1}$$

where ω is the center frequency of the pass band and Q is the quality factor of the filter.

Figure 10 shows the FFT of input and filtered harmonic in which only 23 dB of fundamental is rejected, whereas by proposed approach the fundamental is decreased by 160 dB as shown in Fig. 11. This is done with 2.5 MHz fundamental. Therefore, the proposed method gives better SNR for the signal at the input of the ADC. The proposed system shows improvement with other fundamental frequencies also. Therefore, the proposed filtering method is very well utilized for fetching the harmonic signal information which is very less in amplitude.

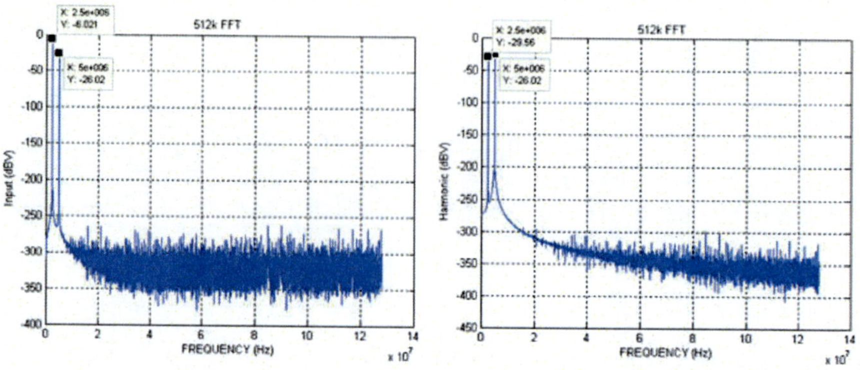

Fig. 10 FFT of input, filtered harmonic, respectively, for 2.5 MHz fundamental in case of conventional filtering method of Fig. 8

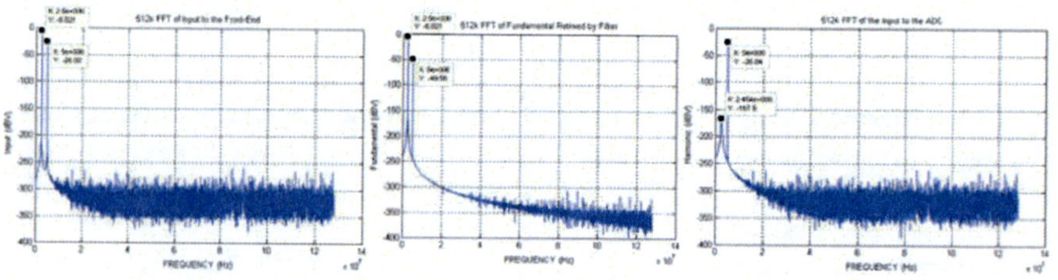

Fig. 11 FFT of input, filtered fundamental and harmonic, respectively, for 2.5 MHz fundamental in case of proposed method

4 Conclusion

We have proposed a Doppler USG system for detecting second harmonic and compared with various existing USG systems for harmonic signal measurement. The proposed USG system is advantageous in terms of its power consumption. Also, the UGC system is proposed in view to make the requirements of the ADC relaxed. As the harmonic signal is quite week in comparison with the fundamental, it is used to make precise visualization of the tissues under blood flow. The proposed filtering approach has the less order of the filter compared to the existing method. The simulation results have also been given for this system and compared with the existing method.

References

1. Hoskins P, Martin K, Thrush A (2010) Diagnostic ultrasound—physics and equipment, 2nd edn. Cambridge University Press, New York
2. Chang PH et al (1995) Second harmonic imaging and harmonic Doppler measurements with Albunex. IEEE Trans Ultrasonics Ferroelectrics Freq Control 42(6):1020–1027
3. Ultrasound technology update: harmonic imaging, GE Medical Systems. http://www.soundvet.com/library/media/pdf/THI_imaging.pdf. Last accessed 20 Nov 2020
4. Kollmann C (2007) New sonographic techniques for harmonic imaging-Underlying physical principles. Eur J Radiol 64(2):164–172
5. Broad RW et al (2003) Ultrasound harmonic signal acquisition. U. S. Patent. Pub. No.: US 6516667 B1
6. Brock-Fisher et al (1996) Means for increasing sensitivity in non-linear ultrasound imaging systems. U. S. Patent. Pub. No.: 5577505
7. Criton AL et al (2000) Ultrasonic harmonic Doppler imaging. U. S. Patent. Pub. No.: 6036643
8. Chapman CS, Lazenby JC (1997) Ultrasound imaging system employing phase inversion subtraction to enhance the image. U. S. Patent, Pub. No.: 5632277
9. Hossack JA et al (2003) Medical diagnostic ultrasound system and method for versatile processing. U. S. Patent, Pub. No.: 6511426 B1
10. Norman O (1996) A band-pass delta-sigma modulator for ultrasound imaging at 160 MHz clock rate. IEEE J Solid-State Circuits 31(12):2036–2041
11. Qin L (2004) Design and validation of a Gm-C bandpass sigma-delta modulator dedicated to front-end ultrasonic receiver. M. S. dissertation, Ecole Polytechnique de Montreal, Canada

MonoLayer Graphene-Based Plasmonic Biosensor for Urine Glucose Detection

Archana Yadav, Anil Kumar, and Preeta Sharan

Abstract In this proposed work, a plasmonic biosensor based on graphene has been presented to detect the biosample consisting of urine glucose. The proposed biosensor is comprised of five layers in the order of prism/Au/Si/graphene-sensing medium. P-polarized monochromatic light of 633 nm has been used for the excitation of the plasmons at the metal–semiconductor interface. This simulation study shows, by optimizing the thickness of gold (Au), silicon (Si), and graphene, the proposed biosensor can provide the sensitivity up to 219°/RIU (Refractive Index Unit) and gives the distinct shift in the resonance angle for a quite small variation in the value of refractive indices (1.335, 1.336, 1.337, 1.338, 1.341, 1.347) corresponding to the glucose concentration level in non-diabetic person (0–15 mg/dl) and diabetic person (0.625 gm/dL, 1.25 gm/dL, 2.5 gm/dL, 5 gm/dL, and 10 gm/dL), respectively. A comparison is also made with, a bare gold (Au) layer and combination of gold–silicon (Au–Si) layer-based structure, and it is found that monolayer graphene plays a major role and enhances the sensitivity remarkably better than the other two structures which are having a sensitivity of 150°/RIU and 180°/RIU, respectively. We expect this novel work, which would be helpful in the diagnosis of the sugar concentration level with high sensitivity and high accuracy.

Keywords SPR · Sensitivity · Silicon · Graphene · Reflectance intensity

1 Introduction

Glucose is an important biomolecule and source of energy in humans, but the heightened values of glucose concentration result in many health problems related to the

A. Yadav (✉) · A. Kumar
Department of ECE, ASET, Amity University, Uttar Pradesh, Noida, UP 226010, India

A. Kumar
e-mail: akumar3@lko.amity.edu

P. Sharan
Department of ECE, The Oxford College of Engineering, Bengaluru 560068, India

M. S. Kaiser et al. (eds.), *Proceedings of Trends in Electronics and Health Informatics*, Lecture Notes in Networks and Systems 376,
https://doi.org/10.1007/978-981-16-8826-3_39

heart, kidney, eyes, etc. [1]. Nowadays, monitoring blood glucose concentration is quite common and easy as well. However, it is also important to diagnose and control the urine glucose level to prevent kidney-related problems at the initial stage [2]. This heightened glucose concentration level in urine results in renal glycosuria [3]. According to WHO, the number of patients having this medical condition is increasing day by day [4]. Therefore, detection of glucose concentration levels and monitoring is very much needed. To date, many researchers have reported so many studies; however, surface plasmon resonance-based (SPR) sensors are much popular since the last decades for finding the various components in the blood, glucose, cholesterol, etc. [5].

In this proposed work, theoretical simulation based on SPR has been done for real time, and label-free detection of the glucose concentration in urine samples has been presented. SPR is an optical phenomenon that arises by the involvement of the p-polarized light with the free electrons at the metal surface [6]. The configuration of the SPR usually consists of the Otto configuration and the Kretschmann configuration. In Otto configuration, there exists an air gap layer between the surface of the prism and the metal layer. Due to this, it will become a little complicated structure, and it is not easy to make a portable one [7], whereas the Kretschmann configuration is much more popular because of its portability as in this configuration; a metal layer is pasted to the base of the prism [8]. This paper deals with the Kretschmann configuration of light coupling for biosensors using the angle interrogation method.

Energy and the momentum of the p-polarized incident light are being conserved at the resonance condition, and reflectance becomes minimum because of the maximum excitation of the surface plasmons. At this point, the incident wave vector becomes equal to the propagation constant of the generated plasmons. This can be presented by Eq. 1 [9].

$$k_i = k_p. \tag{1}$$

where $k_i = \frac{\omega}{c} \text{n1} \sin\theta_i$, incident wave vector, and

$$k_p = \frac{\omega}{c}\sqrt{\frac{\varepsilon_{\text{metal}}\varepsilon_{\text{dielectric}}}{\varepsilon_{\text{metal}} + \varepsilon_{\text{dielectric}}}}$$

ε is the dielectric permittivity constant, and n1 is the refractive index of the first layer.

SPR curves are used for measuring the resonance shift by the change in refractive indices of the sensing medium, and this shift is directly associated with the sensitivity of the biosensor.

Further, the selection of the metal layer and the materials involved in the proposed biosensor is based on the optical and plasmonic properties owns by these materials. In this study, Au metal is used because of having it better optical properties than silver and other metals [10]. Silicon layer because of having the high real value of the dielectric constant gives better sensitivity of the biosensor [11]. Two-dimensional material graphene has some unique and extraordinary optical and electrical properties and provides the promising result in enhancement of the sensor's sensitivity [12]. Hence, the use of the graphene layer over the Au and Si layer demonstrates a significant improvement in the sensitivity of the proposed biosensor.

2 Design Methodology

The schematic diagram of the proposed multilayer biosensor prism/Au/Si/graphene-sensing medium is shown in Fig. 1, for the diagnosis of the glucose levels in the urine samples. Monochromatic light of wavelength 633 nm is used for the excitation of the plasmons.

Prism BK 7, because of its high refractive index, is used as the first layer, and this value of the refractive index can be calculated by Eq. 2.

$$n = \left(1 + \frac{1.03961212\,\lambda^2}{\lambda^2 - 0.00600069867} + \frac{1.01046945\lambda^2}{\lambda^2 - 103.560653} + \frac{0.231792344\lambda^2}{\lambda^2 - 0.0200179144}\right)^{1/2} \tag{2}$$

where λ is the wavelength of incident light [13].

The second layer has been used of Au, and the refractive index can be calculated by the Drude—Lorentz model expressed by Eq. 3.

$$n = \left(1 - \frac{\lambda^2 * \lambda_c}{\lambda_p^2(\lambda_c + \lambda * i)}\right)^{1/2} \tag{3}$$

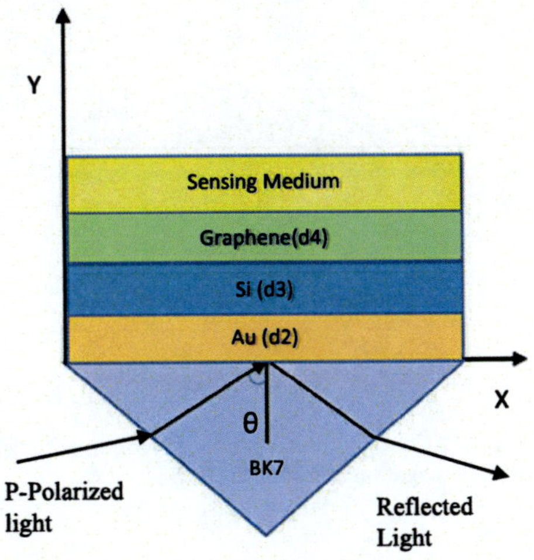

Fig. 1 Multilayered schematic of proposed biosensor for the glucose level detection

Table 1 Refractive indices of the proposed materials and their optimized thickness

Layers	Refractive index values	Thickness of the layers
Prism (BK7)	1.5151	–
Au	$0.14330 + 3.6080i$	50 nm
Si	3.9160	03 nm
Graphene	$3 + 1.149i$	0.34 nm (monolayer)
Sensing medium	[1.335, 1.336, 1.337, 1.338, 1.341, 1.347]	–

where λ is an incident wavelength, λ_p (Plasma wavelength) is 1.6826×10^{-7} m, and λ_c (Collision wavelength) is 8.9342×10^{-6} m [14].

Table 1 shows the layers and corresponding values of refractive indices and the thickness. The optimized thickness of the Au layer is 50 nm. The third layer of silicon is of the thickness of 03 nm, and the refractive index is 3.9160 [15]. The fourth layer is added of graphene, which provides strong interactions with the biomolecules, is having the refractive index value $3 + 1.149i$ [16] with the thickness of 0.34 nm of each layer. Sensing layer consisting of the biosample of urine with the glucose concentration of 0–15 mg/dl, 0.625 gm/dl, 1.25 gm/dl, 2.5 gm/dl, 5 gm/dl, 10 gm/dl and corresponding refractive indices are 1.335, 1.336, 1.337, 1.338, 1.341, 1.347 [17]. Here, we have simulated all the results by using the finite element method by COMSOL Multiphysics v.5.5 (Fig. 2), and the obtained numerical data have been plotted by using MATLAB.

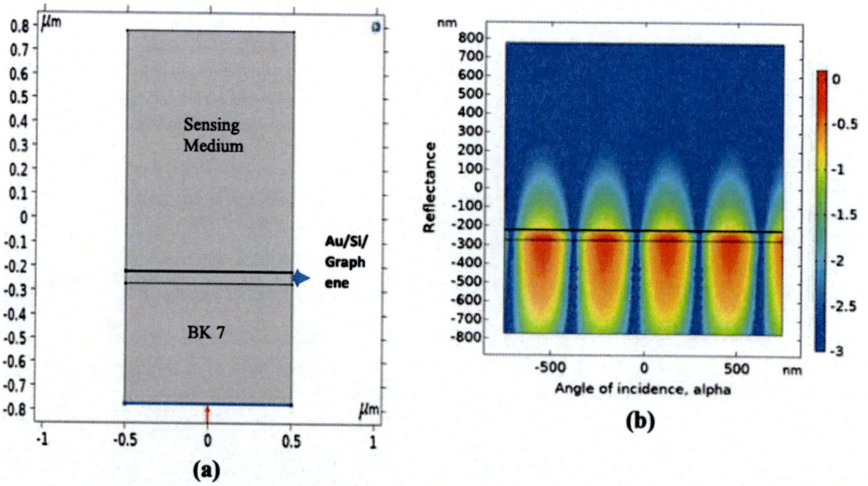

Fig. 2 **a** Configuration of proposed biosensor by using COMSOL multiphysics. **b** Surface magnetic field propagation at resonance angle

3 Mathematical Modeling of Proposed SPR Biosensor

Simulation modeling of biosensor has been done by using the Fresnel equations employing the transfer matrix method for n layer structure. The relationship between the tangential electrical and magnetic field at the boundary of the first layer and the boundary of the final layer is expressed by Eq. 4

$$\begin{matrix} X \\ Y \end{matrix} = Z_1 Z_2 Z_3 \ldots Z_{n-1} \begin{matrix} X_{n-1} \\ Y_{n-1} \end{matrix} = Z \begin{matrix} X_{n-1} \\ Y_{n-1} \end{matrix} \tag{4}$$

Also,
For polarized waves at the boundary,

$$X_m = H_Y^T + H_Y^R \tag{5}$$

$$Y_M = E_Y^T + E_Y^R \tag{6}$$

Further, solving Maxwell's equations for the n layer structure, solution can be obtained in the terms of the magnetic field for the incident light [18]

$$Hy = \left\{ \begin{matrix} Ace^{(-ik_c z)} e^{i(\omega t - k_x x)} & \text{Sensing Layer} \\ \left\{Aae^{(ik_{m2} z)} + Bae^{(-ik_{m2} z)}\right\} e^{i(\omega t - k_x x)} & \text{Graphene} \\ \left\{Age^{(ik_g z)} + Bge^{(-ik_g z)}\right\} e^{i(\omega t - k_x x)} & \text{Silicon Layer Dielectric} \\ \left\{Ame^{(ik_{m1} z)} + Bme^{(-ik_{m1} z)}\right\} e^{i(\omega t - k_x x)} & \text{Inner metal Layer (Au)} \\ Ase^{(ik_p z)} e^{i(\omega t - k_x x)} & \text{Prism} \end{matrix} \right\} \tag{7}$$

Skipping the intermediate steps in the calculation, reflection coefficient r_p obtained is [19]

$$r_p = \left| \frac{r_{sm} + r_{m\text{fac}} e^{2ik_m d_m}}{1 + r_{sm} r_{m\text{fac}} e^{2ik_m d_m}} \right|^2 \tag{8}$$

And reflection intensity R is

$$R = \left| r_p \right|^2 \tag{9}$$

In addition, the sensitivity of the biosensor can be defined by the following equation:

$$S = \frac{\Delta\theta_{res}}{\Delta n_s} \tag{10}$$

where $\Delta\theta_{res}$ represents the difference in resonance angle, and Δn_s is the difference in the refractive index of the biosample.

4 Numerical Analysis and Discussion

In this proposed work, simulation of an enhanced sensitive SPR-based biosensor has been done using the transfer matrix method for angle interrogation. Sensing medium is used as biosample of having refractive indices 1.335, 1.334, 1.335, 1.336, 1.337, 1.338, 1.341, and 1.348 correspondingly glucose concentration level 0–15 mg/dl (normal person) and for diabetic person 0.625 gm/dl, 1.25 gm/dl, 2.5 gm/dl, 5 gm/dl, 10 gm/dl. This sensing layer is placed on the top of the biosensor. Due to the fluctuations of the glucose level in the urine sample of a diabetic person, refractive indices vary and that can be detected by the biosensor and shows as the shift in the angle in SPR curve.

High refractive index prism BK 7 is considered as the first layer, to couple the incident light. Plasmonic material gold (Au) is pasted on the surface of the prism that works as the second layer of the biosensor. We have optimized the thickness of the Au layer at 50 nm for the better response of the sensor of sensitivity 150°/RIU (Fig. 4a). The third layer is used in the proposed biosensor is the silicon semiconductor to get the sensitivity better than the conventional biosensor (only metal layer). For this purpose, optimization of thickness of the Si layer is done. Resonance angle shift and minimum reflectance values are considered by changing the thickness of the Si layer from 01 to 06 nm which is shown in Fig. 3a. We have found it gives better results at 03 nm and the structure prism/Au/Si-sensing medium gives the sensitivity of 180°/RIU (Fig. 4b). Furthermore, we added one more layer of graphene due to its extraordinary electrical and optical properties, for the better performance of the proposed biosensor. We have checked the performance of the biosensor by adding one 0.34 nm layer of graphene. The result shows a single layer of graphene enhances the sensitivity up to 219°/RIU and a remarkable shift in the resonance angle in SPR curves for the variation of 0.001 in refractive index of the sensing medium. In addition, we have also checked by changing the number of layers of graphene up to 06 layers, i.e., the thickness of 2.04 nm (0.34 * 6) (Fig. 3b); we don't find any significant improvement in the sensitivity or the distinct shift in the SPR curve. Hereby, we have fixed a single layer of graphene over Si layer.

So, the final structure is consisting of a prism/Au/Si/graphene-sensing layer with the optimized thickness of 50 nm, 03 nm, and 0.34 nm, respectively.

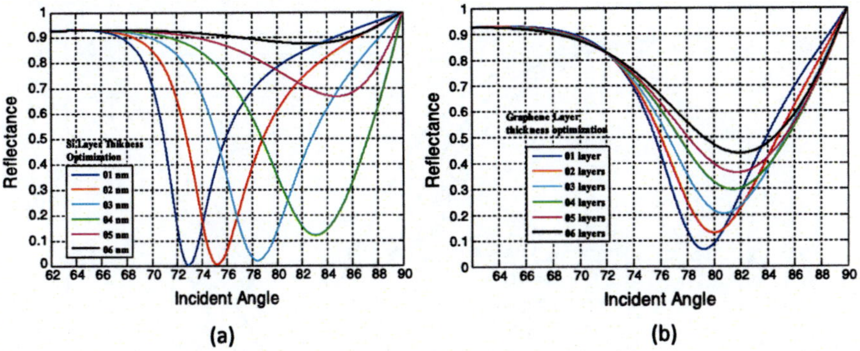

Fig. 3 Thickness optimization for **a** Si layer, **b** graphene layer

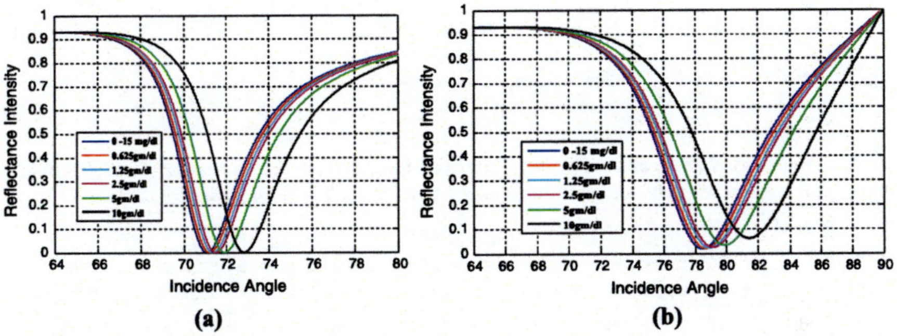

Fig. 4 Reflectance SPR curve for the urine glucose concentration level **a** Au–Si-based structure, **b** bare metal, (Au) structure

For urine sample 0–15 mg/dl (normal person) to 0.625 gm/dl (diabetic person), the difference in refractive index is 0.001, and a corresponding change in resonance angle is from 79.2° to 79.4°, i.e., angle shift is 0.2°. Furthermore, the change in glucose level of the next urine sample is from 1.25 to 2.5 gm/dl; again, the refractive index difference is 0.001, and the corresponding angle shift is 0.2 for 79.7° and 79.9°.

Additionally, for the change in glucose level from 5 to 10 gm/dl, refractive index changes to 0.006, and the corresponding change in resonance angle is 1.5° for variation from 80.7° to 82.2°. Figure 5 clearly shows, for a very small change in the refractive indices of the glucose concentration level of the diabetic person, we get the significant shifts in the SPR curve and lower the values of reflectance intensity. Consequently, higher value of sensitivity is achieved. Table 2 shows the numerical values of the analysis and the comparison for the conventional biosensor (prism/metal layer/sensing layer), Si added layered structure and final structure Si, and graphene based.

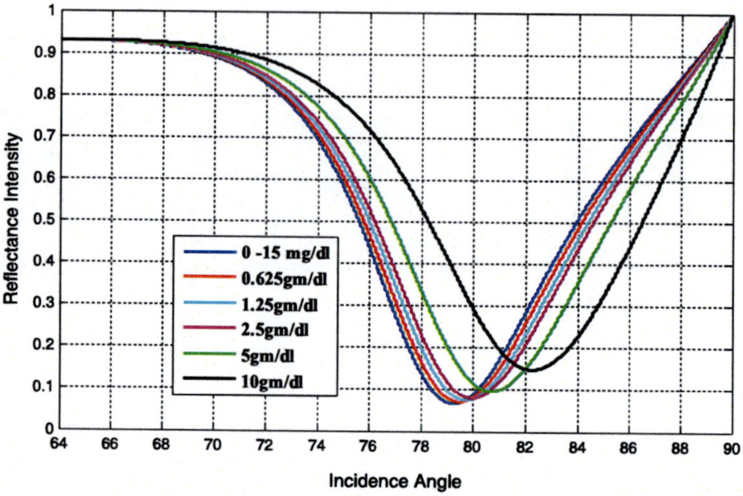

Fig. 5 Reflectance SPR curve for the proposed biosensor

Table 2 Resonance angle and reflectivity intensity for the proposed biosensor (Au/Si/graphene) and its comparison with conventional biosensor (Au) and Au/Si-based biosensor

Glucose level concentration	Ref. index	Au/Si/Graphene		Au/Si		Conventional	
		Resonance angle	Reflectance intensity	Resonance angle	Reflectance intensity	Resonance angle	Reflectance intensity
0–15 mg/dl	1.335	79.26355	0.06694	78.47688	0.01947	71.10521	0.00042
0.625 gm/dl	1.336	79.49732	0.0709	78.70206	0.02131	71.24444	0.00047
1.25 gm/dl	1.337	79.73395	0.07521	78.93124	0.02334	71.38367	0.00052
2.5 gm/dl	1.338	79.97402	0.0799	79.16386	0.02559	71.52461	0.00058
5 gm/dl	1.341	80.71486	0.0967	79.88579	0.03389	71.95204	0.00077
10 gm/dl	1.347	82.27617	0.14868	81.45053	0.06149	72.83726	0.00134
Sensitivity		219°/RIU		180°/RIU		150°/RIU	

5 Conclusion

Detection of glucose levels in urine biosamples is proposed by employing a monolayer of graphene over the plasmonic material Au and Si. Graphene has been proven as one of the best materials for the enhancement of sensitivity and is very promising to provide the best performance parameters for the biosensor. In this paper, monolayer graphene provides the sensitivity up to 219°/RIU consequently gives the lower values of reflectance values that help in the better confinement and better resonance shift in the SPR curve in comparison to the conventional biosensor. This optimized biosensor can be fabricated at nanoscale for the non-invasive techniques also. So, we can expect, this is going to be quite helpful for the fabricators for the easy detection of the glucose concentration with high accuracy.

References

1. Oliver NS et al (2009) Glucose sensors: a review of current and emerging technology. Diabetic Med 26(3):197–210
2. World Health Organization (WHO). Diabetes. Available online: http://www.who.int/news-room/factsheets/detail/diabetes. Accessed on 3 Oct 2018
3. Karim MN, Anderson SR, Singh S, Ramanathan R, Bansal V (2018) Nanostructured silver fabric as a free-standing NanoZyme for colorimetric detection of glucose in urine. Biosens Bioelectron 110:8–15. https://doi.org/10.1016/j.bios.2018.03.025
4. Wild S, Roglic G, Green A, Sicree R, King H (2004) Global prevalence of diabetes: estimates for the year 2000 and projections for 2030. Diabetes Care 27:1047–1053
5. Zhang S, Wang N, Yu H, Niu Y, Sun C (2005) Covalent attachment of glucose oxidase to an Au electrode modified with gold nanoparticles for use as glucose biosensor. Bioelectrochemistry 67:15–22
6. Choi SH, Kim YL, Byun KM (2011) Graphene-on-silver substrates for sensitive surface plasmon resonance imaging biosensors. Opt Express 19:458–466
7. Kim M, Park K, Jeong E-J, Shin Y-B, Chung BH (2006) Surface plasmon resonance imaging analysis of protein–protein interactions using on-chip-expressed capture protein. Anal Biochem 351:298–304
8. Kretschmann E, Reather H (1968) Radiative decay of non-radiative surface plasmons excited by light. Zeitschrift fur Nature forschung 23:2135–2221
9. Hayashi S, Okamoto T (2012) Plasmonics: visit the past to know the future. J Phys D Appl Phys 45:433001. https://doi.org/10.1088/0022-3727/45/43/433001
10. Vibisha GA, Nayak JK, Maheswari P, Priyadharsini N, Nisha A, Jaroszewicz Z, Jha R (2020) Sensitivity enhancement of surface plasmon resonance sensor using hybrid configuration of 2D materials over bimetallic layer of Cu-Ni. Optics Comm 463:125337
11. Tabasi O, Falamaki C (2018) Recent advancements in the methodologies applied for the sensitivity enhancement of surface plasmon resonance sensors. Anal Methods 10:3906–3925. https://doi.org/10.1039/C8AY00948A
12. Wang J, Xiao Y, Cecen V, Shao C, Zhao Y, Qu L (2019) Tunable-deformed graphene layers for actuation. Front Chem 7:725. https://doi.org/10.3389/fchem.2019.00725
13. Lin Z, Jiang L, Wu L, Guo J, Dai X, Xiang Y, Fan D (2016) Tuning and sensitivity enhancement of surface plasmon resonance biosensor with graphene covered Au-MoS2-Au films. IEEE Photonics J 8(6):4803308
14. Rahman MM, Rana MM, Rahman MS, Anower MS, Mollah MA, Paul AK (2020) Sensitivity enhancement of SPR biosensors employing heterostructure of PtSe2 and 2D materials. Opt. Mater. **107**, 110123
15. Aspnes DE, Studna AA (1983) Dielectric functions and optical parameters of Si, Ge, GaP, GaAs, GaSb, InP, InAs, and InSb from 1.5 to 6.0 ev. Phys Rev B **27**(2):985
16. Prabowo BA, Alom A, Secario MK, Masim FCP, Lai HC, Hatanaka K et al (2016) Graphene-based portable SPR sensor for the detection of *Mycobacterium tuberculosis* DNA strain. Procedia Eng 168:541–545. https://doi.org/10.1016/j.proeng.2016.11.520
17. Wu L, Guo J, Wang Q, Lu S, Dai X, Xiang Y, Fan D (2017) Sensitivity enhancement by using few-layer black phosphorusgraphene/TMDCs heterostructure in surface plasmon resonance biochemical sensor. Sens. Actuators B 249:542–548

18. Markos P, Soukoulis C (2008) "Wave propagation," in from electrons to photonic crystals and left-handed materials. Princeton University
19. Yadav A, Sharan P, Kumar A (2020) Surface plasmonic resonance based five layered structure-biosensor for sugar level measurement in human. Results in Optics 1:100002. https://doi.org/10.1016/j.rio.2020.100002

Modeling and Simulation Based Investigation of SiGe Heterojunction Dopingless Vertical TFET for Lower Power Biomedical Application

Shailendra Singh, Raghvendra Singh, and Sanjeev Kumar Bhalla

Abstract This research proposes a SiGe heterojunction based dopingless Vertical tunnel field effect transistor (SiGe-DV-TFET). To obtain high sensitivity for biomedical applications, a cavity is added to the gate metal side of the proposed device. Fluctuation in surface potential is caused by the immobilization of biomolecules within the cavity. Various aspects impacting the device's electrical characteristics, such as spacer length, applied voltages (V_{ds} and V_{gs}), and channel material, have been investigated in this study. To validate the results, the modeling output features were compared to simulated outcomes. The surface potential of each segment is determined using Poisson's equation in one and two dimensions, respectively. In the Silvaco ATLAS tool, multiple outcomes of charge density and dielectric constant are employed to recreate biomolecules for simulation.

Keywords Sensitivity · Biosensor · Modeling · Dopingless vertical tunnel FET · Charged density · Plasma · Amino acids

1 Introduction

Due to their beneficial qualities, such as their plentiful existence with sensitivity, dependability, speed, and compactness, silicon-oriented biosensors have piqued the interest of bio-analytical applications. Biological-sensors based on FETs have showed great promise in a variety of domains, including medicine, nanotechnology, biotechnology, pharmaceuticals, agriculture, and a variety of other industries [1–3]. Biosensors are analytical instruments that detect the target biomolecule entity and generate a stimulus/signal. First, receptors such as enzymes, antibodies, nucleic acids, and cells use a biochemical mechanism to interact/bind with the target analyte [4]. Labeled or label-free detection is possible in biosensors. In the label-free technique, whereas the label method involves the use of external biomolecules.

S. Singh (✉) · R. Singh · S. K. Bhalla
Department of Electronics and Communication Engineering, PSIT-Pranveer Singh Institute of Technology, Kanpur, India

M. S. Kaiser et al. (eds.), *Proceedings of Trends in Electronics and Health Informatics*, Lecture Notes in Networks and Systems 376,
https://doi.org/10.1007/978-981-16-8826-3_40

In comparison to labeled methodology, this label-free technology has higher sensitivity, leverage inherent features of the analyte, and use just one reagent, resulting in reduced analysis time and cost [5–7], and are thus frequently chosen. Several immobilization strategies have been proposed in the literature, including adsorbent, covalent binding, inter-linked, and trapping [8–10]. The absorbed biomolecules will not interface with executed molecule's function. As a result, the reusability of the device has enhanced. Traditional ISFET (Ion sensitive field effect transistor) device difficulties can be resolved with Dielectric Modulated (DMFET) devices, which can detect both charged and uncharged biomolecules, give improved detection sensitivity, quick screening, and need a small sample volume [11–14]. Evolution of expertise, gadgets are being shrunk in order to improve efficiency. Short channel effect (SCEs) has been introduced into nanotechnology devices as a result of their miniaturization, which eventually degrade device features. Device manufacture becomes more difficult when device downsizing approaches 50 nm. Alternative device structures, such as Vertical TFET, and other unique devices, are being created every day to reduce the problem of SCEs [15–18]. The heterojunction structure is used in between source and channel in order to reduce the tunneling distance from 1.1 to 0.7 eV. This will enhance the tunneling speed and also can be controlled by varying the mole fraction value "m" in $Si_{1\text{-}m}Ge_m$.

A novel SiGe heterojunction based dopingless Vertical tunnel field effect transistor (SiGe-DV-TFET) biosensor is introduced to this paper in order to remove the various shortcomings of SCE (Short Channel effect). Label-free biosensing [10–13] offers a lot of potential for being manufactured into providing higher-efficient sensor very versatile. High specificity and sensitivity, increased variables are all characteristics of an effective biosensor [19–21]. This draft presents two-dimensional depletion width calculation of source-channel and channel drain with SiGe layer in between heterojunction based dopingless Vertical tunnel field effect transistor (SiGe-DV-TFET). The gate underlap area is also considered for the analytical model region under doping less condition. It also improves surface potential while reducing tunneling distance [22, 23].

2 Device Architectures and Simulation Methodology

The basic proposed structure heterojunction based dopingless Vertical tunnel field effect transistor (SiGe-DV-TFET) structure is shown in Fig. 1. The corresponding Model schematic diagram with define depletion region is shown in Fig. 2. The charge plasma method was utilized to create a "P + " source area with platinum and an "N + " drain region with a hafnium electrode MG1 = ϕm1 = 3.9 eV (WF1) with platinum MG2 = ϕm1 = 5.8 eV (WF2).

The device channel doping concentration (n_i) = $1 \times 10^{15}/cm^3$. The proposed structure model variables are comparable to those found in conventional devices, with the exception of a nanocavity region for biological molecule recognition. The

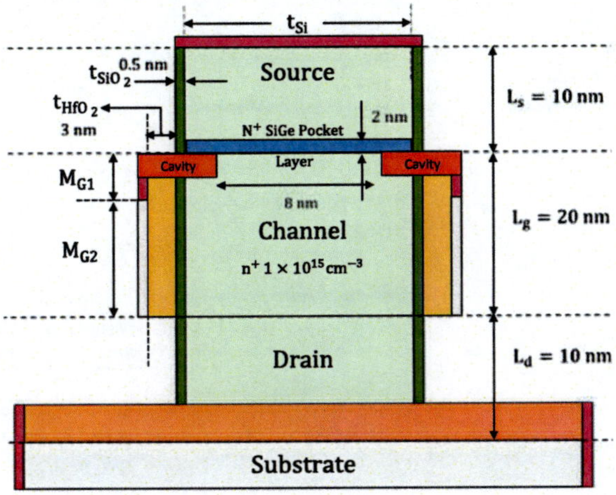

Fig. 1 Schematic diagram of basic proposed structure heterojunction based dopingless vertical tunnel field effect transistor (SiGe-DV-TFET)

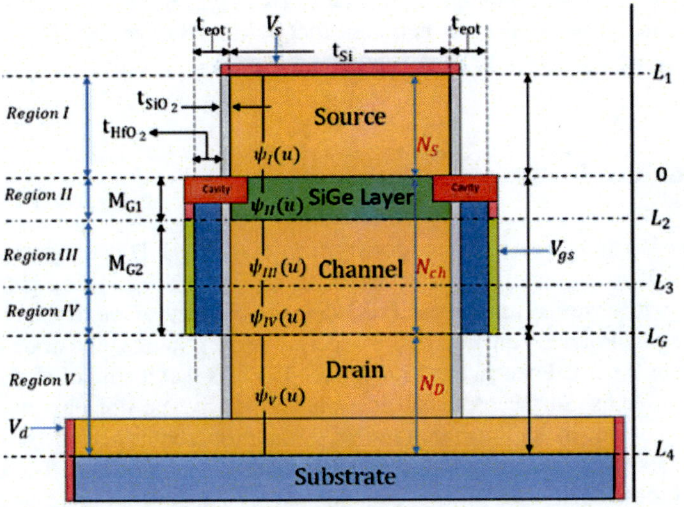

Fig. 2 Corresponding model schematic diagram with define depletion region

model of heterojunction based dopingless Vertical tunnel field effect transistor (SiGe-DV-TFET) biosensors uses Fermi–Dirac model, field dependent model. This draft used a non-local BTBT and doping dependent model. To account for the high doping concentration of the source and drain, a band gap narrowing model is also engaged. The SRH recombination mechanism is considered for the recombination mechanism. Only one type of biomolecule is thought to be immobilized in the cavities at any given moment. Table 1 lists the structural variables that will be used in the simulation. The

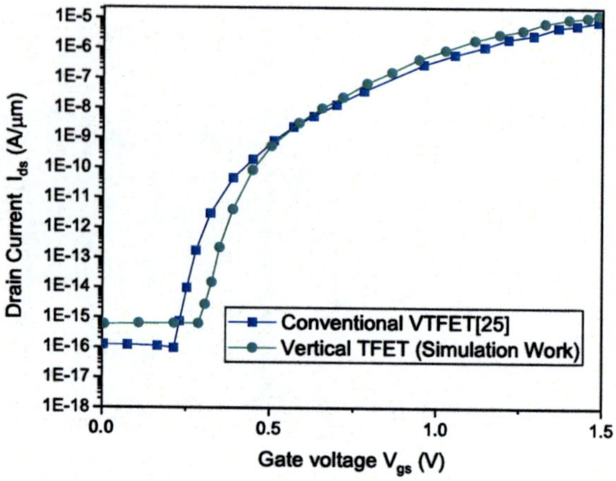

Fig. 3 The calibrated vertical TFET drain characteristics in comparison to the conventional vertical TFET

Silvaco Atlas tool [24] is used to simulate the SiGe-DV-TFET biosensor. With a value of 1, the dielectric constant (k) indicates that dielectric constant increases as the cavity is filled with biological molecules (K > 1). Figure 3 refers to the drain characteristics curve for the conventional silicon material of vertical TFET structure [25] calibrated at $V_{ds} = 1$ V.

3 Modeling Analysis and Its Findings

The under-lap area is explored to identify the possibility 1-D heterojunction based dopingless Vertical tunnel field effect transistor (SiGe-DV-TFET). The impact of the underlap part is viewed as increased resistance in the study. One of the advantages of using a 1-D Poisson equation in the underlap region, source, and drain depletion section over the 2-D Poisson equation in DG-TFET is that it simplifies the computational problems. Surface potential is evaluated for five portions by investigating the proposed gadget. As illustrated in Fig. 2, the proposed device's region is separated into six parts, including the source/drain side depletion width. The following is a list of these areas. The Poisson equation expression is determined by following equations:

$$\Psi_r(u) = -\frac{QN_r}{2.\epsilon_{Si}}.u^2 + C_r u + D_r \tag{1}$$

The parts I, II, VI, and VII are denoted by the letter "r." The Eq. 1 is finally out by integrating the 1D Poisson equation twice. For device the surface potential for section I and section II can be found by executing boundary equation.

$$\Psi_I(-L_s - L_1) = -\Psi_b \tag{2}$$

$$\frac{d\Psi_I}{du} = (-L_s - L_1) = 0 \tag{3}$$

We discovered section I's potential. by replacing Eqs. (3) and (4) into Eq. (1).

$$\Psi_I(u) = -\Psi_b - \frac{qN_a}{2\epsilon_{Si}}(u + L_s + L_1)^2 \tag{4}$$

L_s is the defined length of source side spacer. The first intersection equation at $u = -L_s$ is used for estimating the surface potential in 2nd section.

$$\Psi_I|(u = -L_s) = \Psi_{II}|(u = -L_s) \tag{5}$$

$$\frac{d\Psi_I(u)}{du}|(u = -L_s) = \frac{d\Psi_{II}(u)}{du}|(u = -L_s) \tag{6}$$

We may calculate the potential of section II by using Eqs. (6) and (7).

$$\Psi_{II} = -\Psi_b - \frac{qN_a}{2\epsilon_{Si}}(L_1)^2 - \frac{qN_a}{\epsilon_{Si}}L_1(L_s + u) \tag{7}$$

Exploring the 2-dimensional Poisson equation, the intersecting at x = 0 at L_2.

$$\frac{d^2\Psi_n(u, v)}{du^2} + \frac{d^2\Psi_n(u, v)}{dv^2} = -\frac{qN_n}{\epsilon_{Si}} \tag{8}$$

In a distinct section specifies the electrostatic surface potential. The potential of a heterojunction based dopingless Vertical tunnel field effect transistor (SiGe-DV-TFET) is indicated in the diagram below. The energy bandgap, electron affinity and permittivity of SiGe material can be calculated using following equation

$$E_{SiGe} = \begin{cases} 1.17 - 0.47m + 0.24m^2 m < 0.85 \\ 5.88 - 9.58m + 4.43m^2 m > 0.85 \end{cases} \tag{9}$$

$$\varepsilon_{SiGe} = 11.9(1 + 0.35m) \tag{10}$$

For equivalent oxide thickness following equation can be written as:

$$\Psi_n(u) = E_I \exp\frac{u - u_n}{D_l} + F_I \exp(-\frac{(u - u_n)}{D_l}) + \Psi_{gn} - \frac{q.Nn.Tch}{C_{ox}} \tag{11}$$

where, $\Psi_n(u)$ is defined for other regions onwards from the third section (n = III, IV and V).

$$D_l = \sqrt{\frac{\varepsilon_{si} t_{ch} t_{ox}}{2.\varepsilon_{ox}}} \tag{12}$$

At the interjection of section III and IV with boundary condition

$$\Psi_{III}(L_2) = \Psi_{IV} - \frac{q.N_n.T_{ch}}{C_{ox}} \tag{13}$$

$$\frac{d\Psi_{III}(L_2)}{du} = 0 \tag{14}$$

E_I, F_I are constants, and D_l is the device's characteristic length. The gate potential over the depletion area is denoted by Ψ_{gn}, with subscript n denoting the substrate section. As a result, in a TFET, the body doping $N_n = N_D$ is low. Section III's surface potential is equivalent to

$$\Psi_{III}(u) = (\Psi_t - \Psi_{GIII})\cosh\frac{\{u - L_2\}}{D_l} + \Psi_{GIII} - \frac{q.N_n.Tch}{C_{ox}} \tag{15}$$

For determining the potential in the drain side, we have to look for the potential in section IV and VI.

$$\Psi_{IV}(u) = \Psi_t - \frac{q.Nn.Tch}{C_{ox}} \tag{16}$$

$$L_2 \leq u \leq \left(\frac{L_{ch}}{2} - L_3\right) \tag{17}$$

$$(\frac{L_{ch}}{2} + L_4) \leq u \leq (L_{ch} - L_5) \tag{18}$$

The zone below the tunneling gate, section IV, is denoted "t" while at section VII, it is denoted by the subscript "s." Eq. (9) yields the universal potential for section V and VI, where L_3 and L_4 are the depletion length corresponding to length V.

$$\Psi_V(u) = A_V \exp\frac{u - (\frac{L_{ch}}{2} - L_3)}{D_l} + B_{VI}\exp\frac{-(u - (\frac{L_{ch}}{2} - L_3))}{D_l} + \Psi_{GV} - \frac{Q.Ni.Tch}{C_{ox}} \tag{19}$$

Though the channel's inversion charges, which were previously in section V, will now be in section VI. In section VI, we assume a charge density of p/cm^3. Different boundary conditions are used to determine the indefinite parameters. The lengths of the depletion layers is L_3 and L_4 corresponding to section IV and V potential at the intersections of numerous sections. The flat band voltage at the source and channel boundaries is V_{fbs}. The Potential at $u = -L_3 \text{and} L_4$ is equal to

$$\Psi_{IV}(-L_3) = \Psi_t - \frac{q.Ni.Tch}{C_{ox}} \tag{20}$$

$$\Psi_V(L_4) = \Psi_s - \frac{q.Ni.Tch}{C_{ox}} \tag{21}$$

Electric field at $u = -L_3$ and L_4. The surface potential and electric field are constant at sections V and VI, as define the boundary condition mentioned below. $u = \frac{L_{ch}}{2}$.

$$\Psi_V\left(\frac{L_{ch}}{2}\right) = \Psi_V\left(\frac{L_{ch}}{2}\right) \tag{22}$$

$$\frac{d\Psi_V}{du}|\left(u = \frac{L_{ch}}{2}\right) = \frac{d\Psi_V}{du}|\left(u = \frac{L_{ch}}{2}\right) \tag{23}$$

In order to solve boundary condition (Eq. (29) and (31)), $E_V \text{and} F_V$.

$$E_V = F_V = (\Psi_V - \frac{q.Ni.Tch}{C_{ox}} - \Psi_{GV} + \frac{qN_i D_l^2}{\epsilon_{si}})/2 \tag{24}$$

By solving two boundary conditions (Eq. (30) and (32)), $E_{VI} \text{and} F_{VI}$ are obtained.

$$E_V = F_V = \{\Psi_V - \frac{Q.Ni.Tch}{C_{ox}} - \Psi_{GV} + \frac{q(N_i + p)D_l^2}{\epsilon_{si}}\}/2 \tag{25}$$

To find the depletion length of unknown parameter of L_3 and L_4.

$$\left(\frac{\left((\Psi_t - \Psi_{\mathrm{GV}})\left(\exp\frac{L_3}{D_l} + \exp\frac{-L_3}{D_l}\right) + \Psi_{\mathrm{GV}} - \frac{q\cdot\mathrm{Ni}\cdot\mathrm{Tch}}{C_{\mathrm{ox}}} + \frac{q\cdot(\mathrm{Ni}+p)\cdot\mathrm{Tch}}{C_{\mathrm{ox}}}\right)}{\left(\Psi_s - \frac{q\cdot\mathrm{Ni.Tch}}{C_{\mathrm{ox}}} + \frac{q\cdot(\mathrm{Ni}+p)\cdot\mathrm{Tch}}{C_{\mathrm{ox}}}\right)}\right)^2 - \left(\frac{(\Psi_t - \Psi_{\mathrm{GV}})\left(\exp\frac{L_3}{D_l} + \exp\frac{-L_3}{D_l}\right)}{\left(-\Psi_s + \frac{q\cdot\mathrm{Ni}\cdot\mathrm{Tch}}{C_{\mathrm{ox}}} - \frac{q\cdot(\mathrm{Ni}+p)\cdot\mathrm{Tch}}{C_{\mathrm{ox}}}\right)}\right)^2 = 1 \tag{26}$$

4 Result Analysis

For validation, the demonstrated outcomes are compared to simulated results. The silvaco 2D-ATLAS simulator [24] is used to generate simulated results. Figure 4 shows the energy diagram of a SiGe layer in between heterojunction based dopingless Vertical tunnel field effect transistor (SiGe-DV-TFET). At $K = 6$, $V_{ds} = 0.60$ V, and $V_{gs} = 0.60$ V.

Figure 5 and Fig. 6 show how the potential of neutral ($K = 1$ to 12) and charged ($N_f = -2e^{15}$ to $5e^{15}$) biomolecules varies with respect to the horizontal axis. Because of the high current conduction, this increases the likelihood of tunneling. The fluctuation in the surface potential is caused by the immobilization of biological molecules [24]. In comparison to previous models that do not incorporate source and drain depletion

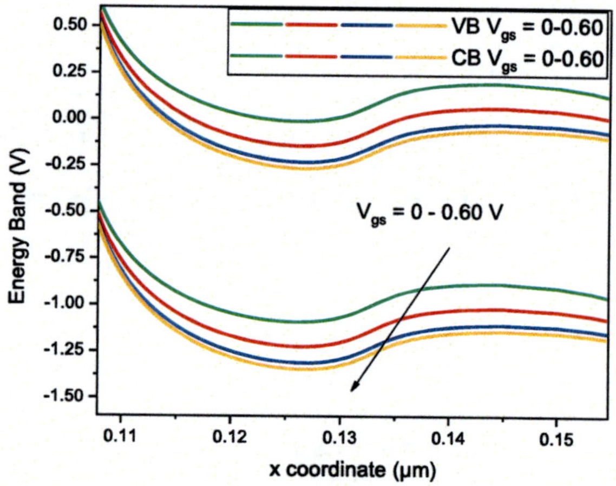

Fig. 4 Schematic Energy band diagram of SiGe-DV-TFET at $V_{ds} = 0.5$ V and $V_{gs} = 0$ to 0.6 V

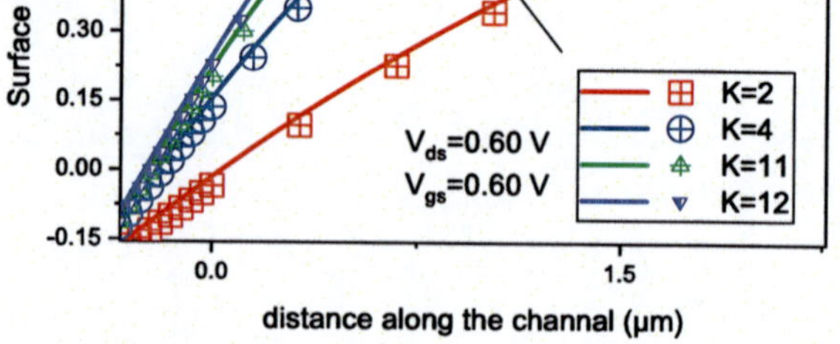

Fig. 5 Variation of different dielectric constant ($K = 1$ to 5) equivalent to different neutral biomolecules

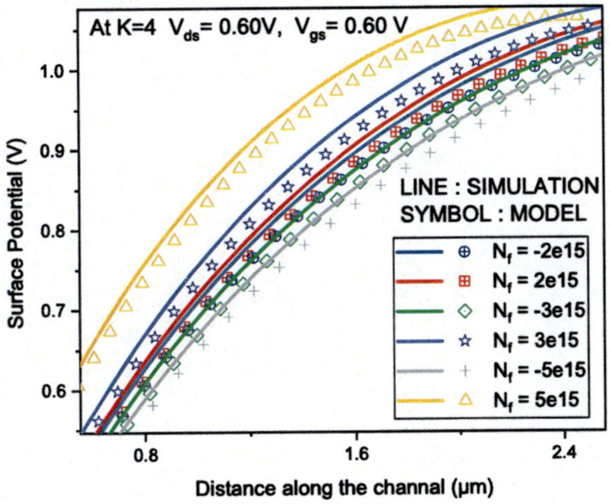

Fig. 6 Variation of charged ($N_f = -6e^{15}$ to $6e^{15}$) with respect to the surface potential

regions, the DM-GUD-TFET shown structural model is a better model. According to Fig. 7, an increase in V_{gs} leads to an increase in potential. When the gate voltage is increased while the drain voltage remains constant, the surface potential is directly proportional to V_{gs}.

Due to the rise in electric-field at the channel drain junction, the source charge is minimally changed when the drain side spacer length (L_d) increases. The breadth of the depletion region on the source side is determined by the amount of doping present. When L_d is increased, the real tunneling and E.F. (electric field) lowers slightly, affecting the potential more.

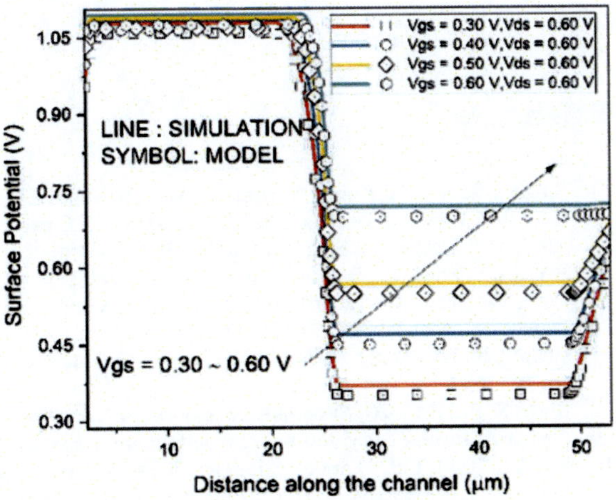

Fig. 7 Variation of charged ($N_f = -6e^{15}$ to $6e^{15}$) with respect to the surface potential

Table 1 Device specification of SiGe-DV-TFET

Device Parameters	Values
Channel doping concentration (L_{ch})	$1 \times 10^{15}/cm^3$
Device thickness (t_{Si})	10 nm
Channel thickness	20 nm
Cavity thickness	4 nm
Work function (WF1)	$M_{G1} = \phi m1 = 3.9$ eV
Work function (WF2)	$M_{G2} = \phi m2 = 5.8$ eV
Electron affinity of SiGe	4.025 kJ/mol
Energy band Gap of Ge	0.76 eV
Electron mobility of SiGe	1538 cm^2/Vs

5 Conclusion

In this paper a compact model analysis is done of novel SiGe heterojunction based dopingless Vertical tunnel field effect transistor (SiGe-DV-TFET) for biosensor applications. With this analysis the proposed device is suppressed with the major impact of short channel effect and leakage current also with cost efficiency in the basic development of the biosensor. With correct biassing circumstances, the proposed model performs better with a modest choice of spacer region width (L_s and L_d) and tunneling gate length thickness. Furthermore, this device is divided with five individual sections in accordance with its depletion region. The final outcome of TCAD simulation is found to be in good agreement with the proposed model.

Acknowledgement We would like to thank Dr. S. K. Bhalla Director, PSIT Kanpur for providing for lab facilities and research environment to carry out this work.

References

1. Singh S, Sharma A, Kumar V, Umar P, Rao AK, Singh AK (2021) Applied Physics A 127(9):1
2. Choi WY, Park BG, Lee JD, Liu TJK (2007) IEEE Electron Device Lett 28(8):743
3. Zhi J, Yiqi Z, Cong L, Ping W, Yuqi L (2016) Journal of Semiconductors 37(9):094003
4. Brocard S, Pala MG, Esseni D (2013) IEDM Tech Dig 5(4):1
5. Wang P-Y, Tsui B-Y (2016) IEEE Trans Nanotechnol 15(1):74
6. Dubey, PK, Kaushik BK (2017) IEEE Transactions on Electron Devices 64(8):3120
7. Chen F, Ilatikhameneh H, Tan Y, Klimeck G, Rahman R (2018) IEEE Trans Electron Devices 65(7):3065
8. Singh S, Raj B (2020) Superlattices and Microstructures 142:106496
9. Kumar A, Raj B (2015) Journal of Computational Electronics 14:820
10. Singh S, Raj B (2020) Superlattices and Microstructures 147:106717
11. Khatami Y, Banerjee K (2009) IEEE Trans Electron Devices 56(11):2752
12. Lee H, Park J-D, Shin C (1827) IEEE Trans Electron Devices 63(5):2016
13. Singh S, Raj B (2021) and Balwinder Raj. In Nanoelectronic Devices for Hardware and Software Security, CRCPress, pp 61–83

14. Brocard S, Pala MG, Esseni D (2013) Electron Devices Meeting (IEDM), 5.
15. Bhuwalka KK, Schulze J, Eisele I (2005) IEEE Trans Electron Devices 52(5):909
16. Kamata Y, Kamimuta Y, Ino T, Nishiyama A (2005) Jpn J Appl Phys 44:2323
17. Bhuwalka KK, Sedlmaier S, Ludsteck AK, Tolksdorf C, Schulze J, Eisele I (2004) IEEE Trans Electron Devices 51(2):279
18. Wang W (2014) IEEE Trans Electron Devices 61:193
19. Sentaurus User's Manual (2017), Synopsys 09
20. ATLAS Device Simulation Software (2016) Silvaco Int., Santa Clara, CA, USA
21. Nigam K, Kondekar P, Sharma D (2016) Micro Nano Letters 11(6):319
22. Sant S, Schenk A (2015) IEEE J Electron Devices Soc 3(3):164
23. Kumar S, Raj B (2016), Handbook of Research on Computational Simulation and Modeling in Engineering. IGI Global 640
24. Singh S, Raj B (2020) J Comput Electron 19(3):1154
25. Singh S, Raj B (2019) Journal of Electronic Materials 48.10, 6253

A Complete Analysis: From Model to Device Level of Tunnel Field Effect Transistors

Rupali Gupta and Saima Beg

Abstract In this manuscript, the tunnel field effect transistors (TFETs) are explored and analyzed completely starting from the tunneling models to various device structures. Initially, the need of quantum mechanical tunneling and its tunneling principle is discussed with the help of Schrodinger equation. Then, various tunneling models local as well as nonlocal tunneling models which are incorporated in the TFETs to support tunneling are briefed. In addition, the conventional TFETs device structure and its fundamental principle of operation are examined with the support of energy band diagrams in the ON condition and ON condition. Finally, to achieve more energy efficient technology, double gate TFET, carbon nanotube TFET, graphene-based TFET, and nanowire TEFT structures and their benefits are examined.

Keywords Tunnel field effect transistor (TFET) · Quantum mechanical tunneling · Carbon nanotube (CNT) TFETs · Silicon nanowire TFET

1 Introduction

With the advent of field effect transistor (FET) and complementary metal oxide semiconductor (CMOS) in 1960 and 1963, respectively, the semiconductor technology/IC design geared up [1, 2]. Such advancement in these industries is possible because CMOS technology supports continuous scaling and thus Moore's principle [3]. But, the scaling in CMOS below 10 nm regime, the gate control on the channel get reduces and faces several short channel effects (SCEs). Due to SCEs, the threshold voltage starts decreasing with channel length and drain-source voltage [4]. The ability of the transistor to work as a switch is get restricted, since it causes large power dissipation because of SCEs [5]. The current transport mechanism of conventional transistor imposes several limitations and thus further scaling of the supply voltage in the digital

R. Gupta (✉) · S. Beg
Department of Electronics and Communication Engineering, Integral University, Lucknow, India

S. Beg
e-mail: saimabeg@iul.ac.in

M. S. Kaiser et al. (eds.), *Proceedings of Trends in Electronics and Health Informatics*, Lecture Notes in Networks and Systems 376,
https://doi.org/10.1007/978-981-16-8826-3_41

IC is not possible [6]. Therefore, at the constant voltage range, further miniaturization of the FETs do not lead an energy efficient IC [7, 8, 9]. In addition, sustained need of novel silicon devices to keep Moore's alive, need of low power in the complex and dense IC design, and requirement of cost-effective methods are other challenges, which require more attention.

So, to implement energy efficient IC, the idea of new materials may be silicon of non-silicon-based materials, novel devices which rely on the new operating principles, energy efficient architectures are need to be investigated [10, 11, 12]. In this regard, the quantum mechanical tunneling-based tunnel field effect transistors came in to consideration and show excellent switching behavior beyond the conventional FETs [13, 14, 15].

2 Quantum Mechanical Tunneling

There are basically two ways by which an electron can pass a potential barrier and render current. In the first one, if the electron possesses sufficient energy then it can jump and overcome the barrier. Whereas in the second way, if the barrier is very thin and the electron does not have sufficient energy to jump, then the electron can penetrate through the barrier and reach to the other side of the barrier is called tunneling. Quantum mechanical tunneling is basic operational principle of the tunnel field effect transistors (TFETs), therefore it is essential to first discuss the idea of quantum mechanics and quantum tunneling phenomenon to capture the institutive understanding of TFETs.

The analogy between quantum mechanics with the classical mechanics is realized by Schrodinger equation and Newton's lay. The Schrodinger equation has the same role in quantum mechanics to that of Newton's law in the classical mechanics [16, 17]. The Schrodinger equation is partial differential equation, which is useful to determine the quantum state of any system and its variation with time. The quantum state of any system is also known as wave function of the system, which is used to represent the expectation values or the probabilities of any physical quantity. The Schrodinger equation for a particle constrained in the x-axis is estimated as Eq. (1).

$$i\hbar\frac{\partial\Psi}{\partial t} = -\frac{\hbar^2}{2m}\frac{\partial^2\Psi}{\partial x^2} + V\Psi \tag{1}$$

Here, ψ represents the wave function of the system, i and $\hbar$ denote the imaginary quantity and Planck constant in reduced form, respectively, m and x denote the mass of the particle and position of the particle along x-axis, V represents the potential energy function. Primarily, it is required to determine the wave function ψ by using the Schrodinger equation because it is primary variable and basically used to estimate the probabilities of the physical quantity in the quantum mechanics [18]. The probability or expectation value of a particle situated in the x-axis can be determined by the following relation (2).

$$\langle x \rangle = \int_{-\infty}^{+\infty} x|\Psi(x,t)|^2 dx \tag{2}$$

The solution $\psi(x, t)$ of the Schrodinger equation can be obtained by variable separable method if the potential energy function (V) is time independent and can be given by Eq. (3), which is product of spatial component $\varphi(x)$ and temporal component of the $\varnothing(t)$.

$$\Psi(x,t) = \psi(x)\varphi(t) \tag{3}$$

Further, with the help of Schrodinger equation, the following relations (4) and (5) can be estimated.

$$\varphi(t) = e^{-\frac{iEt}{\hbar}} \tag{4}$$

$$\frac{\hbar^2}{2m}\frac{\partial^2\Psi}{\partial x^2} + (E - V)\Psi = 0 \tag{5}$$

The expression (5) represents steady state form of the Schrodinger equation in which potential function (V) is time independent, where E represents the particle energy. Expression (5) is generally used to evaluate the solution of the Schrodinger Eq. (1). The energy values E_n for which the solutions of the Schrodinger equation can be obtained are called eigenvalues, and the respective wave function is known as eigenfunction.

3 Tunneling Models

Since the potential profile of the TFETs is complex geometrical form, so the derivation of the tunneling analytical relations to compute the tunneling probability is quite difficult. Therefore, to analyze the behavior of the TFETs, numerical simulations are found to be an essential tool. Since, tunneling in the TFETs is a quantum mechanical phenomenon so that meticulous computational methods which involve non-equilibrium green function formalism are required to achieve the precise results. The consideration of full quantum treatment is computationally complex and expensive, hence semi classical models which are governed by drift–diffusion mechanism are widely used and acceptable in the simulation environment of the TFETs [19, 20]. The development of appropriate models of TFETs is essential for their circuit application. The accurate models give the physical insight of any device as well as beneficial in the optimization and analysis circuits. The TFETs employ band to band tunneling model. In which the electrons tunneling occurs from the valance band to the conduction band and results in generation of electron–hole pair. The electron is generated in the conduction band, and the hole is created in the valance band. Local and nonlocal tunneling models are categorized in the TFETs depending upon the nature of the electric field.

3.1 Local Tunneling Models

Here, the local electric field at a particular location is responsible for the generation rate of the carriers at that location. Kane's model and Hurkx's model are the main local tunneling model in the TFETs devices.

Kane's model: This model is first local band to band tunneling model derived by E. O. Kane and it is developed for the uniform electric field. Kane gives the relation (6) for the generation rate (GBTBT) because of band to band tunneling for the direct band gap materials.

$$G_{BTBT} = AE_{ext}^{\alpha} exp\left(-\frac{B}{|E_{ext}|}\right) \tag{6}$$

where E_{ext} is the uniform electric field, and A, B, and α are the fitting parameters which are needed calibration to show good agreement with the experimental data of the TFETs.

Hurkx's model: Hurkx's model considers recombination and reduces the non-aero current at the VDS = 0, which appears in the Kane's model. In this model, a pre-factor is incorporated with generation rate of the local tunneling model and the pre-factor is given as (7)

$$D = \frac{np - n_i^2}{(n + n_i)(p + p_i)} \tag{7}$$

Here, n_i and p_i represent the intrinsic level concentration of the electrons and holes, and n and p represent the electron and the hole concentrations in the device.

3.2 Nonlocal Tunneling Models

Since, the band to band tunneling relies on the positionally separated quantities, and hence, local tunneling models are insufficient to capture full insight of the device. Moreover, the local tunneling models are developed for the uniform electric field in the tunneling which is not always true, so for the non-uniform electric, these models give non-physical results. In the nonlocal tunneling models, the BTBT tunneling rate is evaluated after accounting positional variation of the energy bands. Node pair base BTBT model and tunnel path-based BTBT are two basic nonlocal tunneling models.

4 Device Structures

The TFETs device structure consist of reversed biased P-I-N structure; the two highly doped "N" region, and highly doped "P" regions are separated by an intrinsic layer or by the low doped channel layer. Figure 1 shows the simple structure of n-type TFETs and p-type TFET. If the drain is doped with (n+) and source is doped with (p+), then TFET is n-type TFET as shown in Fig. 1(a) while if the drain is doped with (P+) and source is doped with (n+), then it is known as p-type TFET as depicted in the Fig. 1(b). The remaining structure is similar to that of conventional MOSFET; i. e., the gate is separated from the channel by a dielectric material. The biasing of the TFET is also represented in the Fig. 1, in the n-type TFETs, the gate and the drain are biased with the positive voltage, whereas for the n-type TFETs, the gate and drain are biased with negative voltage for their correct operation. So, depending upon the nature of the carriers in the channel, the TFETs can also be classified means, if the channel carriers are electrons, then it is n-type and if the channel carriers are holes, the TFET is known as p-type.

Fig. 1 **a** Schematic structure of n-type TFET. **b** Schematic structure of p-type TFET

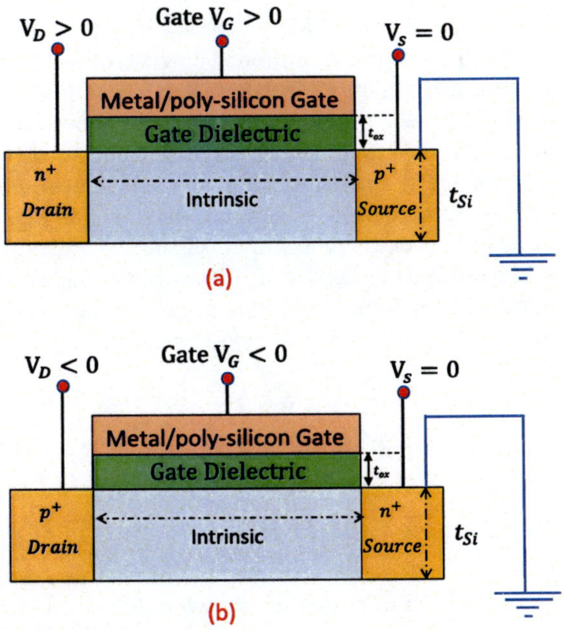

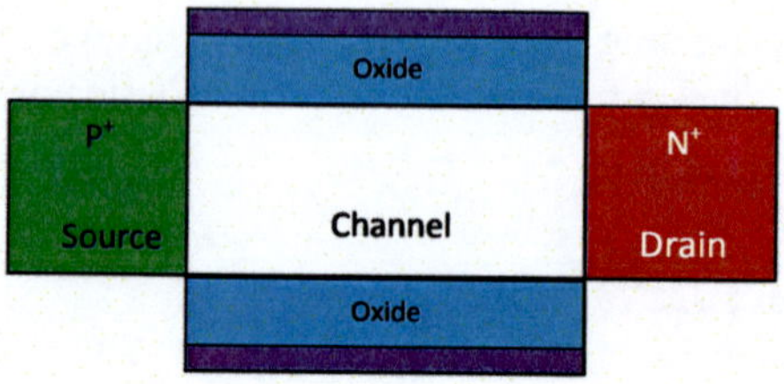

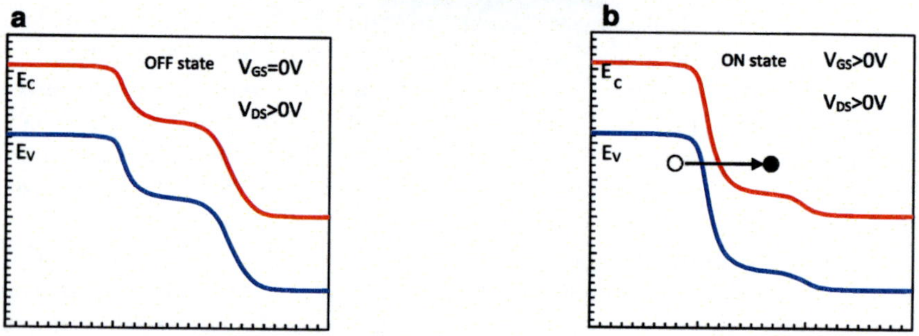

Fig. 2 **a** Energy band diagram of TFET in OFF state. **b** Energy band diagrams of TFET in ON state

4.1 Operation of TFETs

The operation of the TFETs can be easily understandable with the help of energy band diagrams. The energy band diagram of n-type TFET is shown in the Fig. 2(a) and Fig. 2(b). In the OFF state (when Vgs = 0 V) Fig. 2(a), it can be seen that the conduction band of the channel lies well above the valance band of the source so that electron do not find any available energy state to tunnel. But, when a positive gate voltage is applied to the gate, the conduction band of the channel is aligned with the valance band of the source as shown in Fig. 2(b), and therefore, the source electrons can easily tunnel to the channel and they swept to the drain region where positive voltage is applied. In this way, the tunneling or ON current will achieved in the TFETs. Similar operation occurs for the p-type TFETs, the only difference is that the whole phenomena occur at negative gate and drain supply.

5 Classification of TFETs on the Basis of Device Structures

5.1 Double Gate TFETs

The normal TFETs structure shown in Fig. 1 provides small ON current since the gate has less control over the channel, and therefore, it leads some modifications. In the double gate TFET, two gate electrodes are employed; one is at the top and

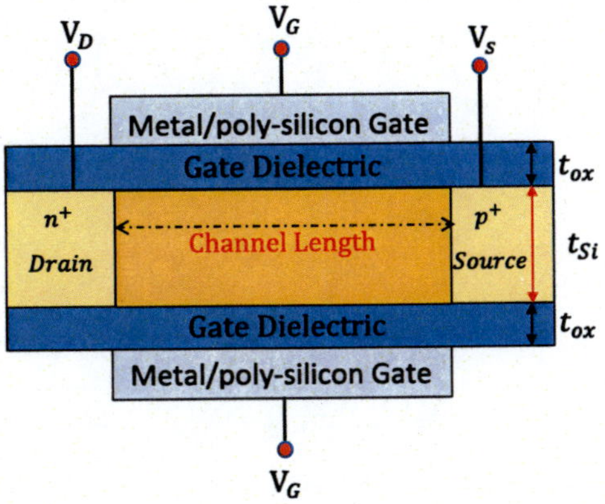

Fig. 3 Schematic diagram double gate TFET

another is at the bottom as shown in Fig. 3. The employment of dual gate enhances the electrostatic gate control over the channel and render large drive current. The doping of the drain region is kept lower than that of source region to ensure reduced ambipolar current. Ambipolar current came in to account when holes of (p+) region of n-type TFETs start tunneling in to channel from the drain at the negative Vgs and constitute reverse current. Similarly, in p-type TFET, the electrons start tunneling from the drain side at the positive Vgs.

5.2 *Carbon Nanotube (CNT) TFETs*

Carbon nanotube is an allotropic form of the carbon which exhibits excellent carrier mobility and geometric size. Moreover, CNT is direct band gap material and shows the tunable energy bands which make CNT more promising; these properties of the CNT are exploited in the fabrication of the TFETs. CNT supports one-dimensional carrier transport and thus provides good control of the gate voltage over the bands of the channel. Figure 4 shows diagram of gate all-around CNT TFET, in which the channel material is replaced with the intrinsic CNT material and CNT of the drain and source is doped with linear p-type and n-type, respectively. The gate is overlapped all around to enhance the gate control over the channel.

5.3 *Graphene TFET*

TFET with the graphene as channel material is shown in Fig. 5, the graphene material shows excellent properties like atomic layer thickness enables high scaling and superior electrostatic gate control on the channel, it exhibits very small short channel effects and high carrier mobility. Thus, the graphene is current and future attraction

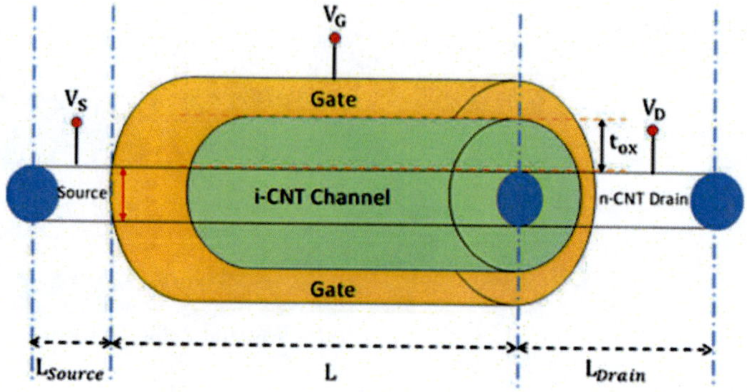

Fig. 4 Schematic diagram of carbon nanotube TFET

Fig. 5 TFET with the graphene as channel material

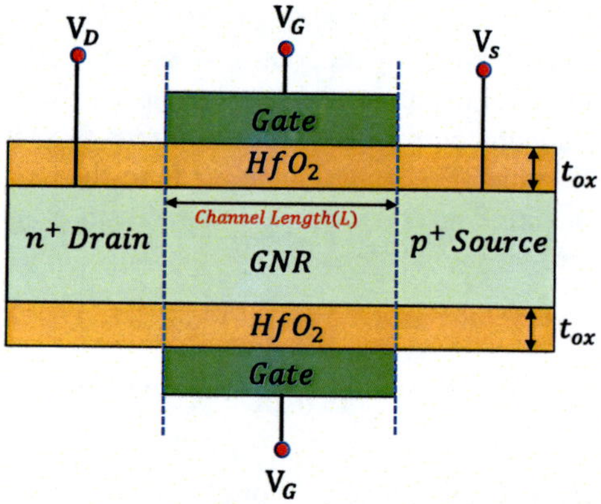

for the transistor design. However, the absence of the band gap in the graphene does not allow completely switched-off condition in the FET and also give small ON–OFF current ratio.

5.4 Silicon Nanowire Vertical TFET

Nanowire is a one-dimensional system having single crystal material and its length is in microns and diameters are few nanometers. The cylindrical geometry along with small diameter of the nanowire facilitates high gate control on channel. The 1D systems of the nanowire enable high tunneling and hence high ON current. A vertical silicon nanowire TFET is shown in Fig. 6, in which the source and drain are doped asymmetrically to achieve low ambipolarity.

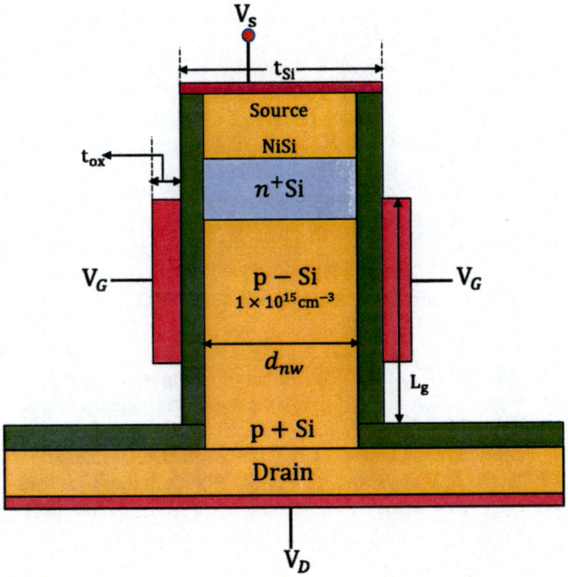

Fig. 6 Schematic diagram of silicon nanowire-based vertical tunnel field effect transistor

6 Conclusion

Here, tunnel field effects transistor which relies on the quantum mechanical tunneling is examined to achieve energy efficient designed in the analog and in the digital domain as well so that the limitations of the conventional MOSFET can be omitted. In this regard, the basic of quantum mechanical tunneling and various local and nonlocal tunneling models which support electron tunneling from the valance band, the source to the conduction band of the channel is discussed. Besides tunneling principle, the basic TFET device structure along with some more advance structures like carbon nanotube TFET, double gate TFET, graphene TFET, and silicon nanowire TFET are incorporated in this study with their working principles.

Acknowledgement We would like to thank **Dr. Saima Beg** for providing lab facilities and research environment to carry out this work.

References

1. Frank DJ, Dennard RH, Nowak E, Solomon PM, Taur Y, Philip Wong H-S (2001) Proceedings of the IEEE 89(3):259 (2001)
2. Koswatta SO, Lundstrom MS, Nikonov DE (2009) IEEE Transactions on Electron Devices 56(3):456
3. Choi WY, Park B-G, Lee JS, King Liu T-J (2007) IEEE Electron Device Letters 28(8):743

4. Singh S, Raj B, Raj B (2021) Nanoelectronic Devices for Hardware and Software Security. CRC Press, pp 61–83
5. Khatami Y, Banerjee K (2009) IEEE Trans Electron Devices 56(11):2752
6. Ionescu AM, Riel H (2011) Nature 479(7373):329
7. Singh S, Raj B (2020) Journal of Computational Electronics 19(3):1154
8. Singh S, Raj B (2019) Journal of Electronic Materials 48(10):6253
9. Choi WY, Park BG, Lee JD, Liu TJK (2007) IEEE Electron Device Letters 28(8):743
10. Zhi J, Yiqi Z, Cong L, Ping W, Yuqi L (2016) Journal of Semiconductors 37(9):094003
11. Brocard S, Pala MG, Esseni D (2013) IEDM Tech Dig 5(4-1), (2013).
12. Wang P-Y, Tsui B-Y (2016) IEEE Transactions on Nanotechnology 15(1):74
13. Dubey PK, Kaushik BK (2017) IEEE Transactions on Electron Devices 64(8):3120
14. Chen F, Ilatikhameneh H, Tan Y, Klimeck G, Rahman R (2018) IEEE Transactions on Electron Devices 65(7):3065
15. Singh S, Raj B (2020) Superlattices and Microstructures 142:106496
16. Kumar S, Raj B (2015) Journal of Computational Electronics 14:820
17. Singh S, Raj B (2020) Superlattices and Microstructures 147:106717
18. Sun MC, Kim SW, Kim G, Kim HW, Lee JH, Shin H, Park BG (2010) Nanotechnology Materials and Devices Conference (NMDC), p 2264
19. Gupta S, Wairya S, Singh S (2021) Superlattices and Microstructures 157: 106992
20. Singh S, Sharma A, Kumar V, Umar P, Rao AK, Singh AK (2021) Applied Physics A 127(9):1

Charge Pump-Phase Frequency Detector based Phase-Locked Loop for Modern Wireless Communication—A Review

Mohammad Amir Ansari, Syed Hasan Saeed, and Deepak Balodi

Abstract Performance and comparison of several architecture topologies involve low phase noise and high-speed phase frequency detector. Phase frequency detector is essential in Phase-Locked Loop. Phase frequency detector has many advantages over Phase detector (PD) and Frequency detector (FD) by detecting frequency and phase simultaneously. Charge pump based phase frequency detector is an important block for signal generation in the PLL. At higher frequencies, the challenges like phase noise, jitter, power consumption, and area arise. This article discusses these design challenges of phase frequency detector at higher frequencies. Parameters of different design topologies have been compared. This comparative study will help the researchers to choose the best design out of the given topologies.

Keywords Phase frequency detector · Charge pump · Phase-locked loop

1 Introduction

One of the major challenges in wireless communication applications is to generate stable output high-frequency signals. Due to the unique property, PLL is used to produce stable high-frequency signals from a low-frequency signal. This article aims to analyze the various topologies of a high phase noise detector and the performance of a high-speed charge pump based phase frequency detector.

The comparison between phase and frequency of the two clocks is done by phase frequency detector and produces either a pump-up or pump-down signal depending on whether the phase of the on-chip clock is lagging or leading the external reference

M. A. Ansari (✉) · S. H. Saeed
Integral University, Lucknow, India
e-mail: mamir@iul.ac.in

S. H. Saeed
e-mail: ssaeed@iul.ac.in

D. Balodi
BBD Engineering College, Lucknow, India

M. S. Kaiser et al. (eds.), *Proceedings of Trends in Electronics and Health Informatics*, Lecture Notes in Networks and Systems 376,
https://doi.org/10.1007/978-981-16-8826-3_42

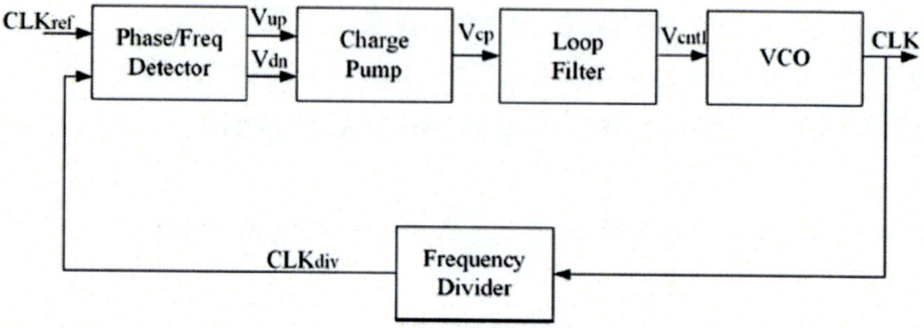

Fig. 1 Design architecture of a charge pump based phase-locked loop

clock. The charge pump increases the voltage on the loop filter capacitor when given a pump-up signal and decreases this voltage when given a pump-down signal. The low-pass filter is used to block the high-frequency components of the charge pump output and set the bandwidth of the PLL feedback loop [1].

The VCO produces an output signal the frequency of which is equal to its input voltage. The frequency divider divides down the VCO output frequency of the clock to produce a clock signal with a frequency in the same range as that of the reference clock. In Fig. 1, CLKref represents the external reference signal, CLK represents the high-frequency output clock, and CLKdiv represents the frequency divided version of the VCO clock that can be compared with the lower frequency reference clock, CLKref [2].

2 Early Developments of PLL

In the modern electronic system, one of the important constituents is Phase-Locked Loop, which is also known as PLL [3]. PLL has become one of the most essential elements due to having a wide range of applications over a broad frequency spectrum [4] like in wireless and wired communication systems, microprocessor board of complex systems, and many other systems. In practical PLL circuit, there are so many imperfections always there. Due to these imperfections, high ripple may appear in the control voltage while the loop is in locked condition. These high ripples change the frequency of VCO, which results in waveform with non-uniformity. Non-ideal effect in PLL has been covered in this section [3, 4]. The low power consumption and small size devices are the main concerns of the new technology's development. Recently, research on digital video broadcasting for portable devices is underway [5, 6].

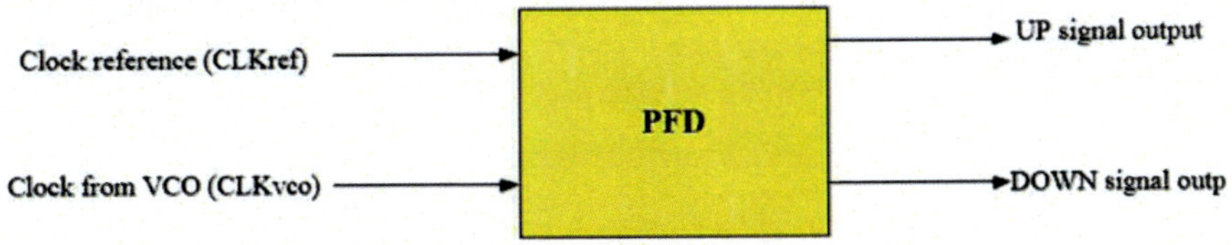

Fig. 2 Phase/frequency detector

3 Conventional PFD

The PFD uses sequential logic to give the difference between the phase and frequency of two inputs. When the signal fed back from the loop lags the reference signal, the output of the pump-up goes high [7, 8]. This indicates that the frequency of oscillation needs to be increased. In the same way, the pump-down output goes high when the feedback clock leads the reference clock, this indicates that the oscillation frequency needs to be decreased. According to the difference between phase and frequency of the input signals the phase frequency detector has two outputs that work accordingly. A PFD is shown in Fig. 2.

4 Design Challenges in PFD-CP

The PFD is a digital circuit that uses sequential logic to detect differences in the phase or frequency between its two input clocks. Phase detector and frequency detector are usually used for detecting phases and frequency. However, with PFD, the former can also be used to simultaneously detect both phases and frequency. The main problem associated with detection of phase change because it degrades the performance of PLL [9]. The charge pump is the core component of the Phase-Locked Loop. In Fig. 3, the charge pump (CP) enabled PLL is the widely used architecture. The name CP- PLL stems from the fact that the output of phase detector (PD) works as a current source that drives current in and out of the loop filter, not a voltage source. This type of PLL is very famous due to its suitability to integrate into microelectronics devices. This form of charge pump is known as CP-PLL.

One of the disadvantages that PFD suffers from is dead zone. Small difference in the phase of the input signals that cannot be detected by a phase-frequency detector is a dead zone [10]. Dead zone appears due to the time delay of the logic components and feedback path of the flip flops. Second problem is due to the short-term fluctuation of a signal relative to its ideal time is called jitter. Jitter is a phenomenon that can be induced by a clock from various sources and are dissimilar across all frequencies. Another issue with the phase frequency detector is phase noise [11]. Phase noise is a frequency domain representation of random fluctuations in the phase of a waveform. It is due to the time-domain instability known as "jitter" [12].

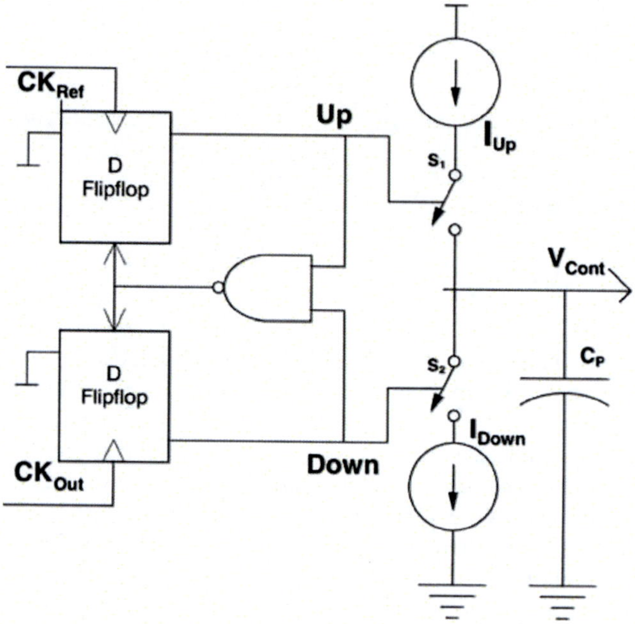

Fig. 3 PFD succeeded by a charge pump topology in conventional PLL

5 Review of Available PFD-CP Architectures

Many architecture approaches depend on the concept of D-Flip Flop phase frequency detector which has three steps. General phase frequency detector architecture has developed with two Delay Flip Flop and feedback taking a NAND gate. Due to the mismatch, DFF-PFD has a problem with dead zone [13]. D-FF-dependent design becomes more complicated and did not get fully discharge, leading to more power consumption. Effect of phase noise pulls down the D-Flip Flop phase frequency detector performance.

The Gain Boosting charge pump having low jitter has been proposed to reduce the current mismatching problem due to high output impedance. The designed phase frequency detector gets zero dead zones [21]. True single-phase clock (TSPC) logic brings down the complexity of conventional phase-frequency detectors. Only16 transistors are used in this new structure to achieve minimum power consumption and delay in the reset path allows the phase-frequency detector to work at high frequency [22]. A High-Speed Phase Frequency Detector Multi Threshold CMOS with power gating technique has better phase noise as compared to DFF-PFD and also it consumes low power consumption and gives high frequency. This design is also free from dead zone (Table 1).

Table 1 Comparative analysis on different topologies

References	Technology/operating voltage	Topology	Phase noise (dBc/Hz)/jitter	Maximum operating frequency (Hz)	Power consumption	No. of transistors/area	Dead zone	Topology specifications
[5]	0.35 μm CMOS3V	Double-edge-checking PFD	Not given	4.78 GHz	Not given	Not given	3 ps	Difference phase-frequency detector (DD-PFD)
[6]	0.35 μm CMOS-3.3v	Standard CMOS (S-PFD)	−24.64	420 MHz	7.4 mW	1750 μm^2	Free	Standard CMOS (S-PFD)
[12]	0.065 μm CMOS-0.7v	Dickson Charge Pump (DCP)	Not given	1.8 MHz	27 μW	0.17 mm^2	Free	Low-leakage enhanced DCP
[13]	0.18 μm CMOS-1.8v	GainBoo sting Charge Pump	3 ps	2.4 GHz	0.4 mW	18	Free	GainBoosting-charge pump
[14]	0.065 μm CMOS-1.2v	CP-PFD	Not given	3.44 GHz	324 μW	322.61 $\mu\ m^2$	Free	True single-phase clock logic
[15]	0.13 μm CMOS- 1.2v	symmetric Structure of PFD	Not given	4.1 GHz	90 μW	250 μm^2	25 ps	Delay lockloop (DLL) logic
[16]	0.18 μm CMOS-1.8v	DLL-PFD	4.1 ps	3.33 GHz	110 μW	16	Free	TSPC and GDI logic
[17]	0.13 μm CMOS-1.2v	Latch-based PFDs	Not given	2.94 GHz	496 μW	Not given	61 ps	PVT variation
[21]	0.13 μm CMOS-1.2v	High-Speed PFD	Not given	1.26 GHz	0.116 μW	1423 μm^2	Free	HSPFD MTCMOS
[22]	0.13 μm CMOS-1.3v	Nano-meter CMOS PLL	−96.01	1 MHz	10.7 mW	0.31 mm^2	Free	Nano-meter CMOS PLL

6 Conclusion

This paper consists of a comparative study of the different topologies of high-speed Charge Pump-Phase Frequency Detectors. There are various parameters to judge the performance of the PFD. The different parameters are power consumption, maximum operating frequency, phase noise and jitter, etc. There exists trade-off between these parameters of phase-frequency detector and there is an uncertainty if the particular PFD architecture is efficient or not. It all depends on the application where we are using the architecture. However, based on our comparative study among the various design, Gain Boosting Charge Pump (GB-CP) can be more practically useful for different proposed designs methodologies, and this design provides optimized values for the application in modern wireless communication.

Acknowledgements We acknowledge this work as intellectual property of Integral University, Lucknow, India vides the Manuscript Communication no. **IU/R&D/2021-MCN0001280**. We are thankful to Integral University for giving us an opportunity to carry out this research work.

References

1. Yu H, Inoue Y, Han Y (2005) A new high-speed low voltage charge pump for PLL applications. In: ASICON2005, 6th international conference on ASIC, October 2005. IEEE
2. Heedley P (2015) EEE232 Class Notes (Unpublished). California State University Sacramento
3. Razavi B (2002) Design of analog CMOS integrated circuits, Chap. 15. Tata-McGraw Hill, pp 532–578
4. Wolaver DH (2015) Phase locked loop circuit design, Chap. 4. Prentice Hall, pp 47–80
5. Chou C-P, Lin Z-M, Chen J-D (2004) A 3-PS dead-zone double- edge-checking phase-frequency-detector with 4.78 GHz operation frequency. In: The 2004 IEEE Asia-Pacific conference on circuits and systems conference, vol 2, 937–940
6. Arshak K, Abubaker O, Jafer E (2004) Design and simulation difference types CMOS phase frequency detector for high speed and low jitter PLL. In: Proceedings of the fifth IEEE international Carcas conference on devices, circuits and systems, vol 1, pp 188–191
7. Vassiliou I, Vavelidis V, Bouras S, Kavadias S, Kokolakis Y, Kamoulakos G, Kyranas A, Kapnistis C, Haralabidis N (2006) A 0.18 μm CMOS dual-band direct-conversion DVB-H receiver. In: IEEE international solid-state circuits conference, vol 33.1, pp 606–607
8. Dickson J (1976) On-chip high-voltage generation in MNOS integrated circuits using an improved voltage multiplier technique. IEEE J Solid-State Circ SC-11:374–378
9. Witters J, Groeseneken G, Maes H (1989) Analysis and modeling of on-chip high voltage generator circuits for use in EEPROM circuits. IEEE J Solid-State Circ 24:1372–1381
10. Tanzawaand T, Tanaka T (1997) A dynamic analysis of the Dickson charge pump circuit. IEEE J Solid-State Circ 32:1231–1240
11. Arul Murugan C, Banuselvasaraswathy B, Gayathree K (2019) High-voltage gain CMOS charge pump at subthreshold operation regime for low power applications. Springer Nature Singapore Pte Ltd. https://doi.org/10.1007/978-981-13-3765-9_44
12. Mahmoud A, Alhawari M, Mohammad B, Saleh H, Ismail M (2019) A gain-controlled, low-leakage Dickson charge pump for energy-harvesting applications. IEEE Trans Very Large-Scale Integr (VLSI) Syst, 1063–821

13. Kailuke A, Agrawal P, Kshirsagar RV (2019) Design of low power, low jitter PLL for WiMAX application in 0.18 μm CMOS process. In: International conference on pervasive computing advances and applications- Per CAA, pp 390–397
14. Lad Kirankumar H, Rekha S, Laxminidhi T (2020) A dead-zone-free zero blind-zone high-speed phase frequency detector for charge-pump PLL. Circ Syst Signal Process 39:3819–3832
15. Sofimowloodi S, Razaghian F, Gholami M (2019) Low-power high-frequency phase frequency detector for minimal blind-zone phase-locked loops. Circ Syst Signal Process 38:498–511
16. Rezaeian A, Ardeshir G, Gholami M (2020) A low-power and high- frequency phase frequency detector for a 3.33-GHz delay locked loop. Circ Syst Signal Process 39:1735–1750
17. Chen W-H, Inerowicz ME, Jung B (2010) Phase frequency detector with minimal blind zone for fast frequency acquisition. IEEE Trans Circ Syst—ii: Express Briefs 57(12)
18. He Y, Cui X, Lee CL, Xue D (2014) An improved fast acquisition PFD with zero blind zone for the PLL application. Key Lab of Integrated Microsystems, Peking University Shenzhen Graduate School Shenzhen, China
19. Abrar M, Chaudhry SM (2016) Design of a low noise, low power and spurious free phase frequency detector and charge pump for phase-locked loops. J Eng Appl Sci 35(2). ISSN 1023-862X -eISSN 2518-4571
20. Maiti M, Saw SK, Nath V, Majumder A (2019) A power efficient PFD-CP architecture for high-speed clock and data recovery application. Springer-Verlag GmbH Germany, part of Springer Nature, Microsystem Technologies, (0123456789()-volV) (0123). https://doi.org/10.1007/s00542-019-04458-4
21. Al Amin FBN, Ahmad N, Hairol Jabbar M (2018) A low power CMOS phase frequency detector in high frequency PLL system. IOP Conf Ser J Phys Conf Series 1049:012059
22. Manikandan RR, Amrutur B (2015) A zero charge-pump mismatch current tracking loop for reference spur reduction in PLL. Microelectron J 46(6), 422–430

Communication

Compact Printed Multiband Fractal Antenna for C, X and Ku Band Applications: Design and Analysis

Ruchi Kadwane and Jaikaran Singh

Abstract The objective of this paper is to design and analyze compact size multiband fractal patch antenna suitable for multiband applications. The proposed fractal antenna consists of a main patch, a ground plane and a 50 Ω feed line. The dielectric material selected for the design is Epoxy FR4, which has dielectric constant of 4.4 and height of the substrate is 1.57 mm. The antenna is occupying an area of 20×24 mm^2 for the ground plane. A parametric study of the proposed fractal patch antenna is carried out to achieve multiband performance. The effects of addition of self-similar shapes with smaller dimensions in step by step iterative process have been investigated based on the antenna performance. The study also includes design methodology, frequency setting, 3D polar plot, radiation patterns, gain and directivity parameter analysis of proposed antenna design. The geometry is simulated using Ansoft HFSS software.

Keywords Bandwidth · Beamwidth · Directivity · Fractal · Gain · Multiband · Patch · Radiation pattern · Resonant frequency · Return loss · VSWR

1 Introduction

Today, due to increase in multimedia application, several communication systems require multiple frequency bands for various different communication services. Conventionally, single band antenna cannot operate at all the frequency bands and also so many mobile communication devices may be of pocket size, demands to shrink the size of the entire device or circuits. As to fulfill the above two requirements of multiple frequency bands and small size of device, there is need to design a compact size device i.e. antenna, which can cover joint bands simultaneously, known as multiband antenna.

A multiband antenna, in telecommunication, is a communication device which supports multiple radio frequency bands. Multiple bands in mobile device supports

R. Kadwane (✉) · J. Singh
Department of Electronics and Communication Engineering, LNCTU, Bhopal, Madhya Pradesh, India

M. S. Kaiser et al. (eds.), *Proceedings of Trends in Electronics and Health Informatics*, Lecture Notes in Networks and Systems 376,
https://doi.org/10.1007/978-981-16-8826-3_43

roaming between different regions where different standards are used for mobile telephone services. Patch antenna with fractal design is one of the best choice for this multiband application.

Fractal antenna is an antenna that uses self-similar designs which maximize the effective length or increase the perimeter of the material, thus it can send or receive electromagnetic radiations within a given total surface area or volume.

Fractal antenna also referred to as multilevel or space filling curves with repetition of a motif over two or more scale sizes or iterations. They have compact size with multiband or wideband property, which has useful applications in cellular telephone or microwave telecommunication applications.

Fractals have been created in antennas since 1988. Fractal nature of the antenna shrinks its size without the use of any component, such as inductor or capacitor. It also gives good multiband performance, wide bandwidth and small area and reference shows that the gain with small size results from constructive interference with multiple current maxima, afforded by the electrically long structure in a small area.

This paper presents compact size pentaband microstrip patch antenna design which has a simple fractal geometry. Numerous fractal antenna design approaches have been proposed for various wireless applications. Wide research has been made to improve the performance parameters of a MPA (microstrip patch antenna) in the previous years. Some research carried out by researchers in this field are summarized in next section.

2 Literature Survey

There have been numerous design changes of antenna with thousands of published documents relating to its design, analysis and optimization. The present study is based on design and parametric analysis of multiband fractal patch antenna for various wireless applications. The following designs have been useful references in our work on fractal antennas.

Paper [1] presents microstrip patch antenna with a hexagonal fractal pattern for ground based surveillance radar applications. In this paper multiple slots have been added to the ground plane and a stepped pattern has been implemented to increase the current density and the gain. In paper [2] compact dual band circular face fractal antenna is designed and fabricated with return loss ($S11$) below -10 dB of 1.84 GHz (2.2–4.07 GHz) and 2 GHz (6–8 GHz) which can be applied to wireless local area network (WLAN) and ultra-wide band applications. In paper [3] flexible Sierpinski carpet fractal antenna has been presented which is more tolerant to folding than its conventional patch counterpart. In paper [4] planar multiband fractal antenna based on Sierpinski triangle is presented, which is suitable for wireless power transmission applications. The paper [5] focuses on design and analysis of hexagon inspired fractal geometry and defected ground plane to evaluate the performance of patch antenna for wireless applications. Reduced fractal UWB microstrip antenna is displayed in the paper [6] for future versatile advancements. It is used for wide band applications like

WiMAX, WLAN. In paper [7], a new fractal antenna has been proposed by combining Minkowski and Sierpinski carpet antennas with area 45 × 38.92 mm^2 and exhibits multiband characteristics. The simulated antenna covers five bands while fabricated antenna covers four bands for wireless communication. In paper [8] two designs of fractal antennas have been studied. 4NEC2 software is used to simulate the designs. Simulated results present that the triangular KOCH curve design shows multiband behavior whereas the Serpinski gaskets design resonates at single frequency.

3 Antenna Geometry

In this section design of a low-profile compact printed fractal antenna for fixed bands is presented. The proposed fractal antenna consists of a main patch, a ground plane and a 50 Ω feed line. Epoxy FR4 dielectric material is selected for the design which has dielectric constant 4.4 and height of the substrate is 1.57 mm. The antenna is occupying an area of 20 × 24 mm^2 for the ground plane. Figure 1 shows fractal geometry of proposed antenna.

The fractal geometry is the best suited for its self-similar structures. This iterative geometry can be best conveyed pictorially Fig. [1], the antenna design starts with single rectangle patch as main radiator as shown in Fig. 2a. Further iteration is carried out by adding smaller and smaller rectangles to the previously obtained geometry, which produces the design of first iteration as shown in Fig. 2b. Similarly, the second iteration is obtained by adding further rectangles to each corner of previously obtained design as shown in the Fig. 2 c. The third iteration is carried out by adding still more number of rectangles to the previously obtained geometry. In the designed rectangle-shape fractal, surface area of the radiating patch increases with increase in the number of iterations.

The analysis and software simulated results of different iterations are discussed in next section. A parametric study of the proposed patch antenna design was carried out to achieve multiband performance. The effects of different iterations of rectangle-shape fractal have been investigated based on the antenna performance. The first iteration is done by adding four rectangles in the main rectangle; second iteration

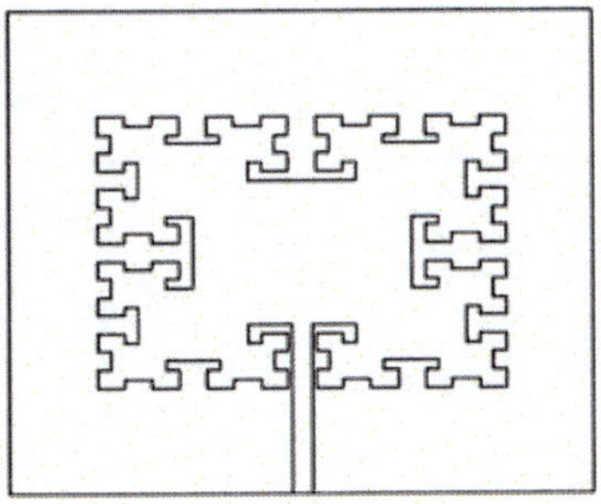

Fig. 1 Structure of proposed antenna. Total Volume = 20 × 24 × 1.57 mm^3

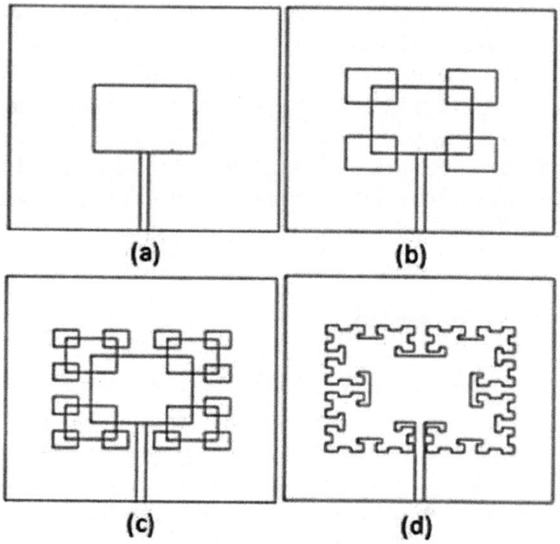

Fig. 2 Iterative geometry

is done by addition of twelve rectangles again. Similarly next iteration is done by addition of thirty six smaller size rectangles in previously obtained geometry. At each step, copy of the initiator is added with a scaled copy of the generator. This process is repeated to form step 5.

4 Parametric Analysis

Antennas are made for efficient radiation or reception of electromagnetic signals. There are several parameters which describe performance of the antenna. Some of the parameters are,

4.1 Radiation Pattern

When a signal is fed into an antenna, the antenna will emit radiation distributed in space in a certain way. A graphical representation of the relative distribution of the radiated power in space is called radiation pattern.

4.2 VSWR

Full form of VSWR is Voltage Standing Wave Ratio and it is also referred to as Standing Wave Ratio (SWR). In standing wave pattern VSWR is the ratio of maximum voltage to minimum voltage. VSWR varies from +1 to infinite. VSWR parameter is a measure that numerically describes how well the antenna is impedance matched to the radio or transmission line it is connected to. VSWR is a function of the reflection coefficient, which describes the power reflected from the antenna. For antennas VSWR is always a real and positive number. Smaller the VSWR better the antenna matched to the transmission line and more power is delivered to the antenna. Minimum value of VSWR is 1.0 which means no power is reflected from the antenna, it is ideal case. For practical antennas VSWR should be < 2.

4.3 Gain

Antenna gain is the ability of the antenna to radiate more or less in any direction compared to a theoretical antenna. Gain is calculated by comparing the measured power transmitted or received by the antenna in a specific direction to the power transmitted or received by a hypothetical ideal antenna in the same situation.

4.4 Bandwidth

Bandwidth is defined as 'the range of frequencies within which the performance of the antenna, with respect to some characteristic, conforms to a specified standard'. Bandwidth can be defined as the range of frequencies, on either side of a center frequency, where the antenna characteristics (such as radiation pattern, VSWR, gain etc.) are within an acceptable value of those at the center frequency.

4.5 Directivity

Directivity of an antenna is a measure of the concentration of the radiated power in a particular direction. It may be considered as the ability of the antenna to direct radiated power in a given direction. It is usually a ratio of radiation intensity in a given direction to the average radiation intensity.

4.6 Return Loss

It is a logarithmic ratio measured in dB that compares the power reflected by the antenna to the power that is fed into the antenna from the transmission line. In other words, it is the difference in dB between forward and reflected power measured at any given point in an RF system. The parameter return loss is a measure of the reflected energy from a transmitted signal. Larger the value of return loss less is the energy that is reflected. For good impedance matching resonant frequency must lie below −10 dB.

4.7 Beamwidth

The beamwidth of a pattern is defined as the angular separation between two identical points on opposite side of the pattern maximum. There are a number of beamwidths in an antenna pattern. In a plane containing the direction of the maximum of a beam, the angle between the two directions in which the radiation intensity is one-half value of the beam is known as Half-Power Beamwidth (HPBW). Another beamwidth is the angular separation between the first nulls of the pattern and it is referred to as the First-Null Beamwidth (FNBW). The beamwidth of an antenna is a very important figure of merit and often used as a trade-off between it and the side lobe level; that is, as the beamwidth decreases, the side lobe increases and vice versa.

5 Simulated Results and Discussion

In the design of multiband antennas, it is desirable to have the ability to set the frequency bands independently from each other, but it is very challenging to achieving this ability. Very often, when some parameters are adjusted to set a band to a particular frequency, the frequencies of all other bands are affected and we have to re-design the antenna.

Fractal is a geometric object which is similar to itself on all scales. On a fractal object if we zoom in, it will look similar or exactly like the original shape. This property is called self-similarity.

A parametric study of the proposed fractal patch antenna is carried out to achieve multiband performance. To validate the above characteristics, the proposed structure is simulated using Ansoft HFSS (High Frequency Structure Simulator) software. The effects of addition of self-similar shapes with smaller dimensions in step by step iterative process have been investigated based on the antenna performance. The design steps can be described as follows:

Step 1: The main radiator is designed to generate single band and its dimensions are optimized in terms of minimizing the reflection coefficient across the band by

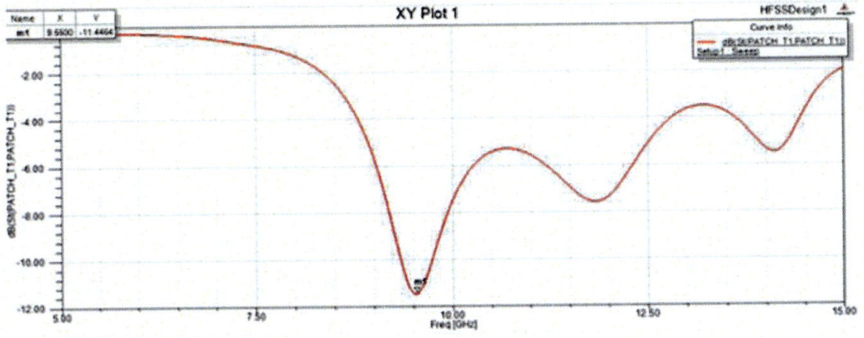

Fig. 3 $S11$ parameter of main patch

simulation. It appears at 9.55 GHz instead of maximum at 10 GHz that may be caused by some resonance effect. Figure 3 shows return loss versus frequency plot for the main radiator, at 9.55 GHz, $S11 = -11.45$ dB.

Step 2: In second step, we reduce size of ground plane and analyze its effect on S parameter. It improves return loss parameter and gives two more resonant frequency bands but, resonant frequency at 9.55 GHz gets collapse. Figure 4 shows return loss versus frequency plot. Simulated result presents two resonant frequencies at 15.63 GHz and 19.05 GHz with $S11 = -15.14$ and -18.04 dB respectively.

Step 3: Now, we start design of fractal geometry with iterative process. Four sub-patches with same shape but smaller dimensions are added to the main radiator. It results frequency band at 19.05 GHz get shifted to 17.91 GHz and one more band generates at 7.84 GHz frequency. This new geometry generates resonant frequency for three bands at 7.84, 15.25 and 17.91 GHz with $S11 = -28.03$, -12.52 and -21.61 dB respectively. Figure 5 shows return loss versus frequency plot for first iteration.

Step 4: Now, twelve sub-patches with same shapes and smaller dimensions are added to each corner of the patch geometry achieved in third step. It generates the

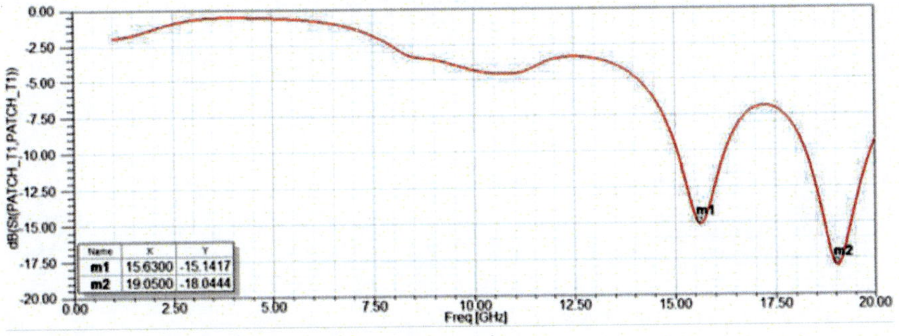

Fig. 4 $S11$ parameter of main patch with reduced ground structure

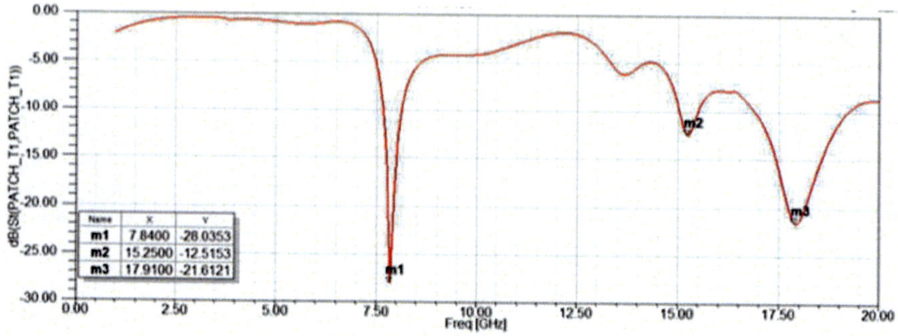

Fig. 5 $S11$ parameter versus frequency: I iteration

resonant frequency for four bands. Frequency bands are generated in step III shifted from 7.84 to 7.27 GHz, 15.15 to 15.53 GHz and from 17.72 to 17.34 GHz. Fourth band at 18.58 GHz frequency is generated with −20.77 dB return loss. Thus, in step IV four resonant frequency bands are achieved at 7.27, 15.54, 17.34 and 18.58 GHz with $S11 = -18.56, -15.23, -16.39$ and -20.77 dB respectively. Figure 6 shows return loss versus frequency plot for second iteration.

Step 5: To continue this iterative process 36 sub-patches with same shapes and smaller dimensions are added to the patch geometry achieved in previous step, in similar manner. Frequency bands generated in step IV slightly detuned and new bands are generated. It generates the resonant frequency for five bands at 6.89, 8.13, 10.03, 16.11 and 17.82 GHz with $S11 = -19.69, -24.95, -25.11, -17.29$ and -19.35 dB respectively. Figure 7 shows return loss Vs frequency plot for fifth step, III iteration.

VSWR, 3D polar plot for directivity, radiation pattern, beamwidth and gain plot for proposed final fractal antenna geometry are shown in Figs. 8, 9, 10, 11 and 12 respectively.

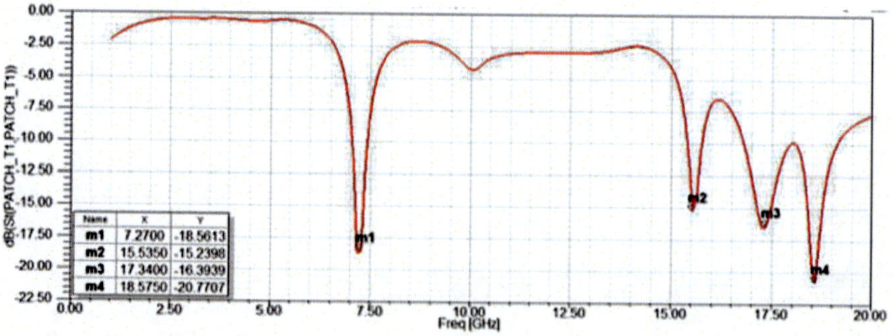

Fig. 6 $S11$ parameter versus frequency plot: II iteration

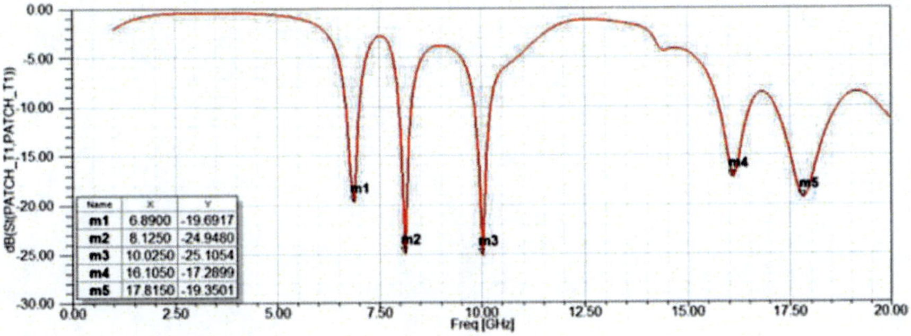

Fig. 7 $S11$ parameter versus frequency plot: III iteration

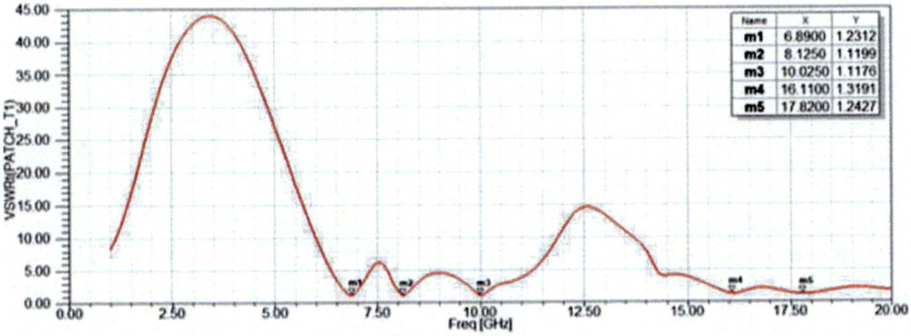

Fig. 8 VSWR curve of proposed antenna

Fig. 9 3D polar plot for directivity of proposed antenna

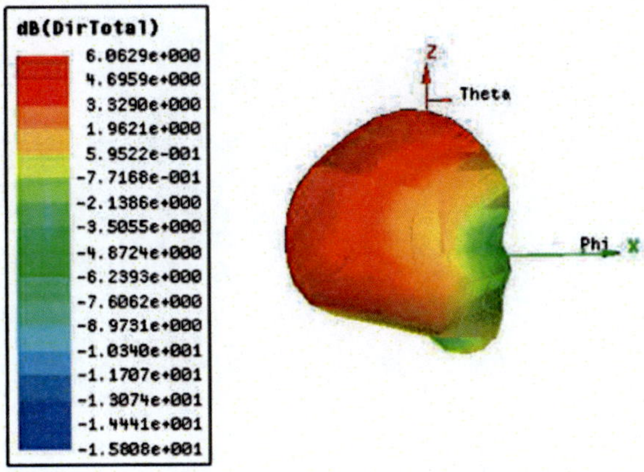

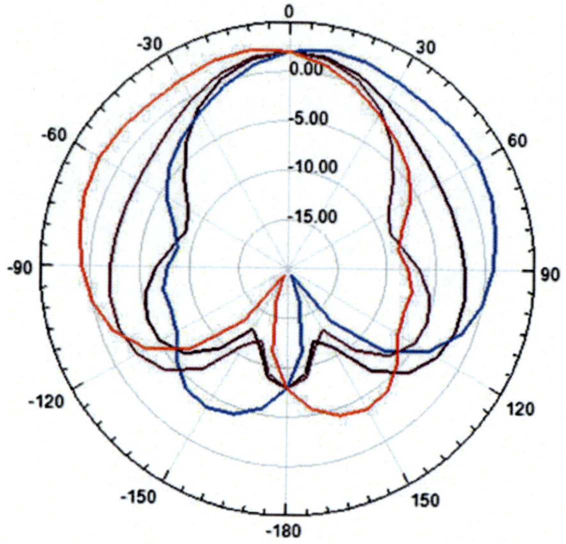

Fig. 10 Radiation pattern curve

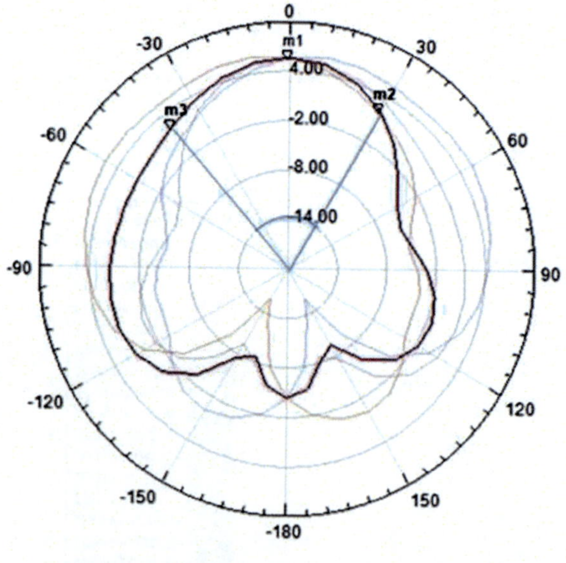

Fig. 11 Beamwidth of proposed antenna

The overall gain and directivity achieved by the antenna is 2.05 dB and 6.06 dB respectively. VSWR curve of proposed antenna shows that VSWR obtained for all five bands at 6.89 GHz, 8.13 GHz, 10.03 GHz, 16.11 GHz and 17.82 GHz are 1.23, 1.12, 1.12, 1.32 and 1.24 respectively; which are between 1 and 2 range. Table 1 summarizes values of Return Loss ($S11$) in dB and their VSWR at all resonant frequencies.

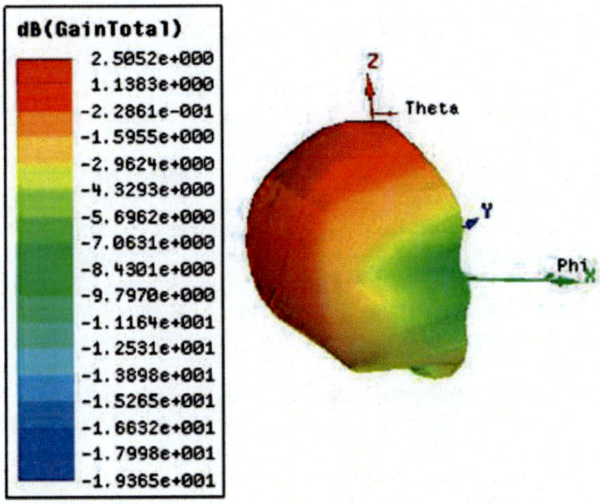

Fig. 12 3D polar plot for Gain of proposed antenna

Table 1 Result summary after simulation

Frequency (GHz)	Return loss ($S11$) (dB)	VSWR	Bandwidth (MHz)
6.89	−19.69	1.23	300
8.13	−24.95	1.12	281
10.03	−25.11	1.12	380
16.11	−17.29	1.32	855
17.82	- 19.35	1.24	1520

6 Conclusion

This paper proposes low profile multiband fractal antenna geometry for various wireless applications. The proposed design has simple configurations and occupying $20 \times 24 \times 1.5\ \text{mm}^3$ volume. It has been shown that the performance of this antenna in terms of its frequency domain characteristics is mostly dependent on fractal geometric iterations. It is demonstrated by simulation that the proposed antenna has five bands of operations at 6.89, 8.13, 10.03, 16.11 and 17.82 GHz resonant frequency. All frequency bands having less than −10 dB return loss with 300, 281, 380, 855 and 1520 MHz bandwidth respectively. All five bands have VSWR less than 1.5 over that range of frequency. This antenna geometry has 6.06 dB directivity and 2.50 dB overall gain. Beamwidth is 70°. Proposed antenna geometry is compact in size and highly suitable for C, X and Ku band applications.

References

1. Dhakad SK, Dwivedi U, Baudha S, Bhandari T (2017) A slotted microstrip antenna with fractal design for X-band based surveillance applications. Int J Control Theory Appl 10. ISSN-0974-5572
2. Zakariyya OS, Sadiq BO, Olaniyan AA, Salami AF (2016) Dual band fractal antenna design for wireless application. Comput Eng Appl 5(3). ISSN: 2252-4274
3. Radoni V, Palmer K, Stojanovi G, Crnojevi´c-Bengin V (2012) Flexible Sierpinski carpet fractal antenna on a hilbert slot patterned ground. Int J Antennas Propag 2012, Article ID 980916, 7 p. ISSN: 2252-5459
4. Benyetho T, Zbitou J, El Abdellaoui L, Bennis H, Tribak A (2018) A new fractal multiband antenna for wireless power transmission applications . Hindawi Active Passive Electron Compon 2018, Article ID 2084747
5. Desai A, Upadhyaya T, Patel R, Bhatt S, Mankodi P (2018) Wideband high gain fractal antenna for wireless applications. Progr Electromagn Res Lett 74:125–130
6. Avula R, Rangarao M, Kumari Y (2019) Fractal ultra wide band antenna for 5G applications. Int J Recent Technol Eng (IJRTE) 7(5S4). ISSN: 2277-3878
7. Sharma N, Sharma V, Bhatia SS (2018) A novel hybrid fractal antenna for wireless applications. Progr Electromagn Res M 73:25–35 (2018)
8. Neetu SB, Bansal RK (2013) Design and analysis of fractal antennas based on Koch and Sierpinski fractal geometries. Int J Adv Res Electr Electron Instrum Eng 2(6). ISSN: 2278-8875

Enhancing Security with In-Depth Analysis of Brute-Force Attack on Secure Hashing Algorithms

Rajat Verma, Namrata Dhanda, and Vishal Nagar

Abstract Brute-force attack is considered one of the oldest attacks in the entire history of cybersecurity. Amid the diverse cyberattacks, the brute-force technique or exhaustive search has always gained its importance when it comes to access data in an unauthorized manner. Slowly and gradually, a lot more variants of brute-force have been released by the cybercriminals as they have also evolved. Alternatively, hashing has also evolved timely as a countermeasure of various cyberattacks. All variants of the SHA are illustrated here in this paper such as SHA-0, SHA-1, SHA-512, and SHA-256. SHA is also very popular as a network peer-to-peer technology blockchain also uses this for its security. The objective of the paper is to attain a measure of enhanced security. This paper discusses the in-depth analysis of brute-force attack on the secure hashing algorithms. Moreover, a study of diverse brute-force attacks is also highlighted in this paper.

Keywords Brute-force · SHA · Secured communication · Privacy preservation · Cryptanalysis

1 Introduction

In cybersecurity, when it comes to guessing passwords by the Hit and Trial [1] method, brute-force has already established its name in the industry many years ago. In passive cybersecurity attacks, brute-force is an attempt of decrypting any kind of encrypted textual matter [2]. Cybercriminals keep on trying diverse combinations again and again to gain access to sensitive information of the user. The sensitive data can be a password, PIN, credit/debit card-sensitive data, etc. The amount of time

R. Verma (✉) · N. Dhanda
Department of Computer Science & Engineering, Amity University Uttar Pradesh, Lucknow Campus, Lucknow, India

V. Nagar
Department of Computer Science & Engineering, Pranveer Singh Institute of Technology, Uttar Pradesh, Kanpur, India

M. S. Kaiser et al. (eds.), *Proceedings of Trends in Electronics and Health Informatics*, Lecture Notes in Networks and Systems 376,
https://doi.org/10.1007/978-981-16-8826-3_44

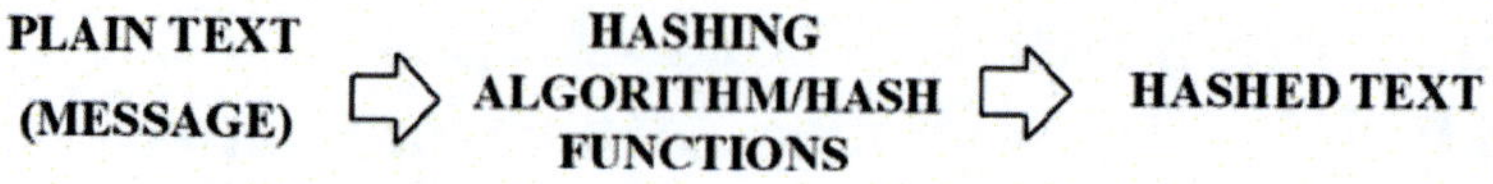

Fig. 1 Simple illustration of hashing

required to perform the cyberattack will depend on the resources that the cybercriminal is having or to what extent the attacker is willing to perform. The attackers can configure the script, code, bots to perform the attacks efficiently when compared to a normal human being [3]. On the other side, secure hashing algorithms play a vital role in enhancing the security of systems by tackling attacks with a huge number of digits. For instance, SHA-256 always gives a fixed output of 64 hexadecimal digits. The possible combinations with 64 hexadecimal digits are numerous that will be depicted along with other variants of SHA in the next sections of the paper.

2 Material and Methods

2.1 *Hashing: The One-Way Encryption*

One of the constituent pillars of cryptography is hashing/hash functions along with the symmetric and asymmetric key cryptography [4]. Hashing is a function (Mathematical) that condenses variable-size inputs to a fixed-size output. If the identical input is given 100 times, the output will be the same for that number of inputs. Hashing is sometimes referred to as "One-Way Encryption" [5]. A diagrammatic representation of hashing is illustrated in Fig. 1.

In Fig. 1, the plain text or message is passed on to the hashing algorithm or function to obtain the hashed text. Message digest is the other name of hashed text.

The hashing algorithms can be configured for a variety of operations depending on the configuration needs and purposes such as security, speed, storing passwords, and databases [6]. Hashed values are a result of one-way encryption and are always original/non-duplicates [7]. A variety of software are available on the cyberspace to perform the brute-force attack such as rainbow crack, hydra, and Ophcrack [8].

2.2 *Digital Signatures*

Digital signature is a technique of cryptography which is attempted to validate the integrity as well as authenticity of the facts and figures that is digitally present [9].

Hashing is a part of the main constituents of the digital signature algorithm. With the evolution of public-key cryptography, the digital signature algorithms became popular around the 1970s [10].

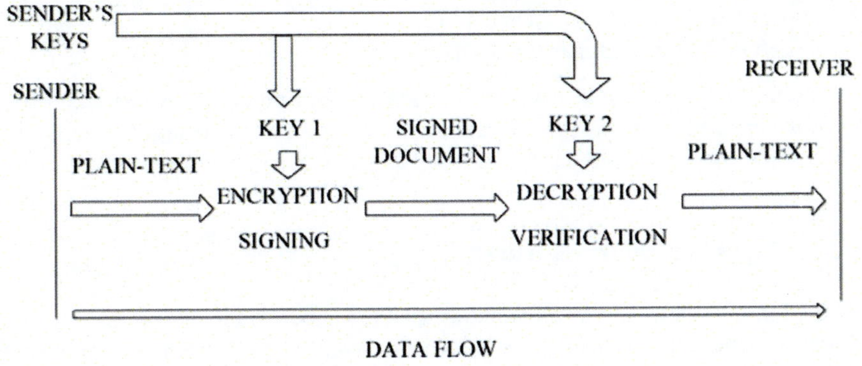

Fig. 2 Simple illustration of digital signature

A quick demonstration of digital signature is depicted below:

Digital signature is applied in the ecosystem of public-key cryptography. The originator make use of his/her private key to the signing rule to perform the signature digitally. The plain text or the message in combination with signature (Digitally) is sent to the recipient. The receiver receives the complete signature and the original message, and applies the public key of the sender and then applies the verification algorithm at the complete message with the purpose of verification [11].

If the output is found to be true, it is accepted, and if not, it is rejected. The working of the digital signature is shown in Fig. 2.

Figure 2 illustrates the operation of a digital signature algorithm. Here, the messages are generally long and require the asymmetric-key architecture [12]. The solution is to use a hashed text/message digest as its length is fixed according to the algorithm that is applied [13].

2.3 *Brute-Force Attack*

Brute-force attacks are the traditional methods to obtain the sensitive or private information of a user. This private information can contain PIN numbers, passwords, usernames, etc. Various scripts and programs are used to achieve the motive of brute-force attacks [14]. The next subsection illustrates the goals of brute-force measures.

2.3.1 Goals of Brute-Force Attacks

The diverse goals of brute-force attacks are highlighted below:

1. Redirecting domains to malicious Web sites [15]
2. Selling sensitive information to un-trusted third parties [16]

3. Spreading fake/malicious content [17]
4. Theft of personal information [18]

Alternatively, there is a constructive side of brute-force attacks as well. The network engineers or the ethical hackers working for reputed organizations use brute-force attacks to test their network standards or encryption standards [19].

2.3.2 Types of Brute-Force Attacks

At the initial stages, only a few varieties used to happen in the market. Slowly and gradually, a variety of brute-force attacks are evolved. Some of them are highlighted below for easy understanding.

1. Simple Brute-Force Attacks: In this attack, the cybercriminals attempt to predict the passwords without the help of any tools or software. [20]
2. Dictionary Attacks: In dictionary attacks, the cybercriminals select a target and runs a script to find the possible sensitive information such as passwords against the target [21]
3. Hybrid Brute-Force Attacks: A hybrid attack combines the features of dictionary and brute-force attacks [22].
4. Reverse Brute-Force Attacks: It starts in reverse order with a known password/leaked password [23].
5. Credential Stuffing: If the cybercriminal has a combination of password and username for one Web site, the same duo will be used for the other profiles as well [24].

2.4 Secure Hashing Algorithms (SHA)

The credit of developing SHA goes to the National Institute of Standards and Technology (NIST) and the National Security Agency (NSA) in around 1993 [25]. If SHA is depicted in one line, it would be taking variable sized inputs and converting them into fixed-sized message digest as outputs by taking the help of a hashing algorithm [26].

Typically, there are four series of SHA that are highlighted below:

1. SHA-0: This gave the fixed output of 160-bit or 20-bytes long. It was taken back pre-maturely. The reason was that it was published with a major flaw and gave birth to its successor, i.e., SHA-1 [27].
2. SHA-1: It was similar to message digest (MD)-5 and also gave a fixed output of 160-bit or 20-bytes long. It was used to support the digital signature algorithms. [28]
3. SHA-2: This version of SHA introduced two major categories, i.e., SHA-256 and SHA-512. The former results in a 64 hexadecimal digits and the latter give an output of 128 hexadecimal digits. [29]

Table 1 Analysis of SHA-0 [Same will be for SHA-1]

SHA	Number of bits	Possible number of combinations	Scientific notation of possible combinations
SHA-0	160	2^160 = 1461501637330902918203684832716283019655932542976	1.461501637330902918203684832716283019655932542976 × 10^48
SHA	**Number length**	**Hexadecimal values**	**Factorial value**
SHA-0	49 decimal digits	40	40! = 815915283247897734345611269596115894272000000000

4. SHA-3: This SHA is performing very appropriately in today's world and makes use of the hash function called Keccak [30].

2.4.1 Analysis of Brute-Force Attacks on Secure Hashing Algorithms

The key length of diverse SHA algorithms considering brute-force algorithm is analyzed over here in this subsection.

1. SHA-0: This SHA produced a fixed output of 160 bit or 20 bytes. This hashed text has 40 hexadecimal digits. But, this was introduced with a flaw, so this was taken back and not currently used. It was introduced in 1993. The detailed analysis of SHA-0 is illustrated below in Table 1.

   If considering 1 possible second for 1 combination and divide the time value by 2.628e + 6.

   Observations:

   - Possible months for decoding possible combinations: 1461501637330902918203684832716283019655932542976/2.628e + 6= 5.56126345390802255e + 41 months.
   - Possible months for decoding factorial value: 815915283247897734345611269596115894272000000000/2.628e + 6 = 3.10469706657207962e+ 41 months.
   - If the decoding of possible combinations is increased by 1000 times: 5.5612635e + 38 months.
   - Result: not feasible!
   - If factorial interpretation is increased by 1000 times: 3.1046971e + 38 months.

2. SHA-1: The entire results of SHA-1 will be identical to SHA-0 (depicted in Table 1) as it also produces 40 hexadecimal digits result. SHA-1 was designed by National Security Agency (U.S.). It was introduced in 1995. [25]
3. SHA-256: This SHA-256 is a very popular algorithm of SHA-2 and produces an output of 64 hexadecimal digits [31] and was first published in 2001. The detailed analysis of SHA-256 is illustrated below in Table 2. This SHA-256 is commonly used in blockchain technology [32]. It is more secured than SHA-1.

Table 2 Analysis of SHA-256

SHA	Number of bits	Possible number of combinations	Scientific notation of possible combinations
SHA-256	256	2^256 = 115792089237316195423570985008687907853269984665640564039457584007913129639936	1.15792089237316195423570985008687907853269984665640564039457... × 10^77
SHA	**Number length**	**Hexadecimal values**	**Factorial value (64!)**
SHA-256	78 decimal digits	64	1.26886932185884164103433389335161480802865516174545192198801... × 10^89

It has 256 bits so provides enhanced security when compared to SHA-1. SHA-2 is more complex when compared to SHA-1. SHA-256 works better on 32-bit processors. SHA-256 is smaller than SHA-512 thus saving bandwidth. SHA-256 is still one of the most secured algorithms of the cryptographical world.

If considering 1 possible second for 1 combination and divide the time value by 2.628e + 6.

Observations:

- Possible months for decoding possible combinations: 115792089237316195423570985008687907853269984665640564039457584007913129639936/2.628e + 6 = 4.4060868471086381e + 70 months.
- Possible months for decoding factorial value: 126886932185884164103433389335161480802865516174545192198801894375214704230400000000000000/2.628e + 6 = 4.82826457883806288e + 82 Months.
- If the decoding of possible combinations is increased by 1000 times: 4.4060868e + 67 months.
- If factorial interpretation is increased by 1000 times: 4.8282646e + 79 months.
- Result: not feasible!

4. SHA-512: This SHA-512 produces a result of 128 hexadecimal digits [33]. The detailed analysis of SHA-512 is illustrated below in Table 3. SHA-512 works better on 64-bit processors. SHA-512 is ahead of SHA-256 with respect to collision resistance [34]. Currently, there are a few systems or no systems that are currently using this measure.

   If considering 1 possible second for 1 combination and divide the time value by 2.628e + 6.

   Observations:

- Possible months for decoding possible combinations: 13407807929942597099574024998205846127479365820592393377723561443721764030073546976801874298166903427690031858186486050853753882811946569946433649006084096/2.628e + 6 = 5.10190001387768583e

Table 3 Analysis of SHA-512

SHA	Number of Bits	Possible Number of Combinations	Scientific Notation of Possible Combinations	Number Length	Hexa-Decimal values	Factorial Value (128!)
SHA-512	512	2^512 = 1340780792 9942597099 5740249982 0584612747 9365820592 3933777235 6144372176 4030073546 9768018742 9816690342 7690031858 1864860508 5375388281 1946569946 4336490060 84096	1.34078 0792994259 7099574024 9982058461 2747936582 0592393377 723... × 10^154	155	128	3.85620 4823625804 2173567706 5923463640 6174931095 9022359027 882... × 10^215

+ 147 months.

- Possible months for decoding factorial value: 385620482362580421735677065923463640617493109590223590278828403276373402575165543560686168588507361534030051833058916347592172932262498857766114955245039357760034644709279247692495585280000000000000000000000000000000/ 2.628e + 6 = 1.46735182559077121e + 209 months.
- If the decoding of possible combinations is increased by 1000 times: 5.1019e + 144 months.
- If factorial interpretation is increased by 1000 times: 1.467352e + 206 months.
- Result: not feasible!

3 Results and Discussion

The numbers obtained from the above textual matter are prodigious; from that it is observed that all the algorithms are very much secure, but the time taken to crack all possible combinations of different SHA algorithms are different as SHA-0 and SHA-1 produce 160-bit result, i.e., 40 hexadecimal digits; SHA-256 produces 256-bit result, i.e., 64 hexadecimal digits, and SHA-512 produces 512-bit result, i.e., 128 hexadecimal digits. SHA-512 is much secured when compared to SHA-256, SHA-0, and SHA-1 in terms of longer hashes in brute-force attack. Similarly, SHA-256 is much secured when compared to SHA-0 and SHA-1 in terms of hash length. The detailed analysis of SHA-0, SHA-1, SHA-256, and SHA-512 highlighted in Tables 1, 2, and 3, respectively. The term not feasible in the result of each SHA depicts that this approach is not a good measure in attacking a system.

4 Conclusion and Future Scope

Both the aspects, i.e., brute-force attacks and SHA are evolving at a rapid speed. The reasons to use brute-force, as well as SHA, are diverse. SHA along with brute-force can have positive as well as negative effects as discussed in this paper. This paper shows the in-depth analysis of diverse SHA algorithms to tackle brute-force attacks. SHA-512 emerges as a better approach when compared to all the preceding versions in terms of brute-force attacks. Moreover, a study of hashing, digital signature, brute-force attacks, types of brute-force, and SHA is highlighted in this paper.

Additionally, it will work on some more techniques to get better results with the objective of enhancing security.

References

1. Shahid M, Qadeer MA (2009) Novel scheme for securing passwords. In: 2009 3rd IEEE international conference on digital ecosystems and technologies. IEEE, pp 223–227
2. Xu Y, Wang H, Li Y, Pei B (2014) Image encryption based on synchronization of fractional chaotic systems. Commun Nonlinear Sci Numer Simul 19(10):3735–3744
3. Azad BA, Starov O, Laperdrix P, Nikiforakis N (2020) Web runner 2049: evaluating third-party anti-bot services. In: International conference on detection of intrusions and malware, and vulnerability assessment. Springer, Cham, pp 135–159
4. Bellare M, Goldreich O, Goldwasser S (1994) Incremental cryptography: the case of hashing and signing. In: Annual international cryptology conference. Springer, Berlin, Heidelberg, pp 216–233
5. Merkle RC (1990) A fast software one-way hash function. J Cryptol 3(1):43–58
6. Archer DW, Bogdanov D, Lindell Y, Kamm L, Nielsen K, Pagter JI, Smart NP, Wright RN (2018) From keys to databases—real-world applications of secure multi-party computation. Comput J 61(12):1749–1771
7. Yang Y, Yu J, Zhang Q, Meng F (2015) Improved hash functions for cancelable fingerprint encryption schemes. Wireless Pers Commun 84(1):643–669
8. Islam S (2020) Security auditing tools: a comparative study. Int J Comput Sci Res 5(1):407–425
9. Al-Haj A (2015) Providing integrity, authenticity, and confidentiality for header and pixel data of DICOM images. J Digit Imaging 28(2):179–187
10. Furht B, Muharemagic E, Socek D (2005) An overview of modern cryptography. Multimedia Encryption and Watermarking, pp 31–51

11. Rivest RL, Shamir A, Adleman L (1978) A method for obtaining digital signatures and public-key cryptosystems. Commun ACM 21(2):120–126
12. Kiah MM, Al-Bakri SH, Zaidan AA, Zaidan BB, Hussain M (2014) Design and develop a video conferencing framework for real-time telemedicine applications using secure group-based communication architecture. J Med Syst 38(10):1–11
13. Saraf KR, Jagtap VP, Mishra AK (2014) Text and image encryption decryption using advanced encryption standard. Int J Emerg Trends Technol Comput Sci (IJETTCS) 3(3):118–126
14. Florêncio D, Herley C, Van Oorschot PC (2014) An administrator's guide to internet password research. In: 28th large installation system administration conference (LISA14), pp 44–61
15. Alzahrani BA, Reed MJ, Vassilakis VG (2015) Resistance against brute-force attacks on stateless forwarding in information centric networking. In: 2015 ACM/IEEE symposium on architectures for networking and communications systems (ANCS). IEEE, pp 209–210
16. Ravi S, Raghunathan A, Chakradhar S (2004) Tamper resistance mechanisms for secure embedded systems. In: 17th international conference on VLSI design. Proceedings. IEEE, pp 605–611
17. Alazab M, Broadhurst R (2016) Spam and criminal activity. Trends Issues in Crime and Criminal Justice (526):1–20
18. Kim I (2012) Keypad against brute force attacks on smartphones. IET Inf Secur 6(2):71–76
19. Sharma K, Singh A, Sharma VP (2009) SMEs and cybersecurity threats in e-commerce. EDPACS The EDP Audit, Control, and Security Newsletter 39(5–6):1–49
20. Huang Z, Ayday E, Fellay J, Hubaux JP, Juels A (2015) Genoguard: protecting genomic data against brute-force attacks. In: 2015 IEEE symposium on security and privacy. IEEE, pp 447–462
21. Narayanan A, Shmatikov V (2005) Fast dictionary attacks on passwords using time-space tradeoff. In: Proceedings of the 12th ACM conference on Computer and communications security, pp 364–372
22. Dave KT (2013) Brute-force attack seeking but distressing. Int J Innov Eng Technol Brute-force 2(3):75–78
23. Cao PM, Wu Y, Banerjee SS, Azoff J, Withers A, Kalbarczyk ZT, Iyer RK (2019) {CAUDIT}: continuous auditing of {SSH} servers to mitigate brute-force attacks. In: 16th {USENIX} symposium on networked systems design and implementation ({NSDI} 19) (2019), pp 667–682
24. Rees-Pullman S (2020) Is credential stuffing the new phishing? Comput Fraud Secur 2020(7):16–19
25. Ghoshal S, Bandyopadhyay P, Roy S, Baneree M (2020) A journey from md5 to sha-3. Trends in Communication, Cloud, and Big Data, pp 107–112
26. Lee J, Nikitin K, Setty S (2020) Replicated state machines without replicated execution. In: 2020 IEEE symposium on security and privacy (SP). IEEE, pp 119–134
27. Chabaud F, Joux A (1998) Differential collisions in SHA-0. In: Annual international cryptology conference. Springer, Berlin, Heidelberg, pp 56–71
28. Wang X, Yin YL, Yu H (2005) Finding collisions in the full SHA-1. In: Annual international cryptology conference Springer, Berlin, Heidelberg, pp 17–36
29. Chaves R, Kuzmanov G, Sousa L, Vassiliadis S (2006) Improving SHA-2 hardware implementations. In: International workshop on cryptographic hardware and embedded systems. Springer, Berlin, Heidelberg, pp 298–310
30. Baldwin B, Byrne A, Lu L, Hamilton M, Hanley N, O'Neill M, Marnane WP (2010) FPGA implementations of the round two SHA-3 candidates. In: 2010 international conference on field programmable logic and applications. IEEE, pp 400–407
31. Pappala S, Niamat M, Sun W (2012) FPGA based trustworthy authentication technique using Physically Unclonable Functions and artificial intelligence. In: 2012 IEEE international symposium on hardware-oriented security and trust. IEEE, pp 59–62
32. Dattani J, Sheth H (2019) Overview of blockchain technology. Asian J Convergence in Technol 5(1):1–3

33. Shankar TN, Sahoo G, Niranjan S (2012) Using the digital signature of a fingerprint by an elliptic curve cryptosystem for enhanced authentication. Inf Secur J Global Perspect 21(5):243–255
34. Ahmad I, Das AS (2005) Hardware implementation analysis of SHA-256 and SHA-512 algorithms on FPGAs. Comput Electr Eng 31(6):345–360

Integration of Back-Propagation Neural Network to Classify of Cybercriminal Entities in Blockchain

Rohit Saxena, Deepak Arora, and Vishal Nagar

Abstract Bitcoin is a decentralized, pseudonymous cryptocurrency that has become one among the most demanded digital assets to date. Because of its uncontrolled nature and users' inherent anonymity, it has seen a significant surge in its use for illegal operations. As a result, numerous systems for characterizing diversified entities across the Bitcoin network must be developed. In this work, we offer a way for breaking Bitcoin anonymity using a revolutionary cascade machine learning model that only utilizes a few features taken straight from Bitcoin blockchain data. We gathered approximately 29 million samples from diverse sources and generated data for four different entities: exchanges, gambling, pools, and services. On a dataset balanced using SMOTE and weight of the entities, the back-propagation neural network (BPNN) model was trained and tested. Cross-validation accuracy has been utilized to evaluate the model's accuracy. On the dataset balanced using the weight of the entities, the BPNN model classified the entities with 71.51%, while with SMOTE, the accuracy of classification is 71.22%.

Keywords Bitcoin · Blockchain · Back propagation neural network

1 Introduction

Bitcoin was coined in 2008, and it has since risen to become the most successful cryptographic money among multiple competitors, boosting the economy by the huge sum of money within only a few years. Bitcoin is a type of cryptocurrency that is made up of a series of computer codes that have a monetary value. All transactions

The original version of this chapter was revised: The affiliation of the volume editors has been updated. A correction to this chapter is available at
https://doi.org/10.1007/978-981-16-8826-3_57

R. Saxena (✉) · D. Arora
Amity University Uttar Pradesh, Lucknow, India

V. Nagar
Pranveer Singh Institute of Technology, Kanpur, Uttar Pradesh, India

M. S. Kaiser et al. (eds.), *Proceedings of Trends in Electronics and Health Informatics*, Lecture Notes in Networks and Systems 376,
https://doi.org/10.1007/978-981-16-8826-3_45

and payments are completed over the Internet in this setting. Bitcoin differs from traditional Internet transactions in that it is based on a peer-to-peer (P2P) network that is not linked to a centralized third-party organization, such as an e-bank, a notary, or any other traditional online financial service provider that supervises, monitors, and approves electronic payment transactions. Instead, Bitcoin users have absolute power over what they want to do with their own money because they may freely order how and when to utilize digital money. Bitcoin has grown in popularity, attracting an increasing number of customers who want to use it as a payment option in numerous organizations. Bitcoin is frequently described as being "quick," "convenient," "tax-free," and "revolutionary."

Bitcoin was, and still is, referred to as an anonymous currency in some contexts. Although Bitcoin addresses, unlike traditional financial systems, has nothing to do with any real-world identity at the protocol level, this fact does not guarantee great anonymity. Bitcoin transactions are broadcast in cleartext over a peer-to-peer network and then stored in a massively replicated shared database after being confirmed by miners. A common technique to improve Bitcoin privacy is to use a different address for each transaction.

Illegal laundering of money and financing terrorism have been linked to Bitcoin and other cryptocurrencies [1, 2], as well as the online drug trade [3]. On the online black marketplaces like Silk Road 3, Alpha Bay, and Valhalla, cryptocurrencies have been linked to cybercriminal behaviors. Consumers can use Bitcoins to buy cybercrime-as-a-service, hacking tools, malware, stolen credit card information, and compromised login and password combinations, for example.

Bitcoin is frequently used to propagate ransomware around the world. WannaCry, a ransomware attack that began in May 2017, spread fast around the world. In a few hours, WannaCry labeled "the worst ransomware outbreak in history," infected over 300,000 machines in 150 countries. This attack was extremely destructive since it was a worm that looked for new computers and systems to infect, rather than just a ransomware application. WannaCry encrypts all files on infected devices, rendering them unreachable to the victim until the culprit is paid at least $300 in Bitcoin (s). The ransomware payments were received using three hardcoded Bitcoin addresses/wallets. A total of 335 payments, totaling 51.91182371 Bitcoin or US$144,010.54, has been sent into the three Bitcoin wallets as of June 20, 2017.

Such obstacles and challenges, unfortunately, still exist today. Due to its features, particularly its pseudo-anonymity, Bitcoin has become the preferred payment system for illicit activities. Bitcoin transactions are linked to public keys or addresses rather than real-world identities, and the latter does not require any verified personal data to create. While some enterprises openly provide their addresses when it is essential to delivering their services, others hide their spending habits by using privacy-enhancing payment channels or mixing services. This is a regular occurrence in entities associated with tor markets, ransom payments, frauds, and thievery.

The purpose of this study is to investigate if an uncovered cluster can be classified into one of the categories of exchange, gambling, hosted wallet, merchant services, mining pool, mixing, ransomware, fraud, tor market, or others. This study will increase the transparency of the ecosystem, encouraging businesses and consumers to utilize Bitcoin as a payment method and expand the economy without resorting to criminal actions. This research works reviewed in this paper focus on the classification of Bitcoin addresses based on their activity.

The remainder of the paper contributes as follows: Sect. 2 reviews the related work, followed by a discussion of conceptual overview of the research in Sect. 3. Section 4 gives an overview of the data preparation procedure; Sect. 5 suggests the methodology adopted in the study. The results obtained are outlined in Sect. 6, followed by the conclusion and future scope in Sect. 7.

2 Related Work

Several publications have attempted to disprove Bitcoin's alleged pseudo-anonymity. The first way of breaking down Bitcoin's anonymity used network analytical techniques over addresses mixed with open-source data from Wikileaks, demonstrating that Bitcoin user addresses can be connected [4]. A subsequent technique required direct interaction with the network by submitting transactions and clustering public keys using co-spend algorithms, which led to the discovery of 1.9 million Bitcoin addresses related to real entities or pseudo-identities [5]. Using an open-source framework, the Bitcoin blockchain was processed; public keys were clustered; clusters were tagged, and the network was shown. The system was able to identify an address holding 111,114 BTC pertaining to a Silk Road cold wallet and precisely estimate ransoms delivered to CryptoLocker using only an address provided by a victim on a forum as a lead [6]. Another technique was to use statistical analysis to figure out how its users behaved when sending, receiving, and keeping money. Unlike large portions of transactions moving minimal quantities of coins and the specific subject of study, countless numbers of transactions sending more than 50,000 BTC all at once, this approach discovered that the vast majority of coins remain hidden in addresses that haven't been associated in outgoing transactions [7]. The k-means algorithm was used to cluster a portion of the Bitcoin blockchain with the purpose of detecting anomalous behavior, uncovering anomalous transactions, and detecting abnormal behavior from some clients suspected of money laundering [8]. In [9], the authors developed a method for correlating Bitcoin users' pseudonyms behind NAT with the public IP address of the host where the transaction is generated. The attack's goal was to use one octet of outbound connections to identify each client. Even if they connect to the Bitcoin network via Tor, the approach outlined in [10] linked the sessions of unreachable nodes. The authors do this by employing a novel method that organizes block requests made by nodes in a Bitcoin session graph. The modified Bitcoin client is likewise vulnerable to this attack [10]. A transaction clustering approach was presented and executed based on the analysis of propagation times on four popular cryptocurrencies: Bitcoin, Zcash, Dash, and Monero [11]. Biryukov and Tikhomirov [12] was the first to analyze the prevalence of cybercriminal entities in the Bitcoin ecosystem. They trained unsupervised machine learning classifiers using the dataset provided by the data provider, which used three methods of clustering Bitcoin transactions to categorize entities: co-spend, intelligence-based, and behavior-based. A multiclass classification on Bitcoin blockchain clusters was carried out with the objective of seeing if supervised machine learning algorithms could be helpful to predict the category of an undiscovered cluster given a set of previously recognized clusters as training data [13]. On the basis of transaction history summarization, a multiclass service identification technique in Bitcoin was presented. For improved identification, the suggested technique gets transaction history and analyses the working of the retrieved transactions [14]. Transaction history summary for Bitcoin addresses and entity classification was included as new features. To create a model for machine learning classification for detecting abnormalities of Bitcoin network addresses, the transaction history summary was composed of basic statistics, supplementary statistics, and transaction moments [15]. A cascade machine learning model combined with a sufficient collection of input attributes directly extracted from Bitcoin blockchain data was used to demonstrate a technique to challenge Bitcoin anonymity through entity characterization [16].

3 Conceptual Overview

3.1 Cryptocurrencies

Cryptocurrency is conceivably the most secured form of digital money exchange, as it is built on a decentralized network via the Internet and uses cryptography to perform financial transactions. Although the conceptual theory behind the cryptocurrency technology was proposed in 1991 [17], it was only introduced to the world in 2009 as bitcoin [18]. Unlike traditional money exchange systems, bitcoin relies on a dispersed network of nodes known as miners to keep track of transactions. Each mining node maintains a list of transactions in blocks, each of which contains the preceding block's SHA 256 cryptographic hash. Because this process is persistent, and transaction blocks are stored in all nodes, it is almost difficult to change it. Each node checks all transaction history before committing any transaction to validate that the amount to be sent is correct. Following validation, each transaction in a block conducts repeated hashing procedures using the sender's public key and the preceding transaction's hash value.

3.2 Anonymity

Anonymity is defined as a way of obtaining "freedom from identification, concealment, and lack of distinction" [19], and it can also be defined as a phenomenon in which one can conceal one's identity from others [20]. With the advent of the

Internet and subsequent advancements in electronic commerce, communications, and social media, as well as developments like Web 2.0, there is indeed a growing discussion regarding anonymity, particularly in online environments. The proponents of anonymity see online anonymity as an essential tool for preserving information privacy by shielding personal data from untrustworthy platforms and parties [20]. Anonymity, on the other hand, is regularly exploited, creating a climate conducive to hate speech and libelous remarks by those who act irresponsibly with impunity [20, 21]. Communications over the Internet can be formed with a high degree of certainty, hiding the identity of the communication's source, thanks to the development of public-key cryptography and software agents in the 1990s, such as anonymous remailer servers [22]. These techniques cleared the ground for the formation of pseudonymous entities in Internet communication, which can send and receive messages while keeping the originator's identity hidden. Pseudonymity varies from anonymity in that anonymity demands the complete elimination of all identification information, whereas pseudonymity allows for the construction and maintenance of a pseudo/alternate identity, allowing for partial concealing of the true identity information [19, 23].

3.3 Entity Categorization

One of the most active kinds of enterprises is the exchange, which is a global digital marketplace, wherein traders can trade cryptocurrencies using different fiat (money made legal tender by a government edict) or other digital currencies. As stated in [24], exchanges serve as the "front and exit doors" to the bitcoin realm and are perfect for concealing unlawful activities. The **darknet market** is another option. These are online marketplaces where users can buy narcotics, ammunition, and other commodities and services that are prohibited in most nations. These crypto-markets promote legal and illegal transactions among their customers by using electronic currencies [25]. Furthermore, as described in [26], so-called **mixers** are services that allow users to obfuscate processes. Mixed transactions, on the other hand, boost user privacy and can be used to launder unlawful payments. A few more categories are listed in [12] which are **gambling**, an entity that provides Bitcoin-accepting gambling services, such as Lucky Games and Nitrogen Sports. In exchange for a reward proportional to their contribution to a block's solution, **mining pools** are made up of distributed miners that pool their processing power over a mining network. AntPool and BTC Top are two examples.

4 Data Preparation

The dataset for this study was gathered from the Blockchair and WalletExplorer repositories. Samples for three months were chosen for the study, namely December 2020, November 2020, and January 2021.

4.1 Raw Dataset

Blockchair is a blockchain explorer which has the dumps for the cryptocurrencies such as Bitcoin, Ethereum, Bitcoin Cash, Dogecoin, Litecoin, Bitcoin-SV, and ZCash. The transaction dataset collected from the Blockchair comprises of block_id, hash, time, size, weight, version, lock_time, is_coinbase, has_witness, input_count, output_count, input_total, output_total, input_total_usd, output_total_usd, fee, fee_used, fee_per_kb, fee_per_kb_usd, fee_kb_kwu fee_per_kwu_usd, cdd_total. WalletExplorer is a bitcoin explorer with address grouping and wallet labeling. The transaction dataset collected from this repository contains date, received from, received amount, sent amount, sent to, balance, and transaction.

4.2 Data Preprocessing

When considered separately, the features in both the dataset were insufficient for both training and testing. To make the best use of the collected dataset, the features of both datasets were merged on the basis of transaction hash. After merging, 29,228,184 feature-rich samples were obtained. Out of 29,228,184 samples, 427,625 samples were be labeled. The available labeled entities were *exchange, gambling, mining pool, mixing services.*

4.3 Data Cleaning

The labeled dataset thus obtained was cleaned by performing the following tasks:

a .***Handling null and infinite values***: Deep learning models do not handle the null and infinite values; therefore, such samples were dropped.

b .***Encoding string values to integer***: Using the encoder library of scikit-learn, string values were encoded to an integer to make them adaptable for deep learning models.

4.4 Selection of Features

The transaction hash is generated randomly corresponding to the transaction performed by the Bitcoin users. Because of this random nature, they were dropped. Moreover, few features such as block_id were of low co-relation and were not participating in the training and testing of a classification model. Hence, they were also removed. The features which got selected are as follows: label, size, weight, version, lock_time, is_coinbase, has_witness, input_count, output_count, inout_total_usd, output_total_usd, fee_usd, fee_per_kb_usd, fee_per_kwu_usd, cdd_total, rec/sent, amount. At this step, the dataset is now ready for training and testing.

5 Methodology

To classify and predict the accuracy of the classification, the dataset obtained was trained and tested over the back-propagation neural network (BPNN) and evaluated on cross-validation (CV) accuracy.

5.1 Balancing of Classes/Entities

In the dataset of 427,625 samples, the entity exchanged had the majority of samples 335,847, i.e., 78.53%, while the entity gambling had merely 2254 samples which were 0.53% of the total samples. This led to the issue of class imbalance. To handle this issue, SMOTE [27] and the weight of the entities are employed. SMOTE stands for synthetic **m**inority **o**versampling **t**echnique which produces synthetic samples for the minority classes so that the utilization of imbalanced classes can be enhanced. The other technique, i.e., the weight of the entities oversamples the minority classes and under-samples majority classes so that there's a uniform distribution of samples of all four entities. The weight of an entity was calculated using the following formulae:

$$w_i = n/(k * n_i)$$

where.

w_i *the weight of the entity i,*
n number of dataset samples,
k number of dataset entities,
n_i number of dataset samples of entity *i*

With this approach, samples of mining pool, gambling, and mixing services were oversampled while that of exchange was under-sampled.

5.2 *Training and Testing of Model*

In this study, the back-propagation neural network (BPNN) was validated using the SMOTE and weight of entities techniques on balanced dataset samples. The y-axis had the labels (exchange, pool, services, and gaming), whereas the X-axis contains the remaining attributes. Samples from the training and testing datasets are distributed 60% and 40%, respectively. Both approaches were trained and tested using the TensorFlow libraries on Google's colaboratory.

6 Result

The BPNN was trained and tested to classify the entities and predict the CV accuracy. The model was trained for the dataset samples prepared using SMOTE and the weight of the entities. The classification of entities is shown in Fig. 1, while the results obtained on training and testing of the model are as shown in Table 1.

From Table 1, it is evident that the class balancing carried out using the weight of the entities is giving a slightly better prediction than SMOTE strategy with the exception that the number of samples trained using SMOTE is more than that of the weight of the entities.

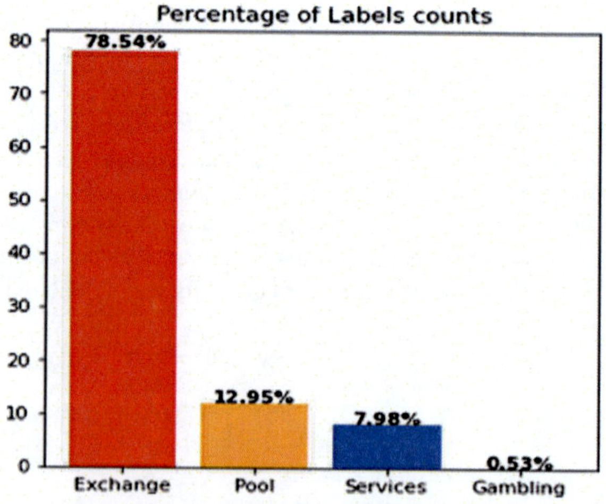

Fig. 1 Classification of entities

Table 1 Comparison of approaches based on CV accuracy

Class balancing strategies	CV accuracy (%)
SMOTE	71.22
Weight of entities	71.51

7 Conclusion and Future Work

Back propagation neural networks were trained on dataset samples of Bitcoin transactions obtained from the Blockchair and WalletExplorer repositories for this study. The transaction hash was then used to merge it. The issue of class imbalance was overcome by carrying out necessary oversampling using SMOTE and oversampling and under-sampling as required using the weight of the entities. The model was evaluated for both the approaches of class balancing on the basis of cross-validation accuracy. The strategy of the weight of the entities seems to be more accurate in comparison to SMOTE.

The accuracy of the model can be enhanced by developing a hybrid approach employing the heuristics on the existing model. Moreover, the availability of cluster is also the limitation of the research; therefore, available datasets can be clustered that can widen the scope of the research.

References

1. Irwin ASM, Milad G (2016) The use of crypto-currencies in funding violent jihad. J Money Laundering Control 19(4):407–425. https://doi.org/10.1108/JMLC-01-2016-0003
2. Pflaum I, Hateley E (2014) A bit of a problem: national and extraterritorial regulation of virtual currency in the age of financial disintermediation. Georgetown J Int Law 45(4):1169–1215
3. Martin J (2014) Lost on the silk road: online drug distribution and the 'cryptomarket.' Criminol Crim Just 14(3):351–367. https://doi.org/10.1177/1748895813505234
4. Reid F, Harrigan M (2013) An analysis of anonymity in the bitcoin system. In: Altshuler Y, Elovici Y, Cremers A, Aharony N, Pentland A (eds) Security and privacy in social networks. Springer, New York. https://doi.org/10.1007/978-1-4614-4139-7_10
5. Meiklejohn S, Pomarole M, Jordan G, Levchenko K, McCoy D, Voelker GM, Savage S (2016) A fistful of bitcoins: characterizing payments among men with no names. Commun. ACM 59, 4 (April 2016):86–93. https://doi.org/10.1145/2896384
6. Spagnuolo M, Maggi F, Zanero S (2014) BitIodine: extracting intelligence from the bitcoin network. In: Christin N, Safavi-Naini R (eds) Financial cryptography and data security. FC 2014. Lecture Notes in Computer Science, vol 8437. Springer, Berlin, Heidelberg. https://doi.org/10.1007/978-3-662-45472-5_29
7. Ron D, Shamir A (2013) Quantitative analysis of the full bitcoin transaction graph. In: Sadeghi AR (ed) Financial cryptography and data security. FC 2013. Lecture Notes in Computer Science, vol 7859. Springer, Berlin, Heidelberg. https://doi.org/10.1007/978-3-642-39884-1_2
8. Hirshman J, Huang Y, Macke S (2013) Unsupervised approaches to detecting anomalous behavior in the bitcoin transaction network, 3rd ed. Technical report, Stanford University
9. Biryukov A, Khovratovich D, Pustogarov I (2014) Deanonymisation of clients in bitcoin P2P network. In: Proceedings of the 2014 ACM SIGSAC conference on computer and communications security (CCS '14). Association for Computing Machinery, New York, 15–29. https://doi.org/10.1145/2660267.2660379
10. Mastan ID, Paul S (2017) A new approach to deanonymization of unreachable bitcoin nodes. In: International conference on cryptology and network security. Springer, Cham, pp 277–298
11. Biryukov A, Tikhomirov S (2019) Deanonymization and linkability of cryptocurrency transactions based on network analysis. 2019 IEEE European symposium on security and privacy (EuroS&P), pp 172–184. https://doi.org/10.1109/EuroSP.2019.00022

12. Sun Yin H, Vatrapu R (2017) A first estimation of the proportion of cybercriminal entities in the bitcoin ecosystem using supervised machine learning. In: 2017 IEEE international conference on big data (Big Data), pp 3690–3699. https://doi.org/10.1109/BigData.2017.8258365
13. Harlev MA, Sun Yin H, Langenheldt KC, Mukkamala R, Vatrapu R (2018) Breaking bad: de-anonymizing entity types on the bitcoin blockchain using supervised machine learning. In: Proceedings of the 51st Hawaii international conference on system sciences. Hawaii international conference on system sciences. https://doi.org/10.24251/hicss.2018.443
14. Toyoda K, Ohtsuki T, Mathiopoulos PT (2018) Multi-class bitcoin-enabled service identification based on transaction history summarization. In: 2018 IEEE international conference on internet of things (iThings) and IEEE green computing and communications (GreenCom) and IEEE cyber, physical and social computing (CPSCom) and IEEE smart data (SmartData), pp 1153–1160. https://doi.org/10.1109/Cybermatics_2018.2018.00208.
15. Lin YJ, Wu PW, Hsu CH, Tu IP, Liao SW (2019) An evaluation of bitcoin address classification based on transaction history summarization. In: 2019 IEEE international conference on blockchain and cryptocurrency (ICBC). IEEE, pp 302–310
16. Zola F, Eguimendia M, Bruse JL, Urrutia RO (2019) Cascading machine learning to attack bitcoin anonymity. In: 2019 IEEE international conference on blockchain (Blockchain). IEEE, pp 10–17
17. Haber S, Stornetta WS (1991) How to time-stamp a digital document. J Cryptol 3:99–111. https://doi.org/10.1007/BF0019679199111
18. Nakamoto S (2008) Bitcoin: a peer-to-peer electronic cash system. Decentralized Bus Rev 21260.
19. Scott SV, Orlikowski WJ (2014) Entanglements in practice: performing anonymity through social media. MIS Q 38(3):873–893
20. Brazier F, Oskamp A, Prins C et al (2004) Anonymity and software agents: an interdisciplinary challenge. Artif Intell Law 12:137–157. https://doi.org/10.1007/s10506-004-6488-5
21. Levmore S (2010) The internet's anonymity problem. In: Lemore S, Nussbaum M (eds) The offensive internet: speech, privacy, and reputation. Harvard University Press, Cambridge
22. Michael FA (1995) Anonymity and its enmities (1995) 1 J Online Law art. 4. Available at SRN: https://ssrn.com/abstract=2715621
23. Michael Froomkin A (1999) legal issues in anonymity and pseudonymity. Inf Soc 15(2):113–127. https://doi.org/10.1080/019722499128574
24. Moore T, Christin N (2013) Beware the middleman: empirical analysis of bitcoin-exchange risk. In: Sadeghi AR (ed) Financial cryptography and data security. FC 2013. Lecture Notes in Computer Science, vol 7859. Springer, Berlin, Heidelberg. https://doi.org/10.1007/978-3-642-39884-1_3
25. Christin N (2013) Traveling the silk road: a measurement analysis of a large anonymous online marketplace. In: Proceedings of the 22nd international conference on World Wide Web (WWW '13). Association for computing machinery, New York, 213–224. https://doi.org/10.1145/2488388.2488408
26. Moser M (2013) Anonymity of bitcoin transactions
27. Chawla NV, Bowyer KW, Hall LO, Kegelmeyer WP (2002) SMOTE: synthetic minority over-sampling technique. J Artif Intell Res 16:321–357

On the Development of Planar Antenna for Wireless Communication Systems

Sushil Kakkar and Shweta Rani

Abstract The work in this paper provides the detailed concept behind the development of rectangular shape planar antenna. Special emphasis is placed on the dimensional parameters, which provide greater impact on the radiation and resonant performance of the antenna. The low priced and easily available FR4 substrate is used to construct the antenna. The dimensions and position of the patch are obtained using numerous simulations. The planar antenna exhibits 52.62% wider bandwidth and reflection coefficient of −44.61 dB at 2.11 GHz.

Keywords Bandwidth · Planar antenna · Reflection coefficient

1 Introduction

Among the earliest inventions of tremendous significance to antenna, design engineering was the invention of planar antennas [1–3]. This invention made it possible for antenna engineers to develop the vast variety of planar antennas with different shapes and sizes. So far in literature, planar antennas have been designed of numerous wireless applications like medical military and commercial [4, 5]. Early versions of these antennas were relatively simple and studied for several years. However, introduction of complex structure such as inverted F antennas, fractal antennas, and antenna with non-Euclidian geometries provides extra degree of freedom in design process [6, 7]. These antennas have limitations of complex designs, comparatively difficult to fabricate and tuning of dimensional parameters require complex computational methods [8–10]. No doubt simple shapes and structures of planar antennas are miles left behind but still there is a wide scope present to analyze them for further improve-

S. Kakkar (✉)
ECE Department, Bhai Gurdas Institute of Engineering and Technology, Sangrur, Punjab, India
e-mail: sushil.kakkar@bgiet.ac.in

S. Rani
ECE Department, GZSCCET, Maharaja Ranjit Singh Punjab Technical University, Bathinda, Punjab, India

M. S. Kaiser et al. (eds.), *Proceedings of Trends in Electronics and Health Informatics*, Lecture Notes in Networks and Systems 376,
https://doi.org/10.1007/978-981-16-8826-3_46

ment in the system performance. In this light, a sincere and efficient effort has been made to analyze and design small size planar antenna for wireless communication application.

2 Antenna Design

During the past two decades, there have been tremendous advances in planar antenna designs. The development of such antennas stems from the hard research work of antenna design engineers. In presented work, antenna is designed using low priced FR4 substrate which is very reliable and easily available. The electrical permittivity of the substrate is 4.4 and height of the antenna is 1.57 mm. The novelty of the proposed work lies in the design of small strip like radiator that has been critically analyzed in conjunction with the comparatively large fixed size ground plane to achieve better resonating parameters. The resonating properties of the antenna are severely depended on its dimensional behavior. Tuning for the required frequency is obtained by varying the dimensions of the antenna, which simultaneously tunes the frequency and impedance matching. Construction of proposed antenna is inspired from rectangular geometry. The length L and width W of the rectangular plane antennas have been optimized using large number of simulations. The dimensions of the ground plane are 47×33 mm. The geometry of the proposed antenna is presented in Fig. 1.

3 Results and Discussion

The simulations of the antenna have been performed on the efficient electromagnetic simulator IE3D. The obtained simulated results show that the proposed antenna possesses wider bandwidth of 52.62% ranging from 1.909 to 3.323 GHz at 2.11 GHz resonating frequency. Proper placement of feed and optimized location of the radiator on the plane of ground is responsible for the good impedance matching and −44.61 dB reflection coefficient at 2.11 GHz resonating frequency. The s-parameters of the presented antenna are depicted in Fig. 2

3.1 *Effect of Location of Patch*

In order to finalize the location of the patch on the ground plane, a critical analysis has been carried out by varying the position of the patch. The achieved result from this analysis is detailed in Fig. 3. It may see that the presented patch when placed closer to the either left or right sides of the plane of ground possess exactly similar resonating properties and perform better than the situation in which the patch is

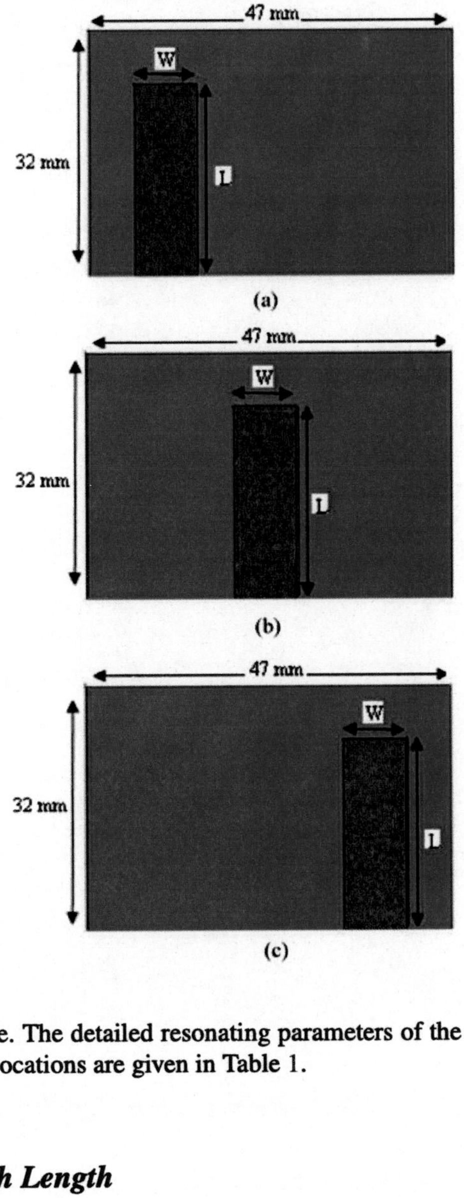

Fig. 1 Geometry of the proposed antenna, **a** patch (p3) close to the left side edge of the ground plane, **b** patch (p2) element at the center of the ground plane, **c** patch (p1) close to the right side of the ground plane

placed at the center of the ground plane. The detailed resonating parameters of the proposed antenna with different patch locations are given in Table 1.

3.2 *Effect of Variation in Patch Length*

Figure 4 gives the graphical comparison of the rectangular planar antenna by varying the patch length. It is very much clear that the patch length of 25 mm outperformed the antennas with other patch lengths.

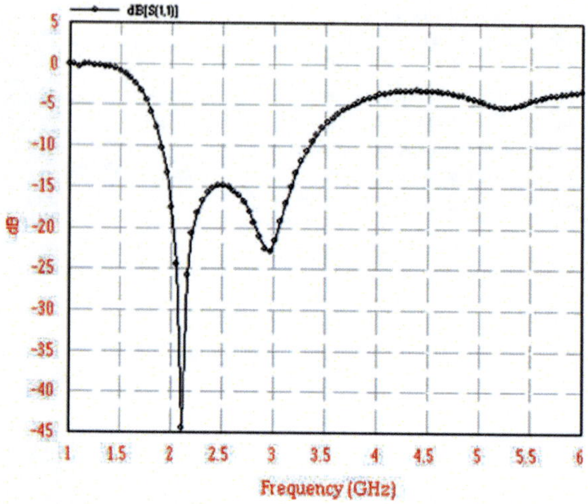

Fig. 2 S-parameters of the presented rectangular planar antenna

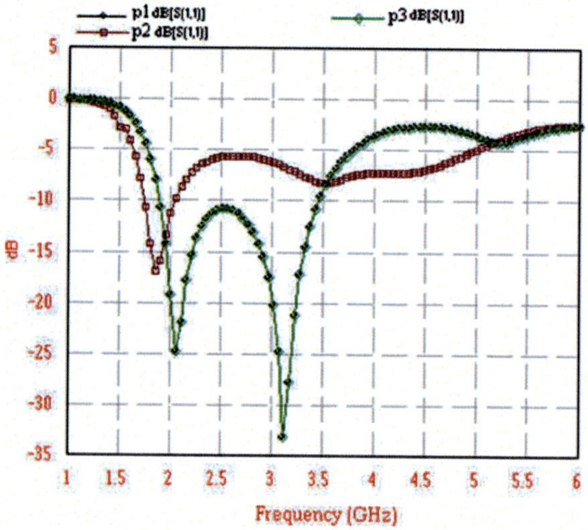

Fig. 3 S-parameters of the planar antenna with varying position

3.3 Effect of Variation in Patch Width

The resonant ability of the proposed antenna is also analyzed by varying the width of the planar radiating element. The effect of the varying patch width is depicted in Fig. 5. It is noticed that the planar antenna is exhibits better resonating properties at patch width of 6 mm in comparison to the other patch widths taken in to consideration here for comparison purpose.

Table 1 Resonating parameters of proposed antenna with different patch location

Antenna patch	Primary resonating frequency (GHz)	Reflection coefficient (dB)	Input impedance (ohms)	VSWR	Bandwidth (%)
Patch closer to left edge of ground plane (p1)	2.061	−24.85	44.70 + j1.116	1.121	59.27
Patch at the center of ground plane (p2)	1.859	−17.04	62.54 + j9.749	1.327	13.44
Patch closer to right edge of ground plane (p3)	2.061	−24.85	44.70 + j1.116	1.121	59.27

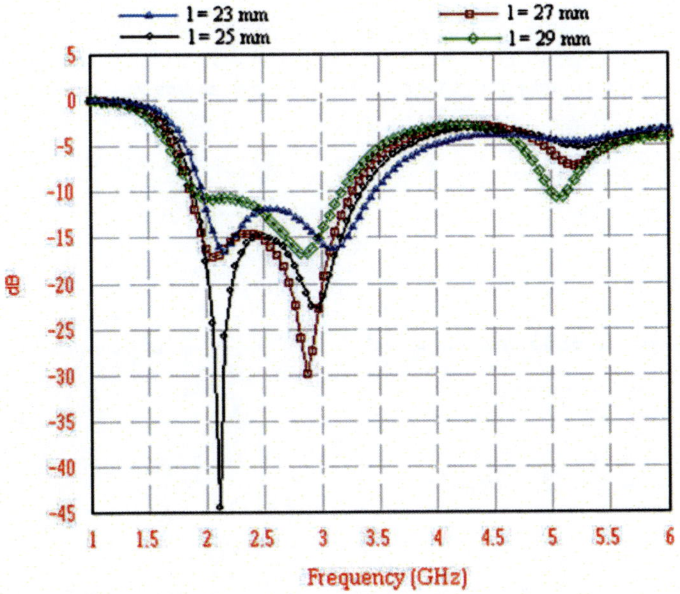

Fig. 4 S-parameters of the presented rectangular planar antenna with varying patch length

3.4 Radiation Patterns

It is here worth mentioning that the antenna radiates efficiently within its wider bandwidth range and more specifically at resonant frequency of 2.11 GHz. The radiation patterns in both principle planes are shown in Fig. 6. The obtained radiation

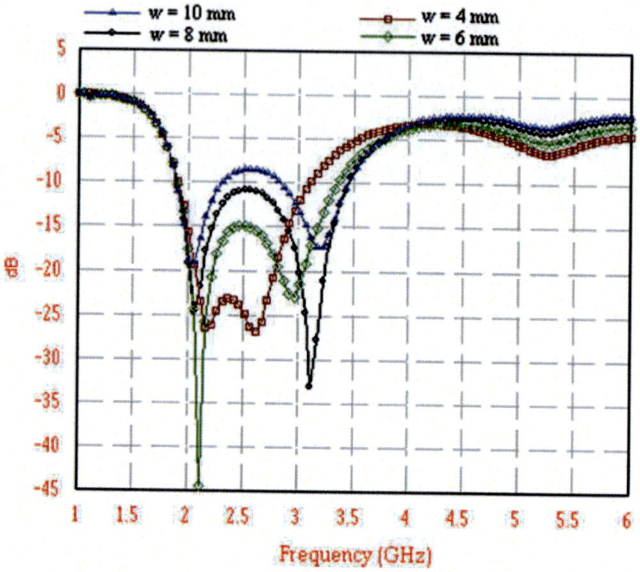

Fig. 5 S-parameters of the presented rectangular planar antenna with varying patch width

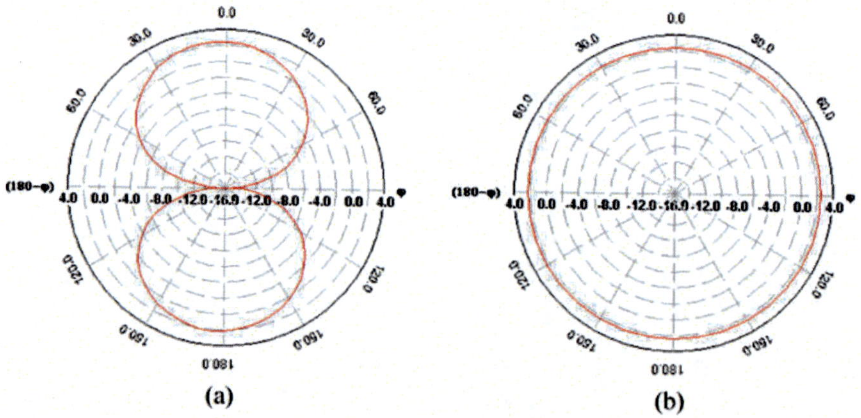

Fig. 6 Radiation patterns of the presented rectangular planar antenna at 2.11 GHz. **a** E-plane, **b** H-plane

patterns reveal that the planar antenna exhibits omni-directional pattern in azimuth plane and directional pattern in elevation plane.

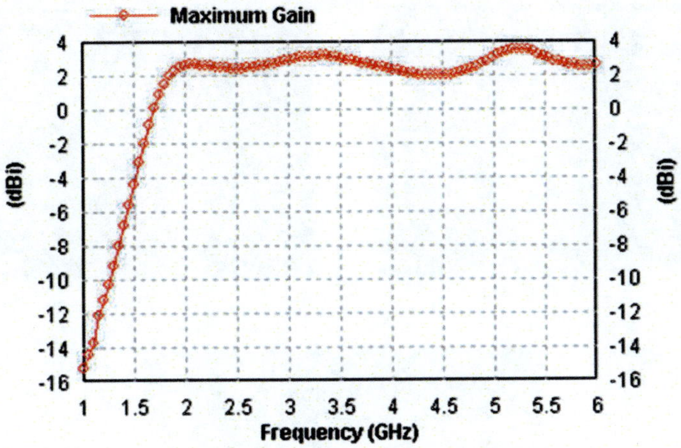

Fig. 7 Gain of the presented rectangular planar antenna

3.5 Gain

Figure 7 depicted the gain versus frequency graphical representation of the proposed antenna. The antenna possesses gain of 2.61 dB at 2.11 GHz resonant frequency. It may also be observed that antenna exhibits almost flat gain which is above than 2 dBi over the whole frequency band of operation (1.901–3.323 GHz).

3.6 Current Distribution

The current distribution characteristics of the presented planar antenna with different patch locations are given in Fig. 8. It is quite clear from the figures that the antenna depicts higher current density at the edges of the antenna.

4 Conclusion

This paper provides an extensive study about the rectangular planar antenna etched on a broader fixed ground plane. The effect of variation in the position of the patch on ground plane and effect of variation in the length and width of the patch is critically examined and validated. The antenna possesses wider bandwidth of 52.62% and significant reflection coefficient of −44.61 dB at 2.11 GHz. These results confirm the suitability of proposed antenna for wireless communication applications. The analysis of the ground plane by implementing defects can be taken as the future scope of this study.

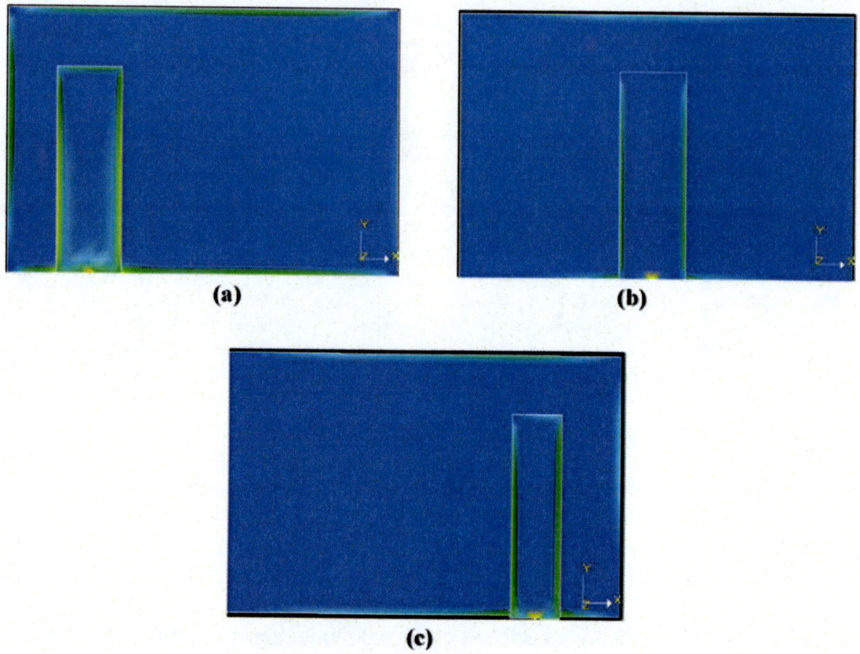

Fig. 8 Current distribution of the presented rectangular planar antenna, **a** patch (p3) close to the left side edge of the ground plane, **b** patch (p2) element at the center of the ground plane, **c** patch (p1) close to the right side of the ground plane

References

1. Balanis A (1997) Antenna theory. Wiley
2. Cheng Y, Liu H (2018) A novel concentric annular-ring slot dual-band circularly polarized microstrip antenna. Hindawi Int J Antennas Propag 1–8
3. Kumar NK, Amala VK, Sri P (2018) Design of concentric circular ring patch with DGS for dual-band at satellite communication and radar applications. Wireless Pers Commun 98:2993–3001
4. Singh AP, Rani S (2011) Simulation and design of broad-band slot antenna for wireless applications. In: Proceedings of the world congress on engineering, WCE 2011, 6–8 July 2011, Imperial College, London, U.K., vol 2, pp 1390–1393
5. Jan JY, Su JW (2005) Bandwidth enhancement of a printed wide slot antenna with a rotated slot. IEEE Trans Antennas Propag 53(6):2111–2114
6. Rani S, Singh AP (2012) On the design and optimization of new fractal antenna using PSO. Int J Electron 100(10):1383–1397
7. Kakkar S, Rani S, Singh AP (2021) Triple band notch microstrip patch antenna with fractal defected ground structure. IETE J Res. https://doi.org/10.1080/03772063.2021.1875894
8. Osman MAR, Rahim MKA, Samsuri NA, Salim HAM, Ali MF (2011) Embroidered fully textile wearable antenna for medical monitoring applications. Progr Electromagn Res 117:321–337

9. Singh G, Kanaujia BK, Pandey VK, Gangawar D, Kumar S (2019) Design of compact dual-band patch antenna loaded with D-shaped complementary split ring resonator. J Electromagn Waves Appl 33(16):2096–2111
10. Kakkar S, Kamal TS, Singh AP (2016) Small patch antenna with DGS for emergency management. MATEC Web Conf J 57:1–3

Energy Efficient Clustering and Optimal Multipath Routing Using Hybrid Metaheuristic Protocol in Wireless Sensor Network

Binaya Kumar Patra, Sarojananda Mishra, and Sanjay Kumar Patra

Abstract Energy Efficiency now a day's becomes a main issues in Wireless sensor Network. Hierarchical Clustering with multipath routing protocol technique is the important to improve packet over head, network lifetime, QOS, and power consumption. There are many such methodssuggested to Improve the Energy efficiency of whole WSN region. Out of these protocols the ad-hoc On demand Distance Vector (AODV) routing protocol is very suitable, as it has more scalable and less overhead. This AODV protocol has two operations to find and maintain routes i.e. Path discovery and path maintenance. By doing the Clustering approach the data packet is shared among members of different clusters by the help of Cluster Head, which ultimately saves energy. Hence Hierarchical clustering algorithm is used in this approach along with Hybrid Genetic Algorithm (GA) with Particle Swarm Optimization (PSO) algorithm.The GA and PSO algorithm creates a hierarchy of cluster heads. The energy saving scheme increases with number of level increase in the Cluster presents in WSN. Therefore Hierarchical Clustering with Hybrid GA and PSO (HC-HGAPSO) methodology performed better Throughput, Network lifetime, and Residual Energy.

Keywords WSN · Clustering · AODV · GA · PSO · Energy efficient

1 Introduction

Wireless Sensor Network consists of sensor nodes having small in size with low-priced and limited supply of power embedded device. Through sensing and monitoring the physical environment, sensor node aggregates the data. Usually node forwards the collected data to the base station by the help of nearest neighbor node in a multi-hop fashion. Due to limited energy supply, the WSN frequently needs a energy efficient routing technique for data transmissions. A reliable path from source to base station is required for efficient transmission which helps in reduce retransmission, decrease congestion, and energy consumption. To survive for long-term sensing

B. K. Patra · S. Mishra (✉) · S. K. Patra
Department of Computer Science Engineering and Applications, Indira Gandhi Institute of Technology, Sarang, India

M. S. Kaiser et al. (eds.), *Proceedings of Trends in Electronics and Health Informatics*, Lecture Notes in Networks and Systems 376,
https://doi.org/10.1007/978-981-16-8826-3_47

over a large wide area, sensor node should preserve energy because of limited battery life. Substitution of sensor battery is impossible as they are deployed in remote and harsh condition. For that it is very prime important to give priority for low energy consumption so that the network lifetime will increase and the network will become energy efficient.

In the cluster-based WSN, many researchers focus on energy efficient and routing protocol. In this approach the energy efficient protocol is adopted with strategy like hierarchical clustering, data aggregation, and multipath routing to optimize network lifetime. Here node energy level and distance between neighbor nodes are key consideration. One of the approaches for optimization is application of bio-inspired algorithm. In this work two bio-inspired hybridized algorithm i.e. Genetic algorithm and Particle swarm optimization is used.

The proposed protocol brings the following input:

1. Hierarchical clustering is applied to improve the transmission distance. Thus improve delay performance.
2. Cluster head (CH) selection method is used to increase the quality of load balancing in different networks types. Latency reduces by using simultaneous operating cluster.
3. Implement an intelligent hybrid bio-inspired routing (GA &PSO) methods to obtain globally optimal chain of shortest distance for transmission of data.

2 Related Work

Ramluckun and Basoo [1] Proposed a energy efficient model by using Ant Colony optimization and cluster chain-based routing. In that clustering method is integrated with PEGASIS with ACO to decrease redundancy in data, distance between nodes, transmission delay in long chain link. With the packet lost more the transmission is stopped. Hence during fault, appropriate methods for relaying information should be addressed further.

Wang et al. [2] have introduced a PSO-based clustering approach with mobile sink for WSN. Cluster Head is evaluated by considering nodes remaining energy and position of the node. The main drawback is that, selection of nodes residual energy and position of nearest neighbor node should be achieved again by using routing protocol.

Barekatain et al. [3] have proposed an energy aware routing technique by using K-mean and genetic Algorithm (GA). The optimal number of CH is selected by implementing improved GA method. K-mean balances the energy distribution and enhances network life time in WSN. Hierachical clustering using K-mean with GA should be used in large-scale WSN and nodes with the BS location in additional.

Gupta et al. [4] proposed genetic algorithm (GA)-based multipath routing having energy efficiency in WSN. In this work, All nodes shared the BS in the network and use a routing fitness function with several parameters used for multipath routing.

Heinzelman et al. [5] have proposed Hirarchical Routing protocol that involves cluster-based structure of the sensor nodes. A node from a cluster selected as cluster head (CH).The CH does the data fusion and aggregation. LEACH is first clustering routing protocol used in WSN. In this protocol a set of randomly selected sensor node considered as CH and the CH task is to maintain consistent energy load among the sensor. LEACH protocol has two phases: The setup and steady state phases. The set up phase is used for cluster construction and cluster head selection. In Steady state phase CH aggregates the information from different nodes. Then the cluster head transmits gathered data to the BS by one hop communication. Various types of LEACH protocol are suggested to overcome some loopholes such as LEACH-C [6], MR-LEACH [7], and HEED [8].

Shankar et al. [9] used a hybrid approach of PSO and HSO for selection of energy efficient CH. Elshrkawey et al. [10] described the various issues in LEACH protocol in his research like inappropriate choice of cluster head, node sends its data in their slot and a improved TDMA is used.

In [11] A two tier PSO protocol is introduced using PSO clustering and routing problems are addressed. In this method encoding technique of particle and fitness value is used for evaluation of optimal best path solution from CH to BS. This technique increases energy efficiency, good cluster quality, and best network coverage. In [12] authors address two issues in clustering and routing by using PSO. Multiobjective fitness function with PSO is used in routing purpose. The network life time, packet delivery ratio, energy used, and dead node detection approach improves by using linear /non-linear math mathematical formulation.

Gao et al. [13] presented PSO-based clustering routing to reduce the energy used for the WSN. The higher residual energy node is considered as CH in clustering. After PSO clustering, the data transmission process was initialized between the nodes to the CH and CH to the BS. The data gathering, aggregation, and allocation of CH was required an extra energy.

In [14], GA is used to optimize neighbor node distance for less energy consumption. Here distance between sensor nodes to the CH and CH to the BS is regarded as objective function. The node having residual energy maximum is considered as CH and helps to minimize the transmission distance between CH and BS. The GA reduces the route distance and hence enhances network lifetime [15]. An improved form of GA is introduced by removing invalid node, hence increases the performance of the system. Hierarchical clustering with bio-inspired hybrid optimization is designed by various clustering algorithm approach [16–18]. The clustering with cluster head selection plays key parameter to decide the optimization techniques. The performance of GA and PSO hybridized with other bio-inspired approach resulting very good improvement performance as compare to other traditional and some other hybride approach.

3 Energy Model

In this research, "n" no of nodes are deployed randomly in a $(m \times n)$ WSN area. In this deployment nodes are static including the sink. Sensor node energy is used for data acquirement, data processing, and packet transmission. The energy consumption in packet transmission is more important as compare to data processing process. Each node is assigned with a unique ID number. Nodes sense the coverage area and communicate with the sink. During packet transmission each node losses some amount of energy and it depends on the distance from sink to node.

In a WSN, at the time of sending and receiving a node losses energy i.e. based on two channel transmission model. It is called free space (d^2 power loss) for direct transmission or one hop. For multipath fading (d^4 power loss) for packet transmission via multi-hop. The energy consumption model can be defined as below:

$$E_{\mathrm{n}}T_{\mathrm{rx}}(k,d) = \begin{cases} kE_{\mathrm{n(elec)}} + k\epsilon_{\mathrm{fres}}\, d^2, & d < d_0 \\ kE_{\mathrm{n(elec)}} + k\epsilon_{\mathrm{mp}}\, d^4, & d \geq d_0 \end{cases}$$

where, $E_{\mathrm{n}}T_{\mathrm{rx}}(k,d)$ electrical energy for transmissions of a k-bit of message over a route Distance d, k is the size of the data packets in bits, ϵ_{fres} is the free space energy loss, ϵ_{mp} is the multipath energy loss, and $E_{\mathrm{n(elec)}}$ is the energy per bit for packet transmission. Both the two ϵ_{fres} and ϵ_{mp} are required in the communication intensifier to send a k-bit data over d^2 and d^4 for free space and multipath transmission. Threshold distance is d_0 which controls the state between ϵ_{fres} and ϵ_{mp} The equation for computing d_0 is as follows:

$$d_0 = \sqrt{\frac{\epsilon_{\mathrm{fres}}}{\epsilon_{\mathrm{mp}}}}$$

The distance between transmitting and receiving end is greater than the distance d_0. Otherwise, this free space technique is used to evaluate energy dissipation.

3.1 Cluster Head (CH) Selection

In this approach, Hierarchical clustering is used. Energy aware threshold function is used for formation of cluster Head (CH). The node which contains more energy will have more probability to become cluster head. If random value is smaller than the Threshold value ($T_h(i)$), then it is selected as CH. $T_h(i)$ and this is calculated as defined below:

$$T_h(i) = \frac{P_{opth}}{1 - P_{opth}\left(r.\bmod\left(1/P_{opth}\right)\right)} \times \frac{E_i(r)}{E_{avg}(r)} \text{ for each nodes if } E_i(r) > 0$$

Here, r is the present round in the WSN lifetime,$E_i(r)$ is the initial energy at node i, and $E_{avg}(r)$ is the remaining energy. The calculation of $E_{avg}(r)$ is as follows:

$$E_{avg} = \frac{\Sigma E_i(r)}{n} \text{ For each node } i.$$

n = Total No of sensor nodes in the network.

4 Proposed HC-HGAPSO Algorithm

PSO algorithm [19] is the societal actions of birds in flocks. The Birds, here it is regarded as particle of a cluster communicate themselves to increase the possibility of acquiring the best position in the flock [20]. Each particle must possess best fitness value in the search space and find the local best position. The best fitness called as global best position obtained so far of the flock [21]. Few drawback of PSO is that slow and less accuracy of convergence rate, which falls in to local minima. GA is a global search algorithm developed by John Holland [22]. The GA includes GA operators, selection, mutation, and cross over to get best solution until end of the condition is touched. Mutation operator in GA [23] is to exclude trapping at local minima but it slows down the convergence.

In this model, a hybrid method of GA-PSO is designed for better solution. The proposed approach improves the convergence accuracy and increases global convergence. Exploitatation and Exploration are two important characteristics in any bio-inspired approach. The suggested approach is a hybrid optimization, having a fusion of the perception of velocity and updating of position in the system of PSO. This also includes the conception of selection, mutation, and crossover of GA.

The GA model is very suitable for simulation of the natural types selection. This computaional model is biological evolution like process. This algorithms initiate a population of some possible solutions to problems. It is a assemble of a number of ancoded gene. This genes are considered as the basic entity of a chromosomes. The GA algorithms obey the rules of survival for the fittest. After the generation of initial population, The GA operator goes through the phase of crossover and mutation to generate next generation population set. Basically the new generation is more suitable than the previous on and is more fittest for solution. It is expressed through the fitness function. It is used as the optimal solution of any problem.

In a WSN,the multipath routing process can be regarded as genetic process. The fact like energy efficiency and fault tolerance of each sensor node are taken to consideration at the time of evaluation of optimal path. For this crossover and mutation operators are used.

4.1 Genetic Algorithm Techniques Used in AODV for Local Optimal Path Selection

GA technique is a efficient to find path optimality WSN. In this work, the basic rule of Genetic Algorithm is included. The main idea of use of GA is to find a shortest path. This method consumes less energy and enhances the network lifetime.

GA Rules Used

- Source to destination route considered as individual population.
- Neighbor node connecting node treated as child
- The route distance from source to destination considered as a chromosome.
- A string of adjoining nodes regarded as gene.
- All the potential route from source to the destination considered as chromosome structure.

4.1.1 Algorithm for AODV_GA

Step-1 Assume Total no of nodes is N, as Initial Population in a WSN.
Step-2 Initialization of all nodes.
Step-3 Basing on the Fitness function, select the neighbor node.

Fitness function calculation is in Eq. (1)

$$\mathrm{FF_T} = \mathrm{FF_R} + \mathrm{FF_D} \tag{1}$$

where

$\mathrm{FF_T}$ Individual node Fitness function.
$\mathrm{FF_R}$ Individual node Fitness function based on Residual energy.
$\mathrm{FF_D}$ N nodes Fitness function based on distance.

$$\mathrm{F\_D} = \frac{D_{\mathrm{N,N}}}{D_{\mathrm{T}}}$$

$D_{\mathrm{N,N}}$ Euclidean distance between two neighbor node.

D_{Total} Source to destination Distance.
Step-4 From source to destination All possible set of paths are created by Crossover and Mutation operators.
Step-5 Apply FF to GA until a complete path to find. It stops when the entire node runs out of Battery.
Step-6 The set of all path having best P value (shortest distance) is picked out and selected as initial solution for PSO.
Step-7 Now the PSO comes to action for further minimization of path cost.

4.2 *Particle Swarm Optimization (PSO) Algorithm Techniques for Global Best Path Selection*

The PSO algorithm generally used for optimization where problem is non-linear and continuous. The PSO algorithm based on population improves better solution for such types of issues. To find the global optimality of a distance functions defined in a given space. The PSO contains a swarm of a predefined size of the particles.

Each particle is responsible for storing information i.e. used for getting the optimality route solution from the present best particles.ng patterns of candidate, which is generated randomly. The GA and PSO hybridization, where "*N*" is a discriminate pattern of particles. All the patterns are covered in all the dimension. Here basing on the generation of order each patterns takes after to one grid. The particle "*N*" agents are formed and extend to the search-space. Every particles agent evaluates the Objective function and stored. Current optimum particles fitness value i.e. P_{best}. Among total populations results, the best value is measured as the global best i.e. G_{best}. In this work minimum route cost is considered as fitness function. Changes in velocity of each particle are done by the PSO. PSO manages the information of results i.e. global best value, objective value, and termination value.

1. Each CHs should considered as particles having two characteristics, velocity and position of the particle.
2. Initiation of the approach starts on random distribution. Each random solution is carried out by population size.
3. The minimum path distance is accepted as fitness function and the fitness value will be calculated by taking the fitness function. Euclidean distance is used to find the neighbor nodes distance and will be evaluated as:

$$D = \sqrt{(x_2 - x_1)^2 + (y_2 - y_1)^2}$$

Here, (x_1, y_1) and (x_2, y_2) are node1 and node 2 position value. Each solutions fitness value is calculated by the aggregated distance cost. Hence the G_{best} is finding out by considering the least aggregated distance in each result.

4. Creation of new particles: new particles produce from the old one in the random manner from old solution is considered as the creation of a new one.

4.1 Current velocity calculation: the rate of change in the particles positions considered as current velocity. new velocity equation can be defined as:

$$V_{\text{current}} = W \times V_{\text{old}} + W_1 \times (\text{Local } P_{\text{best}} - \text{Current } P_{\text{best}}) + W_2 + W_2(G_{\text{best}} - \text{Current } P_{\text{best}})$$

4.2 The particles new position is evaluated as follows:

$$P_{\text{current}} = P_{\text{old}} + V_{\text{current}}$$

Now the new particle (V_{current} and P_{current}) comes.

5. The $P_{\text{current fitness}}$ value is evaluated by using the path distance.
6. The comparison of Old and Current particles Fitness value results in the selection of best one for next processing of iteration.

   If FV current > FV old.
   Then assign old (FV) as current (FV);
   else.
   Old one acts as current particle for next iteration.
   Iteration Terminate.

7. Heighest fitness value of a particle in the each iteration is considered as P_{best}.
8. From Each P_{best}, the particle with heighest fitness value is regarded as a G_{best} solution. Finally, G_{best} particle is selected for inter cluster data transmission path (Fig. 1).

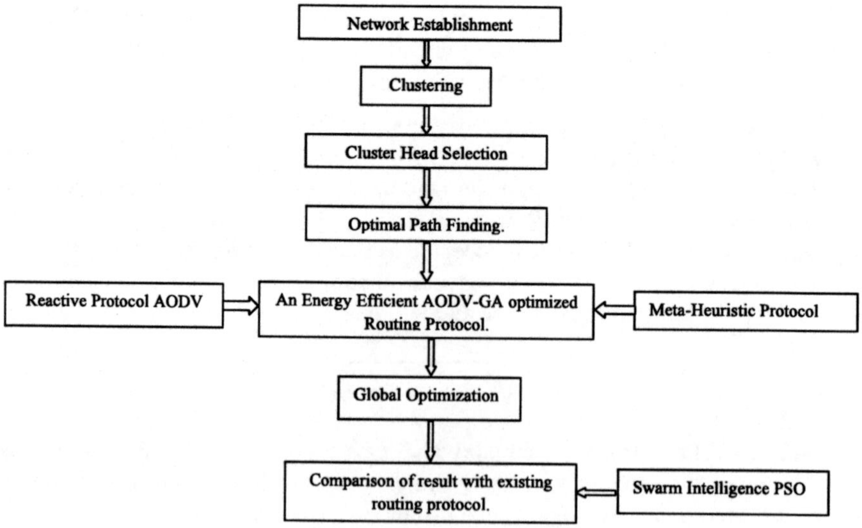

Fig. 1 Flow chart of proposed methodology

5 Experimental Performance Evaluation and Results Discussion

In this implementation work, the simulation tool used is MATLAB for the performance of the planned protocol. The parameter used in simulation is provided in Table 1. In this simulation nodes have been distributed arbitrarily in 100×100 m^2 Area.

5.1 *Throughput*

Figure 2 shows the network Throughput evaluation of HC-HGAPSO with AODV-GA and AODV-PSO. Throughput represents the no of packets that successfully received by the sink. From the figure, it is clear that the Throughput of the proposed work shows significant improvement as compare to other two. With the increase in the no of rounds there is remarkably more changes in the Throughput than existing energy efficient protocols.

5.2 *Residual Energy*

Figure 3 shows the performance results of Residual energy. Residual energy is the time when the last node die in the WSN. This represents the results graph of proposed protocol to other energy efficient protocol. The Residual energy of this HC-HGAPSO approach shows steady and maximized against the other two.

Table 1 Simulation parameters

Parameter	Value
Clustering approach	Hierarchical
Routing method	AODV
Simulation tool	MATLAB
Node coverage area (x, y) in meter	100, 100 m
Base station (x, y) in meter	50, 150 m
Sensor nodes (n)	100 Nos
Initial energy in Joules	0.1
Probability	0.1
Energy (transmitter) in Joules	50×10^{-9}
Energy (receiver) in Joules	50×10^{-9}
Amplifier (multipath) in MHz	0.0013×10^{-13}
Data packet size	4000
Maximum lifetime in second	2500

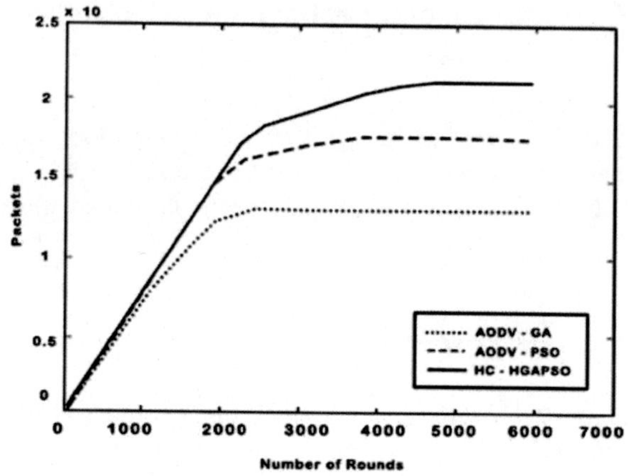

Fig. 2 Comparison of throughput result

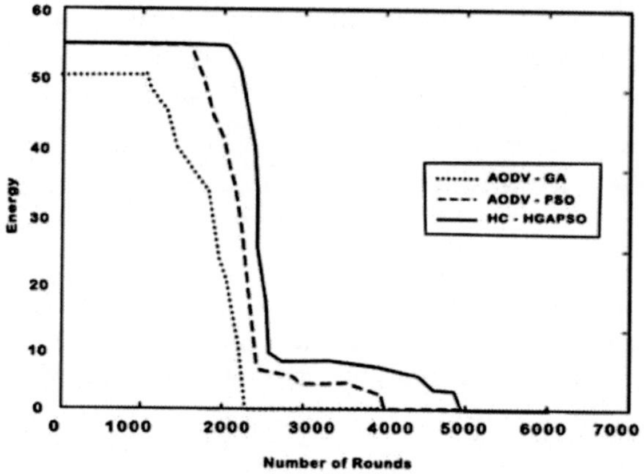

Fig. 3 Comparison of residual energy result

5.3 *Network Lifetime*

Figure 4 shows that the proposed work exhibits the best as against the other, relating to network lifetime. Network life time of a WSN is the time when the first and last node die. The figure shows a significant improvement of network lifetime of the HC-HGAPSO proposed protocol as against the other two protocols. The network life time of this proposed protocol is quit more than the other two protocols.

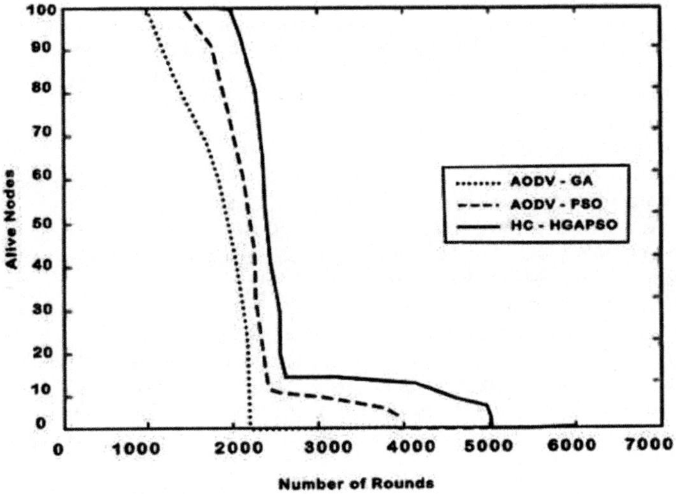

Fig. 4 Comparison of network lifetime result

6 Conclusion

This Paper used a methodology i.e. "HC-HGAPSO" to improve energy consumption by implementing Hierarchical clustering and a hybrid protocol. The hierarchical clustering process creates a number of clusters. The CH selection with optimal multipath route is used for minimum energy consumption by taking residual energy as a key parameter. The CH transmits data to the BS. Then the data packet of each node fused. The transmission of data packet from one node to another is done by AODV. This technique is optimized by HGAPSO methods to find optimal route and hence improve energy Efficiency. From the simulation results, this methodology found to be best one as compare to other two protocols. From this analysis it is concluded that hybrid protocol shows better results efficiently in case of optimal route and energy consumption. The efficiency can be further enhanced with improved clustering methods by including heterogeneity in the WSN.

References

1. Ramluckun N, Basoo V (2018) Energy-efficient chain-cluster based intelligent routing technique for wireless sensor networks. Appl Comput Inf
2. Wang J, Cao Y, Li B, Kim HJ, Lee S. (2017) Particle swarm optimization based clustering algorithm with mobile sink for WSNs. Future Gener Comput Syst, 452–457
3. Barekatain B, Dehghani S, Pourezaferani M (2015) An energy-aware routing protocol for wireless sensor networks based on new combination of genetic algorithm & k-mean .Procedia Comput Sci 72:552–560

4. Gupta SK, Kulia P, Jana PK (2016) Energy efficient multipath routing for wireless sensor networks: a genetic algorithm approach. In: 2016 International conference on advance in computing, communications and informatics (ICACCI). IEEE, pp 1735–1740
5. Heinzelman WR, Chandrakasan A, Balakrishnan H (2000) Energy efficient communication protocol for wireless microsensor networks. In: Proceedings of 33rd annual Hawaii international conference on system sciences, pp 10–19
6. Heinzelman WR, Chandrakasan A, Balakrishnan H (2002) An application-specific protocol architecture for wireless micro sensor networks. Wireless Commun 660–670
7. Dogar AB, Saha GA, Farooq MO (2010) MR-LEACH: multi-hop routing with low energy adaptive clustering hierarchy. In: Fourth international conference on sensor technologies and applications (SENSORCOMM), pp 262–268
8. Younis O, Fahmy S (2004) A hybrid energy-efficient, distributed clustering approach for ad-hoc sensor networks. EEE Trans Mobile Comput 366–379
9. Shankar T, Shanmugavel S, Rajesh A (2016) Hybrid HSA and PSO algorithm for energy efficient cluster head selection in wireless sensor networks. Swarm Evol Comput 30:1–10
10. Mohamed E, Elsherif Samiha M, Elsayed WM (2017) An enhancement approach for reducing the energy consumption in wireless sensor networks. J King Saud Univ Comput Inform Sci. ISSN 1319-1578
11. Elhabyan RS, Yagoub MC (2015) Two-tier particle swarm optimization protocol for clustering and routing in wireless sensor network. J Netw Comput Appl 52:116–128
12. Kuila P, Jana PK (2014) Energy efficient clustering and routing algorithms for wireless sensor networks: Particle swarm optimization approach. Eng Appl Artif Intell 33:127–140
13. Gao F, Luo W, Ma X (2019) Energy constrained clustering routing method based on particle swarm optimization. Cluster Comput 22(3):7629–7635
14. Aziz L, Raghay S, Aznaoui H, Jamali A (2016) A new approach based on a genetic algorithm and an agent cluster head to optimize energy in wireless sensor networks. In: 2016 International conference on information technology for organizations development (IT4OD), pp 1–5
15. Yao G-S, Dong Z-X, Wen W-M, Ren Q (2016) A routing optimization strategy for wireless sensor networks based on improved genetic algorithm. J Appl Sci Eng Technol 19:221–228
16. Wang J, Gao Y, Liu W, Sangaiah AK, Kim HJ (2019) An improved routing schema with special clustering using PSO algorithm for heterogeneous wireless sensor network. Sensors 19(3):671
17. Sambo DW, Yenke BO, Förster A, Dayang P (2019) Optimized clustering algorithms for large wireless sensor networks: a review. Sensors 19(2):322
18. Roy C, Das DK, Srivastava A (2019) Particle swarm optimization based cost optimization for demand side management in smart grid. In: Proceedings of the 2019 international conference on electrical, electronics and computer engineering (UPCON). IEEE, pp 1–6
19. Kennedy J, Eberhart R (1995) Particle swarm optimization (PSO). In: Proceedings of the IEEE international conference on neural networks, Perth, Australia, pp 1942–1948
20. Park JB, Jeong YW, Shin JR, Lee KY (2009) An improved particle swarm optimization for nonconvex economic dispatch problems. IEEE Trans Power Syst 25(1):156–166
21. Logenthiran T, Srinivasan D, Phyu E (2015) Particle swarm optimization for demand side management in smart grid. In: Proceedings of the 2015 IEEE innovative smart grid technologies-Asia (ISGT ASIA). IEEE, pp 1–6
22. Goldberg D (2014) Genetic algorithms in search, optimization, and machine learning. Addison-Wesley, Reading, MA
23. Konak A, Coit DW, Smith AE (2006) Multi-objective optimization using genetic algorithms: a tutorial. Reliab Eng Syst Saf 91(9):992–1007

A Comparative Analysis on Blockchain Technology Considering Security Breeches

CH. Ravikumar, Isha Batra, and Arun Malik

Abstract Nowadays, blockchain technology become a positive pandemic by holding the Internet by storm. Thanks to its free accessibility and safety in nature where the technology of blockchain had emerged as a technology of revolution for the next coming waves of a buzz industrial profile. One is Stuff's network which is sponsored by the company Cloud Infrastructure and Internet things (IoT). To analyze the effect of cyber-attacks in the traditional cyber-framework and study the blockchain cryptocurrency architecture to assess the short comings of blockchain technology. This paper focuses on the various articles of blockchain technology and identified the issues related to security, confidentiality, and accessibility. In this paper, a comparison is done on various articles based on the methodology and merits.

Keywords Blockchain · Cryptocurrency · Cloud of things · Internet of things

1 Introduction

Blockchain technology offers transformative solutions in terms of centralization of power, anonymity, and network stability to tackle cloud problems, though the Internet of Things offers elastic properties and flexible usability to optimize the blockchain efficiency of operations. Therefore, blockchain and the cloud with objects, called the BCoT prototype, are viewed as a promising enabling factor for only a post-set of specific conditions. The cryptocurrency is a secure, open, and useable blockchain. The blockchain concept is based on a peer-to-peer database network on which no centralized agency holds transactions. Block-chain transactions are deep sub open

CH. Ravikumar · I. Batra (✉) · A. Malik
Computer Science and Engineering, Lovely Professional University, Phagwara, Punjab, India
e-mail: isha.17451@lpu.co.in

A. Malik
e-mail: arun.17442@lpu.co.in

M. S. Kaiser et al. (eds.), *Proceedings of Trends in Electronics and Health Informatics*, Lecture Notes in Networks and Systems 376,
https://doi.org/10.1007/978-981-16-8826-3_48

to all blockchain network members. Blockchain utilizes encryption and encryption techniques to verify the authenticity of data transfers, ensuring protection against the linked chains' changes and alterations.

Besides, the blockchain enhances the exciting qualities of federalism, transparency, and protection that often improve customer engagement and substantially save operating expenses. These outstanding capabilities have promoted the use of architecturally based blockchain technological advances. Now could be a really good time to answer to the field of hot analysis. From a technological standpoint, blockchain is a shared service and was first used as the nucleotide lead of the Bitcoin cryptocurrency in commercial activities.

On the other hand, the transition in connectivity and networking has created a variety of possibilities for digital technology, in particular the Internet of Things (IoT) and storage systems, via new construction technology, growth, business processes, and structures. IoT is used in many communications operations like smaller towns, large buildings, livestock, and hospitals. However, due to the lack of IoT computers' resources, energy, and technological capital, they often allocate IoT device operations to cloud computing and thus follow the principle of Cloud of Things (CoT). The Cloud of Things network offers unregulated computing and analytical capabilities to IoT networks, supported by infrastructure. This also offers a flexible, elastic online storage framework that enables the incorporation of allocation of a wide network of IoT applications, demonstrating an enormous capacity to increase user interface quality, device performance, and service delivery capabilities. But the present CoT infrastructures appear to be ineffective due to the above-mentioned concerns. Second, conventional solutions to CoT rely primarily on remote networking technologies, where remote cloud servers connect, control, and maintain IoT devices.

This concept is unlikely to escalate in light of the rising proliferation of IoT networks. Such a unit up in particular not only poses the constraint of key component problems and failure figures that contribute to the destruction CoT network.

Second, deeper integrated CoT capabilities will require a third provider—for example, a cloud provider, to manage IoT devices which raises concerns about data security. Yeah, Internet of Things (IoT) sincerely does the cloud severe, but until then sensitive details can be activated without consumer approval, due to massive disclosure of identity and channel security problems.

Third, IoT users of contemporary CoT processors are losing outcomes. IoT owners do not influence their customer information within modern CoT architectures and consider it challenging to handle data access through cloud IoT universes. Centralized communication network research inevitably results in strong moving image as well as power use it for IoT applications leading to extensive data transmission, which in severe circumstances hamstrings broad-scale CoT formation. A centralized arrangement is not a feasible choice for highly central power, and a decentralized CoT environment with a wide variety of districts, besides. Developing a more open atmosphere is seen as a possible avenue for ensuring economic development and CoT's sin large applications. Centralized code systems are centralized to cloud environments integrating the concepts of closed security that are widely found in graphical interfaces. Nonetheless, with the help of ground-breaking blockchain technologies, the latest phase of IT creation is envisaged to be open and autonomous IoT software ideologies.

Currently, crypto has emerged as a dynamic, secure, but instead, transparent channel to address core issues related to the current central service providers and needs to drive the next step of technologies for CoT technology. The mix of blockchain and CoT particularly contributes significantly to a novel framework that we label as the BCoT framework. Integrating these modern technologies gives all societies immense advantages, drawing expanded interest from academics and industry. The implementation of blockchain will offer significant benefits for the CoT networks that arise.

Benefits of a Blockchain

As one of the first cryptographic keys, RSA (Rivest–Shamir–Adleman) is widely used to store records. In a very cryptographic algorithm, there is the key to encryption that is distinct from either the private secret decryption key. Inside RSA, this asymmetry centered on either the difficulty of computer technology to take into account two of the slightly positive product quality integers, the "factoring issue" [1].

Configurable assistance to cryptocurrencies with blockchain: For broad blockchain networks, the amount of information in the different blockchains may be massive. Therefore, it would be very important to include powerful statistical services to increase the speed procedure of making, so that scalable blockchain services can be made available. The blockchain, along with its dielectric and scalability capabilities, would provide on-demand computing resources for blockchain organizational culture in the maximum context. For instance, the public clouds offer a broader footprint in a federated cloud scenario for blockchain network operators. Besides capturing blockchains across the mesh network and using the urgent virtual machine skills and strategies within each cloud, cloud programs help in these contexts. And cloud computing and blockchain integration make the deployed application highly scalable. Some the benefits which are related to blockchain are listed below.

1. **Decentralization**: Blockchain is a potential solution given its independence, by growing the use of a trustworthy external group within the CoT network to deal effectively with cluster and single-particle failures. Blockchain node instability does not completely affect the BCoT networks. However, blockchain's peer-to-peer approach enables all platform users to verify IoT data validity and maintain the interconnectedness of fair access rights.

2. **Security measures**: The BCoT network can acquire reliable safety by using understanding-enabled technologies to allow both providers and IoT network processes to obtain mandatory consent in business IoT environments. This system should prevent potential risks to computing resources and boost superior IoT data access, thus ensuring strong network security.

3. **Data privacy**: Cryptocurrency application networks are a widely enticing solution to protect adjustments in IoT record keeping, due to the lasting and secure advanced features by blockchain. The constructed using decryption key chains and key exchange of blockchain is to document evidence and sharing of information

instances matters that ensure the integrity and ensures validity which enables us to track their channel connection payments and retain computing and cell phone control.

4. **Corporation**: Without shared confidence, blockchain enables a decentralized system with infinite power for information sharing among distinct entities. Removing external things builds open networks where all IoT users and network service providers can work and collaborate in the BCoT team to achieve the goals. Thus, it allows for the introduction of highly scalable BCoT networks.

5. **Safety Blockchain**: Blockchain algorithm can boost the blockchain platform's safeguard itself by using cloud storage.

6. **Fault tolerance**: Network that helps duplicate blockchain's knowledge via a network of database servers that are closely linked through the software platform. This avoids the standard-failure risks associated with any interruptions in the cloud service and therefore maintains reliable infrastructure. Additionally, the Lazio-cloud environment may allow the blockchain programs to operate simultaneously on that user's device in the event of a disaster (Fig. 1).

On the (in) sustainability of contemporary authentication protocols based on PKI, all available community methodology is based on a public key infrastructure (PKI) where user licenses are provided by a reasonably authority trustworthy, and the auditor will have to handle customer certificates to locate the appropriate strong authentication key. However, authentication company including granting, transportation, distribution, or authorization is quite expensive and tedious. Removing the credentials management problem can also be competitive and, in fact, advantageous [2].

EoS is a block one-built open blockchain network. EoS aims to build a blockchain network that facilitates features and operating system-like applications. EoS uses an efficient feature block with DPoS contract to facilitate a stronger blockchain especially compared to the drawbacks of low availability and lack of traditional blockchain performance. The DPoS nodes must participate in the witness voting,

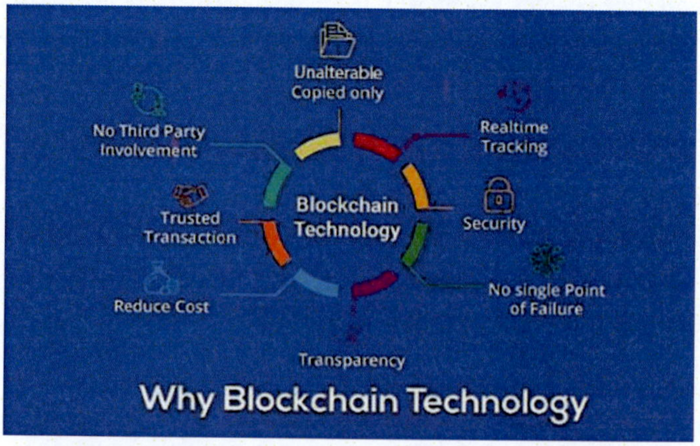

Fig. 1 Importance of blockchain [1]

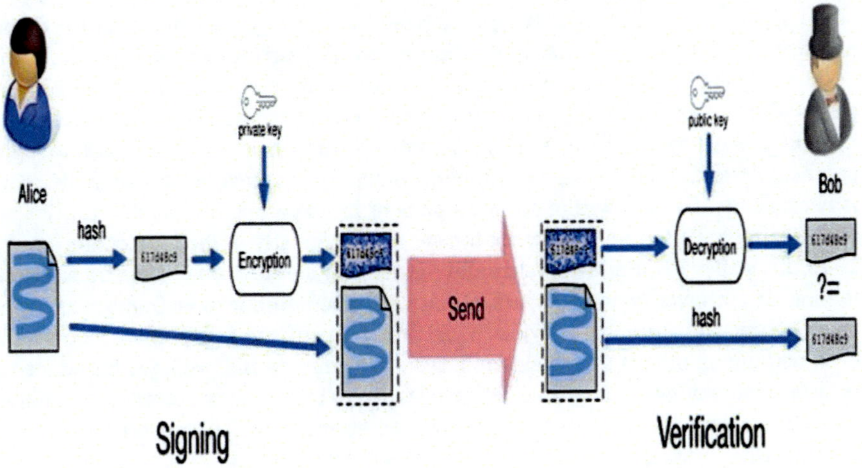

Fig. 2 Digital signature used in blockchain [2]

as opposed to PoW and PoS compromise schemes. Only those nodes winning the general poll (minimum 21 votes) qualify for block generation. Likewise, there are another 100 candidate nodes named as witness jurors. Whether there are issues with the 21 points of the complainant, otherwise they would be treated as substitutions. This EoS block length is approx. 0.5 s [3].

A more effective way of proving a file's existence is to cryptographically encrypt text queries with a time-stamp (Fig. 2).

The symbol uses a trusted provider (TSP) to assist users in trying to stamp their information at night, where a file is sent to TSP after it has been created, and TSP delays it and posts it to the owner of the file with the time-stamp. Incorporate a time-stamp in cloud storage systems to easily outsource results. The blockchain crypto-mechanism and data storage security was employed to determine the data privacy factors. Besides, the summary presents still what are cloud security and privacy breaches, how the performance was carried with the adoption of the blockchain security framework analyze the blockchain concept and base technologies and to review the pattern of studies to date to explore fields to be explored, taking into account cloud storage environments.

2 Related Work

The study analyzes research papers based on various authors' reviews; the authors have clearly described the blockchain into the cloud and described the importance of blockchain technology in the cloud platform and how privacy was achieved in cloud applications. These papers summarized the security mechanism in the cloud platform and how security was evaluated for ensuring privacy mechanism.

In this paper [4], Lin Zhong, Qianhong expanding participates severe network bandwidth and lower entry speeds hinder their widespread use of existing blockchain networks. And to alleviate that illness, he indicated a reliable, ergonomic light payment system (SVLP). Billing and offering refunds approaches are versatile. This is because the division within our arrangement lacks computational complexity, so users do not have to find each week for pre-images mostly in the long chain.

In this paper [5], Satoshi Nakamoto carried out an electronic sales transaction, without any reliance on trust. Organizations with the traditional coin frame made from an electronic signature that provides equal protection of ownership but is incomplete even without an order to reduce double costs. To counter this, we have introduced a peer-to-peer framework that uses proof-of-work to document a common functional context that enables an attacker to alter computationally as faith governs a plurality of computing power.

In this paper [6], Doriane Perard, Lucas Jacque, et al., defined the use of blockchains to build a new, decentralized computer network that has been deemed. The methodology of blockhouses focuses on a method that contains three components: initialization of the storage device, day-audits, and conclusion of the device. It focuses on proofs of retrievability for authenticated messages, allowing contracts to check the data is securely preserved by the server. The main problem that happens in the network may be that the scale of the blockchain is too drastically it is impossible to store. By canceling production, the erasure codes are used to rectify the problem.

In this paper [7], Jin Ho Park, Jong Hyuk Park presented the transaction of P2P network technology. Basic measures such as production proof, but stack proof was introduced to strengthen the credibility of the blockchains. The 51% state of attack that includes problems just of infringed credibility and transaction lack of availability after a violation that concerns 51% of the transaction ledger. Residual identity, however, does not have security, because it does not ensure that the payment information will be completely deleted.

In this paper [8], Huaqun Wang et al. suggested a private PDP program focused on blockchain. The method may even recognize the security of the customer according to a discussion on anonymity. There is also a need to remove the certificate authentication mechanism to further boost efficiency. Hence, the blockchain-based PDP scheme focused on identification is essential for research. Analyzing the keys-evolving blockchain-based PDP system is essential if more strengthening of the private key is necessary.

In this paper [9] Simanta Shekhar Sarmah designed blockchain applications to store their data in their P2P networks, so that efficient utilization of the computing resources is feasible. The two key algorithms, including concrete evidence-of-job and proof-of-stake, blockchain transactions are used primarily to ensure stability. Cloud-storage applications of blockchain are now under study.

In this paper [10] Ivan Damg˚ard, Chaya Ganesh, et al., proposed a unique approach that comes to mind: that is, we might also exchange a trapdoor (say, an RSA key) with such a user party and let them work together again to decide the encoding using the protected trapdoor technology. We should take note of the large body of RSA key generation and distributed signature publications for the coding protocol. Future work is left with the best approach for the mechanism.

In this paper [11], Yong Yu, Yanqi Zhao, et al., proposed a blockchain-based selective disqualification anonymous identity verification for smart processes in the industry (BASS) that endorses data retention personality traits, specific revoke, certification rightness, and tri-speed unlinkability for smart international orders. Point cheval and Hillary recommend a targeted form of revoking that focuses on complex inverters and the signing algorithm as the BASS overlay.

In this paper [12], according to the Sunoo Park, Albert Kwon, et.al, Bitcoin is perhaps the most widely known cryptocurrency ever mobilized, and its more distinctive attribute is its centrally managed nature. This is reached through all of the intrinsic protocol (Nakamoto Consensus) using objective evidence that has the flaw of preventing huge sums of cash spent on the ledger. As a side effect, coal mines in the cryptocurrency are spreading less over time. Applied orbital proof to make use of digital currency, explore future attacks on such a blockchain-like network using spatial proof, and construct a new economic model of router and bank transfer forms to overcome such attacks.

In this paper [13], Ben Fisch, created a functional proof-of-space (PoS), with continually tight safety graphs centered on rigid graphs layered in-depth and constant expander. Real evidence-of- space (PoS) is an engaging balanced choice to make in which a prover displays a particular location used to store the data. PoRep, publicly reliable confirmation of the prover dedicating special buildings to saving one or more replicas of reclaimable data, compliance proofing.

In this paper [14], GuowenXu, Hongwei Li, scope query was used in a variety of ways as a simple database tool, including SQL handovers, location-based tools, and computational geometry. Employees are gradually inclined to save costs for local information storage through cloud services due to the increasing amount of data. In concept, we demonstrate the reliability of our suggested technique as regards spatial data anonymity, indexing and trapdoor secrecy, and trapdoor data unlinkability. Indeed, detailed analyses reveal that our latest model is highly efficient compared to existing schemes.

3 Research Analysis

According to the various authors' contributions and research, the blockchain still has different security breaches due to the lack of trust. Generally, the cloud system is organized with various auditing and assessment tools to audit the various kinds of data, but still the unauthorized users are stealing data. The role-based access control system defined an attribute-based hierarchical system to define accessibility by combining the cryptography techniques, the computation of cryptography hash function needs a different attribute set, which leads to a more computation problem. "They break down exclusively crude data, or, in other words, data should be dissected at a few layers. The data broke down at the lowest layer overburdens cloud security frameworks, overpowers human chiefs, and may not contain enough proof about the expectations of an aggressor. Existing security systems cannot socially dissect data. Fundamentally, data about the connections of occasions is not accessible at prediction time". The authorization case is unclear, since it has the issue of disclosing the keys to attack the blockchain by splitting the private keys; it does not include security for actively supported, because it does not verify the digital signature has been removed completely. The cases of information security do not provide compatibility either owing to malicious interference, the system is inaccessible It does not have data protection, since it does not ensure the deletion of the digital wallet.

As per the blockchain, cloud-based frameworks have problems with both the violated credibility and lack of availability of digital currency after an attack that changes your transaction ledger. The improved blockchain scenario neither ensures confidentiality nor offers accessibility. Subsequently, it does not offer the security of residual details as it does not verify that perhaps the digital asset is completely removed.

4 Comparison Between Different Methods

The following table demonstrates the complete comparison between the different methods of blockchain technology. This comparison is made on the methodology and merits as shown in Table1.

Based on various authors' reviews, the authors have clearly described the blockchain into the cloud and described the importance of blockchain technology in the cloud platform and how privacy was achieved in cloud applications. The above papers summarized the security mechanism in the cloud platform and how security was evaluated for ensuring privacy mechanism.

The blockchain crypto-mechanism and data storage security was employed to determine the data privacy factors. Besides, the summary presents still what are cloud security and privacy breaches and how the performance was carried with the adoption of the blockchain security framework. I analyze the blockchain concept and base technologies and to review the pattern of studies to date to explore fields to be explored, taking into account cloud storage environments.

5 Conclusion

This paper focuses on the different methods used in blockchain technology. It shows analysis of results of state-of-the-art algorithms. The comparison has been done on the basis of the research methodology and merits. The comparison reveals that there is a need to improve the existing methods in terms of confidentiality, accessibility, security, and can be used as a future directions.

Table 1 Comparison between methods of blockchain technology

Author	Methodology	Merit
Yuan et al. [15]	CPVPA	They proposed a certificate less public authentication system
Zehui et al. [16]	Interactions between the miners and edge providers are an algorithm for producing the best output for both miners and providers in a centralized fashion	This is to add, miners purchase and lease quantities of computing capacity from edge providers without any network management difficulties
Mona Taghavi et al. [17]	Proposed a multi-agent process improvement platform based on blockchain to overcome the federations of conventional cloud services, and corrupted QoS	This paper proposes a new, blockchain- based, cooperative collaboration model embodying quality guarantee for cloud service providers leasing each other's computing services
Xiaojun et al. [18]	Introduced an innovative conditional ethnicity-preserving the cloud-based WBAN public audit program	Ethnicity-preserving the cloud-based WBAN public audit program, enabling TPA to monitor external provider validity with diagnostic knowledge
Yuan et al. [19]	An effective and secure PEKS scheme called SEPSE	This paper provides to prevent inaccessible KGA, as other main servers have been used to support encrypt keys and alleviate SEPSE from the issue of any point of failure
Yuan et al. [20]	Chronos+	Chronos+ is a stable time-stamping framework built on blockchains for cloud storage services in which Chronos+ log archive open to cloud service providers allows both data and time-stamping services
Yinghu et al. [21]	Introduced BPay, a blockchain-based payment service network for the procurement	In cloud computing, we to be exact, researchers, recommended goals in terms of machine architecture, theory, adversarial paradigm, concept, and model data For BPay specified
Huang et al. [22]	New BaaS bottleneck model	According to their analysis, the majority in previous cryptocurrencies is the bottleneck, such as bitcoin. Protocol has changed significantly in recent years

(continued)

Table 1 (continued)

Author	Methodology	Merit
Wang et al. [23]	Blockchain	Blockchain-based PDP scheme based on identity is important for analysis. Analysis of key-evolving blockchain-based PDP scheme is important to further enhance security of the private key
Yu et al. [11]	Blockchain anonymous authentication	Anonymous authentication with selective revocation for smart industrial applications (BASS), which supports privacy attributes, selective revocation, credential soundness, and multispeed unlinkability

References

1. Yu J, Wang H (2017) Strong key-exposure resilient auditing for secure cloud storage. IEEE Trans Inf Forensics Secur 12(8):1931–1940
2. Sun SF, Au MH, Liu JK, Yuen TH (2017) RingCT 2.0: a compact accumulator-based (Linkable Ring Signature) scheme for blockchain cryptocurrency Monero. ESORICS 2017:456–474
3. Zhong L, Wu Q, Xie J, Li J, Qin B (2019) A secure versatile light payment system based on blockchain. Futur Gener Comput Syst 93:327–337
4. Zhong L, Wu Q, Xie H, Li J (2020) A secure versatile light payment system based on blockchain. IEEE Syst J
5. Nakamoto S (2020) Bitcoin: a peer-to-peer electronic cash system in 'https://bitcoin.org/bitcoin.pdf
6. Perard D, Gicquel L, Lacan J (2020) BlockHouse: blockchain-based distributed storehouse system, from 'https://www.researchgate.net/publication/338737884_BlockHouse_Blockchainbased_Distributed_Storehouse_System
7. Park J, Park J (2017) Blockchain security in cloud computing: use cases, challenges, and solutions. https://doi.org/10.3390/sym9080164, Symmetry 9, 164
8. Wang H, Wang Q, He D, Blockchain- based private provable data possession. IEEE Trans Dependable Sec
9. Sarmah SS (2019) Application of blockchain in cloud computing. IEEE Syst J. https://www.ijitee.org/wp-content/uploads/papers/v8i12/L35851081219.pdf
10. Damg˚ard I, Ganesh C, Orlandi C (2019) Proofs of replicated storage without timing assumptions. IEEE Syst J
11. Yu Y, Zhao Y, Li Y, Du X, Wang L, Guizani M (2019) Blockchain-based anonymous authentication with selective revocation for smart industrial applications. In: IEEE transactions on cloud computing
12. Park S, Kwon A, Fuchsbauer G, Gaži P, Pietrzak K (2019) SpaceMint: a cryptocurrency based on proofs of space. In: IEEE transactions on cloud computing
13. Fisch B, Tight proofs of space and replication. https://link.springer.com/chapter/https://doi.org/10.1007/978-3-030-17656-3_12
14. Xu G, Li H, Dai Y, Yang K (2019) Enabling efficient and geometric range query with access control over encrypted spatial data. IEEE Syst J
15. Zhang Y, Xu C, Lin X, Shen XS (2019) Blockchain- based public integrity verification for cloud storage against procrastinating auditors. IEEE Trans Cloud Comput. https://doi.org/10.1109/TCC.2019

16. Xiong Z, Kang J, Niyato D, Wang P, Poor V (2019) Cloud/edge computing service management in blockchain networks: multi-leader multi-follower game-based ADMM for pricing. IEEE Trans Serv Comput. https://doi.org/10.1109/TSC.2019
17. Taghavi M, Bentahar J, Otrok H, Bakhtiyari K (2019) A blockchain-based model for cloud service quality monitoring. IEEE Trans Serv Comput. https://doi.org/10.1109/TSC.2019.
18. Zhang X, Zhao J, Xu C, Li H, Wang H, Zhang Y (2019) CIPPPA: conditional identity privacy-preserving public auditing for cloud-based WBANs against malicious auditors. IEEE Trans Cloud Comput. https://doi.org/10.1109/TCC.2019
19. Zhang Y, Xu C, Ni J, Li H, Shen XS (2019) Blockchain-assisted public-key encryption with keyword search against keyword guessing attacks for cloud storage. IEEE Trans Cloud Comput. https://doi.org/10.1109/TCC.2019
20. Zhang Y, Xu C, Cheng N, Li H, Yang H, Shen XS (2019) Chronos+: an accurate blockchain-based time- stamping scheme for cloud storage. IEEE Trans Serv Comput. https://doi.org/10.1109/TSC.2019
21. Zhang Y, Deng R, Liu X, Zheng D, Outsourcing service fair payment based on blockchain and its applications in cloud computing. IEEE Trans Serv Comput. https://doi.org/10.1109/TSC.2018
22. Huang B et al (2015) BoR: toward high-performance permissioned blockchain in RDMA-enabled network. IEEE Trans Serv Comput 14(8)
23. Wang H, Wang Q, He D (2019) Blockchain-based private provable data possession. IEEE Trans Dependable Sec Comput. https://doi.org/10.1109/TDSC.2019
24. Zheng Z, Xie S, Dai H-N, Chen X, Wang H (2018) Blockchain challenges and opportunities: a survey. Int J Web Grid Serv 14(4):352–375

Compact Tapered Shape Wide Slot UWB Antenna with 5. 6 GHz Band-Notched Characteristics

Gaurav Sahu, Vivek Kumar, and Abhishek Singh Rathour

Abstract A printed antenna with a tapered shape wide slot with single band-notched characteristic has been proposed in this paper. Simulation studies show that the proposed antenna has a relative bandwidth of 134% (3.125–15.750 GHz) for S11 ≤ -10 dB which covers the entire UWB. A C-shaped slot has been cut on the conducting patch in order to get single band-notched characteristics in the 5.15–5.825 GHz band. The overall size of the antenna is 22×20 mm^2; an FR4 substrate is used with a dielectric constant of 4.3 (for operating frequencies greater than 1 GHz) and loss tangent 0.025.

Keywords Ultra-wide band (UWB) · Microstrip slot antenna · Single band-notched · EIRP

1 Introduction

In the year 2002, Federal Communication Commission (FCC) has issued a frequency band from 3.1 to 10.6 GHz which is known as Ultra-Wideband (UWB) [1] and it is free to use. Due to a draught of bandwidth, such a step taken by FCC has been welcomed by the industry as well as by the scientific community. An ultra-wideband system transmits very short-duration pulses with relatively very low energy to minimize EM interference with the available present network WLAN (5.15–5.825 GHz), WIMAX, and IEEE 802.16 (3.4–3.69 GHz). If an ultra-wideband system utilizes the all UWB band, then the EIRP cannot exceed −41.3 dBm/MHz for both indoor and outdoor applications both. Due to the limited available power UWB systems are more popular for indoor applications such as short-range data and voice communication between electronic devices for WPAN/WBAN positioning and tracking for the indoor location.

G. Sahu · V. Kumar (✉) · A. S. Rathour
Department of Electronics and Communication Engineering, Pranveer Singh Institute of Technology, Kanpur, India
e-mail: vivekrastogi@ieee.org

M. S. Kaiser et al. (eds.), *Proceedings of Trends in Electronics and Health Informatics*, Lecture Notes in Networks and Systems 376,
https://doi.org/10.1007/978-981-16-8826-3_49

An antenna is an impedance transformer that couples the input or line impedance with the free space impedance. In UWB systems, impedance transformation has a significant impact due to the large available bandwidth. For various applications, a UWB antenna must have a small size (physically and electronically both), be inexpensive, gain flatness, and radiation pattern must be omnidirectional without lowering the antenna performance. Designing a compact antenna with the above necessity is a quite challenging task. Various planar UWB antenna's prototypes have been already produced for wideband applications among which slot antennas are attractive candidates due to their simple structure, ease of design, and good performance, also a wide slot antenna possesses much higher bandwidth as compared to the narrow-slot antenna having less bandwidth.

Recently, various UWB antennas either fed by a coplanar waveguide or by different microstrip tuning stubs have been studied [2–10]. A wide slot antenna with a CPW rectangular excitation stub was introduced in [3]. With proper selection of the size/location of the excitation stub, the bandwidth of an antenna can be increased up to 60%. An E-shaped slot has been introduced on the top side of the material (ground plane) [6] and an E-shaped microstrip tuning stub at the opposite side. This antenna has a bandwidth of 120%. In [8–10] an antenna with a swastika slot with a U slot in a ground plane was developed. This prototype has the highest bandwidth of 138%. To avoid interference with available communication networks/systems various wide bandwidth antenna's prototypes including band-notched characteristics have been proposed. To achieve band-notched properties C-shaped slot, Swastika shape slot, and U-shaped slot [5–14] have been etched while in [14] defected ground structure has been employed. The problem with above-mentioned antennas is their size which varies from 30 × 46 to 26 × 30 mm^2. In [10–14] a small size UWB antenna has been proposed. The dimensions of the proposed prototype were 30 × 30 mm^2. Also, the authors, in [10], did not introduce any properties related to band notch.

In this paper, we have been introducing a tapered shape wide slot antenna fed by a rectangular tuning stub. Moreover, the proposed antenna includes a single band-notch property. The overall size specification of the developed antenna's prototype is 22 mm (width) × 20 mm (length) which is significantly compact than the several antennas as in [2–14]. The proposed antenna also has a relative bandwidth of 134% which is much larger than antennas proposed in [2–6]. We have designed and optimized our antenna using CST-MWS.

2 Antenna Design

The complete antenna's specification has been provided in Fig. 1. We have utilized a less thick substrate FR-4 substrate to design the antenna which has the following specification: thickness–1.6 mm, dielectric constant–4.3, and loss tangent 0.025. To improve the impedance matching, a rectangular slot has been cut on the ground plane under the microstrip feed line. Also, a tapered shape wide slot is etched on the ground plane of the antenna. Studies show that for good mutual coupling between, patch and

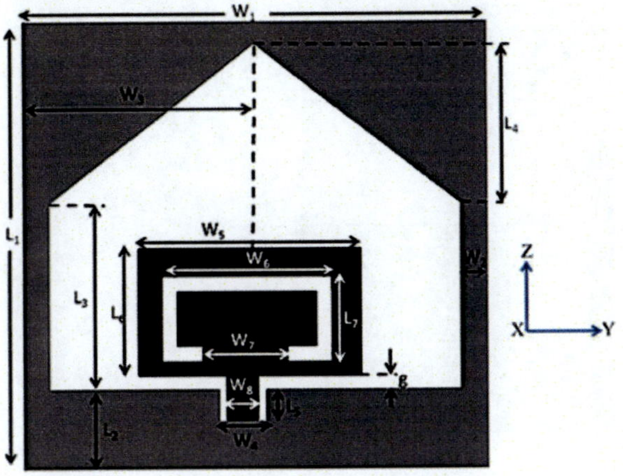

Fig. 1 Rear view of antenna

Table 1 Proposed antenna's specification for optimization

*W*1	*W*2	*W*3	*W*4	*W*5	*W*6	*W*7	*W*8
20	1	10	3	11	8	4.2	3
L1	**L2**	**L3**	**L4**	**L5**	**L6**	**L7**	**g**
22	4.4	10.6	6	0.5	6	4	0.5

the slot, the radiating patch should have an area of at least one-third that of the slot area, and its shape should also be similar to the slot shape which in result provides a wide impedance bandwidth. Also, a rectangular radiation patch is used for excitation on the other side of ground plane. A 50 Ω microstrip line is employed to feed the radiation patch. The parametric specifications of the proposed antenna are shown in Table 1 All values are in millimeters.

To get a single notched centered at a frequency of 5.6 GHz, a C-shaped slot of length λc/2 is etched on the rectangular radiation patch where λc is the wavelength at the center frequency. The length of the antenna is,

$$L = \frac{\lambda_c}{2\left(\sqrt{\frac{\varepsilon_r+1}{2}}\right)}$$

where $L = 2*(W6 + L7) - W7)$ for C-shaped slot, which is 16.5 mm when obtained using (1) but practically obtained length is 19.8 mm.

The surface current density of our antenna at the frequency of 5.6 GHz has been shown in Fig. 2. From the figure, we can clearly visualize that most of the surface current concentrates itself in close proximity of the etched slot.

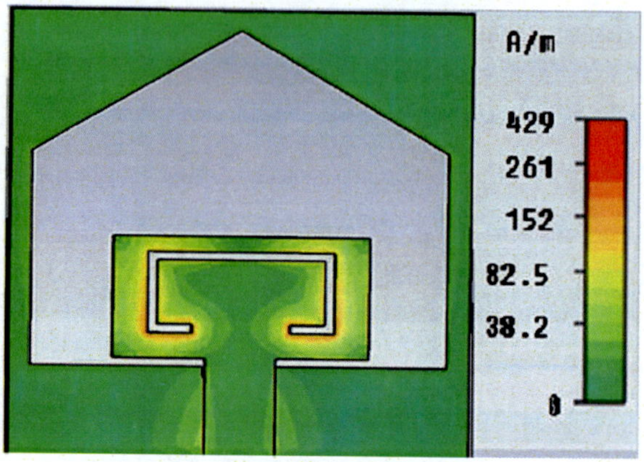

Fig. 2 Simulated surface current density at notched frequency

3 Parametric Study

For the proposed design, numerical studies of some vital parameters have been done to investigate their effect on the performance of antenna.

1. *Effect of Slot Shape:* Studies show that a wide slot antenna is capable of providing large impedance bandwidth. In a slot antenna current mainly flows at the edge of the slot and numerical studies show that this current increases the cross-polarization component in the *yz*-plane. So by reducing the width of the surrounding ground strips, this current can be reduced, and as a result, cross-polarization reduces. The proposed antenna has smaller ground strips which help in making the antenna smaller. Figure 3 shows the VSWR comparison for different slot shapes. It can be seen that with the introduction of a wide slot the bandwidth of the antenna increases significantly. It is because now there are two resonators one is a patch and the other is a slot. These two works together as a coupled resonator. Wide slot also helps in impedance matching at lower frequencies.

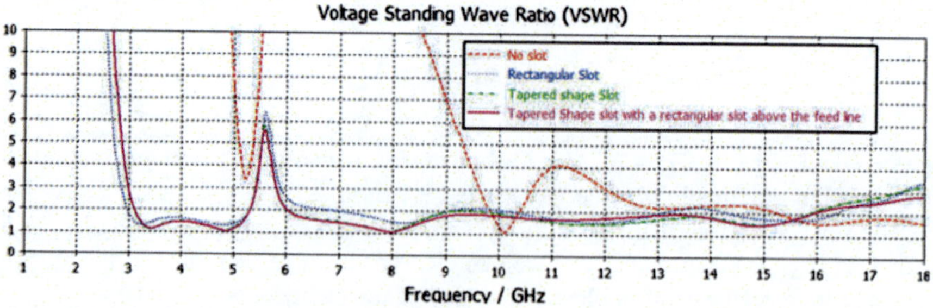

Fig. 3 Simulated VSWR for different slot shape

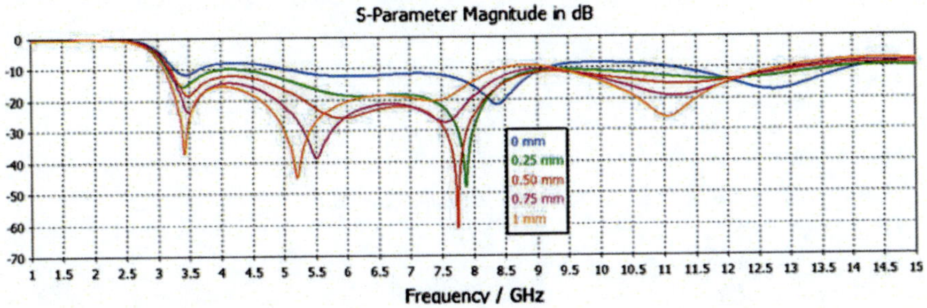

Fig. 4 Simulated return losses for different feed gap values

2. *Effect of feed gap*: It is a key parameter because it provides matching between the wide tapered slot and the feed line. In [5] and [8] effect of the feed gap on antenna, performance has been thoroughly studied. By increasing the coupling between the feed line and wide slot impedance bandwidth can also be increased. For an ideal value of coupling, an ideal impedance bandwidth can also be achieved. But if the coupling further increases from this ideal value it yields poor impedance matching because of over coupling. In Fig. 4, the simulated return losses for different values of the feed gap have been shown.

The influence of the gap '*g*' on the frequency referring to lower part of bandwidth is negligible but on the upper side of bandwidth, it has significant effects. The optimum value $g = 0.5$ mm results largest bandwidth.

4 Result and Discussion

The design, characterization, and optimization of various parameters of this antenna have been done with CST-MWS. It has been fabricated and is under test so we will discuss only simulation-based results. Figure 5 outlined the antenna's bandwidth

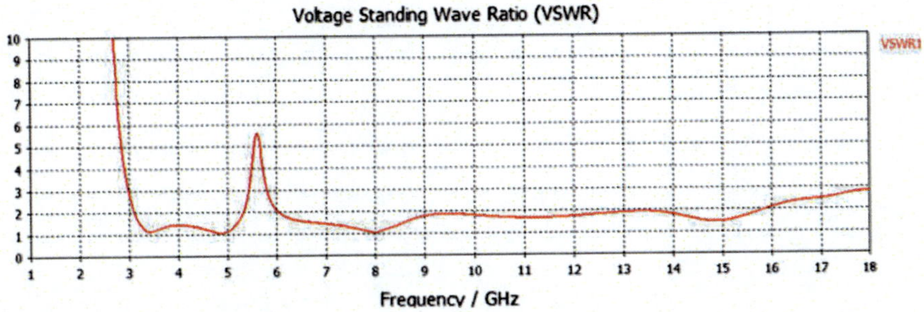

Fig. 5 Simulated VSWR of the proposed antenna

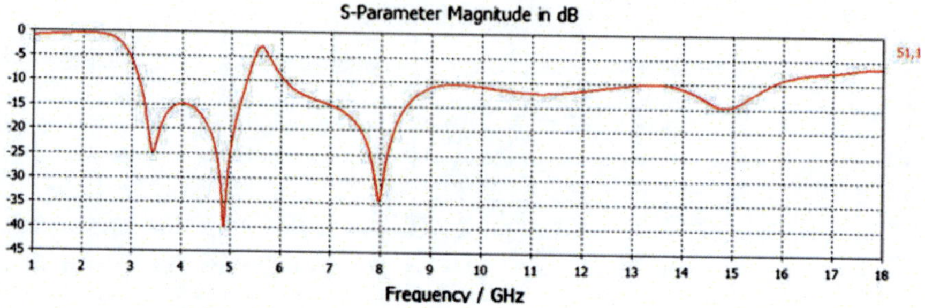

Fig. 6 S11 (Return loss) curve of given antenna

from 3.125 to 15.875 GHz (for VSWR ≤ 2) except for 5.3–6 GHz. The center frequency for this notched band is 5.6 GHz and the maximum value of VSWR is 5.61. Figure 6 shows the S11 curve of the proposed antenna. It gives a wide bandwidth of 3.125–15.750 GHz for $S11 \leq -10$ dB except for 5.3–6 GHz. The $fc = 5.6$ GHz with the maximum value of $S11$ is -3.1 dB has been achieved for the notched band.

Figure 7 shows the simulated co and cross polar-radiation pattern at resonant frequencies of 3.414, 4.86, and 8 GHz. The observed radiation patterns are omnidirectional with very low cross-polarization components.

5 Conclusion

A compact tapered shape wide slot antenna with single band-notched is outlined in this paper. The proposed antenna's prototype has a less complex design with small dimensions of 22×20 mm^2. Simulation results show that the proposed antenna has a frequency span from 3.125 to 15.750 GHz. Also' it has omnidirectional radiation patterns for UWB frequency band. This antenna's prototype has a return loss of −3.1 dB at the center frequency of the notched band which helps to avoid interference with WLAN. Therefore, this antenna can be a good candidate for UWB applications.

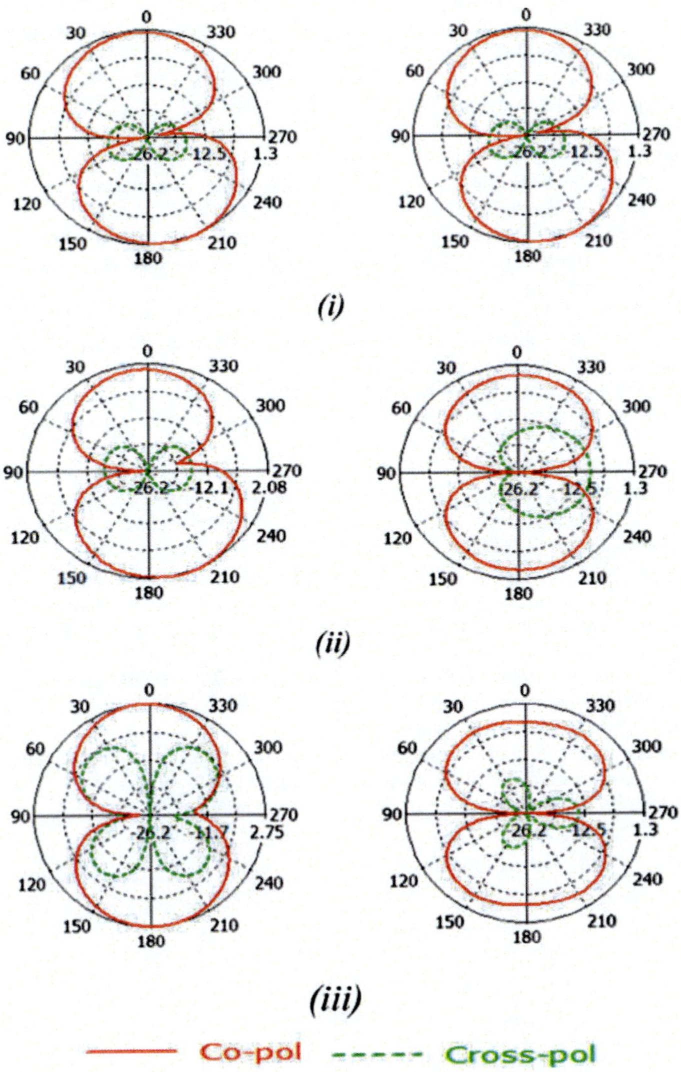

Fig. 7 Co and cross radiation pattern at different frequencies (i) 3.414 GHz (ii) 4.86 GHz (iii) 8 GHz

References

1. Federal Communications Commission (2002) Revision of part 15 of the commission's rules regarding ultra-wideband transmission systems. USA, First Rep. & Order 48-02
2. Lee W-S, Kim K-J, Kim D-Z, Yu J-W (2005) Compact frequency notched wideband planar monopole antenna with an L-shaped ground plane. Microwave Opt Technol Lett 46(4):340–343

3. Singh P, Ray K, Rawat S (2019) Analysis of sun flower shaped monopole antenna. Wirel Pers Commun 104(3):881–894
4. Sze JY, Chang CC (2008) Circularly polarized square slot antenna with a pair of inverted-L grounded strips. IEEE Antennas Wirel Propag Lett 7:149–152
5. Chu QX, Yang Y-Y (2008) A compact ultra wide band antenna with 3.4/5.5 GHz dual band-notched characteristics. IEEE Trans Antennas Propag 56(12):3637–3644
6. Li WT, Shi XW, Hei YQ (2009) Novel planar UWB monopole antenna with triple band-notched characteristics. IEEE Antennas Wirel Propag Lett 8:1094–1098
7. Xiong L, Gao P (2012) Compact ultra-wideband antenna with inverted U-shaped slot and parachute-like radiation patch. International workshop on microwave and millimeter wave systems and technology
8. Kumar V, Kumar S, Gupta B (2014) Performance analysis of Swastika Slot UWB antenna in vicinity of dispersive human layered tissue model. In: IEEE region 10 symposium (TENSYMP 2014), pp 219–223, 14–16 April 2014
9. Kumar V, Gupta B (2014) Swastika Slot UWB antenna for body-worn application in WBAN. In: IEEE 8th international symposium on medical information and communication technology (ISMICT 2014), pp 1–5, 2–4 April 2014
10. Rawat S, Keshwala U, Ray K (2018) Compact design of modified pentagon shaped monopole antenna for UWB applications. Int J Electr Electron Eng Telecommun 7(2):66–69
11. Keshwala U, Rawat S, Ray K (2020) Inverted K-shaped antenna with partial ground for THz applications. Optik 219:165092
12. Singh R, Rathour AS, Kumar V, Seth D, Rawat S, Ray K (2018) Design and analysis of low profile, enhanced bandwidth UWB microstrip patch antenna for body area network. Engineering vibration, communication and information processing. Lecture Notes in Electrical Engineering, vol 478, pp 187–195
13. Singh R, Arora M, Dubey YM, Kumar V, Sahu G (2020) RT/Duroid 5880- based Hook slotted multi frequency low profile patch antenna for WBAN applications. In: Materials today: proceedings, vol 30, Part 1, pp 28–34
14. Toshniwal S, Sharma S, Rawat S, Singh P, Ray K (2016) Compact de- sign of rectangular patch antenna with symmetrical U slots on partial ground for UWB applications. In: Innovations in bio-inspired computing and applications. Springer, Cham, pp 535–542

Isolation Enhancement Using PRSR Technique for Wireless Applications

Manish Deshmukh, Sumit Kumar Gupta, and Akansha Chandravanshi

Abstract This work presents the implementation of parallel rectangular strip resonator (PRSR) in microstrip patch two-element multiple input multiple output (MIMO) antenna for isolation enhancement. PRSR consists of three rectangular strips which are parallel to each other and separated by small distances. The proposed design implemented on FR-4material provides lesser edge-to-edge distance (EtEd) of 3 mm at resonating frequency of 5.14 GHz, and the proposed decoupling structure provides a band stop characteristic over the operating band of 5.05–5.23 GHz. The proposed method helps to improve the antenna parameters. Improved reflection coefficient and isolation obtained is −57.2 dB and −29.4 dB, respectively. Low envelope correlation coefficient (ECC) of less than 0.0005 and diversity gain is of about 10 dB over the operating range. The proposed design is good enough for WIFI, WLAN application.

Keywords Isolation · Edge-to-edge distance (EtEd) · Envelope correlation coefficient (ECC) · Parallel rectangular strip resonator (PRSR) · Multiple input multiple output (MIMO) · Diversity gain (DG)

1 Introduction

Point-to-point communication is considered as the backbone for antennas since they are expected to provide the wireless transmission between devices. Besides being able to achieve good signal to noise ratio and immunity to noise, they should have a compact structure and can be easily constructed and mounted on various devices. Some point- to-point applications that require high performance the weight, size, shape, unit cost, ease of installation are constraints; any antenna is very much required

M. Deshmukh (✉) · S. K. Gupta · A. Chandravanshi
Department of ECE, School of Studies of Engineering & Technology, Guru Ghasidas Vishwavidyalaya Bilaspur (C.G.), Bilaspur, India

S. K. Gupta
e-mail: sgupta@ggu.ac.in

M. S. Kaiser et al. (eds.), *Proceedings of Trends in Electronics and Health Informatics*, Lecture Notes in Networks and Systems 376,
https://doi.org/10.1007/978-981-16-8826-3_50

to meet these needs, so microstrip antenna is preferred [1]. For the requirement of high speed with high quality without any outage issue, it explores the field of multiple input multiple output. MIMO is one of the latest forms of smart antenna technology to improve communication performance [2]. The MIMO antenna system enhance diversity performance while suffers mutual coupling. In the previously published literatures, various technique were explored to enhance the isolation. In the MIMO antenna system [3–9] Sierpinski Knopp fractal geometry loaded with complementary split ring resonator (CSRR) as the radiator, concentric square ring as the radiating patch with CSRR loaded in its ground plane, electromagnetic band gap structure, decoupling array, neutralization line parasitic elements, metamaterials, and defected ground structure (DGS). In order to reduce the mutual coupling normally, the antenna elements are placed farther apart from each other. In paper [10], edge-to-edge distance (EtEd)(mm) is 25 mm to keep isolation performance high by using two port CDRA technique with DGS. In [11], EtEd is 23 mm by adopting parasitic element and DGS. As a result, the size of the structure increased. When working in the compactness of size of the structure, it affects the cost, structure, and fabrication complexity. In paper [12], the decoupling method used neutralization line-based technique by applying metamaterial Rogors RO-4350. Here, the EtEd between the antenna elements is 6mm and isolation is -27 dB at a resonant frequency of 5.15 GHz that increases the cost of manufacturing. In paper [13], metamaterial-based superstrate toward the isolation enhancement of MIMO antenna is initiated, where EtEd is 3.5 mm and isolation is −28 dB at frequency 5.75 GHz, and as we can observe, the cost and structural complexity of the antenna increases.

The proposed 'two-element planer structure antennas' serves additional advantages over the previous studies. This advantage includes

1. This resonator manipulates the current distribution in such a way that it will help to reduce the mutual coupling.
2. Two-elements antenna array is placed in such a way that it aids in achieving high isolation, high diversity gain, low return loss, and low ECC.
3. The unique placement of two-element antennas assists in avoiding the structural complexity.
4. Its uniplanar structure is simple in design, compact in size, and inexpensive. In the present work, the parallel rectangular strip resonator antenna is designed and operated at 4.9–5.25 GHz. For its application in WLAN, WiMAX, Wi-Fi, the parallel rectangular strip resonator is placed between the patches. The placement led to its improved isolation and significantly improved its aforementioned drawbacks.

The research paper presented is structured by introducing MIMO antenna and research areas to improve its performance. Then we discuss the detailed work of proposed MIMO antenna design. In Sect. 2, different stages of antenna design methodology are contributed in the subsequent section. In Sect. 3, the result and discussion of the proposed MIMO antenna is discussed with the various antenna parameters. Section 4 concludes the paper citing the advantages over the similar works that have already been carried out.

2 Antenna Design Methodology

The proposed two-element MIMO antenna is designed in three stages. In the first stage, planar microstrip patch antenna consists of a radiating patch, and the parametric studies have been carried out and optimized to observe better antenna performance. In the next stage, the design is modified to multiple input multiple output (MIMO) for improving the performance of the antenna in terms of antenna diversity performances. Further, 2×1 microstrip patch antennas are taken and placed on a uniquely shaped FR-4 substrate in order to get best isolation between the antenna elements. In the final stage, the technique named PRSR is introduced to improve the antenna performance. In the following subsection, all the stages are discussed in detail.

2.1 *Single Input Single Output Antenna Design*

A microstrip patch antenna is one of most promising antennas nowadays, because of its simplicity in structure. This is a type of printed antenna, in which the antenna patch is printed on an acquired substrate. Microstrip patch antennas find several applications in wireless communication, for example, satellite communication, global positioning satellite (GPS), RFID, mobile communication, etc. The patch is normally made of conducting material such as copper or gold and can take any possible shape. The radiating patch and the feed lines are usually photo etched on the dielectric substrate [14]. For a rectangular patch, the length of the patch L_p is usually $0.3333\lambda o < L_p < 0.5\ \lambda o$, where λo is the free-space wavelength. The patch is selected to be very thin such that $t \ll \lambda o$ (where t is the patch thickness). The height H_s of the dielectric substrate is usually 1.6 mm. The dielectric constant of the substrate (εr) is 4.3. Microstrip patch antennas radiate primarily because of the fringing fields between the patch edge and the ground plane [14]. For good antenna performance, a thick dielectric substrate having a low dielectric constant is necessary since it provides larger bandwidth, better radiation and better efficiency. However, such a typical configuration leads to a larger antenna size. In order to reduce the size of the microstrip patch antenna, substrates with higher dielectric constants must be used which are less efficient and result in narrow bandwidth.

In order to enhance the impedance matching, well below $|S11|<-25$ dB at 5 GHz small variations is initiated in the feed width (W_f) and length of inset (Li) illustrated in Fig. 1. This technique is based on the paper [15] in which feed width is varied for impedance matching and the variation in the length of inset affects the $S1, 1$. The introduced antenna now exhibits $|S11<-10$ dB$|$ bandwidth ranging from 4.8 to 5.0 GHz. With the center frequency of 5 GHz, the $|S11|$ achieved is -59.01 dB. In Fig. 1b, the detailed design dimensions are shown. The optimized dimensions in mm are: $L_s = 27.84$, $W_s = 36.85$, $L_p = 13.92$, W_p=18.42, $W_f = 2.9$, $L_i = 4$, $W_i = 1$.

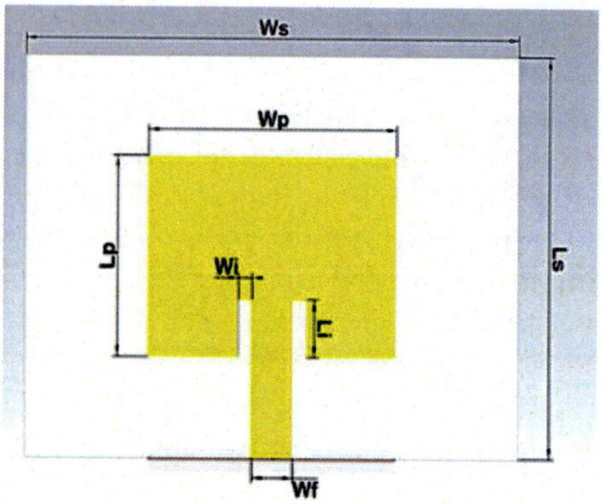

Fig. 1 Single-element microstrip patch antenna

[Note—Here the optimized dimensions means that the antenna is properly designed and analyzed by means of numerical sweeps so the desired *S* parameter could be achieved].

The resonance frequency of the final microstrip patch antenna having patch dimension is calculated using Eqs. (1), (2), (3), (4) given below

$$W_{\mathrm{p}} = \frac{c}{2f\sqrt{\frac{(\varepsilon_{\mathrm{r}}+1)}{2}}} \tag{1}$$

$$\varepsilon_{\mathrm{ref}} = \frac{(\varepsilon_{\mathrm{r}}+1)}{2} + \frac{(\varepsilon_{\mathrm{r}}-1)}{2}\left[1+12\frac{h}{wp}\right]^{\frac{1}{2}} \tag{2}$$

$$\Delta L_{\mathrm{p}} = 0.412h\frac{(\varepsilon_{\mathrm{ref}}+0.3)\left(\frac{w_{\mathrm{p}}}{h}+0.268\right)}{(\varepsilon_{\mathrm{ref}}-0.258)\left(\frac{w_{\mathrm{p}}}{h}+0.8\right)} \tag{3}$$

$$\Delta \mathrm{L}_{\mathrm{p}} = \frac{\lambda_0}{2} - 2\Delta L_{\mathrm{p}} \tag{4}$$

where W_{p} = width of patch, L_{p} = length of patch, f = resonating frequency, εr = dielectric constant (Fig. 2).

2.2 *Array Antenna (Concept of MIMO)*

The concept of MIMO presents a brief introduction to multiple antenna techniques for increasing channel capacity. The MIMO system has some clear benefits over the single-element microstrip patch antenna system and has attracted attention in modern wireless communication systems. The proposed work initiated to improve isolation enhancement and has focused on low cost, low profile, low volume, light in weight and ease to fabrication with maintaining good electrical properties such

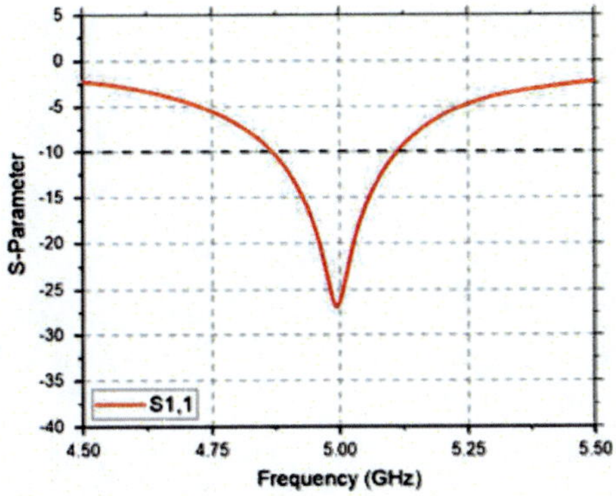

Fig. 2 $S1, 1$ Parameter

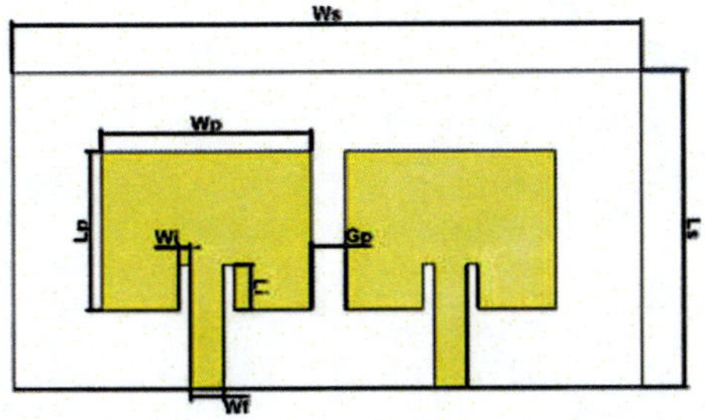

Fig. 3 MIMO antenna without PRSR

as return loss and isolation [16]. High power is transmitted by deploying multiple antennas to achieve an improved mutual coupling, scattering parameter, ECC, and reliability. MIMO antenna systems prefer better isolation between antenna elements and a compact size for application in portable devices [16].

The 20×20 mm^2 microstrip patch antenna is duplicated and placed on a substrate of 55.3×27.8 mm^2 with a separation of 3 mm (0.05λo) between both antenna elements. The reflection coefficient and isolation between the elements of this structure is observed. Both the antennas have a good reflection coefficient of about -26.84 dB but increased mutual coupling of about -12 dB at resonant frequency of 5 GHz. The optimized design and its $|S$-parameters$|$ are depicted in Figs. 3 and 4

2.3 *Parallel Rectangular Strip Resonator (PRSR)*

The parallel rectangular strip resonator (PRSR) technique is introduced in Fig. 5 in order to provide a compact size, high isolation, and ease of integration to the designed antenna with wireless modules. Parallel rectangular strip resonator (PRSR) is implemented between the patches for isolation enhancement. It consists of three parallel rectangular strips separated by a small distance of 0.5 mm. The individual dimensions

Fig. 4 S parameter

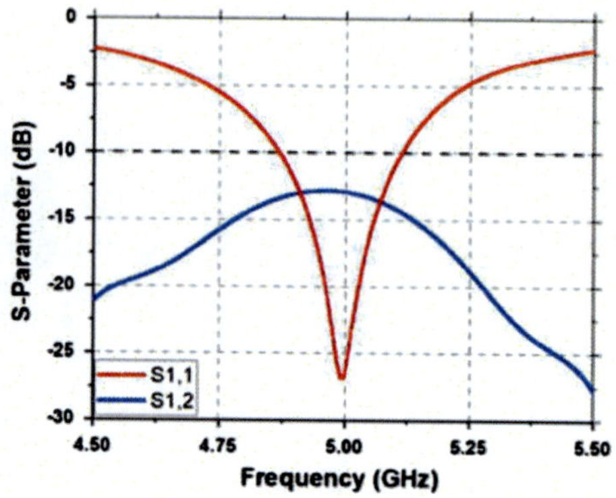

Fig. 5 MIMO antenna with PRSR

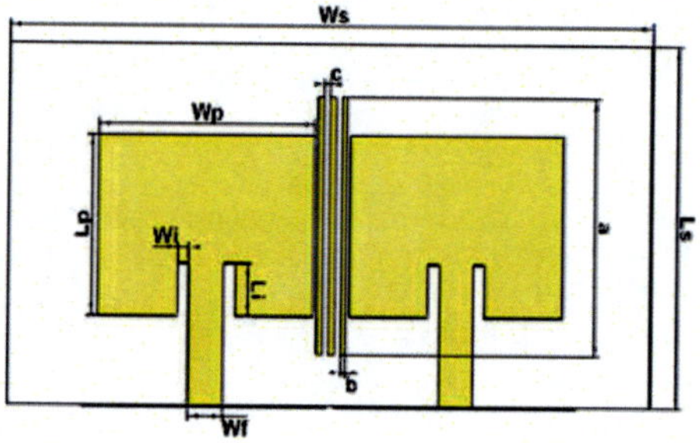

of the following rectangular strips are 19.84 × 0.5 mm. The attempted configuration provides an improved isolation graph depicted in Fig. 6 having return loss of −57.7 dB and isolation of −29.22 dB at the resonating frequency of 5.144 GHz.

Fig. 6 S parameter of MIMO with PRSR

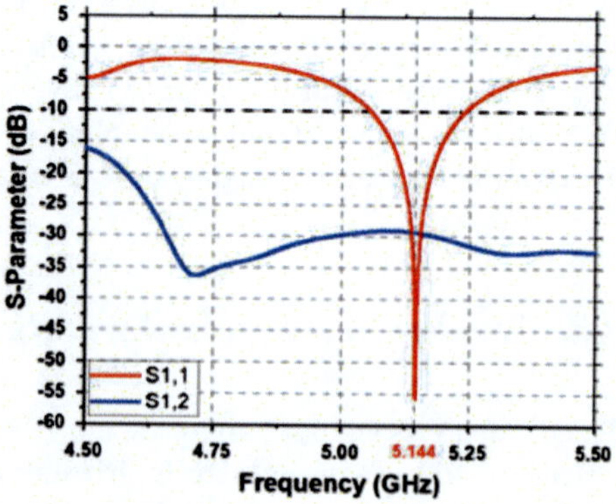

3 Results and Discussions

The reported MIMO antenna system was designed using substrate material FR-4 lossy, and measurements were carried out to validate the antenna efficiency for practical utilization. The simulated S parameters of proposed design PRSR MIMO are shown in Fig. 7. The PRSR MIMO antenna has return loss of −57.7 dB with improved isolation of −29.6 dB at the resonating frequency of 5.144 GHz. The MIMO antenna without PRSR produces a poor return loss of −26.84 and isolation of −12 dB at a resonating frequency of 4.999 GHz. Apart from this, the detailed discussion of evaluated results of the important MIMO parameters like surface current, ECC, DG is discussed in the subsequent section.

3.1 Surface Current

The surface current of MIMO antenna with and without PRSR is shown in Fig. 8. The surface current maximum (A/m) magnitude at ports 1 and 2 is 45.5 dB. The phase of the pattern is 45°.

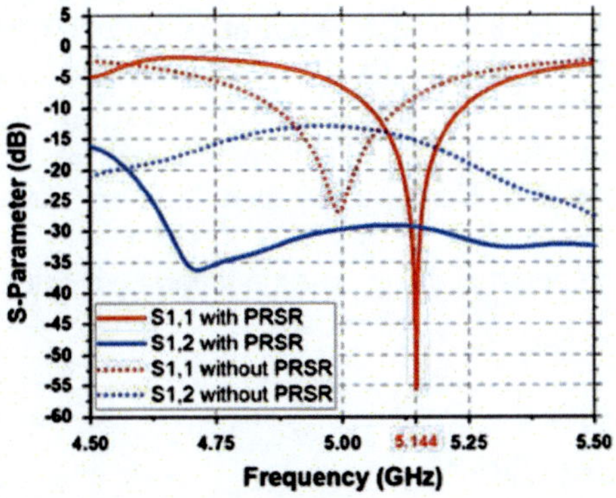

Fig. 7 S parameter with PRSR and without PRSR

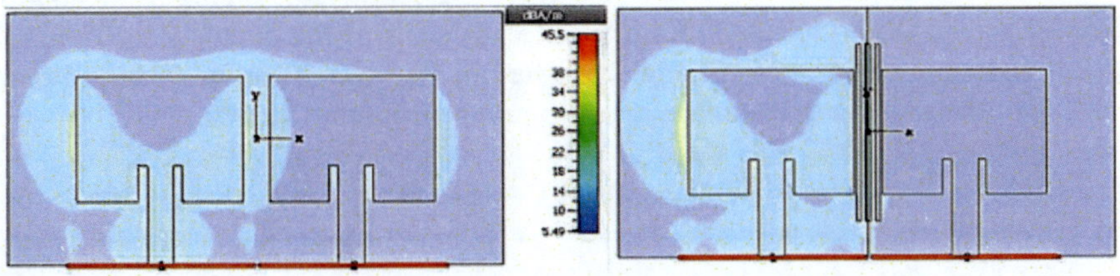

Fig. 8 Surface current of MIMO antenna with PRSR and without PRSR

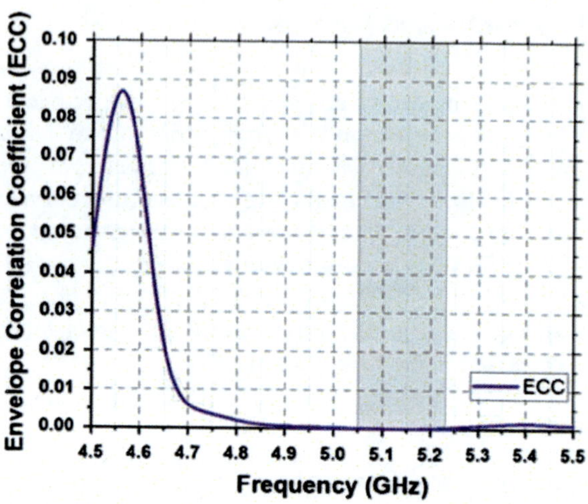

Fig. 9 Envelope correlation constant (ECC)

3.2 *Envelope Correlation Coefficient (ECC)*

ECC is an important diversity performance parameter that describes the isolation and correlation between different antenna elements and how much the radiation pattern in multi antenna systems affect each other when all the ports are working simultaneously [17]. In the presented work, ECC is obtained using *S* parameters; i.e.; ECC is <0.0005 in the whole frequency band from 5.05 to 5.23 GHz, as shown in Fig. 9. The value obtained of ECC is 0.0005 which is very less than its standard value (<0.5). Very low value of ECC shows that there is a very low correlation between the antenna radiators.

In case of ECC computation using far-field parameters, only minute differences are observed [18].

3.3 *Diversity Gain (DG)*

To have good quality and reliability in wireless systems, the DG of the MIMO design has to be high, nearly 10 dB in the operating bandwidth ranging from 5.05 to 5.23 GHz. The DG is calculated from the ECC value using the Eq. (5) [19]. The DG of the discussed MIMO structure is elucidated in Fig. 10b. It can be observed that the DG of the antenna in the entire operating range is around 10 dB.

$$\mathrm{DG} = 10 \times (1 - |\mathrm{ECC}|) \tag{5}$$

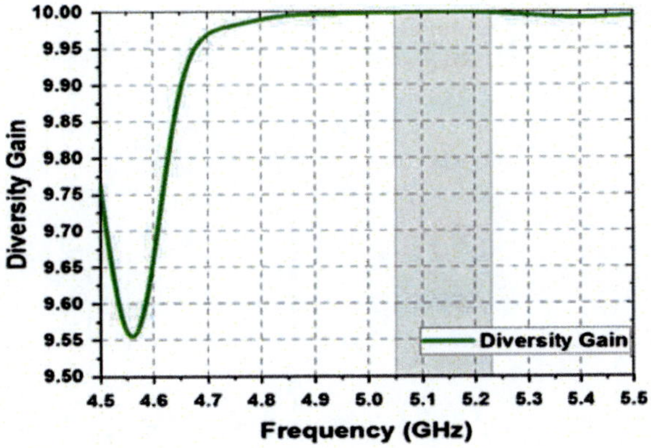

Fig. 10 Diversity gain

4 Conclusion

In this proposed work, analysis and design of two-element MIMO antennas is taken into consideration and comparison with previously published work is shown in the Table 1 which represent the improvement in isolation with other parameters. The main purpose of using PRSR technique is to obtain high mutual coupling reduction and makes the extension of the antenna elements much easier by keeping minimum edge-to-edge distance. It can be easily extended to have a four- and eight-element MIMO design. The MIMO antenna is developed from analyzing a single-element microstrip patch antenna to two-element designs. Considering the ECC and measured isolation between the antenna elements, it can be concluded that the MIMO design has a good separation between the antenna elements as the ECC is well below 0.0005, and the final outcome obtained in peak enhanced isolation is −29.22 dB. Its operating bandwidth ranging from 5.05 to 5.23 GHz increases the data rate which further benefits the MIMO system. The obtained result with isolation enhancement shows that the proposed MIMO antenna system can work well in WLAN applications with high data rate and also shows good diversity performance.

Table 1 Comparative analysis of the proposed structure with some similar antennas

References	Dim. (mm^2)	Reso. frequency (GHz)	EtEd* (mm)	Isolation (dB)	S11 (dB)	No. of port	ECC	C.S.#	Material
[20]	**3200**	3.5	6	−40	−20.1	2	No	Yes	FR-4
[21]	2800	2.55	15.58	−44	−23.5	2	No	Yes	FR-4
[22]	1824	5.75	3.5	−28	−20	2	<0.025	Yes	RT/Duroid 5870
[23]	11,025	5.25	7.4	−28	−44	2	<0.0022	Yes	Rogers RO400C
[14]	4200	5.7	3	−41	−22	4	<0.003	Yes	RT/Duroid 5870
[24]	7200	0.75–7.65	–	<−12	−37	5	<0.243	No	RO-4350
[25]	5625	5.7	–	−15	−41	4	<0.04	No	FR-4
[26]	16,800	2.4, 2.6	–	−12	−20, −25	4	<0.0.08, <0.07	No	FR-4
Pro- posed work	**1500**	**5.14**	**3**	**−29.22**	**−57.7**	**2**	**<0.0005**	**No**	**FR-4**

(EtEd*—Edge-to-edge distance, C.S.#—Complexity of structure)

References

1. Balanis CA, Ioannides PI (2007) Introduction to smart antennas. United States: Morgan & Claypool Publishers
2. Sharawi MS (2013) Printed multi-band MIMO antenna systems and their performance metrics. IEEE Antennas Propag Mag 55(5):218–232. https://doi.org/10.1109/MAP.2013.6735522
3. Rajkumar S, Selvan KT, Rao PH (2018) Compact 4 element Sierpinski Knopp fractal UWB MIMO antenna with dual band notch. Microw Opt Technol Lett 60(4):1023–1030
4. Ramachandran A et al (2015) A four-port MIMO antenna using concentric square-ring patches loaded with CSRR for high isolation. IEEE Antennas Wirel Propag Lett 15:1196–1199
5. KSL Parvathi SR Gupta 2021 Novel dual-band EBG structure to reduce mutual coupling of air gapbased MIMO antenna for 5G application AEU-Int J Electron C 138 153902 https://doi.org/10.1016/j.aeue.2021.153902
6. Kadu M, Rayavarapu N (2021) Compact stack EBG structure for enhanced isolation between stack patch antenna array elements for MIMO application. Int J Microwave Wirel Technol 13(8):817–825. https://doi.org/10.1017/S1759078720001543
7. Jiang W, Cui Y, Liu B, Hu W, Xi Y (2019) A dual-band MIMO antenna with enhanced isolation for 5G smartphone applications. IEEE Access 7:112554–112563. https://doi.org/10.1109/ACCESS.2019.2934892
8. Shiddanagouda FB, Vani RM, Hunagund PV (2020) Miniaturized dual-band printed MIMO antenna with DGS for L-band and C-band wireless applications. In: 2020 IEEE international conference on communication, networks and satellite (Comnetsat), pp 111–116. https://doi.org/10.1109/Comnetsat50391.2020.9328996
9. Yon H, Aris MA, Abd Rahman NH, Nasir NAM, Jumaat H (2019) A design of decoupling structure MIMO antenna for mutual coupling reduction in 5G application. In: 2019 international symposium on antennas and propagation (ISAP), pp 1–3
10. Divya G, Jagadeesh Babu K, Madhu R (2021) Quad-band hybrid DRA loaded MIMO antenna with DGS for isolation enhancement. Int J Microw Wirel Technol 1–10. https://doi.org/10.1017/S1759078721000519
11. Peng H, Zhi R, Yang Q, Cai J, Wan Y, Liu G (2021) Design of a MIMO antenna with high gain and enhanced isolation for WLAN applications. Electronics 10(14):1659. https://doi.org/10.3390/electronics10141659.
12. Li M, Jiang L, Yeung KL (2020) A general and systematic method to design neutralization lines for isolation enhancement in MIMO antenna arrays. IEEE Trans Veh Technol 69(6):6242–6253. https://doi.org/10.1109/TVT.2020.2984044
13. Behera SK (2007) Novel tuned rectangular patch antenna as a load for phase power combining. Ph.D. thesis, Jadavpur University, Kolkata
14. Mark R, Rajak N, Mandal K, Das S (2019) Metamaterial based superstrate towards the isolation and gain enhancement of MIMO antenna for WLAN application. EU Int J Electron Commun 100:144–152. ISSN 1434-8411, doi.org/https://doi.org/10.1016/j.aeue.2019.01.011.
15. Tahir N, Brooker G (2011) A novel approach of feeding, impedance matching and frequency tuning of microstrip patch antenna by single microstrip line. In: IEEE symposium on industrial electronics and applications, pp 593–597. https://doi.org/10.1109/ISIEA.2011.6108784
16. Manuel Prasanna K (2013) Design and analysis of two port MIMO antennas with wideband isolation. Department of Electronics and Communication Engineering National Institute of Technology Rourkela
17. Sharma A, Biswas A (2017) Wideband multiple-input–multiple-output dielectric resonator antenna. IET Microwaves Antennas Propag 11(4):496–502. https://doi.org/10.1049/iet-map.2016.0515
18. Thaysen J, Jakobsen KB (2006) Envelope correlation in (N, N) MIMO antenna array from scattering parameters. Microw Opt Technol Lett 48(5):832–834
19. Kumari T, Das G, Sharma A, Gangwar RK (2019) Design approach for dual element hybrid MIMO antenna arrangement for wideband applications. Int J RF Microwa Comput Aided Eng 29(1):e21486

20. Vishvaksenan KS, Mithra K, Kalaiarasan R, Raj KS (2017) Mutual coupling reduction in microstrip patch antenna arrays using parallel coupled-line resonators. IEEE Ant Wirel Propag Lett 16:2146–2149
21. Jiao T, Jiang T, Li Y (2017) A low mutual coupling MIMO antenna using 3-D electromagnetic isolation wall structures. In: Sixth Asia-Pacific conference on antennas and propagation (APCAP), pp 1–2. https://doi.org/10.1109/APCAP.2017.8420496
22. Mark R, Singh HV, Mandal K, Das S (2019) Reduced edge-to-edge spaced MIMO antenna using parallel coupled line resonator for WLAN applications. Microw Opt Technol Lett 61. https://doi.org/10.1002/mop.31911
23. Hassan T, Khan MU, Attia H et al (2018) An FSS based correlation reduction technique for MIMO antennas. IEEE Trans Antennas Propag 66(9):4900–4905. https://doi.org/10.1109/TAP.2018.2842256
24. Hussain R, Sharawi MS, Shamim A (2018) An integrated four-element slot-based MIMO and a UWB sensing antenna system for CR platforms. IEEE Trans Antennas Propag 66(2):978–983
25. Chouhan, S., & Malviya, L. (2020). Four-port shared rectangular radiator with defected ground for wireless application. International Journal of Communication Systems, 33(9), e4356.
26. MoradiKordalivand A, Rahman TA, Khalily M (2014) Common elements wideband MIMO antenna system for WiFi/LTE access-point applications. IEEE Antennas and Wire- less Propagation Letters 13:1601–1604

Review on a Full-Duplex Cognitive Radio Network Based on Energy Harvesting

Vikas Srivastava and Parulpreet Singh

Abstract Full-duplex (FD) interaction gets anticipated to double spectrum efficiency (SE) with either the growth of self-interference repression methods. The secondary users (sus) may concurrently carry out range signaling and data transfer in cognitive radio (CR) which is FD-based, to attain better detecting quality and higher SU utilization. Recently, another primary performance metric in wireless devices of fifth-generation (5G), excellent efficiency toward energy (EE), may have fascinated increasing attention. An RF energy harvesting (EH) method is planned to extend the battery life of small-power communications appliances. All over the paper, the energy planting complete duplex CR is being talked about.

Keywords Full duplex · Cognitive radio · IoT · Spectrum sensing · Energy harvesting · Spectrum sensing

1 Introduction

A spectrum efficiency (SE) requires to get enhanced in future 5G Wi-Fi networks to achieve sharply increasing data rates [1]. The Time division duplex (TDD) or Frequency division duplex (FDD) methods are using the process of half-duplex (HD), which has intrinsic low. Full-duplex (FD) procedure, in which intelligent devices can convey or receive data that use frequency resources and the identical timeframe, has enormous potential that would twofold the system's capability, in turn enhancing the Wi-Fi network's available SE [2].

Energy efficiency (EE), a further essential quality metric in 5G Wi-Fi networks, has drawn considerable attention over the last few years [3]. Various other researches were dedicated to enhancing the EE, like researching energy-efficient methods, using

V. Srivastava (✉) · P. Singh
Lovely Professional University Jalandhar, Jalandhar, India

V. Srivastava
Pranveer Singh Institute of Technology, Kanpur, India

M. S. Kaiser et al. (eds.), *Proceedings of Trends in Electronics and Health Informatics*, Lecture Notes in Networks and Systems 376,
https://doi.org/10.1007/978-981-16-8826-3_51

renewable energy sources, designing the network procedures, making it energy-aware, and so on [4]. Frequent new battery for one device is always expensive in many commercial applications. Wireless transmission systems to the future, the technique of energy harvesting (EH) is used to power communications devices using green energy like polar, wind, etc. [5]. Radiofrequency (RF) electricity harvested could be utilized for small-power communications devices.

An efficient way is a Cognitive radio (CR) to increase the SE [6]. In a CR scheme, unauthorized users, often known as secondary users (sus), may opportunistically use the licensed spectrum underneath the constraint of intervention with primary users (PU's) are limited to a manageable level. Spectrum signaling is key to CR [7]. In interface mode, data could be transmitted by the sus to the pus identified to be unavailable. FD spectrum sensing can be seen as an efficient method for improving a cognitive radio station system [4]. The tertiary users may simultaneously perform spectrum sensing or data transfer throughout the CR network based on FD. However, the efficiency gets degraded through which it senses self-interference (SI) because all its data transmission can interfere with the received transmitter from the PU of the SU. Digital Interference Cancelation or Antenna Cancelation methods could decrease interference to a signal obtained from PU by the SU. Throughout, the researchers considered the "LAT (listen-and-talk)" protocol to CR and examined LAT-based cooperative range sensing efficiency. Secondary power transmitting becomes optimum to increase the LAT-based CR channel efficiency. The FD spectrum sensing scheme has been proposed in [4] to SU in a multichannel CR system. A protocol for FD cognitive gets examined by media access control (MAC).

The SU's can use either yield energy with the help of the primary signal or just by utilizing the PU's range for data. Cognitive radio related to energy harvesting should enhance EE and SE. In [8], secondary consumers can collect power to the ambient environment from either the PU's natural resources or RF transmissions. The effect of the allocation strategy of power investigated PU's latency and SU's throughput. A 2-D range or strategy of power sensing becomes planned in [9] to enhance the tracking performance and the primary communication power level, which may also get estimated. The quality gain for either the energy harvesting CR network has been achieved through considering the control dimension. Authors regarded a multichannel situation in [9]. The channel choice probability gets designed to optimize the SU throughput through harvesting enough energy or finding adequate opportunities for access to a spectrum.

Since the birth of first-generation (1G) digital communication system, work, lifestyle, or growth trends of different sectors have also been deeply affected. This generation has brought a drastic change in the lifestyle of the people. A fifth-generation (5G) digital communication system is created to cope more efficiently with rapid growth for mobile data traffic, massive connection for devices, the constant development of a novel trade, or even a new future for the application. The main driving force for 5G growth becomes the mobile Internet and also the Internet of Things (IoT). Future 5G not only meets a person's diverse needs in different regions. A true interdependence, like residence, function, leisure, or transportation, with

IoT, can permeate and meet various academic fields like industry, pharmaceutical, transport, and other industries.

With the rapid growth of wireless broadband exposure or terminal tech, the public gets curious about the details or facilities from the Web. In the process of switching at any time, the mobile Internet has also been rapidly created. The main objective was toward public-centric communication, which focuses on offering a great experience. It is forecasted that the demand for communication applications like remote locations, crowded stadiums, or high-speed rail can also be increasingly higher shortly. Thus to meet such kinds of demands, 5G plays an important role.

As one of the most promising innovations, the IoT is obtaining increasing publicity from either the academic or manufacturing circles [9, 10, but get regarded as the essential technology which leads to significant network evolution [11]. The concept for IoT was first proposed by the MIT teacher Kevin Ashton and his friends in 1999. They advocated a successful combination of radiofrequency identification (RFID) tech of Communications technology and afterward identifying or managing product details via the Internet. Its main trick is to create object recognition, sensor systems, interactions among the people, and the Internet, one channel that connects both those objects [11], which are into interactions with the people and get varied details about them all over the place. IoT can communicate almost everything to the Internet. It's excellent for the fast development with reasonable tiny sensors, omnipresent network, well-organized computes, or data management. According to Approach Analytics [10], almost 12 billion web-connected appliances were used internationally until 2014. That is for each person comparable to 1.7 devices. As seen, through 2020, 33 billion systems, such as machine-to-machine (M2M), valuable objects, smartphones, computers, intelligent grids, intelligent home tablets, or wearable devices, are in use [11]. The IoT can penetrate all levels of an economy with the growth of information systems, such as intelligent transportation, protecting the environment, public security, home automation, smart firefighting, manufacturing monitoring, long-term care, health, water system tracking, food traceability, recognition, and intelligent collecting. It makes the work easier and sufficient [12] (Fig. 1).

Mobile Internet may have subverted a traditional telecommunication service model and given users unparalleled knowledge. IoT integrates a physical world and the digital world, and via better connectivity or functionality impacts people's behavior or lifestyle. Due to the fast expansion of portable IoT, a 5G scheme can face new criteria or challenges throughout the four application situations for high coverage areas with great capacity and efficient connectivity, as described throughout the table below. Moreover, these new necessities are not available in 4G or pre-generation technologies. The system will dramatically happen to look for the challenges which arose due to extraordinary performance measures in various situations, like new spectrum discovery, use of dynamic spectrum, or higher energy efficiency (Fig. 2).

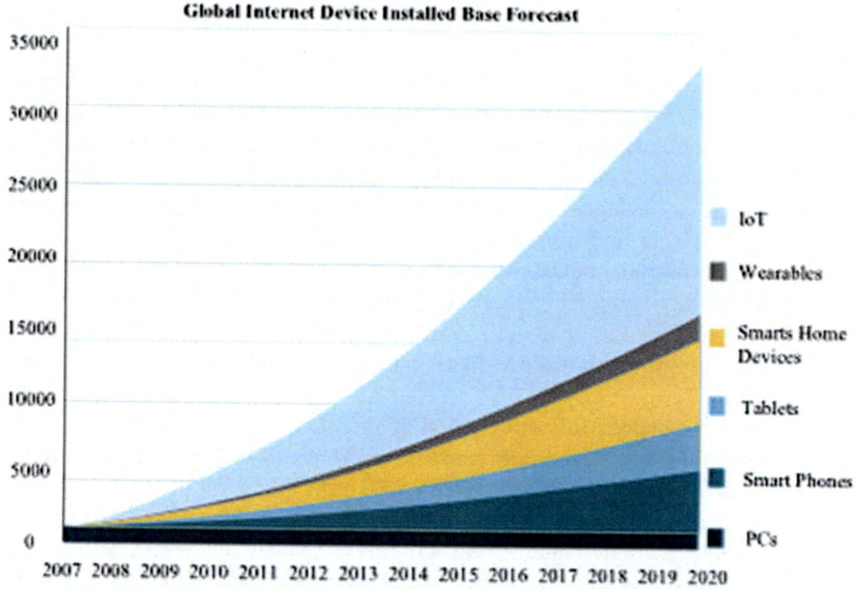

Fig. 1 The IoT and connected devices in 2020 [8]

Fig. 2 The network changes radically in 5G

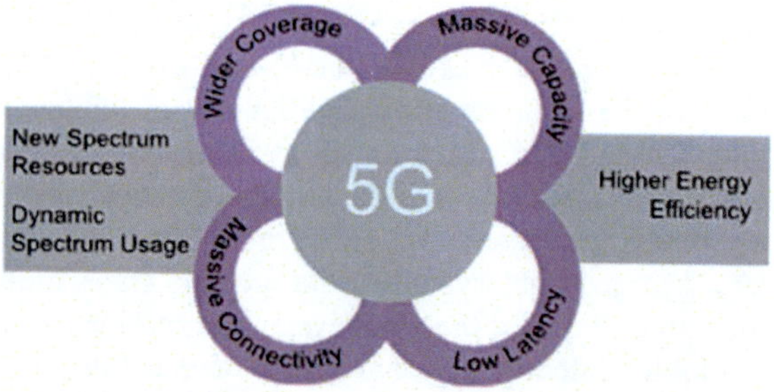

1.1 New Spectrum Exploration

There needs to be a considerable volume for intelligent terminal internet access all over the future. Hence, a data level gathered by IoT is comparatively larger compared to the collected data by mobile interaction to people-to-people communication [12]. Additionally, information about device/user, forwarding, or control gets conducted through bands of a mobile communication network [13] and the Industrial Scientific Medical (ISM). Although the non-licensed signal bands were the band's ISM (such as RFID, Zigbee, NFC, Wireless, Bluetooth, or UWB, etc.), devices may need them for free. Also, ISM bands are more congested as IoT apps rise. For the mobile technology bands (such as 2G, 3G, or 4G networks), the spectrum prerequisite or allocation depends on the objectives of people-to-people interaction. It does not consider the traffic model for human-to-human communication or interaction around things [14]. The result could lead to congestion in the network or unequal allocation of resources. Consequently, a mechanism for variable allocation of the spectrum could not satisfy the increasing demand for the resources from different appliances. When less significance is given to such problems, the shortage of a range would, in the future, be an insurmountable bottleneck to 5G growth.

1.2 Dynamic Spectrum Usage

With the rapid development of IoT customers and connectors, significant challenges face infrastructure and the network framework. Additionally, the device's operating systems conduct the tasks of receiving, processing, and forwarding data throughout the current TCP/IP protocol [15].

1.3 Higher Energy Efficiency

As IoT continues to evolve, there has to be a vast network that links the various aspects of people's lives. Generally speaking, IoT devices were battery-powered, or battery configuration, maintenance, or replacement was complex and costly [16]. Moreover, these systems are sometimes placed in regions challenging to reach or unavailable in some industrial machinery. Energy efficiency is indeed crucial in the face of such unique apps. The optimal electricity leadership algorithm should get intended to understand the lengthy-running or regular operation for devices with a view of the characteristic of IoT devices. With the advancements of the CR, technology has viewed a very effective way of coping with spectrum scarcity or common usage issues, which get dynamically re-using frequencies allocated to get registered users and appear to become the best output for both the difficulties and necessities 5G system. The research community has given a great deal of attention to CR themes. Many aspects from various conventional sensing techniques and collaborative sensing ways are outlined in [17], with the basis for giving space and transmission opportunities to multi-dimensional radio subsets. To meet the requirements of cognitive customers to find the spectrum opportunities over a vast range of frequencies efficiently [18], summed up multiple spectra of wideband sensing procedures or discussed the merits and demerits for every algorithm or their various other issues. [19] A survey was done of the same art of allotment of resources algorithms to underlie the arms (cognitive radio networks) onto the criteria of the procedures, methods, or network interfaces adopted. Based on the optimization criteria, [20] given an overview for recent developments in the allocation for radio resources in CRNS; such allocation schemes were summarized onto the basis for performance optimization criteria such as power consumption, maximization all over, QoS certainty, interference minimization, fairness as well as a priority concern and reduction of hand-offs. Reference [21] provided an updated spectrum judgment survey predicated on spectrum characterization or CR reconfiguration in CRNS. In [21], overlay spectrum access programs get reviewed throughout the cooperative CRNS and the overlay-based CRNS non-cooperative or cooperative game template. The idea for dynamic spectrum exchanging was studied, or other spectrum giving out scenarios investigated of distinct topologies of network, characteristics, or likely use cases. Thus IoT serves many objectives for the industries and proves to be a successful technology.

A paper pattern is as follows: Sect. 2 gives information about RF energy harvesting, Sect. 3 describes half duplex cognitive radio network with energy harvesting. Section 4 describes a full duplex cognitive radio network with energy harvesting. Section 5 gives information about related work. Section 6 is conclusion.

2 RF Energy Harvesting

Energy is one of the fundamental elements in the twenty-first century. Energy cannot be created nor destroyed. It is always converted. But wasted energy is everywhere. We need to find them, convert them (harvesting), transfer them into electrical energy, store them when not used, and recall them when needed. Gathering energy from the natural ambient environment and converting it into usable electrical energy is called energy harvesting. Energy harvesting is essential in reducing dependency on batteries or cells, the need for an energy source for the electronic system, and the self-powered remotely operated sensor network. There are different energy harvesting sources like light/solar, kinetic mechanical, thermal and RF electromagnetic with 60 mW, 20 mW, 0.52 mW and 0.0015 mW harvesting power, respectively. RF energy can be broadcast by billions of equipment, including mobile phones, handheld radios, mobile base stations, Wi-Fi, Wi-Max, and television broadcast stations. With these RF sources, there is a lot of RF energy existing in the environment. Since RF energy is available all time and everywhere, the RF energy harvesting technique would be a good point for a cognitive radio network. Nikol Tesla said, "RF energy is free energy and broadcasts electrical energy without wires. The frequency range of radiofrequency electromagnetic waves is 0.088 GHz to 29.5 GHz. So, an RF energy harvesting system is a system that converts RF energy into electrical energy [22].

The formula for receiving power is found in the FRIIS equation:

$$P_r = \frac{P_t G_t G_r \lambda^2}{4\pi R^2}$$

where P_r is power at receiving antenna, P_t is output power of transmitting antenna, G_t is a gain of transmitting antenna, G_r is a gain of receiving antenna, λ is wavelength, and R is the distance between 2 antennas (Fig. 3).

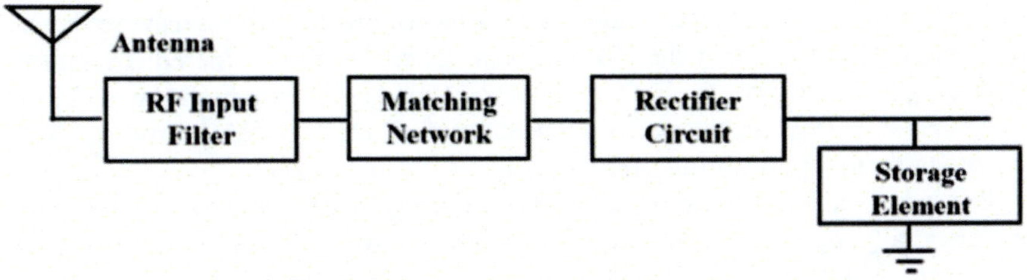

Fig. 3 RF energy harvesting module

The RF energy harvesting system comprises an antenna, RF filter, matched network, rectifier circuit, and storage device. The antenna is a front end element used to capture RF energy from the surrounding atmosphere. A matching circuit is used to transport the maximum receiver power from the antenna to the rectifier circuit, and rectifier circuits convert received RF energy into direct current. The advantage of RF energy harvesting is that it utilizes freely available energy, increases the battery lifetime, predicts input power at the receiver terminal, and harvests power over distance. The disadvantage is that free space path loss is high and has low power density.

3 Half-Duplex Cognitive Radio Network with Energy Harvesting

Owing to the need for higher bandwidth rates for wireless communications caused by the lack of frequency space, the quality of spectrum use needs to be somehow increased [23]. As a result, the wireless technology group plans to develop full-duplex (F-D) communications to enable simultaneous broadcasting and transmission in a single time/range of frequencies, which is projected to increase spatial use performance by a factor of two relatives to H-D communication. Nonetheless, one of the main problems for F-D transmission is minimizing the heavy impact of self-interference and the signal-to-noise ratio (SNR) on both antennas. Therefore, various literature studies have been performed that rely on creating a self-interference cancelation strategy, as shown by Zhang et al. [23], Kim et al. [24], and the references therein. Several researchers have already shown the effectiveness of F-D connectivity in practical applications. Practically, the effect of self-interference on hardware imperfections cannot be fully suppressed; thus, the efficiency of F-D communications depends directly on the suppression factor of self-interference, the channel gain between the communication systems, and the transmitting capacity of both transmitters. Even before working in pseudo-line-of-sight (non-LOS) dwindling networks, the F-D transmitting code of conduct can surpass its H-D counterpart whenever the channel obtains between the communications devices is significant. Unless the channel boost exacerbates, the signals transmitted from the self-interference link overtake transmitted signal of value that has a crucial impact on the F-D link power

[25]. In these cases, the F-D transmitting protocol can not necessarily be the suitable alternative, and hence the H-D protocols must also be considered. Therefore, a switching pattern in both the H-D protocol and the F-D protocol should be established to dynamically leverage the maximum benefits of both H-D and F-D communications by changing the transmitting process [26].

Moreover, in the meantime, the need for wireless communications has grown exponentially, opening up the capacity for modern and effective radio communications networks focused on complex spectrum connectivity and contributing to the idea of cognitive radio (CR) [27]. CR was deemed a feasible solution to spectrum depletion by giving cognitive consumers (CU) timely access to empty approved channels (or main channels). In addition, this is from a study published in the journal, C R-powered energy-harvesting networks (CRN)s have been extensively researched and deployed at various implementation rates. Notwithstanding various attempts to increase energy-production efficiency, the production rate is currently low, and more effort needs to be done in the future [28].

4 Full-Duplex Cognitive Radio Network in Energy Harvesting

Zhang, along with others (2017) had designed a new specification for mutual spectrum allocation for the program under consideration. With its F-D functionality, the proposed protocol would allow the hybrid access protocol (HAP) to receive a signal from the PT and transmit bearings of energy, either to load simultaneous ST or to forward signal from the PT and receive signals from the ST simultaneously. Numerical findings are provided to verify our theoretical study and prove its non-cooperative portion of the proposed protocol [29].

A sub lay of a CRN, which involves a pair of primary nodes, a few secondary nodes, and a wave giver, is considered by Lei and Qaraqe (2016), where the secondary transmitter is powered by renewable energy obtained from the primary transmitter to increase both energy efficiency and spectral quality. The closed-form definitions for correct and asymptotic confidentiality are obtained. Simulations of Monte-Carlo are conducted to show the exactness of the performance. The study reveals that the OAS system is above the SAS system. However, the asymptotic results show that the OAS and SAS schemes may be in the same order of secrecy complexity regardless of which scheme is called. This paper explores the application of the methodology for energy collection (EH) [30].

Chatterjee, Bhowmick, and Verma (2019) have a systematic duplex (FD) cognitive radio network. DF relay technology enables information to flow through a primary user channel (PU), which has been activated by the cognitive radio (CR), the source to the completion node (destination). The efficiency of other parameters has been studied, such as energy transfer configuration, power stream time variable, time monitoring, etc. [31].

A new wireless networking paradigm that boosts spectrum efficiency (SE) and energy efficiency (EE) will be built in Aldhabhani & Alhatmi (2019) with Full-Duplex Energy Harvesting Cognitive Radio Networks (FD EHCRNs). This is a mixture of Full-Duplex Technologies, CR, and RF (Radio Frequency) energy harvesting. FD helps cognitive users to conduct spectrum detection, data transfer, and energy extraction concurrently with the energy harvesting cognitive radio networks (EH-CRN) devices. Consequently, full duplexes in EH CRNs can overcome conventional CRNs' spectrum loss and discontinuing transmission problems. Throughout this publication, a new FD EHCRN proposal model focuses on designing thresholds for identification and the energy harvest model to improve device performance. This journal aims to update the current EHCRN, introducing a new paradigm for spectrum sensing with only two antennas, using full-duplex [32].

5 Related Work

Recently, significant studies have been carried out in FD communications; here, we review the critical articles. To our suggested framework, the first and most important research in the literature focuses on the study of wireless F-D communication's efficiency in comparison with HD counterparts.

In terms [33] of achievable efficiency, they are contrasting the performance of the F-D and H-D transmission protocol. The efficiency for F-D/HD-D2D hybrid communications is studied, and an empirical structure for a [34] D2D-active hybrid duplex network can be monitored. The two devices are often presumed to be the same. The spectrum output goal, expressed as a per-square unit normalized feasible rate. The authors proposed and addressed the issue based on the POMDP Model, emphasizing secondary output, and then analyzed the improvement in efficiency with specific framework parameters. However, in this work, no consideration was given to F-D transmission mode and non-LOS fading interface [35].

Author suggests a scheme for allocating resources to support unmanned aerial vehicles (UAV) networks. The main objective is only to optimize the average UAV network performance. Eventually, the researchers provide a view of the UAV-funded ultra-dense networks (UDNs), demonstrate the broad applications and effective power management in UAV-funded UDNs in networking, cache, and energy transfer. The writers often speak about the prevailing technological problems and available problems in the future [36].

Briefly, works in literature have focused on networks and applications driven by energy harvesting. The latter schemes should then use the greedy algorithm in which transmitter devices attempt to optimize transmitting capacity and determine their associated transmission protocols (H-D or F-D) to increase the imminent output of the current transmission only, without any possible gain being taken into account. The suggested regime would investigate whether the F-D/H-D mode switching schedule can be mutually balanced and the transmission energy assignment for each transmission protocol is upheld [37]. Nasser et al. [38] developed OFDM-based full-duplex CRNs. OFDM-based Full-Duplex Cognitive Radio (FD-CR) was suggested in this paper for Transmitting-Receiving-Sensing (TRS). Subhankar et al. [39]. In an energy harvesting (EH) cooperative cognitive radio network (CCRN), this paper addresses Energy Efficiency (EE) and Spectrum Efficiency (SE) trade-off. Pranabesh et al. [40] performed spectrum sensing in CRN-based on the secrecy and throughput performance.

6 Conclusion

This paper explores the full-duplex cerebral radio with RF energy recovery. Spectrum detection and data transfer can be carried out simultaneously by the secondary transmitter using F-D technologies. There are two types of energy extraction: primary signal RF energy and self-recycled energy from SU. The FD-based CR device has been studied to improve energy efficiency. Both sensing speeds and the transmission capacity of the ST are designed together to increase the EE to ensure sufficient safety of the PU. Furthermore, the balance between energy conservation and bandwidth quality remains.

References

1. Cheng W, Zhang H, Liang L, Jing H, Li Z (2018) Orbital-angular-momentum embedded massive MIMO: achieving multiplicative spectrum-effciency for mmWave communication. IEEE Access 6:2732–2745
2. Towhidlou V, Shikh-Bahaei M (2018) Adaptive full-duplex communications in cognitive radio networks. IEEE Trans Veh Technol 67(9):8386–8395
3. Amjad M, Akhtar F, Rehmani MH, Reisslein M, Umer T (2017) Full-duplex communication in cognitive radio networks: a survey. IEEE Commun Surv Tutorials 19(4):2158–2191
4. Cheng W, Zhang X, Zhang H (2015) Full-duplex spectrum-sensing and MAC-protocol for multichannel nontime-slotted cognitive radio networks. IEEE J Sel Areas Commun 33(5):820–831
5. Sharma SK, Bogale TE, Le LB, Chatzinotas S, Wang X, Ottersten B (2018) Dynamic spectrum sharing in 5G wireless networks with full-duplex technology: recent advances and research challenges. IEEE Commun Surv Tutorials 20(1):674–707
6. Bayat A, Aissa S (2018) Full-duplex cognitive radio with asynchronous energy-effcient sensing. IEEE Trans Wirel Commun 17(2):1066–1080
7. Liao Y, Wang T, Song L, Jiao B (2014) Cooperative spectrum sensing for full-duplex cognitive radio networks. In: Proceeding of IEEE international conference on communication systems, pp 56–60
8. Shi Z, Teh KC, Li KH (2013) Energy-effcient joint design of sensing and transmission durations for protection of primary user in cognitive radio systems. IEEE Commun Lett 17(3):565–568
9. Pratibha M, Li KH, Teh KC (2016) Channel selection in multichannel cognitive radio systems employing RF energy harvesting. IEEE Trans Veh Technol 65(1):457–462

10. Agiwal M, Roy A, Saxena N (2016) Next generation 5G wireless networks: a comprehensive survey. IEEE Commun Surv Tutorial 18:1617–1655
11. Ghanbari A, Laya A, Alonso-Zarate J, Markendahl J (2017) Business development in the Internet of Things: a matter of vertical cooperation. IEEE Commun Mag 55:135–141
12. Höyhtyä M et al (2017) Database-assisted spectrum sharing in satellite communications: a survey. IEEE Access 5:25322–25341
13. Zhou Z, Guo D, Honig ML (2017) Licensed and unlicensed spectrum allocation in heterogeneous networks. IEEE Trans Commun 1815–1827
14. Hortelano D, Olivares T, Ruiz MC, Garrido C, López V (2017) From sensor networks to Internet of Things. Bluetooth low energy, a standard for this evolution. Sensors 17:372
15. Strategy Analytics News & Press Releases. Accessed 14 Oct 2014. [Online]. Available http://www.prnewswire.com/news/strategyanalytics
16. Perera C, Zaslavsky A, Christen P, Georgakopoulos D (2014) Context aware computing for the Internet of Things: a survey. IEEE Commun Surveys Tutorials 16:414–454
17. Whitmore A, Agarwal A, Xu LD (2015) 'The Internet of Things a survey of topics and trends. Inf Syst Front 17:261–274
18. Afzal A et al (2015) The cognitive Internet of Things: a unified perspective. Mobile Netw Appl 72–85
19. Ning H et al (2015) From Internet to smart world. IEEE Access 3:1994–1999
20. Ray BR, Abawajy J, Chowdhury M (2014) Scalable RFID security framework and protocol supporting Internet of Things. Comput Netw 67:89–103
21. Chilipirea C, Ursache A, Popa DO, Pop F (2016) Energy efficiency and robustness for IOT: building a smart home security system. In: Proceedings of IEEE 12th international conference on intelligent computer communication and processing (ICCP), pp 43–48
22. Hoan V-v, Koo I (2018) Joint full-duplex/half-duplex transmission-switching scheduling and transmission-energy allocation in cognitive radio networks with energy harvesting. Sensors 18(7)
23. Zhang L, Xiao M, Wu G, Alam M, Liang YC, Li S (2017) A survey of advanced techniques for spectrum sharing in 5G networks. IEEE Wireless Commun 44–51
24. Kim K, Akbar IA, Bae KK, Um JS, Spooner CM, Reed JH (2017) Cyclostationary approaches to signal detection and classification in cognitive radio. In: Proceedings of 2nd IEEE international symposium on new frontiers in dynamic spectrum access networks (DySPAN), pp 212–215
25. Doost-Mohammady R, Chowdhury KR (2012) Design of spectrum database assisted cognitive radio vehicular networks. In: Proceedings of 7th international ICST conference on cognitive radio-oriented wireless network communication (CROWNCOM), pp 1–5
26. Gregori M, Gomez-Vilardebó J (2016) Online learning algorithms for wireless energy harvesting nodes. In: Proceedings of IEEE international conference on communications (ICC), Kuala Lumpur, Malaysia, pp 1–6
27. Gurakan B, Ozel O, Yang J, Ulukus S (2013) Energy cooperation in energy harvesting communications. IEEE Trans Commun 61:4884–4898
28. Huang X, Han T, Ansari N (2015) On green-energy-powered cognitive radio networks. IEEE Commun Surv Tutorials 17
29. Zhang R, Chen H, Yeoh P, Li Y, Vucetic B (2017) Full-duplex cooperative cognitive radio networks with wireless energy harvesting. pp 1–6
30. Lei H, Xu M, Ansari, IS, Pan G, Qaraqe KA et al (2016) On secure underlay MIMO cognitive radio networks with energy harvesting and transmit antenna selection. IEEE Trans Green Commun Netw 1–1
31. Bhowmick A, Chatterjee A, Verma R (2019) Performance analysis of physical layer security over generalized-K fading channels using a mixture Gamma distribution. IEEE Commun Lett 20:408–411
32. Alhatmi TA, Aldhabhani AM (2019) Full Duplex spectrum sensing and energy harvesting in cognitive radio networks, Access Netw (DySPAN) 212–215
33. Zhang Z, Long K, Vasilakos AV, Hanzo L (2016) Full-duplex wireless communications: challenges, solutions, and future research directions. Proc IEEE 104:1369–1409

34. Naeem M, Illanko K, Karmokar A, Anpalagan A, Jaseemuddin M (2013) Energy-efficient cognitive radio sensor networks: parametric and convex transformations. Sensors 13:11032–11050
35. Wang H, Ding G, Gao F, Chen J, Wang J, Wang L (2018) Power control in UAV-supported ultra dense networks: communications, caching, and energy transfer. IEEE Commun Mag 56:28–34
36. Nguyen VD, Shin OS (2018) Cooperative prediction-and-sensing-based spectrum sharing in cognitive radio networks. IEEE Trans Cogn Commun Netw 4:108–120
37. Fu Y, Yang F, He ZA (2018) Quantization-based multibit data fusion scheme for cooperative spectrum sensing in cognitive radio networks. Sensors 18:473
38. Nasser A, Mansour A, Yao KC (2020) Simultaneous transmitting–receiving–sensing for OFDM-based full-duplex cognitive radio. Phys Commun 39:100987
39. Chatterjee S, Maity SP, Acharya T (2019) Energy-spectrum efficiency trade-off in energy harvesting cooperative cognitive radio networks. IEEE Trans Cogn Commun Netw 5(2):295–303
40. Maji P et al (2020) Secrecy and throughput performance of an energy harvesting hybrid cognitive radio network with spectrum sensing. Wirel Netw 26(2):1301–1314

Performance Analysis and Power Allocation with Joint Sharing in Hybrid Multicarrier-Based Cognitive Radio Network

Sandeep Kumar Jain and Baljeet Kaur

Abstract Limited resources and improper utilization of frequency force us to think about an appropriate approach to frequency and power allocation. In order to provide efficient utilization of available frequency resources, cognitive radio (CR) plays a significant role. Spectrum-sharing capabilities and better adaptability of OFDM which involves multicarrier are measured as potential candidates for the CR system. Reduced capacity due to suppressed subcarriers in OFDM-based CR can be recovered while engaging a greater number of antennas at both ends of the communication system. In this paper, we have proposed a system model and derived mathematical expression for transmit power allocation and ergodic capacity with joint sharing as underlay, overlay, and interweave scenario in hybrid multicarrier-based CR system. Performance analysis for the same is shown in simulation results.

Keywords Ergodic capacity · Spectrum sharing · Multicarrier · Power allocation · Waterfilling

1 Introduction

Mandate of present spectrum band for enhanced data rate, excellent throughput, and higher QoS rising quickly which creates spectrum scarcity problem. Simultaneously, it is also observed that most of the registered allocated bands are not fully utilized and are known as underutilized [1]. In order to resolve issues related to scarcity and utilization of spectrum, Federal Communication Commission (FCC) instigate a smart radio system known as CR system [2, 3], which can be applied to understand Dynamic Spectrum Allocation (DSA) [4] and spectrum sharing in an opportunistic manner. CR is proficient to be alert of the external world in which it is functioning and

S. K. Jain (✉)
ECE, I.K. Gujral PTU, Jalandhar, Punjab, India
e-mail: sandeepjain@svvv.edu.in

B. Kaur
ECE, GNDEC, Ludhiana, Punjab, India
e-mail: baljeetkaur@gndec.ac.in

M. S. Kaiser et al. (eds.), *Proceedings of Trends in Electronics and Health Informatics*, Lecture Notes in Networks and Systems 376,
https://doi.org/10.1007/978-981-16-8826-3_52

can fiddle with its parameters of transmitter accordingly. In this direction, the foremost essential but rendered complicated task of CR is to detect spectrum holes with the help of various spectrum sensing techniques such as detection of primary transmitter, cooperative detection, and detection of interference [5]. In order to manage the simultaneous existence of Primary Users (PU) and Secondary Users (SU), it is recommended that SU should have knowledge about the operating environment and working parameters. Based on assembled information that is requisite for SU for proper functioning in a network, where PU exists and is already being used, hence interference constraint exists.

There are a different number of approaches are available for sharing of spectrum that can be categorized as underlay, overlay, and interweave approach [6, 7]. Following approaches will play an important role to exploit spectrum-related issues like the underutilized and unused spectrum in a DSA mechanism. One of the spectrums sharing approach known as underlay approach worn to overcome spectrum under-utilization, with concurrent existence of PUs and SUs in such a way that interference bound at primary receiver remain tolerable and does not exceed beyond a threshold limit. When PU and SU users subsist in similar spectral regions, although transmission by SU is below the threshold, still there may be a chance of interferences arising due to coexistence [8]. Underlay approach is a much better choice as it allows low power transmission so that interference limits at primary do not cross predefined range. Due to transmission at low power, shorter range and lower data rate applications get good support.

Another sharing approach is overlay which utilizes unused spectrum [9]. Here the existence of PUs and SUs in a side-by-side band in a supportive manner. So, SU gets required information from PU and used it to prevail over interference and provide improvement in the overall performance at PU by relaying. On behalf of that, PU may extend the interference limit. Improved performance achieved in overlay as it contains better collaboration among both types of users. Due to the existence of a side-by-side band, non-orthogonality results in interference [10]. Literatures shows that under certain interference constraints, large amount of power can be transmitted by SU in overlay compared to underlay approach [11, 12].

Interweave approach of spectrum sharing where SUs have to oversee and discover underutilized spectrum bands to use proficiently and establish communications in an opportunistic manner. Only in absence of PUs, vacant slots of spectrum can be accessed by SUs. Under dynamic behavior of PUs, detection of spectrum holes becomes a more vital task that demands agile in switching of frequency band by SUs.

In the overlay approach of spectrum sharing, complete power is allocated to subcarriers lying in unused PU band, due to this rate of transmission may get improved with possibilities of poor channel quality [9]. On the other side in the case of underlay spectrum sharing approach [6], allocation of power to the subcarriers falls in the underutilized spectrum band of PU [13, 14], although it experiences more interference to PU band with better quality of channel. Whereas access of spectrum for SUs will be allowed in interweave approach only when PUs is not working. Following mentioned approaches of spectrum sharing can be used to tackle separate issues related to either unused or underutilized spectrum bands. Now in order to resolve both issues together and provide efficient utilization of resources with optimal power while maximizing capacity and allocation of subcarrier, too much research is going on with a joint or hybrid approach [15, 16].

As OFDM provides reliable broadband communication in longer interval symbols and separates high data rate streams into abundant low data rate streams [17, 18]. With the help of FFT/IFFT, strictly spaced narrowband orthogonal subcarriers, flexibility, and adaptability offered by OFDM to reduce ISI on time-varying Rayleigh fading channel as well as dynamic allocation of spectrum holes efficiently [19]. As subcarrier cancellation reduces capacity in case OFDM-based CR which can be recovered with the use of MIMO [20]. Greater antennas at transmit and receiver offer enhanced beamforming and superior directivity respectively [21]. Such hybrid techniques MIMO-OFDM-based CR [22] shows significant improvement in the overall capacity of system and diversity gains with flat fading channel [23]. As if we want to attain the same capacity, MIMO system required a comparatively lesser amount of transmission power than SISO. As we want the complete advantage of the capacity of CR system in downlink while considering constraint on interference of PU as well as maximum transmit power of SU, in this paper power controlling technique have been put into process with CSI. As channel information attained through training sequence or pilot from PU, for known CSI, waterfilling approach can improve system capacity [24]. Because it allows proper power allocation to each subchannel. While in absence of CSI, power will be allocated equally among each subchannel [25, 26]. In [27], active interference cancellation (ACI)-based spectrum shaping optimal and suboptimal schemes have been presented which allow enhanced transmission rates. In our paper, a system model has been proposed and also derived a mathematical expression for transmitting power allocation and ergodic capacity with joint sharing as underlay, overlay, and interweave scenario in a hybrid multicarrier-based CR system.

The paper is prepared as follows: Sect. 2 describes the proposed system model for hybrid multicarrier-based CR system. Mathematical expression for ergodic capacity and power allocation is obtained in Sect. 3. In Sect. 4, performance analysis has been completed using MATLAB simulation results and finally the conclusions are drawn in Sect. 5.

2 Proposed System Model for Hybrid Multicarrier-Based CR System

As shown in Fig. 1, for the proposed system model we have assumed downlink scenario for SU with concurrent existence of both types of users as PU and SU. We know CSI between secondary users as well as secondary and primary transmitters through user and sensing channels, respectively.

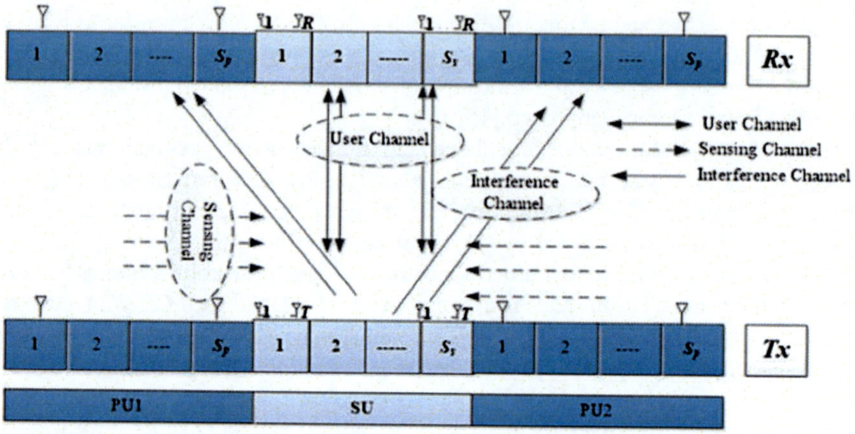

Fig. 1 Proposed system model for hybrid multicarrier-based CR system

Following parameters used in the illustration:

Sp	No. of subcarriers between primary users.
Ss	No. of subcarriers between secondary users.
T	No. of antennas for each subcarrier at transmitter of SU.
R	No. of antennas for each subcarrier at receiver of SU.
$I_{\text{threshold}}$	Interference threshold.
$p_{i,j}$	Transmission power at *j*th antenna of *i*th subcarrier at transmitter of SU.
$\sigma_{i,j}$	Singular value of MIMO channel matrix of secondary users.
σ_0	AWGN variance.
hi, *r*, *t*	User channel gain between *r*th receive antenna and *t*th transmit antenna at SU.
$g_{i,j,t}$	Interference channel gain between *t*th transmit antenna of SU and *j*th PU Rx corresponding to *i*th subcarrier of SU.
Ts	Symbol duration for OFDM.
d_{ik}	Spectral separation between *i*th subcarrier at transmitter of SU and *k*th subcarrier at transmitter of PU.
Δf	Separation among adjacent subcarriers in spectral domain.

3 Expression for Ergodic Capacity and Power Allocation

Maximum channel capacity permits optimal spreading of total transmit power among various number of channels.

General capacity of MIMO system is given as [20]:

$$\mathrm{C} = \sum_{1}^{\text{NumberofChannel}} \log_2\left(1 + H^*\left[\left\{\frac{\text{Total Transmit Power} + \text{Inverse Overall Channel Gain}}{\text{Sum of Channel}}\right\} - \text{Individual Inverse Channel Gain}\right]\right) \tag{1}$$

General steps of waterfilling algorithm [25]:

(1) Assign total amount of transmit power for subcarriers and noise power to each channel corresponding to individual subcarrier.
(2) Calculate water filling area while summing total amount of power and reciprocal of combined channel gain.
(3) Calculate average power allocation to get initial water level.
(4) To get the allocated amount of power as Power = max (0, Power) to each subchannel, perform subtraction of step 2 from step 3.
(5) Under the power and resource constraint for maximizing capacity use the Lagrange function to get a solution of optimization.

MIMO user channel matrix among secondary users given as:

$$H = [H_1, H_2, H_3 \ldots H_i] \tag{2}$$

where,

$$H_i = \begin{bmatrix} h_{i,1,1} & \cdots & h_{i,1,t} \\ \vdots & \ddots & \vdots \\ h_{i,r,1} & \cdots & h_{i,r,t} \end{bmatrix}$$

Each of the subcarriers has a dimension of R × T. Interference channel matrix between the transmitter of SU and receiver of PU given as:

$$G_{i,j} = \left[g_{i,j,1}, g_{i,j,2}, g_{i,j,3} \ldots\ldots g_{i,j,t}\right] \tag{3}$$

With known CSI at transmitter of SU, individual subcarrier channels may be decomposed into parallel self-determining subchannel with the help of singular value decomposition (SVD) method. Singular values of channel matrix on individual subcarriers are assigned as channel gain to individual subchannel.

$$H_{R\times T} = U\varepsilon V^H \tag{4}$$

where,

$$U_{R\times T} = [U_1, U_2, U_3 \ldots U_T]$$

$$\varepsilon_{T\times T} = \begin{bmatrix} \sigma_1 & \cdots & 0 \\ \vdots & \ddots & \vdots \\ 0 & \cdots & \sigma_T \end{bmatrix}$$

$$V_{T\times T}^{H} = \begin{bmatrix} V_1^H \\ \vdots \\ V_T^H \end{bmatrix}$$

Property of singular values such that

$$\sigma_1 \geq \sigma_2 \geq \sigma_3 \ldots \sigma_T \geq 0$$

Capacity of ith subcarrier of SU Tx [24, 25]:

$$C_i = \sum_{j=1}^{\min(T,R)} log_2\left(1 + (p_{i,j})(\sigma_{i,j})^2 \Big/ \sigma_0\right) \quad (5)$$

Due to orthogonality among subcarriers at transmitter of SU, OFDM data transmission is ISI free. But it may be interfering with PU, as PU is not bound to use OFDM. This interference on PU depends on transmit power of transmitter of SU as well as distance between SU subcarrier with PU.

Interference on PU by SU is given as:

$$I_{i,j}(d_i, p_{i,j}) = p_{i.j} T_s \int_{d_{ik}-\Delta f}^{d_{ik}+\Delta f} \left(\frac{\sin \pi T_s f}{\pi T_s f}\right)^2 df$$

For conventional OFDM, allocated optimal power to individual subcarrier given as [28, 29]:

$$p_i = \left\{\left(P_T + \sum_{i=1}^{S_s} \frac{\sigma_0^2}{\sigma_i}\right) - \frac{\sigma_0^2}{\sigma_i}\right\}^{+} \quad (6)$$

For conventional MIMO-OFDM, where initially total transmit power has been estimated using uniform allocation under certain threshold. Then equal amount of power will be allocated to individual subcarrier as [24]:

$$p_i = \frac{I_{\text{threshold}}}{S_s \sum_{i=1}^{S_s} \sum_{k=1}^{S_p} \frac{\partial I_i^k}{\partial p_i}} \quad (7)$$

where p_i is power allocated to each subcarrier under a known interference threshold.

$$P_T = \sum_{i=1}^{S_s} p_i$$

With the help of power allocated to each subcarrier, power for individual MIMO antenna is assigned in the way to maximize capacity of individual subcarrier as well as overall capacity. In order to maximize the capacity of individual subcarriers following optimization problem would be solved.

$$C_{\max} = \sum_{i=1}^{S_s} \sum_{j=1}^{\min(T,R)} \log_2\left(1 + (p_{i,j})(\sigma_{i,j})^2 / \sigma_0\right) \tag{8}$$

Subject to constraint,

$$\sum_{i=1}^{S_s} \sum_{j=1}^{\min(T,R)} p_{i,j} \le P_T$$

$$p_{i,j} \ge 0$$

Water filling solution for the problem mentioned above as:

$$p_{i,j} = \max\left\{0, \gamma - \frac{\sigma_0}{\sigma_{i,j}^2}\right\}^+ \tag{9}$$

where γ is Lagrange's multiplier and can be computed as,

$$P_T = \sum_{i=1}^{S_s} \sum_{j=1}^{\min(T,R)} \max\left\{0, \gamma - \frac{\sigma_0}{\sigma_{i,j}^2}\right\}$$

To get our objective as assigned power in a way that maximizes the capacity of SU under a constraint on interference forced by PU and constraint on maximum transmit power at SU in MIMO-OFDM-based CR system. In order to achieve maximum system capacity of SU, the objective function can be written as [24, 25]:

$$C_{\max} = \sum_{i=1}^{S_s} \sum_{j=1}^{\min(T,R)} \log_2\left(1 + (p_{i,j})(\sigma_{i,j})^2 / \sigma_0\right) \tag{10}$$

Subject to following interference and power constraint:

$$\sum_{k=1}^{S_p} \sum_{i=1}^{S_s} \sum_{j=1}^{\min(T,R)} I_{i,j}^2(d_{i,j}, p_{i,j}) \le I_{\text{threshold}} \tag{11}$$

$$\sum_{i=1}^{S_s} \sum_{j=1}^{\min(T,R)} p_{i,j} \le P_T \tag{12}$$

$$p_{i,j} \geq 0 \tag{13}$$

In order to achieve optimal power allocation solution, apply Lrange multiplier with KKT method in (10) that will provide the result as [30, 31]:

$$p_{i,j} = \left\{ \frac{1}{\alpha \sum_{k=1}^{S_p} \frac{\partial I_{i,j}^k}{\partial p_{i,j}} + \beta_{i,j}} - \frac{\sigma_0}{\sigma_{i,j}^2} \right\}^+ \tag{14}$$

where, $\{Z\}^+ = \max(0, Z)$ and α, β and γ are Lagrange constant multipliers, can be obtained using above mentioned different constraints in (11), (12) and (13) as:

$$\alpha \sum_{k=1}^{S_p} \frac{\partial I_{i,j}^k}{\partial p_{i,j}} + \beta_{i,j} = \frac{1}{\frac{\sigma_0}{\sigma_{i,j}^2} + p_{i,j}} + \gamma_{i,j} \tag{15}$$

$$\beta_{i,j} \left(\sum_{i=1}^{S_s} \sum_{j=1}^{\min(T,R)} p_{i,j} - P_T \right) \geq 0 \tag{16}$$

$$\gamma_{i,j} p_{i,j} = 0 \tag{17}$$

Due to the high level of complexity involved in optimal power control, now in this section we are deriving mathematical expressions for suboptimal power control approach under interference on PU and transmitting maximum amount of power level. Again, convex optimization problem will be solved and will give us two-level water filling approach [24, 25]

$$p_{i,j} = \max \left\{ 0, \frac{1}{\alpha \sum_{k=1}^{S_p} \frac{\partial I_{i,j}^k}{\partial p_{i,j}}} - \frac{\sigma_0}{\sigma_{i,j}^2} \right\}^+ \tag{18}$$

where α is Lagrange's multiplier and obtained using with

$$I_{\text{threshold}} = \sum_{k=1}^{S_p} \sum_{i=1}^{S_s} \sum_{j=1}^{\min(T,R)} \frac{\partial I_{i,j}^k}{\partial p_{i,j}} \max \left\{ 0, \frac{1}{\alpha \sum_{k=1}^{S_p} \frac{\partial I_{i,j}^k}{\partial p_{i,j}}} - \frac{\sigma_0}{\sigma_{i,j}^2} \right\} \tag{19}$$

So, with these expressions allocation of suboptimal power may be obtained so that transmission capacity of cognitive user can be maximized while keeping of interference constraint of PU below threshold level here there is no constraint on transmitting power.

4 Simulation Results and Discussion

To perceive the performance and usefulness of the proposed approach, we used MATLAB software and simulation parameters as given in Table 1. With perfect CSI which will be used for subcarrier and power allocation at transmitter of SU. A MIMO-OFDM-based CR system with Ss is number of subcarriers at SU and Sp is number of subcarriers at PU respectively. MIMO with R × T channel matrix dimension, where number of antennas at transmitter and receiver denoted by T and R, respectively.

Figure 2 shows conventional waterfilling approach for OFDM where subcarriers that have good quality of channel will be assigned with larger amount power and subcarrier with poor channel quality will not be allotted any power.

Joint spectrum sharing will be considered to overcome spectrum-related issues as unused and underutilized spectrum. Figure 3 shows the result for simulation of joint sharing scenario. Here the total number of SU's subcarriers have been presented in four zones such as restricted zone which will not allow transmission from SU in any case. Next one is the interweaving zone, where detection of underutilized spectrum band performed by SU for effective utilization of available resources and establish communications in opportunistic manner. As PU and SU exist simultaneously in side-by-side band but vacant spectrum may be accessed by SU only when PUs is not operating.

Next zone is cooperative zone which allows coexistence of PUs and SUs in alternate bands in a supportive manner. Here SU gets CSI from PU that applied to prevail over interference and provides performance improvement at PU by relaying. On behalf of that, PU may offer a new level of interference threshold comparatively greater than earlier defined interference threshold. Due to high cooperation among primary and secondary users, better performance was achieved in overlay approach.

Table 1 Parameters for simulation

Sr. No	Parameters	Value
1.	Number of sub carrier	(16, 32)
2.	Total power budget	1e−3
3.	Total bandwidth	1 MHz
4.	Density of noise	− 80 dBm, − 90 dBm
5.	OFDM symbol duration	1e−6 s
6.	No. of SU users	4
7.	AWGN noise variance	1e−3
8.	Number of underlay subcarriers	8
9.	Number of overlay subcarriers	8
10.	SNR (dB)	− 20 to 40 dB
11.	Number of iterations	1000

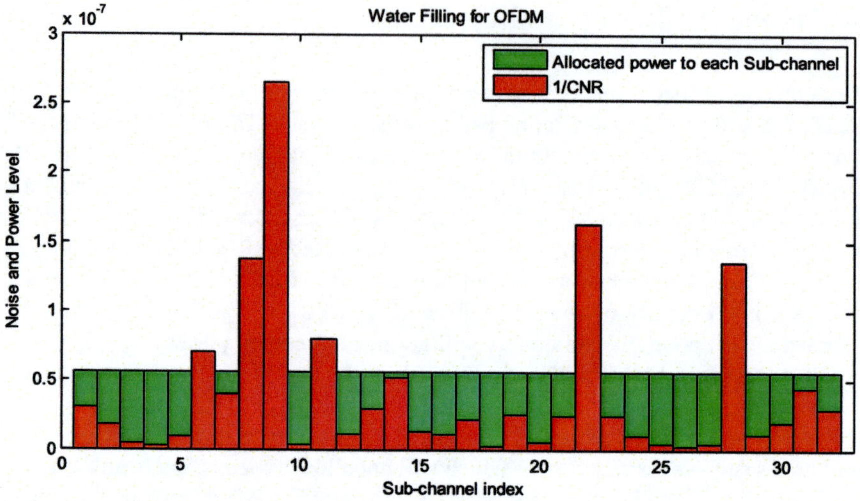

Fig. 2 Conventional water filling for OFDM

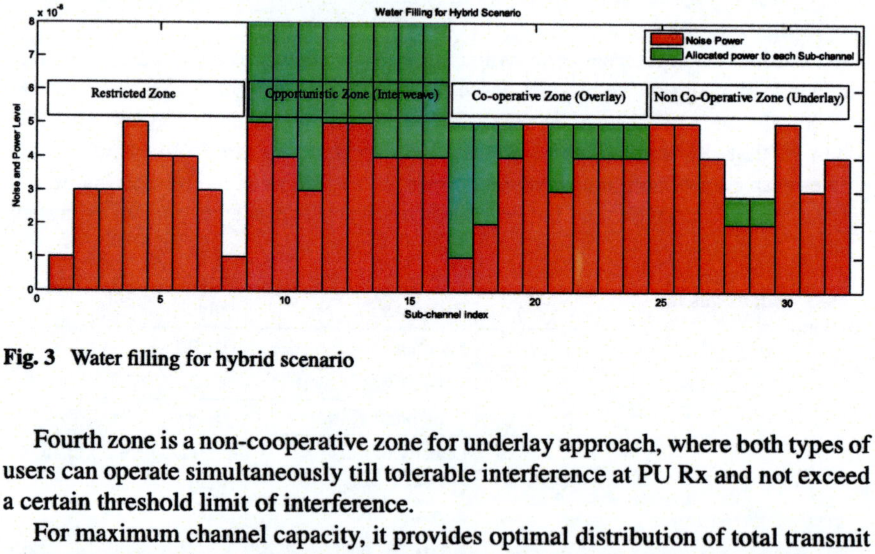

Fig. 3 Water filling for hybrid scenario

Fourth zone is a non-cooperative zone for underlay approach, where both types of users can operate simultaneously till tolerable interference at PU Rx and not exceed a certain threshold limit of interference.

For maximum channel capacity, it provides optimal distribution of total transmit power among various numbers of channels in all cases. To achieve our objective as power allocation in such a way that maximizes SU capacity under constraint on interference level forced by PU and constraint on maximum transmit power at SU expression used for simulation result.

Let us consider deterministic nature of MIMO channel when CSI is unknown at transmitter end, although this channel changes randomly as its channel matrix is not a deterministic matrix which means channel capacity shows random time-varying characteristics. We have considered that time-varying random channel is an ergodic process. Figure 4, shows improvement in channel capacity with respect to SNR and as number of antennas are getting increase at transmitter and receiver end.

In Fig. 5, we have compared ergodic channel capacity for MIMO system with 4 × 4 channel matrix. It shows that closed-loop, when CSI is known, gives us enhanced capacity with respect to SNR due to cooperation and coordination in comparison to open loop when CSI is unknown and we have to go for estimation to get information.

Figure 6 represents the capacity of hybrid multicarrier-based CR systems with underlay, overlay, and joint underlay-overlay spectrum-sharing approaches. So, from simulation, we can say that joint sharing scheme outperforms with individual sharing scheme. In comparison of optimal and suboptimal power allocation techniques, optimal gives better capacity than suboptimal. But due to the high computational complexity involved in optimal power allocation scenario alternative suboptimal power allocation approach can be used.

When we consider conventional OFDM-based CR with and without waterfilling techniques and compare with MIMO-OFDM-based CR with and without water-filling. In both cases, along with waterfilling techniques, we get better capacity. As shown in Fig. 7, reduced capacity due to suppressed subcarriers in OFDM-based CR can be improved while employing a greater number of antennas at transmitter and receiver sides.

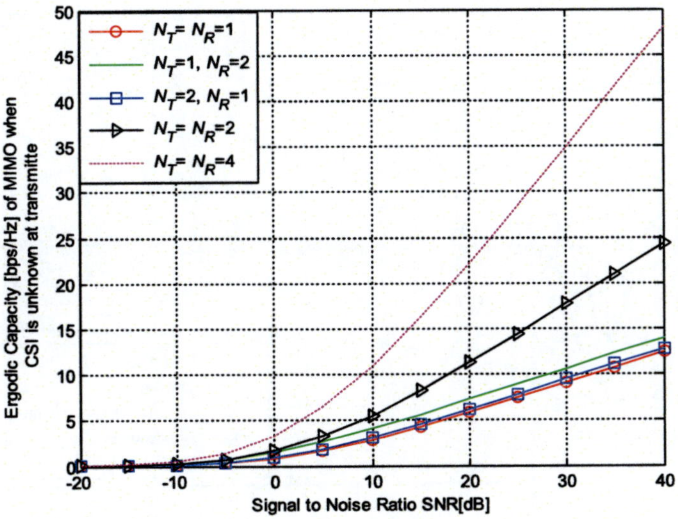

Fig. 4 Ergodic capacity vs SNR when CSI is known at the transmitter side

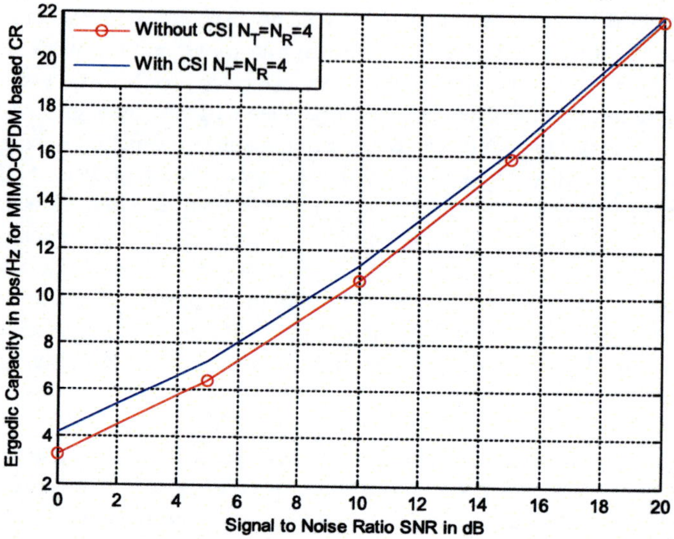

Fig. 5 MIMO capacity vs SNR with and without channel state information

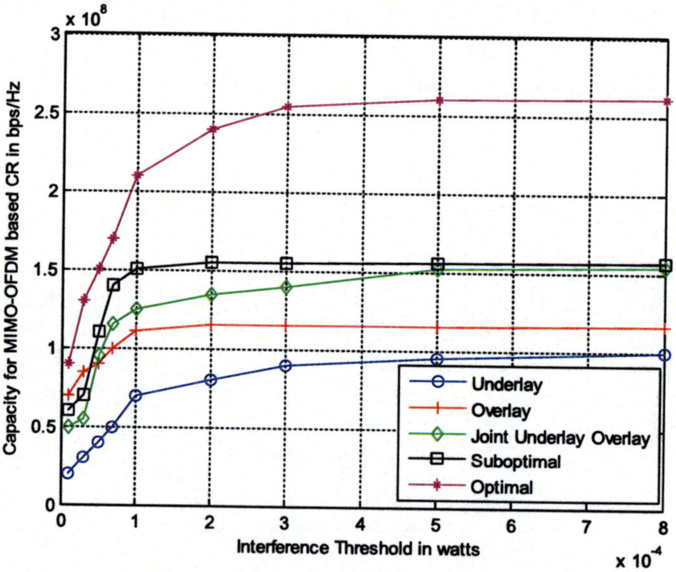

Fig. 6 Capacity of MIMO-OFDM-based CR under various sharing approaches

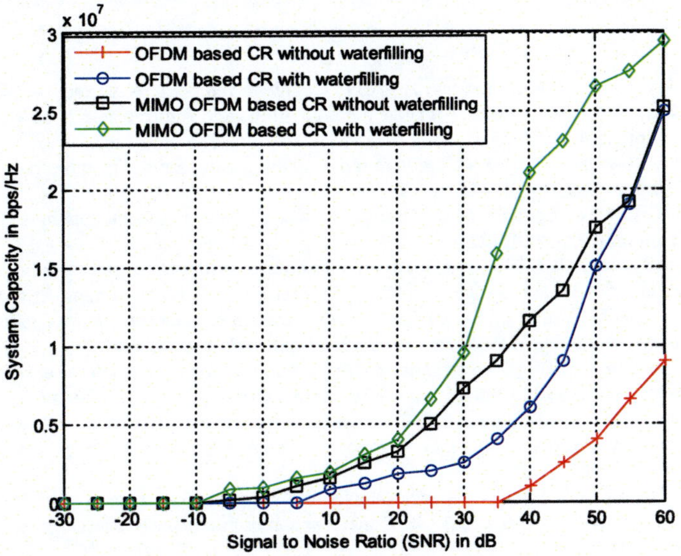

Fig. 7 Capacity of MIMO-OFDM-based CR with and without waterfilling

5 Conclusion

It has been shown that the following mentioned approaches of spectrum sharing can be used to tackle separate issues related to either unused or underutilized spectrum bands. Here in order to resolve both issues together and provide efficient utilization of resources with optimal power while maximizing capacity and allocation of subcarrier, joint or hybrid approach taken into consideration. Proposed hybrid spectrum sharing and optimal power allocation for hybrid multicarrier-based CR network have been illustrated using waterfilling approach accordingly. Through the simulation results, waterfilling techniques for MIMO-OFDM-based CR network with spectral distance between SU to PU subcarriers and other one with joint sharing scheme, have been estimated. It may be extended for a greater number of underlay and overlay subcarrier along with more PUs and SUs in the upcoming paper for better spectrum sharing with efficient and optimal power allocation for massive MIMO-OFDM-based CR system using various techniques.

References

1. Khan AA, Rehmani MH, Rachedi A (2017) Cognitive radio based internet of things: applications, architectures, spectrum related functionalities, and future research directions. IEEE Wirel Commun 4(3):17–25
2. Mitola J, Maguire GQ (1999) Cognitive radio: making software radios more personal. IEEE Pers Commun Mag 6(4):13–18
3. Haykin S (2005) Cognitive radio: Brain-empowered wireless communications. IEEE J Sel Areas Commun 23(2):201–220
4. Gupta MS, Kumar K (2019). Progression on spectrum sensing for cognitive radio networks: a survey, classification, challenges and future research issues. J Netw Comput Appl 143:47–76
5. Sun M., Zhao C., Yan S., Li B. (2017). A novel spectrum sensing for cognitive radio networks with noise uncertainty, IEEE Trans Veh Technol 66(5):4424–4429 (2017)
6. Vu V-H, Koo I (2017) Throughput maximization for cognitive radio users with energy constraints in an underlay paradigm. J Inf Commun Converg Eng 15(2):79–84
7. Srivastava A, Gupta MS, Kaur G (2020) Energy efficient transmission trends towards future green cognitive radio networks (5G): progress, taxonomy and open challenge. J Netw Comput Appl 168:102760
8. Wu Z, Natarajan B (2007, January) Interference tolerant agile cognitive radio: maximize channel capacity of cognitive radio. In: Consumer communications and networking conference, pp 1027–1031
9. Kim D. I., Le L. B., and Hossain E. (2008). Joint rate and power allocation for cognitive radios in dynamic spectrum access environment. IEEE Trans Wirel Commun 7(12):5517–5527
10. Kumar A, NandhaKumar P (2019) OFDM system with cyclostationary feature detection spectrum sensing. ICT Express 5(1):21–25
11. Zhang D, Tian Z, Wei G (2008) Spatial capacity of narrowband vs. ultra-wideband cognitive radio systems. IEEE Trans Wirel Commun 7(11):4670–4680
12. Khoshkholgh MG, Navaie K, Yanikomeroglu H (2009) On the impact of the primary network activity on the achievable capacity of spectrum sharing over fading channels. IEEE Trans Wirel Commun 8(4):2100–2111
13. Yamaguchi H (2004) Active interference cancellation technique for MB-OFDM cognitive radio. 34th European microwave conference, vol 2. The Netherlands, Amsterdam, pp 1105–1108
14. Brandes S, Cosovic I, Schnell M (2006) Reduction of out-of-band radiation in OFDM systems by insertion of cancellation carriers. IEEE Commun Lett 10(6):420–422
15. Bepari D, Mitra D (2015) Improved power loading scheme for orthogonal frequency division multiplexing based cognitive radio. IET Commun 9(16):2033–2040
16. Paulraj AJ (2004) An overview of MIMO communications—a key to gigabit wireless. Proc IEEE 92(2):198–218
17. Gesbert D, Shafi M, Shiu D, Smith PJ, Naguib A (2003) From theory to practice: an overview of MIMO space–time coded wireless systems. IEEE J Sel Areas Commun 21(3):281–302
18. Nee RV, Prasad R (2000) OFDM for wireless multimedia communication. Artech House, London
19. Wang S, Shi W, Wang C (2015) Energy-efficient resource management in OFDM based cognitive radio networks under channel uncertainty. IEEE Trans Commun 63(9):3092–3102
20. Bolcskei H, Zurich E (2006) MIMO-OFDM wireless systems: basics, perspectives, and challenges. IEEE Wirel Commun 13(4):31–37
21. Zhang W, Xia XG, Letaief KB (2007) Space-time/frequency coding for MIMO-OFDM in next generation broadband wireless system. IEEE Wirel Commun 14(3):32–43
22. Shahraki HS, Mohamed-pour K, Vangelista L (2014) Sum capacity maximization for MIMO–OFDMA based cognitive radio networks. Phys Commun 10:106–115
23. Qi Q, Minturn A, Yang Y (2012) An efficient water-filling algorithm for power allocation in OFDM-based cognitive radio system. In: International conference on systems and informatics (ICSAI 2012), pp 2069–2073

24. Kumar K, Singh M (2011). Proposed water filling model in a MIMO system. Int J Emerg Technol Adv Eng.1(2). ISSN 2250-2459
25. Bansal G, Hossain MJ, Bhargava VK (2008) Optimal and suboptimal power allocation schemes for OFDM-based cognitive radio systems. IEEE Trans Wirel Commun 7(11):4710–4718
26. Bansal G, Hossain MJ, Bhargava VK, Le-Ngoc T (2013) Subcarrier and power allocation for OFDMA-based cognitive radio systems with hybrid overlay and underlay spectrum access mechanism. IEEE Trans Veh Technol 62(3):1111–1122
27. Bharti MR, Ghosh D (2016). Hybrid spectral shaping and power loading for OFDM based cognitive radio. In: IEEE international conference on advanced networks and telecommunications systems, IEEE ANTS, pp 1–6
28. Bedeer E, Dobre OA, Ahmed MH, Baddour KE (2013) A novel algorithm for rate/power allocation in OFDM-based cognitive radio systems with statistical interference constraints. In: IEEE global communications conference, GLOBECOM, pp 3504–3509
29. Mathur N, Vamne R (2020) Energy-efficient resource allotment for OFDM-based cognitive radio networks. Int J Adv Comput Technol 9(4):07–09
30. Srivastava A, Kaur G (2021) Resource management for traffic imbalance problem in green cognitive radio networks. Phys Commun 48:101437
31. Jain SK, Kaur B (2020) Optimal power transmission for various spectrum sharing approaches in OFDM based cognitive radio network. ICTACT J Commun Technol 11(3):2228–2233

A Lightweight Cryptographic Scheme to Secure WSNs in Agriculture

Amit Singha, Nasirul Mumenin, Nahid Ibne Akhter, Md. Shahadat Hossain Moon, and Mosabber Uddin Ahmed

Abstract Agriculture, being an important industry, needs the use of contemporary technologies in order to increase production. Wireless sensor networks (WSN) can be used to monitor meteorological factors in an agricultural area in this case. This article offers a safe communication system for WSN where each communication step is encrypted using appropriate cryptographic algorithm. Because a WSN consists of a variety of devices with some constraints, conventional encryption methods are ineffective. MUMAP, an ultra-lightweight mutual authentication protocol, is used in the initial phase of a WSN's connection, when the sensor nodes' collected data are transmitted to the base node, to verify that the data have been obtained from valid sources. The sink nodes then transmit all of the data obtained from the sensor nodes to the main station or base station. TWINE, a lightweight symmetric encryption method, is used to secure the data package at this step. Both of these methods are very safe against a variety of cyber-attacks. As a result, this framework guarantees the WSN's security in two critical communication areas. Because MUMAP and TWINE are both lightweight methods, they may be deployed economically with limited resources.

Keywords Lightweight cryptography · Wireless sensor network · Mutual authentication · Cyber-physical system · Data security

---

A. Singha (✉)
Jahangirnagar University, Dhaka, Bangladesh

N. Mumenin · N. I. Akhter · Md. S. H. Moon
Bangladesh University of Professionals, Dhaka, Bangladesh

M. U. Ahmed
University of Dhaka, Dhaka, Bangladesh

M. S. Kaiser et al. (eds.), *Proceedings of Trends in Electronics and Health Informatics*, Lecture Notes in Networks and Systems 376,
https://doi.org/10.1007/978-981-16-8826-3_53

1 Introduction

Wireless sensor networks (WSNs) are one of the most powerful new technologies, and they, together with the Internet of Things (IoT) [1], are changing the world. The WSN is, in fact, a critical component of the IoT paradigm. WSN was created to provide information to the agricultural industry and therefore enable smart IoT-based farming. Different environmental factors like temperature, humidity, weather station data, leaf wetness, soil temperature/humidity, and many more are relevant in such an application. Monitoring these indicators automatically provides time and cost savings and increased agricultural production (Fig. 1).

WSNs are made up of physically tiny sensor nodes that communicate primarily with the surroundings [2]. The structured network comprises sensing devices connected by a single integrated circuit that contains all of the necessary electrical components. The network's life relies heavily on the energy interface point to the rest of the world since the whole sensor is powered by a tiny battery. However, energy consumption remains one of the significant roadblocks to the widespread use of this technology, particularly in situations where a long network lifespan and excellent service quality are required. WSNs are becoming more popular as a research subject, including their energy consumption, routing algorithms, and sensor placement selection based on a particular premise, resilience, efficiency, and so on. Tracking, transportation, monitoring, surveillance, building automation, military applications, intelligent applications, and agriculture are just a few examples of WSN's application areas [3]. Agriculture production and yields are falling day by day due to a variety of factors. Unpredictable climatic changes, such as temperature, humidity, light, carbon dioxide, soil moisture, acidity, and so on, are the primary causes. Agriculture modernization and environmental protection are required to address the issue of crop failure. With all of the aforementioned problems in mind, we need a new and productive technology that can boost the agricultural system's production, profitability, and sustainability [4]. WSNs are made up of sensor nodes such as temperature sensors, soil sensors, humidity sensors, light sensors, and soil pH sensors, which are all low power, low cost, small volume, and multi-functional. Figure 2a shows the block diagram of a sensor node used in WSN. These sensor nodes are manually installed in the agricultural farm, and they gather climate data before transmitting it to the gateway/sink node. The sink node then transmits this data via the public channel to the user or agricultural expert. The farmer makes a choice and takes necessary action on the agricultural property based on the acquired environmental facts. However, the primary concern for continuous operation is to deliver high-quality service and real-time data securely at the appropriate moment. As a result, while developing a protocol, the first priority should be security. Due to their broadcast nature and hazardous surroundings, WSNs are very vulnerable [5]. As a result, there are many security solutions available, including routing security, key management, and cryptography. The security architecture of WSNs relies heavily on cryptographic methods. WSNs have a number of limitations, including a short battery life and limited memory. WSN is unable to cope with conventional encryption methods due to these

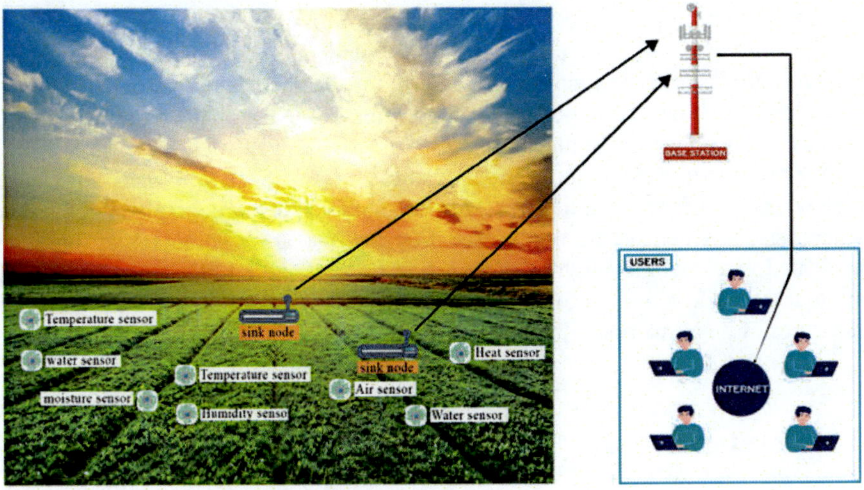

Fig. 1 Application of WSN in agriculture

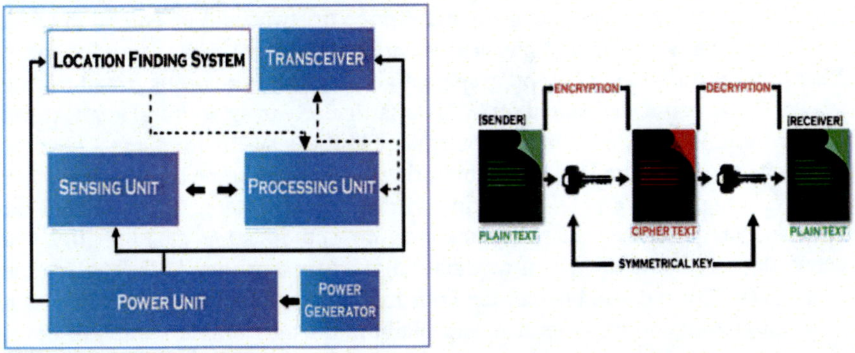

(a) (b)

Fig. 2 **a** Block diagram of a sensor node and **b** Block diagram of cryptography

constraints. Another method dubbed lightweight cryptography (LWC) [6] has been devised to provide more acceptable security with less equipment use and improved results. Although there is no specific criteria to be fit in lightweight algorithms, they often consider lower key sizes, smaller block sizes, smaller code sizes, fewer clock cycles, and so on. There are three types of lightweight cryptographic calculations: block cipher, stream cipher, and hash function. Each lightweight cryptography architect must deal with three important aspects: security, cost, and performance [7]. It is very difficult to accomplish all three main design objectives of security, affordability, and performance at the same time, while any one of these may be easily optimized. Figure 2b presents a block diagram of cryptography.

In this manuscript, a safe WSN communication framework is developed which uses an ultra-lightweight authentication mechanism, modified ultra-lightweight mutual authentication protocol (MUMAP) [8] for sensor node to sink node authentication and a lightweight cryptographic algorithm, TWINE-128 [9] for securing sink nodes to base station communication.

The remainder of the manuscript is laid out as follows: Sect. 2 provides a literature review that includes studies on WSN security, lightweight cryptography, lightweight authentication schemes, and WSNs used in agriculture, among other topics. We have presented an ultra-lightweight authentication method and a lightweight encryption approach for security in WSN in Sect. 3. Section 4 provides features and security measures of these method. Finally, conclusion is drawn in Sect. 5.

2 Literature Review

Despite the fact that numerous research efforts have focused on developing network security protocols and cryptographic solutions for WSN, many problems remain, particularly in terms of data integrity and service trustworthiness. Due to the wide variety of potential cyber and physical security risks, these issues are difficult to address successfully. Many cryptographic algorithms have been suggested to date; however, they are not well suited for WSNs, particularly in agricultural applications. In agriculture, WSNs are becoming increasingly prevalent. Environmental monitoring, precision agriculture [10], and monitoring systems are some of the applications of WSNs in agriculture [11]. As a kind of distributed system, WSNs should satisfy security requirements such as authentication, authorization, data integrity, data trustworthiness, availability, non-repudiation, trust, and privacy [12]. The Internet of Things (IoT) is the backbone of the Fourth Industrial Revolution, contributing to long-term growth and development, especially in the agricultural sectors of developing countries [13]. Potential cyber-physical attacks on different smart agricultural systems may cause serious security issues in today's dynamic and dispersed cyber-physical environment [14]. Threats and attacks of this kind have the potential to cause considerable disruption to connected businesses. The most frequent concerns are cyber security, data integrity, and data loss [15]. A data breach may cause substantial financial and personal damage to farmers as data privacy and ownership are a major security issue in the agriculture sector [16]. Ali et al. [17] investigated the issue of authentication in order to prevent illegal access to the WSN for agriculture. Amin and Biswas [18] suggested a system for user authentication and a key agreement scheme for the WSN environment, based on which a proposed method for user authentication and a key agreement scheme was provided. Naoui et al. [19] published a report that introduced a new security method for LoRaWAN. Shiravale et al. [20] proposed a WSN that has been implemented for precision agriculture, and security measures have also been discussed. The work by Katagi et al.[21] gave an overview of the state-of-the-art technology and standardization status of lightweight cryptography, which could be implemented efficiently in constrained devices. Shah et al. [22] provided a survey on lightweight cryptography for implementation in IoT devices with low resources. A review on implementation of lightweight cryptography was provided by Eisenbarth et al. [23]. Cyber security challenges in the field of Smart farming were investigated by Barreto et al. [24]. Baranwal et al. [25] conducted research on development of IoT-based smart security and monitoring devices for agriculture. It provided very resourceful information to implement a secure WSN for agriculture. IoT in agriculture, recent advances, and future challenges were explored in [26]. Survey on security threats in agricultural IoT and smart farming was conducted by Demestichas et al. [27].

3 Methodology

The main target here is to create a secure communication scheme from sensor nodes to sink nodes and then from sink nodes to the base station, as wireless communication takes place heavily in this part, and it is very vulnerable to various types of cyber-attacks. For our work, we are considering that there are a total n number of clusters, where each cluster has one primary sink node and the number of sensor nodes is m. Each cluster also has an alternative sink node which will act as the primary sink node if for any reason the primary one becomes inactive.

So, here we have an array of clusters of length, n. Then we have two arrays for primary sink nodes and alternative sink nodes, respectively.

1. Clusters, $C_i = C_1, C_2, C_3..., C_n$
2. Primary sink nodes, SPi = SP1, SP2, SP3, ... , SPn
3. Alternative sink nodes, SAi = SA1, SA2, SA3, ... ,SAn

Each cluster has m number of sensor nodes. So, each sensor nodes will be uniquely identified through their numbers.

Sensor nodes under cluster Ci will be, CSij = CSi1, CSi2 , CSi3 , ... , CSim
Our first task is to create an authentication scheme through which each sink node will authenticate the sensor nodes before accepting or sending any data. Then before sending the data to the base station, the sink node will encrypt the data using lightweight symmetric cryptography to ensure security.

Phase—1 (Authentication Scheme) The sensor nodes in a WSN are the whole structure's leaf nodes. They gather information from the sensors and transmit it to the sink node. In the structure, a sink node may have an arbitrary number of leaf nodes underneath it.

The communication link is vulnerable to any kind of attacks. It enables any intruder to interrupt connection with the sink node or alter the data of the sensors while interacting with it. As a result, several authentication methods have been proposed with the goal of safeguarding the communications channel. The authentication mechanism must be extremely lightweight since the sensor nodes have limited computing power, memory, and battery.

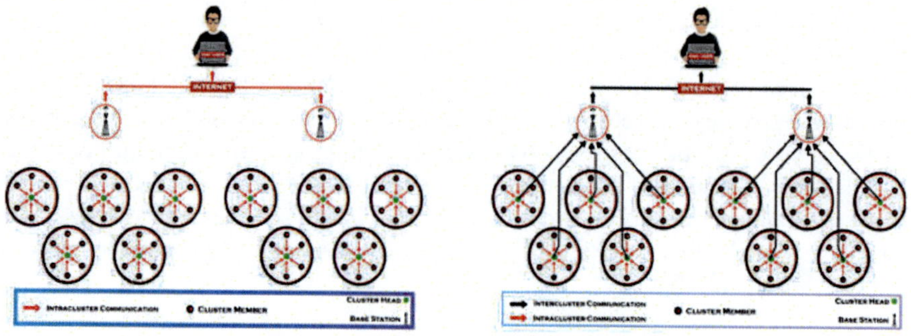

(a) (b)

Fig. 3 **a** Sensor node to sink node communication and **b** Sink node to base station communication

Many authors have offered authentication methods, which we have evaluated. We have chosen to adopt MUMAP: modified ultra-lightweight mutual authentication protocol, an authentication mechanism developed by Raju et al., after studying several protocols. MUMAP is a very light protocol with a high level of security. It just needs a little amount of computing power and uses very little energy. Figure 3a shows the sensor node to sink node communication. It has been cryptanalyzed using the Juel-Weis challenge and shown to be resistant to modular operations. Nodes's identity (ID), pseudonym (IDS), and key (Kr for sink node, Kt for sensor node) are stored in both sink node and sensor node. Kr and Kt are expected to be the same. Algorithm 1 represents the steps of authentication.

$IDS' = ID \oplus IDS;$
$A = IDS \oplus R;$
$B = Rot(Rot(Kr, A), Kr \oplus R;$
$B' = Rot(Rot(Kt, A), Kt \oplus R;$
$C' = Rot(Rot(IDS), R, Kt), Kt \oplus B';$
$C = Rot(Rot(IDS), R, Kr), Kr \oplus B;$
Update
$IDS = Rot(ID \oplus R, K);$
$K = Rot(K \oplus R, IDS);$

Algorithm 1: MUMAP authentication algorithm

Phase—2 (Encryption Scheme) Our second phase starts after receiving the data packets from the sensor nodes. When all the data packets are received, the sink node has to send all the data together to the base station. So, from the individual sink nodes of each cluster, data will be gathered at the base station. The sink node, unlike the sensor nodes, is a small device. Sink nodes have limited computational power and battery life. So, traditional cryptographic algorithms cannot be used here. Researchers have proposed many lightweight cryptographic techniques for these types of applications. Among them, we have selected TWINE-128 for securing this part of communication. Figure 3b shows the sensor node to sink node communication. TWINE has three distinct features: (1) no bit permutation, (2) Feistel-based generalization, and (3) no Galois field matrix. Only one 4-bit S-box and a 4-bit XOR are used. It is the first time these three characteristics have been combined in a method. The steps for TWINE encryption can be written as follows:

1. Take a block of 64-bit data (*P*).
2. Provide the secret key (*K*) (for TWINE-128, key length is 128 bit).
3. Iterate the rotation function. It consists of 4-bit S-boxes and a diffusion layer, which permutes the 16 blocks.
4. Rotation function is iterated 36 times to derive the round key (RK).
5. Encrypt the data using the key.
6. Generate cipher text (*C*).

Using the TWINE encryption scheme, the whole data package is encrypted. And after the encryption, the encrypted data package is sent to the base station. After the package is reached to the base station, it is decrypted. The decrypted file is obtained using the reverse process of encryption.

4 Result Analysis and Discussion

From Sect. 3, we can see that our proposed technique uses two different cryptographic schemes in the most vulnerable communication links to create a secure network. The proposed system provides several functions. Another notable fact is that our system can protect data against various cyber-attacks. An important fact to note here is that the proposed system is a combination of two already proven methods. We have already described them in the previous section. Thus, in this section, we have analyzed the security of the system through the functionality and the security against attacks provided by each algorithms individually.

Functionality The proposed system can provide several key functions, which can be enlisted as follows:

Integrity: Data will be transmitted from sensor nodes to sink nodes based on authentication, so an attacker cannot inject fake data posing as a sensor node beneath that sink node. Furthermore, since the connection between the sink node and the base station is secured by safe, lightweight TWINE, an attacker cannot alter the data.

Mutual authentication: Both the valid sensor node and the sink node should communicate and test each other. The communications conveyed are centered on shared IDs. Specific values are only stored by the actual sensor node and the sink node. As a result, when communicating, the sink node only authenticates the actual sensor nodes.

Confidentiality: The sink nodes' aggregate data packets are encrypted. An attacker must first decrypt the data in order to get it. The encryption method in use is impenetrable to cyber-attacks.

Forward security: If the sensor node is compromised, forward authentication is required to safeguard the sink nodes's previous communication with the sensor node. Suppose the attacker knows the key and ID, but he would not be able to decrypt the previous communication, as the key changes with the random number every time.

Security against Attacks The system provides security against various types of cyber-attacks.They can be enlisted as follows:

Desynchronization attack: To keep the sensor node and sink node synchronized, the protocol changes both the pseudonym and the key in both the sensor node and sink node after each authentication session.

Disclosure attack: To perform complicated computations, every measured value in our method depends on two or more other variables. To compute the swapped values, we utilize the ROT function twice. As a result, even if the attack could compromise A and B (in Algorithm 1), it would not acquire any data.

Replay attack: Different random numbers will be produced for each authentication session in our protocol, and different A, B, and C as mentioned in algorithm 1 will be chosen based on the random value and the local variables. As a result, if an intruder attempts to manipulate R, A, B, or C, communication will be stopped, and replays will not affect our protocol.

Impossible differential attack: In general, one of the most effective attacks against Feistel and generalized Feistel structure-based ciphers is the differential attack. TWINE was built in such a manner that it is impervious to differential attacks [9].

Saturation attack: A strong attack against generalized Feistel structure-based ciphers is the saturation attack. TWINE was put to the test using 4-bit saturations, and it has been proved invulnerable against it [9].

Differential/linear cryptanalysis: Any cryptographic algorithm faces significant danger from differential/linear cryptanalysis. TWINE was tested using differential/linear cryptanalysis to determine whether it could be cracked, but it proved to be unbreakable [9].

5 Conclusions

In this paper, we have proposed an implementation of an ultra-lightweight authentication protocol known as MUMAP in sensor node to sink node communication phase and a lightweight cryptographic algorithm named TWINE in sink node to base station communication phase to create a secure WSN network for the purpose of using in smart agriculture. Use of WSNs in agriculture is becoming popular day by day for its provided advantages. But security is a major issue in this case as if the data gets stolen or modified, the impact or loss can be of huge amount. Thus, we have created a model where the most vulnerable communication parts are being secured. In the first part where the sensor node communicates with the sink node, an authentication scheme is used to ensure that the data is coming from valid nodes under that network. And secondly, while the sink nodes communicate with the base station to send the data package, a lightweight cryptography is used to ensure data security.

The cryptographic techniques used here are very less energy consuming and require less computational power and memory which make them feasible to implement in this case.

References

1. Tzounis A, Katsoulas N, Bartzanas T, Kittas C (2021) Internet of things in agriculture, recent advances and future challenges. Biosyst Eng 164:31-48. ISSN: 1537-5110 (Dec. 2017)
2. Akyildiz IF, Su W, Sankarasubramaniam Y, Cayirci E (2021) Wireless sensor networks: a survey. Comput Netw 38:393–422. ISSN: 1389-1286. (Mar. 2002)
3. Barcelo-Ordinas JM, Chanet JP, Hou K-M, García-Vidal J (2013) A survey of wireless sensor technologies applied to precision agriculture. In: Stafford JV (ed) Precision agriculture '13. Academic Publishers, Wageningen, 2013, 801-808. ISBN: 978-90-8686-778-3
4. Pandithurai O, Aishwarya S, Aparna B, Kavitha K (2017) Agro-tech: a digital model for monitoring soil and crops using internet of things (IOT). In: 2017 third international conference on science technology engineering management (ICONSTEM), 342–346
5. Singh R, Singh DK, Kumar L (2010) A review on security issues in wireless sensor network. J Inf Syst Commun 1. Bioinfo Publications, 1
6. Poschmann A (2009) Lightweight cryptography. Ruhr-University Bochum, Bochum
7. Dhanda SS, Singh B, Jindal P (2021) Lightweight cryptography: a solution to secure IoT. Wirel Person Commun 112:1947–1980. ISSN: 1572-834X(June 2020)
8. Raju MH, Ahmed MU, Ahad MAR (2021) MUMAP: modified ultralightweight mutual authentication protocol for RFID enabled IoT net- works. J Inst Indus Appl Eng 9:33–39
9. Suzaki T, Minematsu K, Morioka S, Kobayashi E (2011) Twine: a lightweight, versatile block cipher. In: ECRYPT workshop on lightweight cryptography
10. Díaz SE, Pérez JC, Mateos AC, Marinescu M-C, Guerra BB (2011) A novel methodology for the monitoring of the agricultural production process based on wireless sensor networks. Comput Electron Agric 76:252–265. ISSN: 0168-1699
11. Oljaca M et al (2021) Wireless sensors in agriculture, Carrent development and future perspective. Accepted: 2015-03-05T18:42:45Z
12. Belapurkar A et al (2009) Distributed systems security: issues, processes and solutions. Wiley, New York
13. Góomez-Chabla R, Real-Avilées K, Moráan C, Grijalva P, Recalde T (2019) IoT applications in agriculture: a systematic literature review. In: Valencia-García R, Alcaraz- Máarmol G, Cioppo-Morstadt Jd, Vera-Lucio N, Bucaram-Leverone M (eds) ICT for agriculture and environment. Springer International Publishing, Cham, 68–76. ISBN: 978-3- 030-10728-4
14. Gupta M, Abdelsalam M, Khorsandroo S, Mittal S (2020) Security and privacy in smart farming: challenges and opportunities. IEEE Access 8. Conference Name: IEEE access, 34564-34584. ISSN: 2169-3536
15. Window M (2019) Security in precision agriculture: Vulnerabilities and risks of agricultural systems
16. El Bilali H, Allahyari MS (2018) Transition towards sustainability in agriculture and food systems: role of information and communication technologies. Inf Process Agric 5:456–464
17. Ali R, Pal AK, Kumari S, Karuppiah M, Conti M (2021) A secure user authentication and key-agreement scheme using wireless sensor networks for agriculture monitoring. Future Gener Comput Syst 84, 200–215. ISSN: 0167-739X (July 2018)
18. Amin R, Biswas GP (2021) A secure light weight scheme for user authenti- cation and key agreement in multi-gateway based wireless sensor networks. Ad Hoc Netw 36:58–80. ISSN: 1570-8705 (Jan. 2016)

19. Naoui S, Elhdhili ME, Saidane LA (2016) Enhancing the security of the IoT LoraWAN architecture. In: 2016 international conference on performance evaluation and modeling in wired and wireless networks (PEMWN), 1–7
20. Shiravale S, Bhagat SM (2014) Wireless sensor networks in agriculture sector- implementation and security measures. Int J Comput Appl 92 Citeseer
21. Katagi M, Moriai S (2008) Lightweight cryptography for the internet of things. Sony Corporation. Citeseer, 7–10
22. Shah AM (2019) A survey of lightweight cryptographic algorithms for IoT-based applications. In: Tiwari S, Trivedi MC, Mishra KK, Misra AK, Kumar KK (eds) Smart innovations in communication and computational sciences (eds). Springer, Singapore, 283–293. ISBN: 9789811324147
23. Eisenbarth T, Kumar S, Paar C, Poschmann A, Uhsadel L (2007) A sur- vey of lightweight-cryptography implementations. In: Conference name: IEEE design test of computers 24. ISSN: 1558-1918, 522–533
24. Barreto L, Amaral A (2018) Smart farming: cyber security challenges. In: 2018 international conference on intelligent systems (IS) ISSN: 1541-1672, 870–876
25. Baranwal T, Pateriya PK (2016) Development of IoT based smart security and monitoring devices for agriculture. In: 2016 6th international conference cloud system and big data engineering (Confluence). IEEE, 597–602
26. Mehta A, Patel S (2016) IoT based smart agriculture research opportunities and challenges. Int J Technol Res Eng 4:541–543
27. Demestichas K, Peppes N, Alexakis T (2020) Survey on security threats in agricultural IoT and smart farming. Sensors 20. Number: 22 Publisher: Multidisciplinary Digital Publishing Institute, 6458

ASER Performance Analysis of Decision Threshold-Based Hybrid FSO-RF Turbulent Link

Deepak Kumar Singh and B. B. Tiwari

Abstract In this paper a novel hybrid Free Space Optical (FSO)-Radio Frequency (RF) model is proposed which is based on the single decision threshold feedback bit technique. The FSO and proposed hybrid FSO-RF link performance is investigated under strong turbulence and misalignment aperture error or pointing error in terms of the average symbol error rate (ASER) and outage probability. Atmospheric turbulence and misalignment aperture are foremost factors that affect the performance of FSO link which entails the requirement of an RF link as a backup to enhance the system performance. The FSO-RF link is preferred in this work over the normal FSO link due to ease in switching among the link established with the help of decision threshold during failure of FSO link. In this proposed hybrid model, Gamma-Gamma distribution is considered as free-space optical turbulence channel and Nakagami-m model is for RF link. The analytical expressions for outage probability, ASER have been derived and results are given for various Subcarrier Intensity Modulation—M-Phase Shift Keying (PSK) schemes. A performance comparative study is reported for FSO link and hybrid FSO-RF link. The obtained result indicates the enhanced system performance whereas the obtained results are validated through Monte-Carlo simulations and results are found in good agreement.

Keywords Average symbol error rate (ASER) · Decision threshold · Free-space optical (FSO) communication · Misalignment error · Subcarrier intensity modulation (SIM)

1 Introduction

The authorized bodies are incapable to handle the growing traffic demands due to existing policy of fixed spectrum allocation strategies. The continuous growth in data traffic originated by mobile users will be witnessed very serious problem in future. By 2021, the number of mobile users connected to the networks is expected

D. K. Singh (✉) · B. B. Tiwari
VBS Purvanchal University, Jaunpur, Uttar Pradesh 222001, India

M. S. Kaiser et al. (eds.), *Proceedings of Trends in Electronics and Health Informatics*, Lecture Notes in Networks and Systems 376,
https://doi.org/10.1007/978-981-16-8826-3_54

to exceed 28.3 billion. This explosive growth of global mobile data traffic attracts global research on cognitive radio networks and OWC technologies [1].

To mitigate the technical challenges like higher bandwidth services where wire-line (fiber/copper cable) solutions and last-mile connectivity problems are difficult to deploy and fulfill the requirement of high speed and large bandwidth applications, Optical Wireless Communication (OWC) is the most suited. Optical wireless communication technologies (OWC) systems (indoor and outdoor) covering a wide unlicensed spectral range of 700–10,000 nm have the potential to offer a cost-effective protocol-free link at data rates exceeding 2.5 Gbps per wavelength up to 5 km range. OWC is a more sensible solution because of its multiple user-sized cells, reduced interference, and improved carrier reuse capabilities due to its intrinsically abrupt boundary [2]. OWC is broadly categorized mainly in four forms, i.e. free space optics (FSO), visible light communication (VLC), optical camera communication (OCC), and light fidelity (Li-Fi), are considered which have potential to fulfill the increasing demands of 5G/6G and Internet of things (IoT) networks for their special features, [3]. Figure 1 shows brief architectures of these technologies. These technologies vary in the type of transmitter (Tx), receiver (Rx), and communication media. Table 1 shows the various technological aspects of OWC technologies.

The visible light communication (VLC) for indoor applications, OCC is Ultraviolet non-line of sight (UV-NLOS) operating at UV frequency for outdoor applications, and FSO normally uses IR for communication but it can also be operated

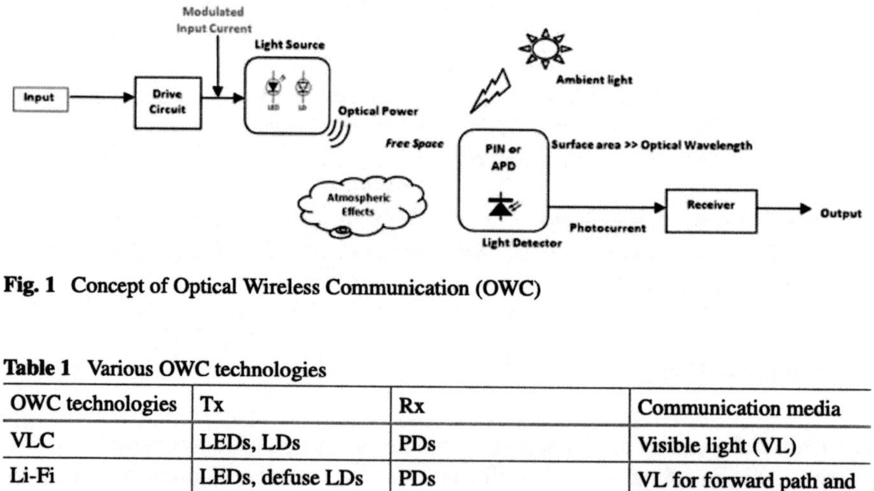

Fig. 1 Concept of Optical Wireless Communication (OWC)

Table 1 Various OWC technologies

OWC technologies	Tx	Rx	Communication media
VLC	LEDs, LDs	PDs	Visible light (VL)
Li-Fi	LEDs, defuse LDs	PDs	VL for forward path and Infra-red (IR) for backward path
OCC	Light or LED array,	Camera or image sensor	VL, IR, and Ultraviolet(UV)
FSO	LDs	PDs or HD	IR, VL, and UV

using VL and UV. It is a short distance and LOS communication operating above 100 GHz near Infra-red (IR) frequency range in EM spectrum.

In the case of FSO Communication, the transmitter aperture and receiver aperture must be aligned, i.e. point to point communication link, mainly for outdoor applications. Since the FSO wavelength range is 700–1600 nm, so bandwidth will be from 100 GHz to a few THz [4].

FSO communication has recently gained a growing interest for both commercial and military applications. Similar to fiber, FSO transmits data in the form of a small conical-shaped beam by means of a low-powered laser or light-emitting diode (LED) in the THz spectrum. Instead of enclosing the data stream in a glass fiber, it is transmitted through the air and operates in a near-infrared (IR) band. FSO becomes attractive technology where fiber installation and RF wireless and wireline solutions are expensive. FSO addresses applications like higher bandwidth services where wireline solutions are difficult, metropolitan networks, inter-building communication, backhaul wireless systems, indoor links, fiber backup, service acceleration, higher security, military purpose, smaller size of transmitting and receiving antennas, higher transmission efficiency, satellite communications, etc. FSO communication is also an emerging alternative to RF communication due to its worldwide compatibility, wide bandwidth, higher capacity in Gbps (data rate), low-cost deployment, low power per bit, high security, and unlicensed optical spectrum [5, 6].

The prominent factors that deteriorate the FSO transmission efficiency performance are atmospheric turbulence and misaligned aperture in clear weather conditions and fog, haze, snow, sandstorms in adverse weather conditions [7]. To overcome the losses and improve the transmission efficiency the RF link is required as a backup in FSO, a hybrid FSO-RF scheme can be used to meet the requirement [8]. So a Hybrid FSO-RF transmission is complementary to the FSO system that is one possible solution for ensuring the availability of links in different weather conditions. FSO is restricted to only Line of Sight (LOS) communication unlike RF communication means the transmitter aperture and receiver aperture should be perfectly aligned that restricted to only a short distance communication over few Km [9, 10]. Since it is operating in the IR range so we can easily go with the bandwidth of a few GHz without much of a problem. In the case of a hybrid FSO-RF link, if the FSO link fails due to NLOS and atmospheric effect then a backup RF link will be utilized.

The earlier work on hybrid FSO/RF system mainly focuses on merging the design of coding and various schemes of FSO and RF link to achieve a soft-switching between two links. In reference [11] hybrid FSO/RF system uses hybrid channel codes. In reference [12] for hybrid FSO/RF system a rate less coded automatic repeat request (ARQA) has been proposed. Reference [13] proposes a bit-interleaved coded modulation scheme for such hybrid systems. The use of short length raptor codes has been proposed in [14]. The link availability of hybrid FSO/RF was investigated in [15] from information theory perspectives. On another front, [16] introduces diversity combining to parallel FSO and RF channels, while assuming both links transmit identical information simultaneously. The performance of a similar hybrid FSO/RF system with non-Gaussian noise has been analyzed in [17]. These hard-switching schemes typically lead to some rate loss compared to soft-switching schemes. Meanwhile, both classes of transmission schemes discussed above require the FSO and RF links to be active continuously, even when experiencing poor quality, which will lead to wasted transmission power and generate unnecessary interference to the environment.

In other investigation [18], the author proposes and implements the hybrid free-space optical (FSO)/radio frequency (RF) wireless communication system without requiring channel state information and hybrid system transmits the same data with the same data rate over both links simultaneously using diversity selection combining scheme.

In this work, the effect of strong turbulence and misaligned aperture error on FSO and proposed hybrid FSO-RF is analyzed and performances are compared for various M-PSK schemes. For the proposed hybrid model Gamma-Gamma distribution is considered for the free-space-optical channel that helps to model strong-to-moderate turbulence and Nakagami-m model is for RF link. The switching among links depends on the decision threshold technique. The system performance is analyzed on the basis of outage probability and average symbol error rate under atmospheric turbulence and misaligned aperture. Closed-form expressions for outage probability and ASER have been derived with/without Pointing Errors and validated using Monte-Carlo Simulations Results are plotted for various SIM/HD—M-PSK schemes and the results indicate an enhanced system performance with hybrid FSO-RF system which means the hybrid FSO-RF system performs better in contrast to the single FSO link due to backup RF link in different fading and weather conditions.

2 System and Channel Models

FSO link performance degrades because of strong attenuation due to fog, snow, pointing error, and atmospheric turbulence. Use of RF link to backup FSO in case of failure, hybrid FSO-RF system is more suited. RF link ensures connectivity thus improves the system reliability. FSO is unstirred by rain while RF is less affected by fog, haze, snow, and pointing errors [19]. Thus FSO and RF will assist each other in different weather conditions.

As given in Fig. 2 the proposed hybrid FSO-RF both FSO and RF links will be available in parallel and only one of them will be active at a particular point of time. Activation of the link will be decided on the basis of decision threshold value. The instantaneous SNR of the FSO link falls below certain threshold SNR, the RF link will be active otherwise FSO link will be active. In this model, the FSO link is the primary link for transmission and the RF link will play the role of secondary link. The outage is defined when the SNR of both FSO and RF links fall below the threshold SNR. For this hybrid FSO-RF system modeling the assumptions are made that receiver has the perfect CSI and feedback bits are received without any error. At the transmitter of the proposed hybrid FSO-RF system, SIM-MPSK digital modulation schemes are used to modulate the bit streams; then modulated signal is

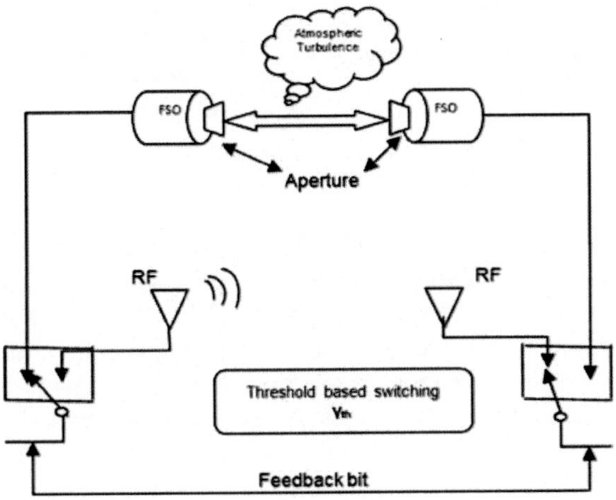

Fig. 2 Proposed hybrid FSO-RF model [7]

fed with a hybrid FSO-RF subsystem and the FSO subsystem used the SIM/HD at the receiver.

2.1 *FSO Subsystem Model*

The probability distribution function (PDF) of Gamma-Gamma FSO channel turbulence I_a is [20]:

$$f_{I_a}(I) = \frac{2(\alpha\beta)^{\frac{\alpha+\beta}{2}}}{\Gamma(\alpha)\Gamma(\beta)} I^{\frac{\alpha+\beta}{2}-1} \kappa_{\alpha-\beta}\left(2\sqrt{\alpha\beta I}\right) \tag{1}$$

where α and β are small-scale (shape) and large-scale parameters of the scattering environment respectively, $\kappa_v(.)$ is the modified Bessel function of the second kind of order (α–β) and $\Gamma(.)$ is the Gamma function $\Gamma(z) = \int_0^\infty x^{z-1} e^x \mathrm{d}x$, α and β are closely related to atmospheric conditions through the following relationship:

$$\alpha = \left[\exp\left(\frac{0.49\delta^2}{\left(1 + 0.18d^2 + 0.56\delta^{12/5}\right)^{7/6}}\right) - 1\right]^{-1}$$

$$\beta = \left[\exp\left(\frac{0.51\delta^2\left(1 + 0.69\delta^{12/5}\right)^{-5/6}}{\left(1 + 0.9d^2 + 0.62d^2\delta^{12/5}\right)^{5/6}}\right) - 1\right]^{-1}$$

Table 2 Values of α, β, and δ^2 for different turbulence regimes [2]

Regimes\parameters	α	β	δ^2
Weak turbulence	11.6	10.1	0.2
Moderate turbulence	4	1.9	1.6
Strong turbulence	4.2	1.4	3.5

where $d = \sqrt{kD^2/4L}$, K is optical wave number ($k = 2\pi/\lambda$) and D is optical receiver's aperture diameter, λ is optical wavelength, and L is distance between transmitter and receiver of optical link. The Rytov variance with atmospheric turbulence strength (C_n^2) that is altitude-dependent, is defined as $\delta^2 = 0.5C_n^2k^{7/6}L^{11/6}$.

Gamma-Gamma distribution parameters of large-scale eddies (α) and small-scale eddies (β) are characterized by received irradiance (I) fluctuations for different atmospheric turbulence conditions such as weak, moderate, and strong turbulence regimes. The value of α and β is less and δ^2 is larger than strong turbulence while the value of α and β is large and δ^2 is lesser than weak turbulence regimes (Table 2).

In this work, we have considered the FSO link under strong turbulence regimes.

The received signal γ_{FSO} of the FSO subsystem is [21]:

$$y_{\text{FSO}} = P_F\eta I_a + n$$

then the instantaneous signal to noise ratio (SNR) of the FSO channel is:

$$\gamma_{\text{FSO}} = \frac{(P_F\eta I_a)^2}{N_0}$$

where P_F is transmitted optical power, $N_0/2$ is additive white Gaussian noise (AWGN) noise variance, and η is responsivity of the detector.

The PDF of the instantaneous SNR γ_{FSO} of the FSO channel without pointing error is:

$$f_{\gamma_{\text{FSO}}}(\gamma) = \frac{1}{2\Gamma(\alpha)\Gamma(\beta)}\gamma^{-1}G_{0,2}^{2,0}\left(\frac{\alpha\beta\sqrt{\gamma}}{\sqrt{\bar{\gamma}_{\text{FSO}}}}\Big|_{\alpha,\beta}^{-}\right) \tag{2}$$

Here $G_{1,3}^{3,0}\left(z/^{a_p}_{b_q}\right)$ is Meijer G-function [22].

Then the cumulative distribution function (CDF) of the instantaneous SNR γ_{FSO} of the FSO channel without pointing error is:

$$F_{\gamma_{\text{FSO}}}(x) = \frac{1}{\Gamma(\alpha)\Gamma(\beta)}G_{1,3}^{2,1}\left(\frac{\alpha\beta\sqrt{x}}{\sqrt{\bar{\gamma}_{FSO}}}\Big|_{\alpha,\beta,0}^{1}\right) \tag{3}$$

2.2 Combination of Irradiance, Misalignment Aperture Error/Pointing Error, and Atmospheric Loss in FSO Subsystem

Misalignment aperture or pointing errors are due to misalignment of detector and laser beam hence the attenuation due to geometric spread with pointing error is [23, 24]: The PDF of pointing error I_p is given by random variable transformation:

$$f_{I_p}(I_p) = \frac{g^2}{A_0^{g^2}}(I_p)^{g^2-1}, 0 \le I_p \le A_0 \tag{4}$$

where $g = \frac{w_{Leq}}{2\sigma_s}$ is called as pointing error coefficient and σ_s is the jitter standard deviation.

The signal loss of a link is defined B-lammbert' law $I_l = \exp(-\alpha_1 L)$ where α_1 (dB/Km) is attenuation coefficient due to fog, haze, etc. and L is the link distance.

Hence the composite channel irradiance is $I_{FSO} = I_a.I_p.I_l$.

The CDF of instantaneous SNR of FSO link with hetero-detection (HD) technique is:

$$F_{\gamma_{HD}}(x) = \frac{g^2}{\Gamma(\alpha)\Gamma(\beta)} G_{2,4}^{3,1}\left(D\frac{x}{\overline{\gamma}_{HD}}\middle|_{g^2,\alpha,\beta,0}^{1,g^2+1}\right) \tag{5}$$

2.3 RF Subsystem

The PDF of the small-scale fading of RF channel with Nakagami-m distribution is [25]:

$$f_{\|h\|}(t) = \frac{2m^m t^{2m-1}}{\Gamma(m)\Omega_p^m} e^{-\frac{m}{\Omega_p}t^2}$$

where $\Omega_p = \mathrm{E}\left[\|h\|^2\right]$, $\|h\| \ge 0$.

The CDF of instantaneous SNR of RF link using Gamma distribution is [26, 27]:

$$F_{\gamma_{RF}}(x) = \frac{x}{\Gamma(m)}\gamma\left(m, \frac{mx}{\overline{\gamma}_{RF}}\right) \tag{6}$$

where $\gamma(a, b)$ is a lower incomplete Gamma function.

3 Performance Analysis

3.1 Outage Probability

Outage Probability for FSO without pointing error, when instantaneous SNR of FSO link becomes lesser than the decision threshold SNR, γ_{th}^{F}:

$$P_{out}^{FSO} = \Pr\left(\gamma \le \gamma_{th}^{F}\right) = F_{\gamma_{FSO}}\left(\gamma_{th}^{F}\right)$$

$$P_{out}^{FSO} = \frac{1}{\Gamma(\alpha)\Gamma(\beta)} G_{1,3}^{2,1}\left(\alpha\beta\sqrt{\frac{\gamma_{th}^{F}}{\overline{\gamma}_{FSO}}}\Big|_{\alpha,\beta,0}^{1}\right) \tag{7}$$

Outage Probability for RF, when the instantaneous SNR of RF link becomes lesser than the decision threshold SNR, γ_{th}^{R}:

$$P_{out}^{RF} = \Pr\left(\gamma \le \gamma_{th}^{R}\right) = F_{\gamma_{RF}}\left(\gamma_{th}^{R}\right)$$

$$P_{out}^{RF} = \frac{\gamma_{th}^{R}}{\Gamma(m)}\gamma\left(m, \frac{m\gamma_{th}^{R}}{\overline{\gamma}_{RF}}\right) \tag{8}$$

Outage Probability for hybrid FSO-RF, if the instantaneous SNR of both FSO and RF links falls below the decision threshold γ_{th}, then outage is declared:

$$P_{out}^{hybrid} = F_{\gamma_{FSO}}\left(\gamma_{th}^{F}\right) \times F_{\gamma_{RF}}\left(\gamma_{th}^{R}\right) \tag{9}$$

Outage Probability for the FSO channel with pointing error is:

$$P_{out}^{FSO^{pe}} = \Pr\left(\gamma \le \gamma_{th}^{F}\right) = F_{\gamma_{FSO}}^{pe}\left(\gamma_{th}^{F}\right)$$

$$\Rightarrow F_{\gamma_{FSO}}^{pe}\left(\gamma_{th}^{F}\right) = \frac{g^2}{\Gamma(\alpha)\Gamma(\beta)} G_{2,4}^{3,1}\left(D\frac{\sqrt{\gamma_{th}^{F}}}{\sqrt{\overline{\gamma}_{FSO}}}\Big|_{g^2,\alpha,\beta,0}^{1,g^2+1}\right) \tag{10}$$

Similarly, the outage probability for hybrid FSO-RF with pointing error is:

$$P_{out}^{hybrid^{pe}} = F_{\gamma_{FSO}}^{pe}\left(\gamma_{th}^{F}\right) \times F_{\gamma_{RF}}\left(\gamma_{th}^{R}\right) \tag{11}$$

where $F_{\gamma_{RF}}\left(\gamma_{th}^{R}\right)$ is the (CDF) outage probability of RF channel.

3.2 Average Symbol Error Rate (ASER)

Using general formula for calculating ASER of FSO system without PE is:

$$P_e^{\mathrm{FSO}} = \int_0^{\infty} p(e/\gamma) f_{\gamma_{\mathrm{FSO}}}(\gamma) \mathrm{d}\gamma \tag{12}$$

After evaluating the integral in Eq. (13) we get:

$$P_e^{\mathrm{FSO}} = \frac{A 2^{\alpha+\beta-3}}{\pi^{3/2}\Gamma(\alpha)\Gamma(\beta)} G_{2,5}^{4,2}\left(\frac{(\alpha\beta)^2}{16B^2\overline{\gamma}_{\mathrm{FSO}}} \middle| \begin{matrix} 1, \frac{1}{2} \\ \frac{\alpha}{2}, \frac{\alpha+1}{2}, \frac{\beta}{2}, \frac{\beta+1}{2}, 0 \end{matrix} \right) \tag{13}$$

Average symbol error rate (ASER) of RF system is:

$$P_e^{\mathrm{RF}} = \frac{A}{2} - \frac{AB}{2\sqrt{\pi}} \sum_{l=0}^{m-1} \frac{C^l \Gamma\left(l+\frac{1}{2}\right)}{\left(B^2 + C\right)^{l+\frac{1}{2}}} \tag{14}$$

where $C = \frac{m}{\overline{\gamma}_{\mathrm{RF}}}$.

ASER for FSO system with pointing error is:

$$P_e^{\mathrm{FSO^{pe}}} = \int_0^{\infty} p(e/\gamma) f_{\gamma_{\mathrm{FSO}}}^{\mathrm{pe}}(\gamma) \mathrm{d}\gamma$$

After evaluating above integral the final expression for ASER of FSO with PE is:

$$P_e^{\mathrm{FSO^{pe}}} = \frac{A g^2 2^{\alpha+\beta-3}}{\pi^{3/2}\Gamma(\alpha)\Gamma(\beta)} G_{4,7}^{6,2}\left(\frac{D^2}{16B^2\overline{\gamma}_{\mathrm{FSO}}} \middle| \begin{matrix} 1, \frac{1}{2}, \frac{g^2+1}{2}, \frac{g^2+2}{2} \\ \frac{g^2}{2}, \frac{g^2+1}{2}, \frac{\alpha}{2}, \frac{\alpha+1}{2}, \frac{\beta}{2}, \frac{\beta+1}{2}, 0 \end{matrix} \right) \tag{15}$$

ASER for hybrid FSO-RF system including pointing error is:

$$P_e^{\mathrm{hybrid^{pe}}} = B_{\mathrm{FSO}}^{\mathrm{pe}}(\gamma_{\mathrm{th}}) + F_{\gamma_{\mathrm{FSO}}}^{\mathrm{pe}}(\gamma_{\mathrm{th}}) P_e^{\mathrm{RF}} \tag{16}$$

where $B_{\mathrm{FSO}}^{\mathrm{pe}}(\gamma_{\mathrm{th}})$ is the ASER of FSO with pointing error during non-outage period and $B_{\mathrm{FSO}}^{\mathrm{pe}}(\gamma_{\mathrm{th}}) = \int_{\gamma_{\mathrm{th}}}^{\infty} p(e/\gamma) f_{\gamma_{\mathrm{FSO}}}^{\mathrm{pe}}(\gamma) \mathrm{d}\gamma$.

4 Results and Discussion

The closed-expressions obtained in Sect. 2 and 3 are taking here in this section for the analysis of the performance of FSO and hybrid FSO-RF links such as outage probability and ASER under various SIM—M-PSK.

The novel Gamma–Gamma distribution model to quantitatively describe strong atmospheric turbulence, the interference caused by misalignment aperture error or pointing error. The receiver employs SIM/HD to obtain the performance of the FSO and hybrid FSO-RF transmission links.

In Figs. 3 and 4 the outage probability is presented using analytical expression found from the Eq. (7) and (8) for the FSO system over Gamma-Gamma fading channels without pointing errors and for RF system over Nakagami-m model respectively. It is seen that for different outage thresholds of 5 dB, 10 dB, and 15 dB as shown, the outage probability is reduced respectively for an average SNR of 40 dB for various M-PSK schemes.

The comparative average SER performance of RF and FSO systems is showed in Figs. 5 and 6 respectively. These Figs. 5 and 6 are representing the Eqs. (13) and (14) simultaneously. Whereas these RF and FSO systems are associated with BPSK, 4-PSK, 8-PSK, and 16-PSK modulation schemes.

The FSO system is considered under strong turbulence conditions ($C_n^2 = 5 \times 10^{-14}\ \text{m}^{-2/3}$). Both systems with the BPSK modulation scheme perform better than the system with the 4-PSK, 8-PSK, and 16-PSK modulation schemes. The degradation of the SER performance of RF and FSO system with an increase in modulation order. This is because of the increase in phase errors in higher-order modulation schemes under the similar channel conditions. The BPSK schemes show better SER over the 4-PSK, 8-PSK, and 16-PSK modulation schemes.

The analytical and simulation results with various PSK schemes are shown in Figs. 7 and 8 which follow the Eqs. (13) and (16) respectively. The comparative analysis for average SER performance of proposed hybrid RF-FSO system with and without misaligned aperture error or pointing error.

The FSO link is considered under strong turbulence condition with BPSK, 4-PSK, 8-PSK, and 16-PSK modulation schemes. The analytical and simulation study

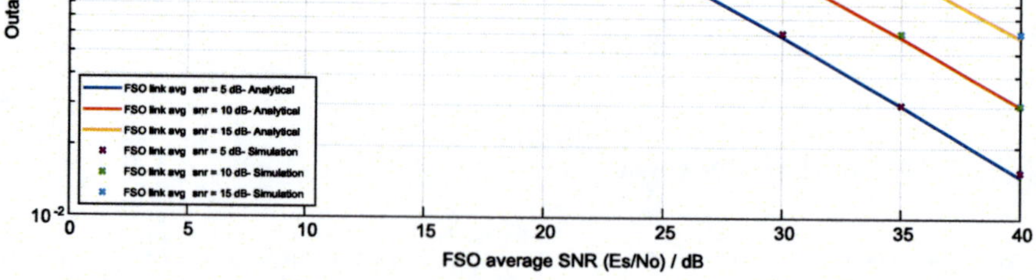

Fig. 3 Outage probability of FSO system without PE

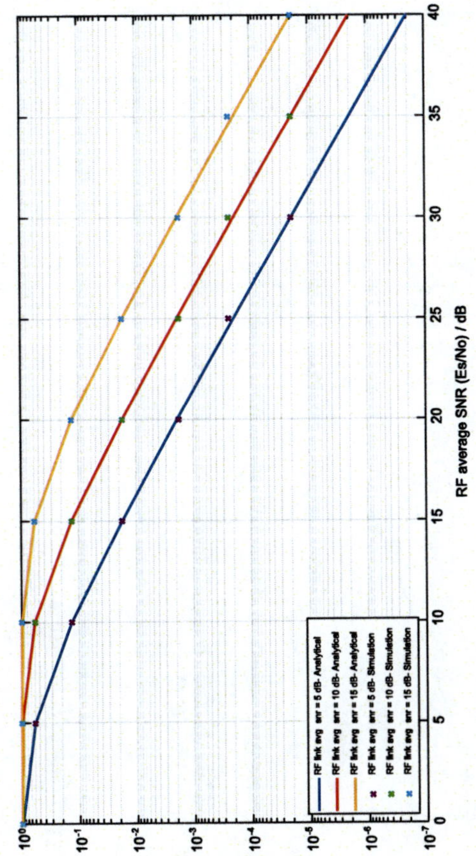

Fig. 4 Outage probability of RF system over Nakagami fading

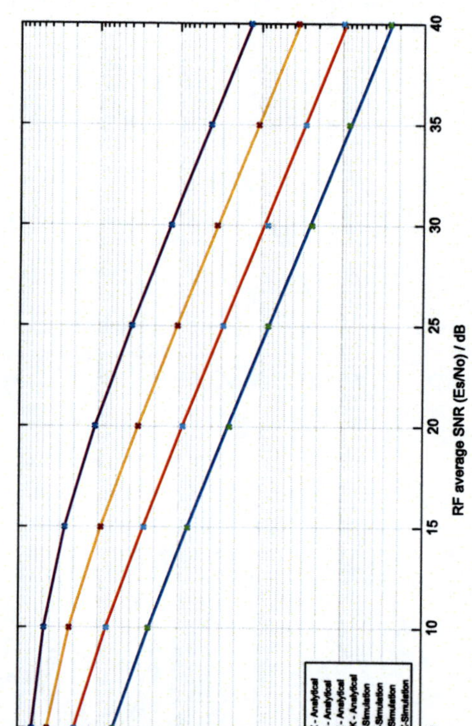

Fig. 5 Comparative average SER performance of RF system

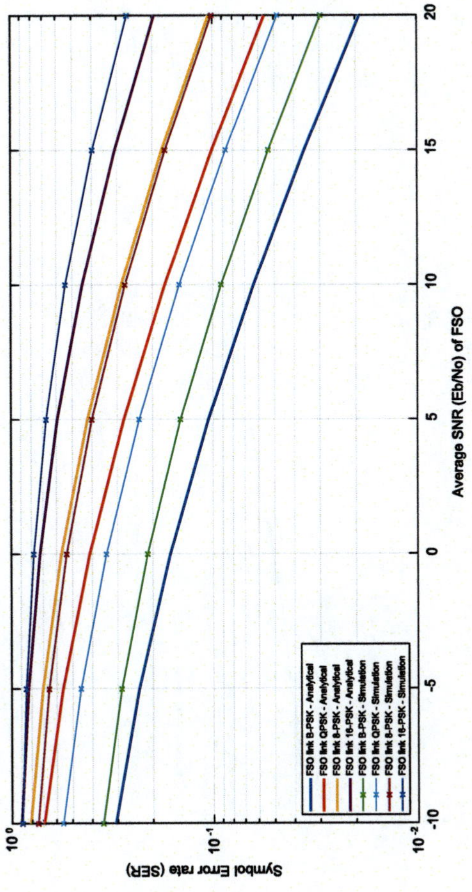

Fig. 6 Comparative average SER performance of FSO system

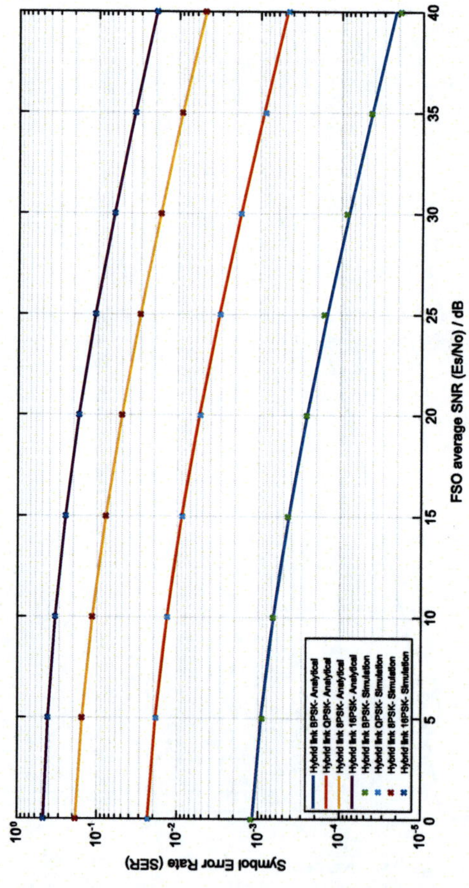

Fig. 7 Average SER of hybrid FSO-RF system without PE

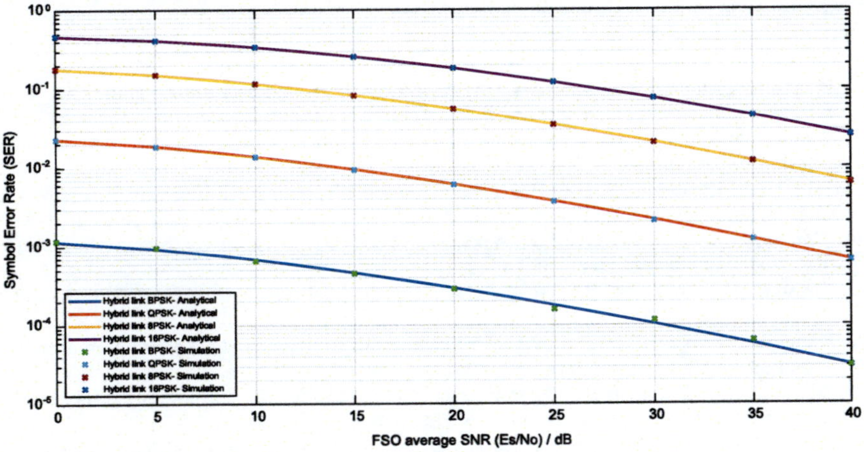

Fig. 8 Average SER of hybrid FSO-RF system with PE

depicted that the results obtained in Figs. 5, 6, 7, and 8 are in good agreement and performance of the system is enhanced as compared to single FSO link and hybrid FSO-RF link without pointing error.

5 Conclusion

The performance of FSO and hybrid FSO links with decision threshold-based switching and various M-PSK modulation schemes has been investigated. Using the precise Meijer's G function, the closed mathematical expressions are derived. Observations show that the proposed hybrid FSO-RF system under pointing error is outperforming compared to single FSO link under said channel conditions.

The performance results showed the superiority of the hybrid system over the FSO system in both cases with pointing error and without pointing error. The results of our investigations prove that the average SER performance could be enhanced by adopting proposed hybrid FSO-RF system in place of single FSO system.

Further, this work will be extended in the investigations using some more generalized channel models for FSO such as Malaga, K-distribution, etc. with spatial diversity techniques such as MIMO, SIMO, etc. The further study may be carried on to evaluate other performance parameters such as ergodic capacity, secrecy outage probability, power allocation strategies for FSO and hybrid FSO-RF using some novel modulation techniques.

References

1. Gupta MS, Kumar K (2019) Progression on spectrum sensing for cognitive radio networks: a survey, classification, challenges and future research issues. J Netw Comput Appl 143:47–76
2. Ghassemlooy Z, Popoola W, Rajbhandari S (2013) Optical wireless communications. CRC Press, T&F Group
3. Li CY, Lu HH, Chou CU, Hsia HM, Feng CY, Chen YH, Huang YT, Nainggolan A (2021) A flexible bidirectional fiber-FSO-5G wireless convergent system. J Lightwave Technol 39(5)
4. Raj AB, Majumdar AK Historical perspective of free space optical communications from early dates to today's developments. IET J 8(2)
5. Safari M, Uysal M (2008) Relay-assisted free-space optical communication. IEEE Trans Wirel Commun 7(12):5441–5449
6. Gappmair W (2011) Further results on the capacity of free-space optical channels in turbulent atmosphere. IET Commun 5(9):1262–1267
7. Sharma S, Madhukumar AS, Swaminathan R et al (2019) Effect of pointing errors on the performance of hybrid FSO/RF networks. IEEE Trans 4(1)
8. Nath S, Sengar S, Shrivastava SK et al (2019) Impact of atmospheric turbulence, pointing error and traffic pattern on the performance of cognitive hybrid FSO/RF system. IEEE Trans Cognitive Commun Netw 6(2)
9. Al-Gailani SA, Salleh MZM, Salem AA, Shaddad RQ, Sheikh UU, Algeelani NA, Almohamad TA (2021) A survey of free space optics (FSO) communication systems, links, and networks. IEEE J 9
10. Kashif H, Khan MN, Altalbe A (2020) Hybrid optical-radio transmission system link quality: link budget analysis. IEEE J 8
11. Vangala S, Pishro-Nik H (2007) A highly reliable FSO/RF communication system using efficient codes. In: Proceedings of IEEE GLOBECOM, pp 2232–2236
12. Abdulhussein A, Oka A, Nguyen TT, Lampe L (2010) Rateless coding for hybrid free-space optical and radiofrequency communication. IEEE Trans Wirel Commun 9(3):907–913
13. He B, Schober R (2010) Bit-interleaved coded modulation for hybrid RF/FSO systems. IEEE Trans Commun 57(12):3753–3763
14. Zhang W, Hranilovic S, Shi C (2009) Soft-switching hybrid FSO/RF links using short-length raptor codes: design and implementation. IEEE J Sel Areas Commun 27(9):1698–1708
15. Letzepis N, Nguyen K, Fabregas AG, Cowley W (2009) Outage analysis of the hybrid free-space optical and radio-frequency channel. IEEE J Sel Areas Commun 27(9):1709–1719
16. Chatzidiamantis N, Karagiannidis G, Kriezis E, Matthaiou M (2011) Diversity combining in hybrid RF/FSO systems with PSK modulation. In: Proceedings of IEEE ICC, pp 1–6
17. Shakir WMR (2018) Performance evaluation of a selection combining scheme for the hybrid FSO/RF system. IEEE Photonic J 10(1)
18. Gupta R, Singh P (2014) Hybrid FSO-RF system: a solution to atmospheric turbulences in long haul communication. Int J Sci Eng Res 5(11), ISSN 2229-5518
19. Nadeem F, Geiger B, Leitgeb E, Muhammad S, Loeschnig M, Kandus M (2011) Comparison of link selection algorithms for free space optics/radio frequency hybrid network. IET Commun J 5(18):2751–2759
20. Majumdar A (2015) Advanced free space optics (FSO): a systems approach. Springer, New York
21. Uysal M, Li J, Yu M (2006) Error rate performance analysis of coded free-space optical links over gamma–gamma atmospheric turbulence channels. IEEE Trans Wirel Commun 5(6):1229–1233
22. Trott M (2021) The wolfram functions site. Accessed [Online]. Available http://functions.wolfram.com/2021/06/03
23. Nistazakis H, Tsiftsis T, Tombras G (2009) Performance analysis of free-space optical communication systems over atmospheric turbulence channels. IET Commun J 3(8):1402–1409
24. Borah DK, Voelz DG (2009) Pointing error effects on free-space optical communication links in the presence of atmospheric turbulence. J Light Wave Technol 27(18):3965–3973

25. Kenneth S, Alouini M (2005) Digital communication over fading channels, 2nd edn. Wiley-Inter science, NJ, USA
26. Gradshteyn I, Ryzhik I (2000) Table of integrals, series and products. Academic Press, New York
27. Prudnikov A, Brychhkov Y, Marichev O (1999) Integral and series, vol. 3: more special functions. CRC, New York, USA

The V-Band SIW Slot Antenna for Millimeter Wave Application

Shailendra Kumar Sinha and Raghvendra Singh

Abstract Substrate integrated waveguide (SIW) technology can be used to design high-speed 5G wireless communication system for 3–300 GHz millimeter frequency range. Nowadays, 5G technology is a promising technology for Internet of things. In millimeter wave communication, substrate integrated waveguide (SIW) has various advantages over the conventional waveguide due to its characteristics and ease of design. In this article, substrate integrated waveguide slot antenna is created in RT/duroid 5870 having permittivity 2.33 and dielectric loss tangent 0.0012. The operating frequencies are 51 and 43 GHz. Antenna resonates at 43 and 51 GHz with peak directivity 4.4126 and peak gain 4.2395 with radiation efficiency 96%.

Keywords SIW cavity · Resonant frequency · Bandwidth · Dual frequency · Slot antenna

1 Introduction

A substrate integrated waveguide (SIW) is a manufactured rectangular waveguide formed in a dielectric by closely arranging metallized ports or via holes which combine upper and lower metal plates. The substrate integrated waveguide (SIW) is a good contender for millimeter wave and terahertz application. It was first introduced in 1994 [1]. Various SIW components like oscillator, coupler, power divider, antenna, and filters have already studied [2]. There are three main components for a substrate integrated waveguide (SIW) slot antenna to operate at a given frequency, width of SIW antenna (w), diameter of SIW antenna (d) and distance between two metallic vias(s). Width of substrate integrated waveguide (SIW) antenna control cutoff frequencies of substrate integrated waveguide (SIW) transmission. The value of d, s shows the similarity of substrate integrated waveguide(SIW) antenna with rectan-

S. K. Sinha (✉)
Pranveer Singh Institute of Technology, Kanpur, India

R. Singh
A.P.J Abdul Kalam Technical University, Lucknow, India

M. S. Kaiser et al. (eds.), *Proceedings of Trends in Electronics and Health Informatics*, Lecture Notes in Networks and Systems 376,
https://doi.org/10.1007/978-981-16-8826-3_55

gular waveguide. The substrate integrated waveguide (SIW) V-band slot antenna is one of the strong contenders to design dual-band antenna. There have been number of substrate integrated waveguide (SIW) slot antenna designs proposed recently that show dual-band application. This type of substrate integrated waveguide (SIW) antenna has a built-in disadvantage of producing multidirectional radiation features that restrict its application. Above 10 GHz, the microstrip and coplanar technologies have high losses, so they are not useful at these frequencies [3]. Substrate integrated waveguide(SIW) technology is reliable, low cost, compact and compatible with high frequencies. Over the last few years, dual-band antenna has attracted considerable attention to satisfy the need of wireless technology [4, 5]. In this paper, to overcome the difficulty of impedance matching in a wide frequency range at millimeter wave bands, the tapered profile and substrate integrated waveguide (SIW) technology is combined [6–11]. The ease in the design of an substrate integrated waveguide (SIW) structure makes the addition of a tapering profile cost effective and reliable [12, 13]. The conventional rectangular waveguide and substrate integrated waveguide (SIW) antenna have similar characteristics except modes of propagation. Substrate integrated waveguide (SIW) supports only TE mode while conventional rectangular waveguide supports TE and TM mode both. The approximate relation of frequency and substrate integrated waveguide (SIW) width (w) is given by Eqs. 1 and 2 for TE_{10} [14–20]

$$f_c(TE_{10}) = C_o/2\sqrt{\epsilon}(w - d^2/0.95s) \quad (1)$$

$$w_{eff} = w - d^2/0.95\,s \quad (2)$$

In this Paper, we have designed V-band SIW slot antenna that works in frequency range of 40–50 GHz which used in millimeter wave radar research and other kind of scientific research. Proposed V-band SIW slot antenna is based on rectangular waveguide structure. In rectangular waveguide, radiation losses are negligible if wall thickness is much thicker than skin depth of the signal. The losses are dominated by dielectric behavior of substrate.

2 Design of Proposed V-Band SIW Slot Antenna

The substrate integrated waveguide antenna is described by its basic criterion like vias diameter (d), vias separation distance and vias neighboring distance (s). The distance between two vias depends on waveguide structure and substrate characteristics. In this paper, substrate integrated waveguide (SIW) antenna is formed by replacing the metallic side wall by vias. Figure 1 consists the geometry of proposed V-band SIW slot antenna. To overcome the impedance matching, the tapering profile is used. The structure of antenna is inspired from [6]. Substrate integrated waveguide (SIW) antennas can either single band or multiband as given . The slots that are etched on metallic plate are radiating elements in the plane of substrate integrated waveguide

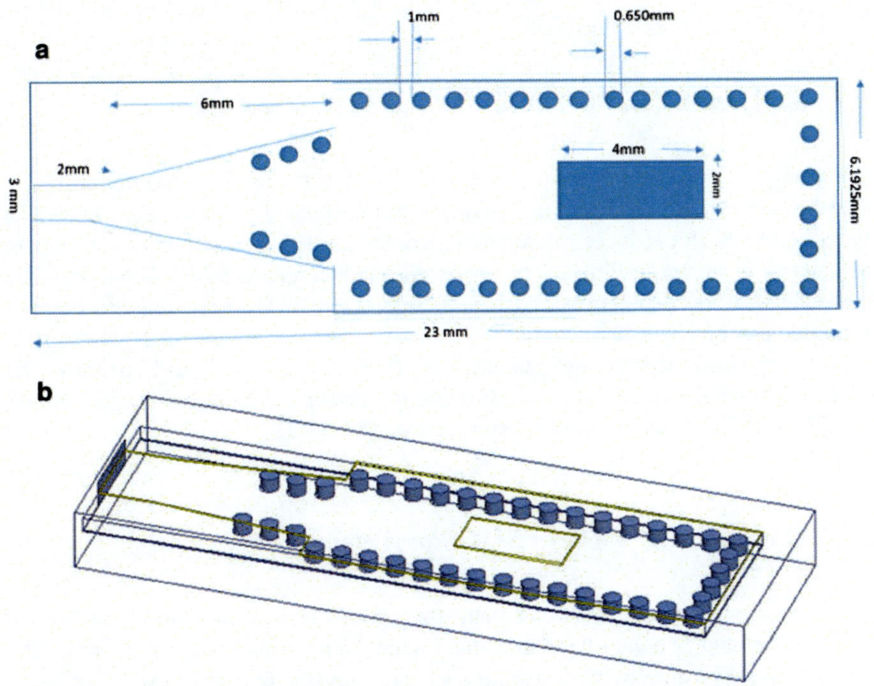

Fig. 1 **a** 2D view of V-band SIW slot antenna, **b** 3D view of V-band SIW slot antenna

Table 1 Dimensions of proposed structure at V-band

Definitions	Value (mm)
Substrate width	6.1925
Substrate length	23
Width of the slot	2
Length of the slot	4
Diameter of vias	0.65
Height of vias	0.508
Separation between two vias	1

(SIW) cavity. The resonant frequency can be changed by location of slot within the substrate integrated waveguide (SIW).

Figure 1a, b shows 2D and 3D models of V-band SIW slot antenna. The parameters such as substrate length, width and height are shown in Table 1. In Table 1, the separation between two vias (*s*) is greater than diameter of vias. To reduce radiation losses, s is taken smaller than 2 times of diameter of vias. To avoid over performance, the ratio of *s* and cutoff wavelength should be greater than 0.05.

3 Results and Discussion

3.1 *Reflection Coefficient of V-Band SIW Slot Antenna*

The design is simulated and analyzed using HFSS software. The minima in Fig. 2 is at 51 and 43 GHz representing the dual-band frequency of SIW cavity [12]. The introduction of slot reduces the reflection coefficient [3]. The reflection coefficient of antenna is shown in Fig. 1. The proposed antenna resonates at 51 and 43 GHz. The reflection coefficient obtained at 51 GHz is −31 dB. The radiation efficiency of proposed antenna is 96%.

Figure 2 shows variation of reflection coefficient with respect to frequency. The proposed V-band SIW slot antenna shows good performance at two frequencies 43 and 51 GHz. The bandwidth of antenna is around 1.5 GHz.

3.2 *Directivity of V-Band SIW Slot Antenna*

The denticity of an antenna shows field strength in specified direction. The V-band SIW slot antenna is a dual-band antenna. Figure 3 shows directivity of V-band SIW slot antenna. The directivity of antenna is maximum at $\theta = +30°, -30°$ (Fig. 4).

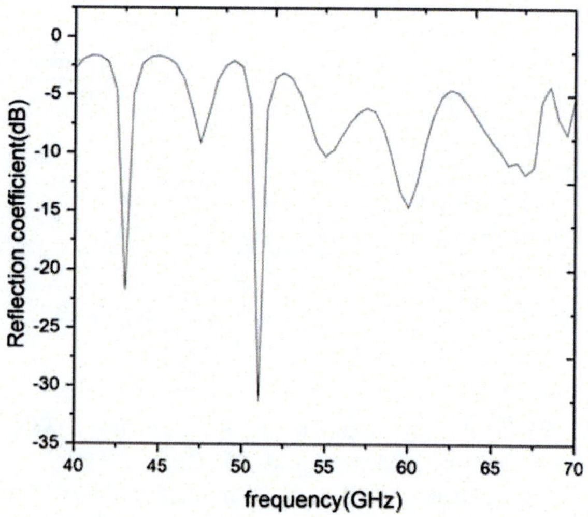

Fig. 2 Reflection coefficient of V-band SIW slot antenna

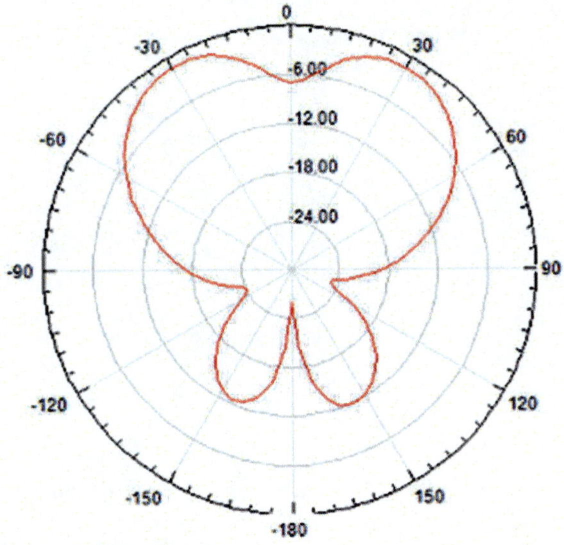

Fig. 3 Directivity of V-band SIW slot antenna

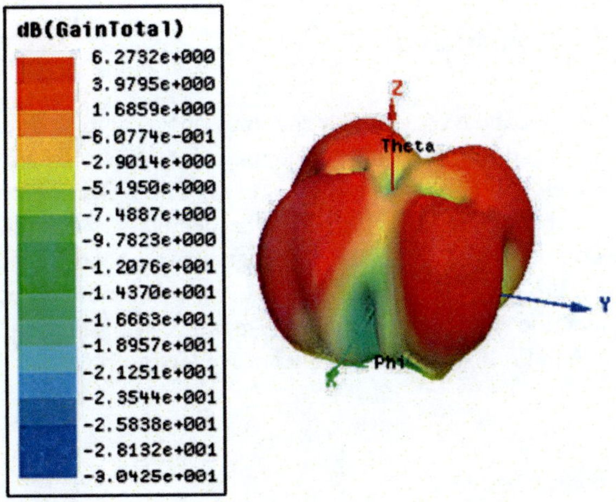

Fig. 4 Gain of V-band SIW slot antenna

3.3 Radiation Pattern of V-Band SIW Slot Antenna

The radiation pattern describes how strongly an antenna radiates in any direction. The shape of radiation determines the application of antenna. Figure 5 shows that the proposed V-band SIW slot antenna radiates maximum field at two directions. It shows the dual-band nature of antenna.

Fig. 5 E-plane radiation pattern of V-band SIW slot antenna

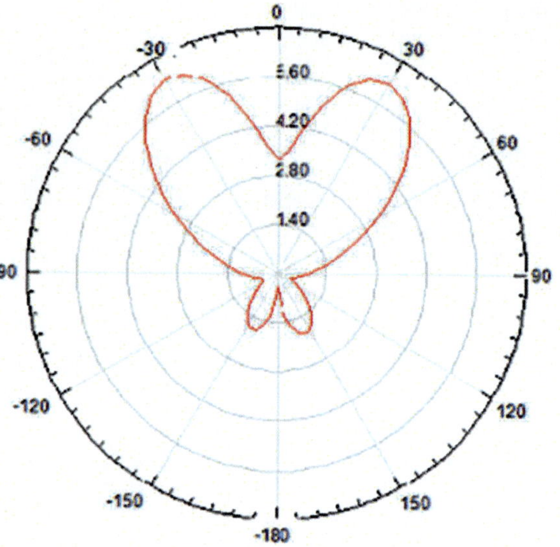

4 Conclusion

The V-band SIW slot antenna, introduced in this paper, is a dual-band antenna operating at millimeter wave frequency 40-60 GHz. To achieve dual-band characteristics, the slot antenna technology is used. The reflection coefficient of −31 and −22 dB is achieved at 51 and 43 GHz, respectively, with high radiation efficiency of 96%. The peak directivity and peak gain of V-band SIW slot antenna are 4.44126 and 4.2396 dB. The gain and directivity can be enhanced by changing the position of metallic vias. This proposed V-band SIW slot antenna is a promising candidate at V-band for 5G and millimeter wave technology.

References

1. Shigeki F (1994) Waveguide line. Japan Patent 06-053 711, Feb. 25, 1994 (in Japanese)
2. Deslandes D, Wu K (2006) Accurate modeling , wave mechanisms, and design considerations of a substrate integrated waveguide. IEEE Trans Microwave Theory Tech 54(6)
3. Hamid N, Omran AH (2020) Dual band substrate integrated waveguide slot antenna for 5G applications. ICATAS-MJJIC
4. AL-Fadhali1 N, Majid HA, Omar R, Dahlan SH, Ashyap AYI, Shah SM, Rahim MKA. Substrate integrated waveguide cavity backed frequency reconfiguration antenna for cognitive radio applies to internet of things applications. Int J RF Microwave Willey
5. Mukherjee S, Biswas A, Srivastava KV. Substrate integrated waveguide cavity backed slot antenna for dual-frequency application. In: Proceedings of the 44th European microwave conference

6. Nair PS, Patnaik A, Kartikeyan MV (2018) Millimeter wave antenna for 5G applications. In: IEEE Indian conference on antenna & wave propagation (InCAP). 978-1-5386-7070-6/18
7. Ashraf N, Vettikalladi H, Alkanhal MAS (2014) A DR loaded substrate integrated waveguide antenna for 60 GHz high wireless communication systems. Int J Antennas Propag
8. Khalichi B, Nikmehr S, Pourziad A, Ebrahimpouri M (2015) Designing wide band tapered-slot antennas. IEEE Antennas Propag Mag
9. Ashraf N, Vettikalladi H, Alkanhal MAS (2013) Substrate integrated wave-guide antennas/array for 60 GHz wireless communication systems. In: 2013 IEEE international RF and microwave conference (RFM), pp 56, 61, 9–11 Dec 2013
10. Hong W, Baek KH, Lee Y, Kim Y (2014) Study and prototyping of practically large scale mm wave antenna system for 5G cellular devices. IEEE Commun Mag 52(9):63–69
11. Kordiboroujeni Z, Bornemann J (2013) Designing the width of substrate integrated waveguide structures. IEEE Microwave Wirel Components Lett 23(10)
12. Deslandes D (2010) Design equations for tapered microstrip-to-substrate integrated waveguide transitions. In: Proceedings IEEE MTT-S international microwave symposium, pp 704–707
13. Wang H, Fang DG, Zhang B, Che WQ (2010) Dielectric loaded substrate integrated waveguide H-plane horn antennas. IEEE Trans Antennas Propag 58(3):640–647 Mar
14. Oraizi H, Jam S (2003) Optimum design of tapered slot antenna profile. IEEE Trans Antennas Propag 51(8):1987–1995 Aug
15. Deslandes D (2010) Design equations for tapered microstrip-to-substrate integrated waveguide transitions. In: Proceedings of IEEE MTT-S international microwave symposium, pp 704–707
16. Xu F, Wu K (2005) Guided-wave and leakage characteristics of substrate integrated waveguide. IEEE Trans Microwave Theory Tech 53(1):66–72 Jan
17. Bozzi M, Georgiadis A, Wu K (2011) Review of substrate-integrated waveguide circuits and antennas. IET Microw. Antennas Propag 5(8):909-920
18. Chen X, Hong W, Cui T, Chen J, Wu K (2005) Substrate integrated waveguide (SIW) linear phase filter. IEEE Microwave Wireless Components Lett 15(11):787–789. https://doi.org/10.1109/LMWC.2005.859021
19. Singh R, Seth D, Rawat S, Ray K (2019) Performance investigations of multi-resonance microstrip patch antenna for wearable applications. Soft Comput: Theories Appl
20. Singh R, Seth D, Rawat S, Ray K. In body communication: assessment of multiple homogeneous human tissue models on stacked meandered patch antenna. Int J Appl Evol Comput (IJAEC)

Performance Analysis of MC-CDMA-Based Cognitive Radio Network Under Rayleigh Fading Channel

Md. Alomgir Kabir and M. Shamim Kaiser

Abstract Higher rate of mobile data traffic demand is increased with the advent of the Internet of things (IoT) and advanced network services (ANS) operators that have begun to develop fifth generation (5G) cellular networks in order to overcome the limitations of the current fourth generation (4G) cellular network. In order to solve the bandwidth scarcity and effective allocation of spectrum resources and also provide higher demand of bandwidth, a multi-carrier code division multiple access (MC-CDMA)-based cognitive radio network (CRN) is proposed and the performance of this system is investigated in this research. MC-CDMA-based CRN improves the channel capacity of the cognitive cooperative network (CCN). Moreover, CCN enhances the spectrum utilization efficiency. Signal to noise plus interference ratio (SNIR) and the bit error rate (BER) are explored, as well as analytical derivations are investigated for performance analysis of our proposed model under Rayleigh fading channels. The comparison between our proposed model and conventional decode and forward (DAF) relaying is also included in the research and MC-CDMA-based cooperative relaying system with multiple receiving antenna schemes to show that the recommended approach is effective. The simulation as well as the numerical results are presented to demonstrate that the suggested cooperative relaying spectrum sharing technique is efficient.

Keywords MC-CDMA · CRN · SNIR · BER · Outage capacity · Outage probability

Md. A. Kabir (✉)
Department of Electrical, Electronic and Communication Engineering, Military Institute of Science and Technology, Dhaka, Bangladesh

M. S. Kaiser
Institute of Information Technology, Jahangirnagar University, Dhaka, Bangladesh
e-mail: mskaiser@juniv.edu

M. S. Kaiser et al. (eds.), *Proceedings of Trends in Electronics and Health Informatics*, Lecture Notes in Networks and Systems 376,
https://doi.org/10.1007/978-981-16-8826-3_56

1 Introduction

The presents of limitation in number of spectrum allocation policies establishing a wireless spectrum for a new network are extremely difficult because the majority of the bandwidth has already been allotted. [1, 2] To solve the problem of spectrum scarcity, cognitive radio (CR) is a novel paradigm that allows users to share or utilize spectrum in a flexible and opportunistic manner as well as utilize the spectrum efficiency. Cognitive radio network (CRN) consists of primary user (PU) as well as secondary user (SU) where PUs use a fix or specified licensed bandwidth provided by Government policy. Those who are use unlicensed bandwidth or share the PUs spectrum are called SU [3]. Establishing high data rate over traditional wireless communication, transmission cause interference due to multipath fading. To achieve the target data rate, the best choice is multi-carrier (MC)-based systems. As a consequence, MC code division multiple access (MC-CDMA) is spreading the original data stream in different subcarrier by different code in the frequency domain. Every network hole consists of MC-CDMA-based primary transmitter (PT) or primary receiver (PR) as well as secondary transmitter (ST) or secondary receiver (SR), respectively.

In wireless communication systems, the proper measure of channel capacity for a slowly varying fading channel is outage capacity and it is also more practical systems performance metric. Furthermore, as a result of multipath fading or shadowing, the link gain between PT and PR over the direct link transmission decreases or the interference gain between ST (active) to PR and ST (active) to ST (inactive) increases then the PUs chance of going outage. As a result, we take outage capacity into account.

As a result, interference management is a major concern for CRNs in the context of spectrum sharing technology and several interference avoidance methods have been suggested in the context of CRNs due to their spectrum sensing or sharing features [4, 5]. If the data rate in between PT-PR does not satisfy the achievable data rate, then the primary systems (PS) use inactive SU for relay to transmit data PT-PR. As a result, cooperative relays have been used in CRNs to improve system performance and spectrum efficiency [6, 7]. In [7–9], a dual-hop DAF relaying network is introduced into PS using spectrum sharing methods. However, a closed form outage capacity and outage probability are investigated for MC-CDMA-based CRN [10]. Performance of a cognitive cooperative relay aided downlink MC-CDMA system is analyzed [11].

As a more general situation is considered, we offer an interference-limited spectrum sharing protocol in which PR is equipped with multiple antennas and MC-CDMA is used at all nodes (e.g., PT, ST, SR, and PR). The performance of PR is examined in terms of outage probability, outage capacity, and BER over Rayleigh fading environment. We compare our suggested system model to conventional cooperative spectrum sharing approach to demonstrate its effectiveness [7] and in an MC-CDMA-based CRN wireless communication, it has been shown that there is a considerable improvement owing to receive diversity, higher order code length, and OFDM subcarrier.

The remainder of this paper is structured as follows. Section II introduces the MC-CDMA cooperative relay-based system and channel models. Sections III provides the suggested system's theoretical analysis and performance assessment. Section IV presents the numerical results in terms of outage probability, SNIR, outage capacity, and BER, and Section V concludes this study.

2 System and Channel Model

We consider a cooperative relay-based CRN is shown in below Fig. 1 where a similar approach for sharing the radio frequency spectrum was also suggested in [10]. The scenario of the system consists of MC-CDMA-based CRN. There are two systems in this network as PS and SS. Primary network contains a source and destination for transmitting their data are called PT and PR, respectively. It is assumed NN number of SU can communicate with each other by sharing PUs spectrum under interference-limited environment. In this study, all nodes are equipped with a multiple antenna and operated in a half-duplex mode. Because of poor channel conditions and/or channel shadowing, the direct link between PT and PR is presumed to be weak for data transfer. As a result, the link is improper for communication and has been

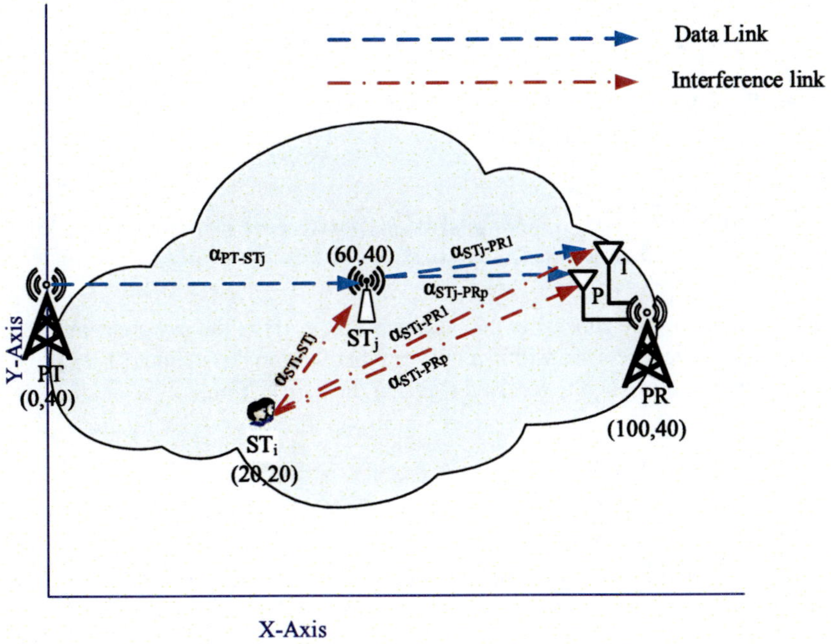

Fig. 1 Proposed system model

neglected as a result. However, to study the performance of such system, we consider different coordinates for fixing the user's location (both PU and SU) environment where wireless network channels experience Rayleigh fading.

The medium that connects between the transmitting and receiving antennas is referred to as the channel. For this communication channel, a Rayleigh fading channel is considered, in which the magnitude of a signal flowing through this medium varies randomly or fades according to Rayleigh distribution. Fading parameters over the link $\mathrm{PT}-\mathrm{ST}_j, \mathrm{ST}_j-\mathrm{PR}_\chi, \mathrm{ST}_i-\mathrm{ST}_j$, and $\mathrm{ST}_i-\mathrm{PR}_\chi$ are $\alpha_{\mathrm{PT}-\mathrm{ST}_j}, \alpha_{\mathrm{ST}_j-\mathrm{PR}_\chi}, \alpha_{\mathrm{ST}_i-ST_j}$, and $\alpha_{\mathrm{ST}_i-\mathrm{PR}_\chi}$, respectively, which is shown in Fig. 1. All of them are distributed as random variables, having mean values of $\lambda_{\mathrm{PT}-\mathrm{ST}_j}, \lambda_{\mathrm{ST}_j-\mathrm{PR}_\chi}, \lambda_{\mathrm{ST}_i-\mathrm{ST}_j}$, and $\lambda_{\mathrm{ST}_i-\mathrm{PR}_\chi}$ sequentially where $\lambda_{i-j,P} = \frac{1}{(d_{i-j,P})^\ell}$ and $d_{i-j,P}$ are the distance between PT $-$ $\mathrm{ST}_{i,j} - \mathrm{PR}_\chi$, therefore, the path loss components between different link $\ell = 2$ are considered for our proposed model [12].

3 Problem Formulation

Suppose that the proposed systems contain k number of cognitive links. The transmission bits of $a_k(n)$, where n is the number of time sequence and the corresponding spreading code sequence, are given below:

$$C_k(t) = \left[C_1, C_2, \ldots C_{N_c}\right] \tag{1}$$

Let, P_T be the normalized transmitted power, then the transmitted symbol on the kth link can be expressed as [10],

$$S_{\mathrm{MC-CDMA}}(t) = \sum_{i,k=1}^{N_c} \sum_{n=-\infty}^{\infty} \sqrt{2P_T} a_k(n) C_k(t) \mathrm{rect}(t - nT) \cos\{(\omega_i t + \varphi_n(t)\} \tag{2}$$

where N_c denotes the subcarrier and assumes that $\varphi_n(t)$ is the instantaneous phase angles of all subcarriers are within a uniform distribution throughout $[0, 2\pi]$.

When there is no SU, the received signal at the base station, can be characterized by

$$r(t) = \sum_{k=1}^{K} \sum_{l=1}^{N} \sum_{n=-\infty}^{\infty} \sqrt{2P_r}\, \alpha_{n,l}(t)\, h_{l,n}(t - nT_C) a_k(t - nT_C)$$
$$C_{k,l}(t - lT_c)\, \cos\{\omega_l t + \varphi_n(t)\} + \zeta_n(t) \tag{3}$$

where P_r is the signal power that was received at PR, $\zeta_n(t)$ is the component of additive white Gaussian noise (AWGN), T_C is the time period between one slot of the chip, and whereas considering this cognitive situation, the fading parameter is $\alpha_{n,l}(t)$.

Due to fading, the data rate between PT − PR is considered to be lower than the target data rate. As a result, the data transmission is processed with the help of cooperative relay. The transmission of PUs data is accomplished via two phases $\mathrm{PT}-\mathrm{ST}_j$ and $\mathrm{ST}_j-\mathrm{PR}$. The received power P_{ST_j} at inactive ST (cooperative relay) and the received power strength P_{PR_χ} at PR are expressed as [12],

$$P_{\mathrm{ST}_j} = \frac{\alpha_{\mathrm{PT}-\mathrm{ST}_j} P_{\mathrm{PT}}}{\left(d_{\mathrm{PT}-\mathrm{ST}_j}\right)^{\mathcal{L}}} \tag{4}$$

$$P_{\mathrm{PR}_\chi} = \frac{\alpha_{\mathrm{ST}_j-PR_\chi} P_{\mathrm{ST}_j}}{\left(d_{\mathrm{ST}_j-\mathrm{PR}_\chi}\right)^{\mathcal{L}}} \tag{5}$$

where $\chi = [1, 2, \ldots P]$, P is the number of receiving antenna at PR, P_{PT}, and 0_{ST_j} are the transmitted power by PT and ST_j sequentially. Also, the interference power P' caused by active SUs at ST_i at as well as PR_χ, it can be determined as follows,

$$P'_{\mathrm{ST}_i-\mathrm{ST}_j} = \frac{\alpha_{\mathrm{ST}_i-\mathrm{ST}_j} \mathrm{P}_{ST_i}}{\left(d_{\mathrm{ST}_i-\mathrm{ST}_j}\right)^{\mathcal{L}}} \tag{6}$$

$$P'_{\mathrm{ST}_i-\mathrm{PR}_\chi} = \frac{\alpha_{\mathrm{ST}_i-\mathrm{PR}_\chi} \mathrm{P}_{\mathrm{ST}_i}}{\left(d_{\mathrm{ST}_i-\mathrm{PR}_\chi}\right)^{\mathcal{L}}} \tag{7}$$

So, in terms of signal power, interference power, and noise power, the SNIR may be expressed for two phases $\mathrm{PT}-\mathrm{ST}_j$ and $\mathrm{ST}_j-\mathrm{PR}_\chi$,

$$\mathrm{SNIR} = \frac{P_s}{\sigma^2_{\mathrm{MAI}} + \sigma^2_n} \tag{8}$$

$$\mathrm{SNIR}_{\mathrm{PT}-\mathrm{ST}_j} = \frac{\sum_{k=1}^{N} |\alpha_k|^2 P^2_{\mathrm{ST}_j}}{\sum_{k=1}^{N} |\alpha_k|^2 \mathrm{MAI} + \sum_{k=1}^{N} |\beta_k|^2 P'_{\mathrm{ST}_i-\mathrm{ST}_j} + \sigma^2} \tag{9}$$

$$\mathrm{SNIR}_{\mathrm{ST}_j-\mathrm{PR}_\chi} = \frac{\sum_{k=1}^{N} |\alpha_k|^2 P^2_{\mathrm{PR}_\chi}}{\sum_{k=1}^{N} |\alpha_k|^2 \mathrm{MAI} + \sum_{k=1}^{N} |\beta_k|^2 P'_{\mathrm{ST}_i-\mathrm{PR}_\chi} + \sigma^2} \tag{10}$$

Hence, finally, the SNIR equation in closed form can be written as follows,

$$\mathrm{SNIR} = \gamma(\alpha) = \frac{\sum_{k=1}^{N} |\alpha_k|^2 P^2_{\mathrm{PR}_\chi}}{\sum_{k=1}^{N} |\alpha_k|^2 \mathrm{MAI} + \sum_{k=1}^{N} |\beta_k|^2 P'_{\mathrm{ST}_i-\mathrm{ST}_j-\mathrm{PR}_\chi} + \sigma^2} \tag{11}$$

Now, the conditional BER for a binary phase shift keying (BPSK) modulated signal may be calculated using the formula,

$$\mathrm{Ber}(\alpha) = \frac{1}{2}\mathrm{erfc}\left[\sqrt{\frac{\gamma(\alpha)}{2}}\right] \tag{12}$$

The joint probability density function (PDF) for the Rayleigh distribution considering two random variables with expected mean value λ_p and λ_s for PS as well as the secondary system (SS), respectively, is given,

$$f(\alpha) = \frac{4\lambda_s^2\lambda_p^2}{\left(\lambda_s^2 + \lambda_p^2\alpha\right)^2} \tag{13}$$

In this way, the average BER may be calculated as shown below,

$$\mathrm{BER} = \int_0^\infty \mathrm{Ber}(\alpha) f(\alpha) \mathrm{d}\alpha \tag{14}$$

$$\mathrm{BER} = \int_0^\infty \frac{1}{2}\mathrm{erfc}\left[\sqrt{\frac{\gamma(\alpha)}{2}}\right] \frac{4\lambda_s^2\lambda_p^2}{\left(\lambda_s^2 + \lambda_p^2\alpha\right)^2} \mathrm{d}\alpha \tag{15}$$

$$\mathrm{BER} = \int_0^\infty \frac{1}{2}\mathrm{erfc}\left[\sqrt{\frac{\frac{\sum_{k=1}^N |\alpha_k|^2 P_{\mathrm{PR}_\chi}^2}{\sum_{k=1}^N |\alpha_k|^2 \mathrm{MAI} + \sum_{k=1}^N |\beta_k|^2 P'_{\mathrm{ST}_i-\mathrm{ST}_j-\mathrm{PR}_\chi} + \sigma^2}}{2}}\right] \frac{4\lambda_s^2\lambda_p^2}{\left(\lambda_s^2 + \lambda_p^2\alpha\right)^2} \mathrm{d}\alpha \tag{16}$$

So, the outage capacity [10] correlated with particular outage probability is represented by the expression

$$C_\epsilon^{\mathrm{DAF}} = \log_2(1 + \gamma(\alpha))(1 - \varepsilon) \tag{17}$$

where the given outage probability [10] can be expressed mathematically as follows.

$$\epsilon' = \sqrt[N]{\epsilon} = 1 - \left(1 - \frac{4\alpha_{\mathrm{PT}-\mathrm{ST}_j-\mathrm{PR}_P}\lambda_{\mathrm{ST}_i-\mathrm{ST}_j}^2}{\lambda_{\mathrm{PT}-\mathrm{ST}_j}^2 + \alpha_{\mathrm{PT}-\mathrm{ST}_j-\mathrm{PR}_P}\lambda_{\mathrm{ST}_i-\mathrm{ST}_j}^2}\right) \left(1 - \frac{4\alpha_{\mathrm{PT}-\mathrm{ST}_j-\mathrm{PR}_P}\lambda_{\mathrm{ST}_j-\mathrm{ST}_P}^2}{\lambda_{\mathrm{ST}_j-\mathrm{PR}_P}^2 + \alpha_{\mathrm{PT}-\mathrm{ST}_j-\mathrm{PR}_P}\lambda_{\mathrm{ST}_i-\mathrm{PR}_P}^2}\right) \tag{18}$$

4 Results and Discussion

This paper presents the numerical findings of the outage capacity, outage probability, and BER for evaluating the performance of a cooperative relaying wireless network architecture. In this case, let us assume that PT and PR are situated at the coordinates (0, 40) and (100, 40), respectively, as well as active ST and inactive ST are situated at (20, 20) and (60, 40), respectively, in between PT to PR. Furthermore, in accordance with the CRN design concept, we must know where the PT is located and its transmission range. The simulation results are used to establish the best values for system parameters including the number of OFDM subcarriers, spreading code, code length, modulation scheme, and outage probability. Table 1 shows the parameters that were used in the numerical simulations, which are summarized below.

4.1 Systems Performance Metric

Figure 2 shows that the outage probability reduces as the SNIR and the number of cooperating relays rise. It can be observed that, the suggested cooperative relaying system has a lower outage probability than the direct link transmission method. Moreover, the theoretical analysis and simulation outcomes clearly demonstrate that the suggested transmission scenario improves as the number of cooperating relays increase.

Increasing the SNIR and the number of cooperative relays improves the outage capacity, as shown in Fig. 3 of this work. It is also observed that the overall system performance is improved.

Figure 4 compares the performance with and without received diversity in terms of BER curves where number of received antenna P = 4, it is found that when the number of receiving antenna P increases, the BER decreases significantly. Also noticed is that the BER decreases enormously with an increase in the number of cooperative relays.

Table 1 Parameters of the system

Parameters	Attributes
The total number of subcarriers, N_c	16
Number of users, K	100, 200, 300, 400
Code length, L	16, 32, 64, 128
Number of receiving antenna, p	4
Outage probability, ϵ	0.1, 0.01, 0.001

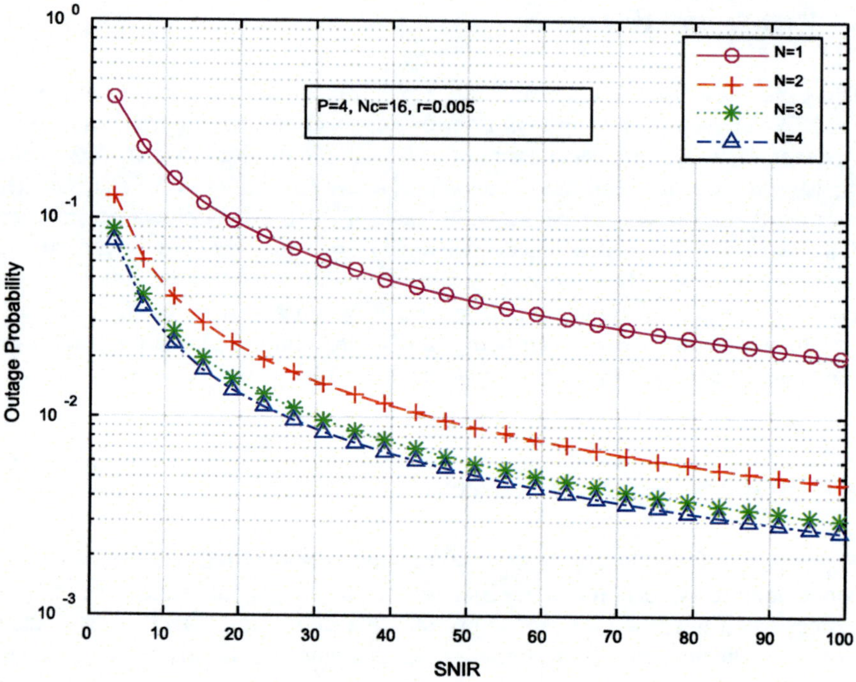

Fig. 2 SNIR versus outage probability of the proposed network scenario considering receives diversity

4.2 Comparison with the Previous Research

The outage capacity has been observed considering SNIR from 2 to 18 dB and varying the given probability $\in = 0.1, 0.01, 0.001$ for $N = 4$ relays. However, the outage capacity of the proposed system with the existing system is also analyzed considering the same number of relays for same SNIR shown in Fig. 5. Comparing this figure, it is noticed that at 12 dB SNIR in Fig. 5 shows outage capacity of the proposed system is 1, 0.6, 0.25 while these values are about 0.9, 0.54, 0.23 in referred research for $\in = 0.1, 0.01, 0.001$, respectively. Hence, it is concluded that the new proposed scheme shows with increasing SNIR improves the outage capacity.

On the contrary, Fig. 6 depicts the outage capacity for a given outage probability as the active ST position changes. It is found from Fig. 6 when the position of active ST is far away from the PR, then outage capacity increases as interference effect decreases with the increase of distance between ST and PR. For the nearest location of ST (20, 20) to PR, the outage capacity of a research [7] has been found almost 0.9 at 10 dB SNIR while for new proposed system, it has been evaluated to be about 1 for the same location and same SNIR. Hence, proposed designed model shows better performance in terms of outage capacity compared to [7].

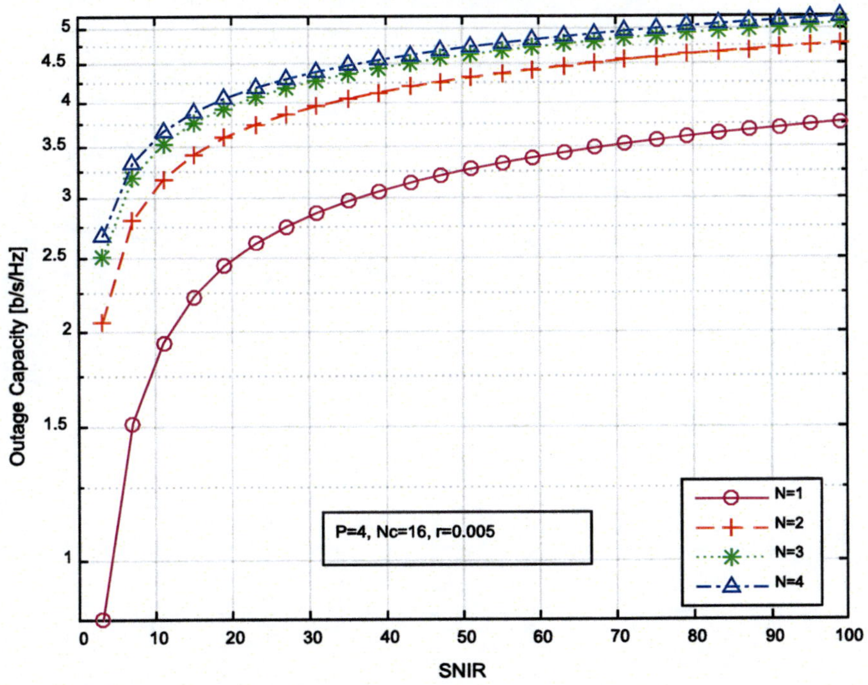

Fig. 3 SNIR versus outage capacity, when active STs are situated at (20, 20) while inactive STs serve as a relay between PT and PR at (60, 40)

Observing the simulation results, it is found that better outage probability has been investigated in the new proposed system shown in Fig. 7. For instance, at 8 dB SNIR, [7] outage probability of the previous research is approximately 0.013 for four relays while for the same condition, the outage probability is 0.004 in the proposed network shown in Fig. 7. Hence, the proposed scheme can be considered as improved version in terms of outage probability.

5 Conclusion

The expressions of SNIR and BER of MC-CDMA-based CRN wireless communication systems with OFDM subcarriers over Rayleigh fading channels are analyzed in this article as well as the multiple receivers are included in the study. This system's performance has been examined of proposed cognitive systems in terms of BER, outage probability, and outage capacity. Therefore, BER performance is assessed for a variety of systems parameters.

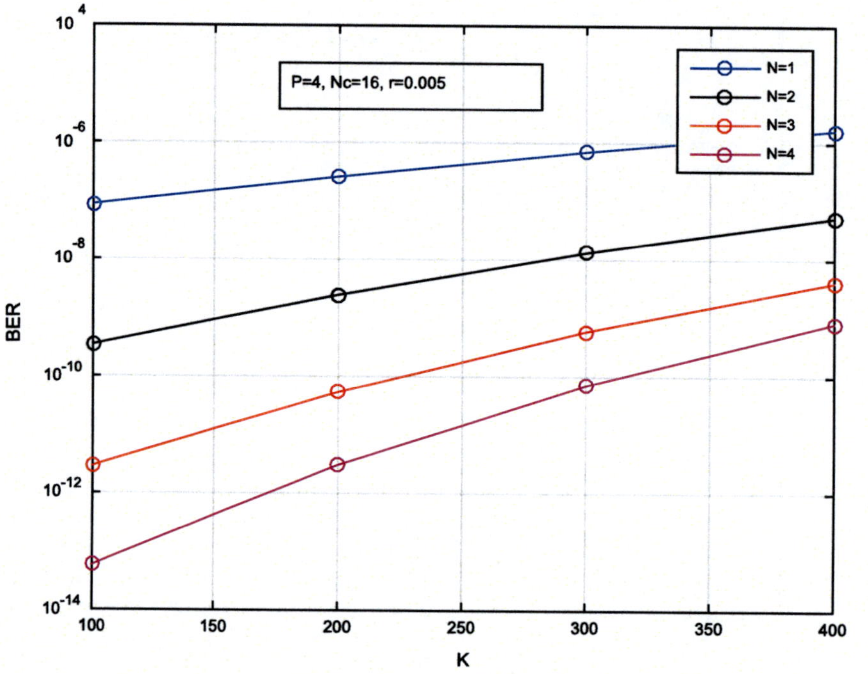

Fig. 4 BER versus K number of users for MC-CDMA-based CRN wireless network with receive diversity at a fixed SNR = 10 dB and number of subcarrier $N_c = 16$

Fig. 5 SNIR versus outage capacity for different values of ε and with $N = 4$ number of STs (cooperative relays)

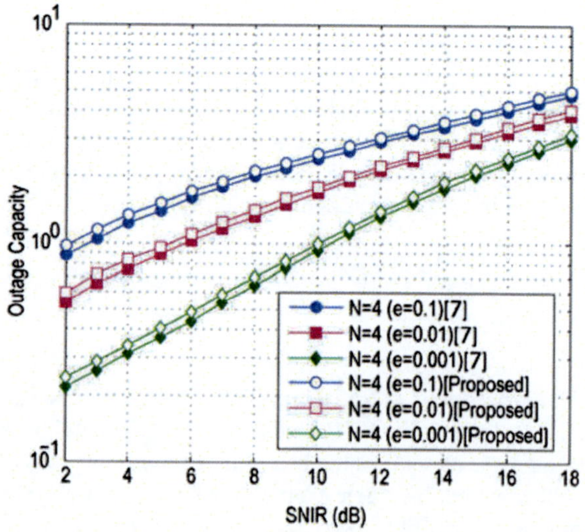

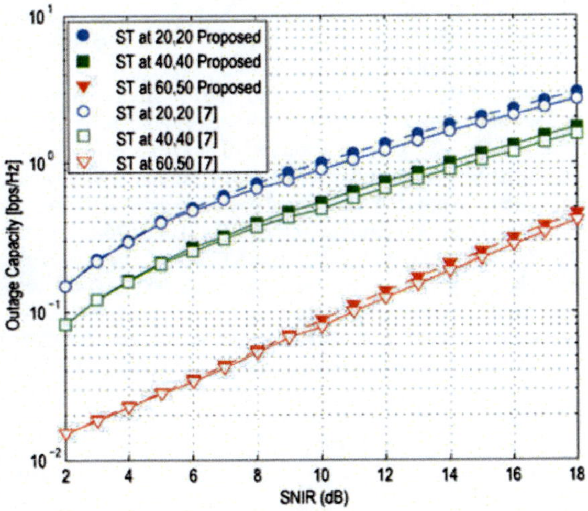

Fig. 6 SNIR versus outage capacity when the ST is moved around but the relay location remains constant

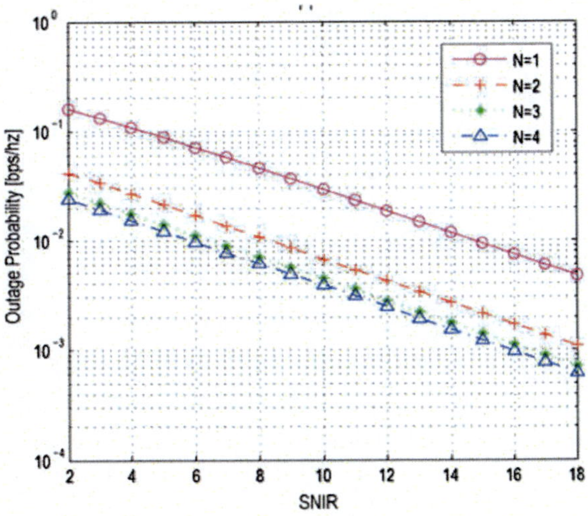

Fig. 7 SNIR vs Outage probability for different values of nodes (cooperative relays)

References

1. Mitola J, Maguire G (1999) Cognitive radio: making software radios more personal. IEEE Pers Commun 6(4):13–18. https://doi.org/10.1109/98.788210
2. Chen K-C, Prasad R (2009) Cognitive radio networks. Wiley, Chichester
3. Devroye N, Vu M, Tarokh V (2008) Cognitive radio networks. IEEE Signal Process Mag 25(6):12–23
4. Chen Z, Wang C-X, Hong X, Thompson J, Vorobyov SA, Zhao F, Ge X (2013) Interference mitigation for cognitive radio MIMO systems based on practical pre-coding. Phys Commun 9:308–315. https://doi.org/10.1016/j.phycom.2012.04.007

5. Kaiser MS, Mamun SA, Ahmed KM (2013) Interference temperature constraint-based radio resource allocation for the network coded cognitive cooperative network (NCCCN). Int J Comput Appl 67(7)
6. Kader MF, Asaduzzaman MM (2013) Hoque, hybrid spectrum sharing with cooperative secondary user selection in cognitive radio networks. KSII Trans Internet Inf Syst (TIIS) 7(9):2081–2100. https://doi.org/10.3837/tiis.2013.09.001.
7. Kader MF, Asaduzzaman MM (2014) Hoque, outage capacity analysis of a cooperative relaying scheme in interference limited cognitive radio networks. Wirel Personal Commun 79(3):2127–2140. https://doi.org/10.1007/s11277-014-1976-8
8. Han Y, Ting SH, Pandharipande A (2012) Cooperative spectrum sharing protocol with selective relaying system. IEEE Trans Commun 60(1):62–67. https://doi.org/10.1109/TCOMM.2011.100411.100469
9. Kaiser MS, Iqbal A, Baseer S, Ali F, Ahmed KM (2010) Performance analysis of network coded bidirectional relaying in OFDM networks. In: International conference on electrical & computer engineering (ICECE 2010). https://doi.org/10.1109/icelce.2010.5700553
10. Kabir MA, Kaiser MS (2015) Outage capacity analysis of MC-CDMA based on cognitive radio network. In: 2015 international conference on electrical engineering and information communication technology (ICEEICT). https://doi.org/10.1109/iceeict.2015.7307463
11. Kabir MA, Ali HM, Antara FA, Kaiser MS (2019, June) Performance of a cognitive cooperative relay aided downlink multi-carrier code division multiple access (MC-CDMA) system. Int J Sci Eng Res 10(6). ISSN 2229-5518
12. Kader MF, Asaduzzaman, Chowdhury M (2012) Cooperative secondary user selection as a relay for the primary system in underlay cognitive radio networks. In: 2012 15th international conference on computer and information technology (ICCIT). https://doi.org/10.1109/iccitechn.2012.650973

Correction to: Proceedings of Trends in Electronics and Health Informatics

M. Shamim Kaiser, Anirban Bandyopadhyay, Kanad Ray, Raghvendra Singh, and Vishal Nagar

Correction to:
M. S. Kaiser et al. (eds.), *Proceedings of Trends in Electronics and Health Informatics*, Lecture Notes in Networks and Systems 376, https://doi.org/10.1007/978-981-16-8826-3

The original version of the book was inadvertently published with the below errors.

Chapter 1 was published without the figures 5c and 5d. which have now been included in the updated version. Chapter 45 was published with incorrect affiliation of the volume editors. This has been corrected.

Correct Affiliations: Rohit Saxena and Deepak Arora are affiliated with Amity University Uttar Pradesh, Lucknow, and Vishal Nagar is affiliated with Pranveer Singh Institute of Technology, Kanpur

The erratum chapters and the book have been updated with the changes.

The updated versions of these chapters can be found at
https://doi.org/10.1007/978-981-16-8826-3_1
https://doi.org/10.1007/978-981-16-8826-3_45

M. S. Kaiser et al. (eds.), *Proceedings of Trends in Electronics and Health Informatics*, Lecture Notes in Networks and Systems 376,
https://doi.org/10.1007/978-981-16-8826-3_57

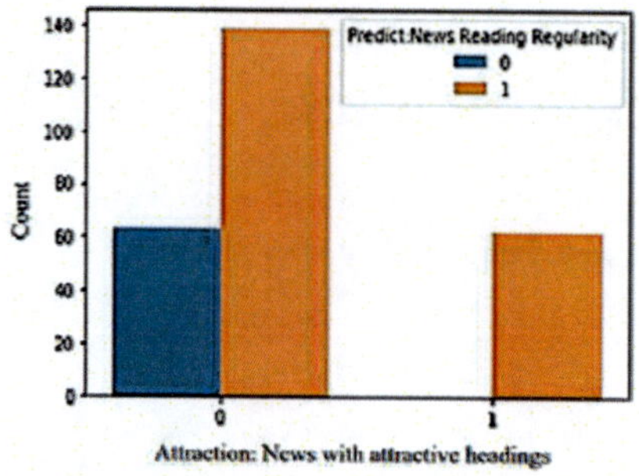

(a) Bar chart for news reading regularity under news with attractive headings: real vs. prediction

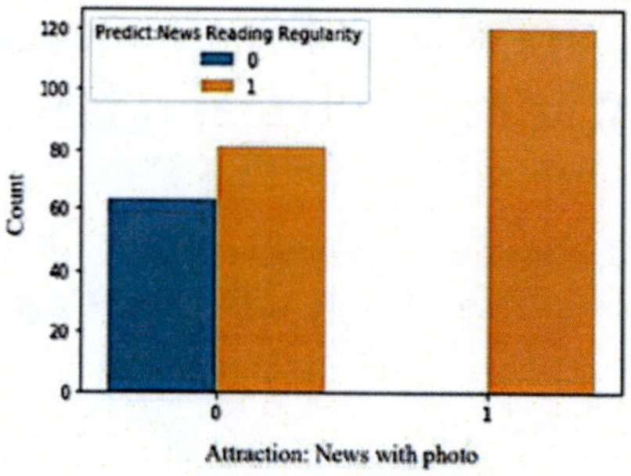

(b) Bar chart for news reading regularity under news with photo: real vs. prediction

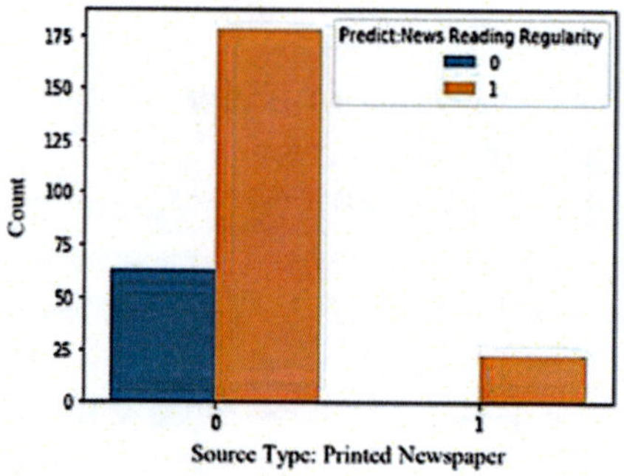

(c) Bar chart for news reading regularity under printed newspaper: real vs. prediction

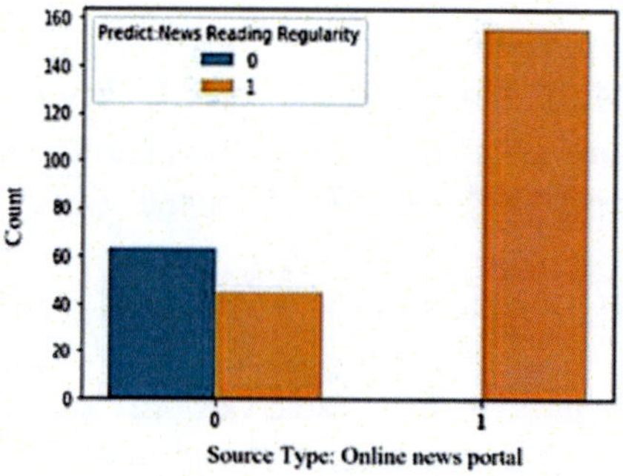

(d) Bar chart for news reading regularity under online news source: real vs. prediction

Fig. 5 Different bar chart analyses of predicted data

Author Index

M. S. Kaiser et al. (eds.), *Proceedings of Trends in Electronics and Health Informatics*, Lecture Notes in Networks and Systems 376,
https://doi.org/10.1007/978-981-16-8826-3